THOMSON DELMAR LEARNING'S
NURSING REVIEW SERIES

Medical-Surgical Nursing

THOMSON DELMAR LEARNING'S
NURSING REVIEW SERIES

Medical-Surgical Nursing

Content taken from:
NCLEX-RN® Review

By:
Alice M. Stein EdD, RN
Retired
Senior Associate Dean for Student and Business Affairs
Drexel University
College of Nursing and Health Professions
Philadelphia, Pennsylvania

THOMSON
DELMAR LEARNING Australia Canada Mexico Singapore Spain United Kingdom United States

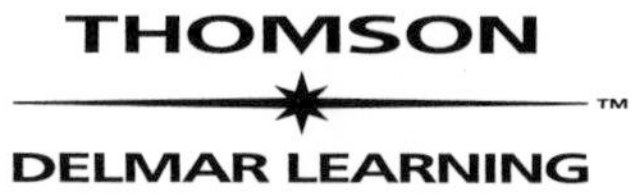

Nursing Review Series: Medical-Surgical Nursing

by Alice M. Stein

Vice President, Health Care Business Unit:
William Brottmiller

Director of Learning Solutions:
Matthew Kane

Acquisitions Editor:
Tamara Caruso

Product Manager:
Patricia Gaworecki

Editorial Assistant:
Jenn Waters

Marketing Director:
Jennifer McAvey

Marketing Channel Manager:
Michele McTighe

Marketing Coordinator:
Danielle Pacella

Technology Director:
Laurie Davis

Technology Project Manager:
Mary Colleen Liburdi
Patricia Allen

Production Director:
Carolyn Miller

Production Manager:
Barbara Bullock

Art Director:
Robert Plante
Jack Pendleton

Content Project Manager:
Dave Buddle
Stacey Lamodi
Jessica McNavich

Production Coordinator:
Mary Ellen Cox

Printed in the United States
1 2 3 4 5 6 7 8 XXX 09 08 07 06 05

For more information, contact
Thomson Delmar Learning,
5 Maxwell Drive,
Clifton Park, NY 12065
Or find us on the World Wide Web at
http://www.delmarlearning.com

Library of Congress Cataloging-in-Publication Data
ISBN 1-4018-1176-0

Contents

Contributors

Margaret Ahearn-Spera, RN, C, MSN
Director, Medical Patient Care Services
Danbury Hospital
Danbury, Connecticut
Assistant Clinical Professor
Yale University School of Nursing
New Haven, Connecticut

Mary Mescher Benbenek, RN, MS, CPNP, CFNP
Teaching Specialist
School of Nursing
University of Minnesota
Twin Cities, Minnesota

Cynthia Blank-Reid, RN, MSN, CEN
Trauma Clinical Nurse Specialist
Temple University Hospital
Philadelphia, Pennsylvania
Clinical Adjunct Associate Professor
Drexel University College of Nursing and Health Professions
Philadelphia, Pennsylvania

Elizabeth Blunt, PhD (c), MSN
Assistant Professor and Director, Graduate Nursing Programs
Drexel University College of Nursing and Health Professions
Philadelphia, Pennsylvania

Margaret Brenner, RN, MSN
Senior Consultant, Pinnacle Healthcare Group, Inc.
Paoli, Pennsylvania

Margaret Brogan, RN, BSN
Registered Nurse/Expert
Children's Memorial Hospital
Chicago, Illinois

Mary Lynn Burnett, RN, PhD
Assistant Professor of Nursing
Wichita State University
Wichita, Kansas

Corine K. Carlson, RN, MS
Assistant Professor
Department of Nursing
Luther College
Decorah, Iowa

Nancy Clarkson, MEd, RN, BC
Professor and Chairperson
Department of Nursing
Finger Lakes Community College
Canandaigua, New York

Nancy Clarkson, RN, C, MEd
Associate Professor of Nursing
Finger Lakes Community College
Canandaigua, New York

Gretchen Reising Cornell, RN, PhD, CNE
Professor of Nursing
Utah Valley State College
Orem, Utah

Vera V. Cull, RN, DSN
Former Assistant Professor of Nursing
University of Alabama
Birmingham, Alabama

Deborah L. Dalrymple, RN, MSN, CRNI
Associate Professor of Nursing
Montgomery County Community College
Blue Bell, Pennsylvania

Laura DeHelian, RN, PhD, APRN, BC
Former Assistant Professor of Nursing
Cleveland State University
Cleveland, Ohio

Della J. Derscheid, RN, MS, CNS
Assistant Professor
Department of Nursing
Mayo Clinic
Mayo Clinic College of Nursing
Rochester, Minnesota

Judy Donlen, RN, DNSc
Executive Director, Southern New Jersey Perinatal Cooperative
Pennsauken, New Jersey

Judith L. Draper, APRN, BC
Assistant Professor
Drexel University College of Nursing and Health Professions
Philadelphia, Pennsylvania

Theresa M. Fay-Hillier, MSN, RN, CS
Adjunct Faculty
Drexel University College of Nursing and Health Professions
Philadelphia, Pennsylvania

Marcia R. Gardner, MA, RN, CPNP, CPN
Assistant Professor
Drexel University College of Nursing and Health Professions
Philadelphia, Pennsylvania

Ann Garey, MSN, APRN, BC, FNP
Carle Foundation Hospital
Urbana, Illinois

Jeanne Gelman, RN, MA, MSN
Professor Emeritus, Psychiatric-Mental Health Nursing
Widener University
Chester, Pennsylvania

Theresa M. Giglio, RD, MS
Instructor, LaSalle University
Philadelphia, Pennsylvania

Beth Good, RN, MSN, BSN
Teaching Specialist
University of Minnesota
Minneapolis, Minnesota

Samantha Grover, RN, BSN, CNS
Psychiatric Mental Health Clinical Specialist
MeritCare Health System
Moorhead, Minnesota

Judith M. Hall, RNC, MSN, IBCLC, LCCE
Lactation Consultant and Childbirth Educator
Mary Washington Hospital
Fredericksburg, Virginia

Judith M. Hall, RNC, MSN, IBCLC, LCCE, FACCE
Mary Washington Hospital
Fredericksburg, Virginia

Jeanne M. Harkness, RN, BA, MSN, BSN, AOCN
Clinical Practice Specialist
Jane Brattain Breast Center
Park Nicollet Clinic
St. Louis Park, Minnesota

Marilyn Herbert-Ashton, RN, C, MS
Director, Wellness Center
F. F. Thompson Health Systems, Inc.
Adjunct Professor of Nursing
Finger Lakes Community College
Canandaigua, New York

Marilyn Herbert-Ashton, MS, RN, BC
Virginia Western Community College
Roanoke, VA

Holly Hillman, RN, MSN
Assistant Professor
Montgomery County Community College
Blue Bell, Pennsylvania

Lorraine C. Igo, RN, MSN, EdD
Assistant Professor
Drexel University College of Nursing and Health Professions
Philadelphia, Pennsylvania

Linda Irle, RN, MSN, APN, CNP
Coordinator, Maternal-Child Nursing
University of Illinois
Urbana, Illinois
Family Nurse Practitioner, Acute Care,
Carle Clinic,
Champaign, Illinois

Amy Jacobson, RN, BA
Staff Nurse
United Hospital
St. Paul, Minnesota

Nancy H. Jacobson, MSN, APRN-BC, CS
Staff Development Coordinator
Rydal Park
Rydal, Pennsylvania

Nancy H. Jacobson, RN, CS, MSN
Senior Manager
The Whitman Group
Huntington Valley, Pennsylvania

Nadine James, RN, PhD
Assistant Professor of Nursing
University of Southern Mississippi
Hattiesburg, Mississippi

Lisa Jensen, CS, MS, APRN
Salt Lake City VA Healthcare System
Salt Lake City, Utah

Ellen Joswiak, RN, MA
Assistant Professor of Nursing
Staff Nurse
Mayo Medical Center
Rochester, Minnesota

Charlotte D. Kain, RN, C, EdD
Professor Nursing, Health Care of Women
Montgomery County Community College
Blue Bell, Pennsylvania

Roseann Tirotta Kaplan, MSN, RN, CS
Adjunct Faculty
Drexel University College of Nursing and Health Professions
Philadelphia, Pennsylvania

Betsy Ann Skrha Kennedy, RN, MS, CS, LCCE
Nursing Instructor
Rochester Community and Technical College
Rochester, Minnesota

Robin M. Lally, PhD, RN, BA, AOCN, CNS
Teaching Specialist; Office 6-155
School of Nursing
University of Minnesota
Twin Cities, Minnesota

Penny Leake, RN, PhD
Luther College
Decorah, Iowa

Barbara Mandleco, RN, PhD
Associate Professor & Undergraduate Program Coordinator
College of Nursing
Brigham Young University
Provo, Utah

Mary Lou Manning, RN, PhD, CPNP
Director, Infection Control and Occupational Health
The Children's Hospital of Philadelphia
Adjunct Assistant Professor
University of Pennsylvania School of Nursing
Philadelphia, Pennsylvania

Gerry Matsumura, RN, PhD, MSN, BSN
Former Associate Professor of Nursing
Brigham Young University
Provo, Utah

Alberta McCaleb, RN, DSN
Associate Professor
Chair, Undergraduate Studies
University of Alabama School of Nursing
University of Alabama at Birmingham
Birmingham, Alabama

Judith C. Miller, RN, MSN
President, Nursing Tutorial and Consulting Services
Clifton, Virginia

Eileen Moran, RN, C, MSN
Clinical Educator
Abington Memorial Hospital
Abington, Pennsylvania

JoAnn Mulready-Shick, RN, MS
Dean, Nursing and Allied Health
Roxbury Community College
Boston, Massachusetts

Patricia Murdoch, RN, MS
Nurse Practitioner
University of Illinois, Chicago
Urbana, Illinois

Jayme S. Nelson, RN, MS, ARNP-C
Adult Nurse Practitioner
Assistant Professor of Nursing
Luther College
Decorah, Iowa

Janice Nuuhiwa, MSN, CPON, APN/CNS
Staff Development Specialist
Hematology/Oncology/Stem Cell Transplant Division
Children's Memorial Hospital
Chicago, Illinois

Kristen L. Osborn, MSN, CRNP
Pediatric Nurse Specialist
UAB School of Nursing
UAB Pediatric Hematology/Oncology
Birmingham, Alabama

Marie O'Toole, RN, EdD
Associate Professor, College of Nursing
Rutgers, The State University of New Jersey
Newark, New Jersey

Faye A. Pearlman, RN, MSN, MBA
Assistant Professor
Drexel University College of Nursing and Health Professions
Philadelphia, Pennsylvania

Karen D. Peterson, RN, MSN, BSN, PNP
Pediatric Nurse Practitioner
Division of Endocrinology
Children's Memorial Hospital
Chicago, Illinois

Kristin Sandau, RN, PhD
Bethel University's Department of Nursing
United's John Nasseff Heart Hospital
Minneapolis, Minnesota

Elizabeth Sawyer, RN, BSN, CCRN
Registered Nurse
United Hospital
St. Paul, Minnesota

Lisa A. Seldomridge, RN, PhD
Associate Professor of Nursing
Salisbury University
Salisbury, Maryland

Janice Selekman, RN, DNSc
Professor and Chair
Department of Nursing
University of Delaware
Newark, Delaware

Robert Shearer, CRNA, MSN
Assistant Professor
Drexel University College of Nursing and Health Professions
Philadelphia, Pennsylvania

Constance O. Kolva Taylor, RN, MSN
Kolva Consulting
Harrisburg, Pennsylvania

Magdeleine Vasso, MSN, RN
Assistant Professor
Drexel University College of Nursing and Health Professions
Philadelphia, Pennsylvania

Janice L. Vincent, RN, DSN
University of Alabama School of Nursing
University of Alabama at Birmingham
Birmingham, Alabama

Margaret Vogel, RN, MSN, BSN
Nursing Instructor
Rochester Community & Technical College
Rochester, Minnesota

Anne Robin Waldman, RN, C, MSN, AOCN
Clinical Nurse Specialist
Albert Einstein Medical Center
Philadelphia, Pennsylvania

Mary Shannon Ward, RN, MSN
Children's Memorial Hospital
Chicago, Illinois

Virginia R. Wilson, RN, MSN, CEN
Assistant Professor, Graduate Nursing Programs
Drexel University College of Nursing and Health Professions
Philadelphia, Pennsylvania

Preface

Congratulations on discovering the best new review series for the NCLEX-RN®! Thomson Delmar Learning's Nursing Review Series is designed to maximize your study in the core subject areas covered on the NCLEX-RN® examination. The series consists of 8 books:

Pharmacology

Medical-Surgical Nursing

Pediatric Nursing

Maternity and Women's Health Nursing

Gerontologic Nursing

Psychiatric Nursing

Legal and Ethical Nursing

Community Health Nursing

Each text has been developed expressly to meet your needs as you study and prepare for the all-important licensure examination. Taking this exam is a stressful event and constitutes a major career milestone. Passing the NCLEX is the key to your future ability to practice as a registered nurse.

Each text in the series is designed around the most current test plan for the NCLEX-RN® and provides a focused and complete content review in each subject area. Additionally, there are up to 400 review questions in each text: questions at the end of most every chapter and three 100 question review tests that support the chapter content. Each set of review questions is followed by answers and rationales for both the right and wrong answers. There is also a free PDA download of review questions available with the purchase of any of these review texts! It is this combination of content review and self assessment that provides a powerful learning experience for you as you prepare for you examination.

ORGANIZATION

Thomson Delmar Learning's unique Pharmacology review book provides you with an intensive review in this all important subject area. Drugs are grouped by classification and similarities to aid you in consolidating this pertinent but sometimes overwhelming information. Included in this text are:

- A section on herbal medicines, now being tested on the exam.
- Case studies that apply relevant drug content
- Prototypes for most drug classifications
- Mechanism of drug action
- Uses and adverse effects
- Nursing implications and discharge teaching
- Related drugs and their variance from the prototype

The review texts for Medical-Surgical Nursing, Pediatric Nursing, Maternity Nursing, Gerontological Nursing and Psychiatric Nursing follow a systematic approach that includes:

- The nursing process integrated with a body systems approach
- Introductory review of normal anatomy and physiology as well as basic theories and principles
- Review of pertinent disorders for each system including: general characteristics, pathophysiology/psychopathology
- Medical management
- Assessment data
- Nursing interventions and client education

Community Health Nursing and Legal and Ethical Nursing are unique review texts in the marketplace. They include aspects of community health nursing and legal/ethical subject matter that is covered on the NCLEX-RN® exam. Community Health topics covered are: case management, long-term care, home health care and hospice. Legal and ethical topics include: cultural diversity, leadership and management, ethical issues and legal issues for older adults.

FEATURES

All questions in each text in the series are compliant with the most current test plan from the National Council of State Boards of Nursing (NCSBN). All questions are followed by answers and rationales for both right and wrong choices. Included are many of the alternative format questions first introduced to the exam in 2003. An icon identifies these alternate types. The questions in each of these texts are written primarily at the application or analysis cognitive levels allowing you to further enhance critical thinking skills which are heavily weighted on the NCLEX.

In addition, with the purchase of any of these texts, a free PDA download is available to you. It provides you with up to an additional 225 questions with which you can practice your test taking skills.

Thomson Delmar Learning is committed to help you reach your fullest professional potential. Good luck on the NCLEX-RN® examination!

To access your free PDA download for Thomson Delmar Learning's Nursing Review Series visit the online companion resource at **www.delmarhealthcare.com** Click on Online Companions then select the Nursing discipline.

Reviewers

Judy Bourrand, RN, MSN
Ida V. Moffett School of Nursing
Samford University
Birmingham, Alabama

Mary Kathie Doyle, BS, CCRN,
Instructor
Maria College
Troy, New York

Mary Lashley, PhD, RN, CS
Associate Professor
Towson University
Towson, Maryland

Melissa Lickteig, EdD, RN
Instructor, School of Nursing
Georgia Southern University
Statesboro, Georgia

Darlene Mathis, MSN, RN APRN, BC, NP-C, CRNP
Assistant Professor
Ida V. Moffett School of Nursing
Samford University
Birmingham, Alabama

Barbara McGraw, MSN, RN
Instructor
Central Community College
Grand Island, Nebraska

Carol Meadows, MNSc, RNP, APN
Eleanor Mann School of Nursing
University of Arkansas
Fayetteville, Arkansas

Maria Smith, DSN, RN, CCRN
Professor, School of Nursing
Middle Tennessee State University
Murfreesboro, Tennessee

1

Multisystem Stressors

CHAPTER OUTLINE

■ STRESS AND ADAPTATION

Definitions

A. Stress: tension resulting from changes in the internal or external environment; either physiologic, psychologic, developmental, or social

B. Stressors: agents or forces threatening an individual's ability to meet his or her needs

C. Adaptation: an individual's (or the body's) reaction to and attempt to deal with stress

General Characteristics

A. A certain amount of stress is necessary for life and growth, but excessive and continuous stress can be detrimental.

B. Success of adaptation depends on perception of stressor(s), the individual's coping mechanisms, and biologic adaptive resources.

C. Types of stressors: physical, chemical, microbiologic, psychologic, social, and age-related growth and development.

General Adaptation Syndrome (Hans Selye)

Response to Stress

A. Caused by release of certain adaptive hormones

B. Three Stages

  1. Alarm Reaction

    a. Sympathetic nervous system is activated (fight-or-flight response)

    b. Results in increased heart rate, blood pressure, and respirations; dilated pupils; increased state of alertness; increased blood sugar and coagulability; increased tension of skeletal muscles

  2. Resistance: body adapts to stressor; uses physical, physiologic, and psychologic coping mechanisms.

CLIENT TEACHING CHECKLIST

Suggest that the client explore tools to cope with stress, such as:

- Assertiveness training
- Journal writing
- Workshops dealing with stress management in the workplace

3. Exhaustion: adaptive resources are depleted, overwhelmed, or insufficient; if stress is excessive and continues, death will occur without support.

Stress Management/Nursing Responsibilities

A. Instruct the client concerning ways to manage stress
   1. Eat a well-balanced diet.
   2. Get sufficient amount of rest.
   3. Exercise regularly.
   4. Use relaxation methods and techniques: e.g., deep breathing, guided imagery, progressive muscle relaxation, relaxation response, meditation, yoga, biofeedback.
   5. Engage in a social support system.

INFLAMMATORY RESPONSE

A reaction of the body at the cellular level in response to injury or noxious stimuli.

Causes

A. Physical irritants (e.g., trauma or a foreign body)
B. Chemical irritants (e.g., strong acids or alkalis)
C. Microorganisms (e.g., bacteria and viruses)

Components

A. Vascular response: transitory period of localized vasoconstriction, followed by vasodilatation, increased capillary permeability, and blood stasis
B. Formation of inflammatory exudate
   1. Composition: water, colloids, ions, and defensive cells
   2. Functions: dilution of toxins, transportation of nutrients to area of injury for tissue repair, transportation of protective cells that phagocytize and destroy bacteria

C. Defense cell response: migration of leukocytes to affected area for phagocytosis of foreign bodies and dead cells

D. Healing: resolution of inflammation and regeneration of tissue or replacement with scar tissue

Assessment Findings

A. Local: pain, swelling, heat, redness, and impaired function of part (five cardinal signs of inflammation)

B. Systemic (appear with moderate to severe response): fever, leukocytosis, chills, sweating, anorexia, weight loss, general malaise

IMMUNE RESPONSE

The essence of the immune system response is recognition, neutralization, elimination, and metabolism of foreign substance with or without injury to the body's own tissue.

Functions of the Immune System

A. Defense: protection against antigens. An *antigen* is a protein or protein complex recognized as nonself.

B. Homeostasis: removal of worn out or damaged components (e.g., dead cells).

C. Surveillance: ability to perceive or destroy mutated cells or nonself cells.

Alterations in Immune Functioning

See Table 1-1.

Types of Immunity

There are two major types of immunity: natural (or innate) and acquired.

A. *Natural (innate) immunity:* immune responses that exist without prior exposure to an immunologically active substance. Genetically acquired immunity is natural immunity.

B. *Acquired immunity*
   1. Immune responses that develop during the course of a person's lifetime.
   2. Acquired immunity may be further classified as naturally or artificially acquired, active or passive. Active immunity results when the body produces its own antibodies in response to an antigen. Passive immunity results when an antibody is transferred artificially.
      a. *Naturally acquired active immunity:* results from having the disease and recovering successfully
      b. *Naturally acquired passive immunity:* antibodies obtained through placenta or breast milk

TABLE 1-1 Alterations in Immune Functioning

Immune Function	Hypofunction	Hyperfunction
Defense	Immunosuppression with increased susceptibility to infection; includes disorders such as neutropenia, AIDS, immunosuppression secondary to drugs and hypo- or agammaglobulinemia.	Inappropriate and abnormal response to external antigens; an allergy.
Homeostasis	No known effect	Abnormal response where antibodies react against normal tissues and cells; an *autoimmune disease*.
Surveillance	Inability of the immune system to perceive and respond to mutated cells, suspected mechanism in cancer.	No known effect.

    c. *Artificially acquired active immunity:* conferred by immunization with an antigen
    d. *Artificially acquired passive immunity:* antibodies transferred from sensitized person (e.g., immune serum globulin [gamma globulin])

Components of Immune Response

A. Located throughout the body

B. Organs include thymus, bone marrow, lymph nodes, spleen, tonsils, appendix, Peyer's patches of small intestine.

C. Main cell types are WBCs (especially lymphocytes, plasma cells, and macrophages); all originate from the same stem cell in bone marrow, then differentiate into separate types.

1. Granulocytes
    a. Eosinophils: increase with allergies and parasites
    b. Basophils: contain histamine and increase with allergy and anaphylaxis
    c. Neutrophils: involved in phagocytosis

2. Monocytes (macrophages) (e.g., histiocytes, Kupffer cells): involved in phagocytosis
3. Lymphocytes (T cells and B cells): involved in cellular and humoral immunity

Classification of Immune Responses

Cellular Immunity

A. Mediated by T cells: persist in tissues for months or years
B. Functions: transplant rejection, delayed hypersensitivity, tuberculin reactions, tumor surveillance/destruction, intracellular infections

Humoral Immunity

A. Mediated by B cells
   1. Production of circulating antibodies (gamma globulin)
   2. Only survive for days
B. Functions: bacterial phagocytosis, bacterial lysis, virus and toxin neutralization, anaphylaxis, allergic hay fever and asthma

■ NUTRITION

Basic Concepts

Principles

A. Essential nutrients: carbohydrates, fats, proteins, minerals, vitamins, and water that must be supplied to the body in specified amounts.
B. Foods: the sources of nutrients, provide energy to help build, repair, and maintain tissue and regulate body processes.
C. Malnutrition: results from deficiency, excess, or imbalance of required nutrients.

Carbohydrates (Sugars and Starches)

A. Major source of food energy; 4 kcal/g; composed of carbon, hydrogen, and oxygen
B. Classification
   1. Monosaccharides: simplest form of carbohydrate
      a. Glucose (dextrose): found chiefly in fruits and vegetables; oxidized for immediate energy
      b. Fructose: found in honey and fruits
      c. Galactose: not free in nature; part of milk sugar
   2. Disaccharides: double sugars
      a. Sucrose: found in table sugar, syrups, and some fruits and vegetables
      b. Lactose: found in milk
      c. Maltose: intermediate product in the hydrolysis of starch
   3. Polysaccharides: composed of many glucose molecules

   a. Starch: found in cereal grains, potatoes, root vegetables, and legumes
   b. Glycogen: synthesized and stored in the liver and skeletal muscles
   c. Cellulose, hemicellulose, pectins, gums, and mucilages: indigestible polysaccharides
4. Dietary fiber: includes several polysaccharides plus other substances that are not digestible by GI enzymes.
   a. Dietary fiber (roughage) holds water so that stools are soft and bulky; increases motility of the small and large intestine and decreases transit time; reduces intraluminal pressure in the colon.
   b. Sources: wheat bran, unrefined cereals, whole wheat, raw fruits and vegetables, dried fruits

C. Functions of carbohydrates
   1. Cheapest and most abundant source of energy; only source of energy for central nervous system
   2. To spare protein for tissue building when sufficient carbohydrate is present
   3. Necessary for the complete oxidation of fats (to prevent ketosis)

D. Dietary sources: grains, fruits, vegetables, nuts, milk, sugars (“empty calories,” contain few nutrients)

Lipids (Fats)

A. Most concentrated source of energy in foods; 9 kcal/g; contain carbon, hydrogen, oxygen

B. Include fats, oils, resins, waxes, and fatlike substances such as glycerides, phospholipids, sterols, and lipoproteins

C. Fatty acids
   1. Saturated fatty acids: usually solid at room temperature; predominantly present in animal fats
   2. Monounsaturated fatty acids: present in oleic acid found in olive oil, peanut oil
   3. Polyunsaturated fatty acids: usually liquid at room temperature; predominantly present in plant fats and fish
   4. Essential fatty acids: cannot be manufactured by the body (e.g., linoleic fatty acid)
   5. Nonessential fatty acids: can be synthesized by the body

D. Functions of lipids
   1. Most concentrated source of energy
   2. Insulation and padding of body organs
   3. Component of the cell membrane
   4. Carrier of the fat-soluble vitamins A, D, E, K
   5. Help maintain body temperature

E. Dietary sources: oil from seeds of grains, nuts, vegetables; milk fat, butter, cream cheese; fat in meat; lard, bacon fat; fish oil; egg yolk

F. *Cholesterol:* essential constituent of body tissues
   1. A component of cell membranes
   2. A precursor of steroid hormones
   3. Can be manufactured in the body
   4. Present in animal fats
   5. Dietary sources: egg yolk, brains, liver, butter, cream, cheese, shellfish

G. Indications for low-fat diet
   1. Cardiovascular disease
   2. Gallbladder disease
   3. Malabsorption syndromes, cystic fibrosis, pancreatitis

Proteins

A. Organic compounds that may be composed of hundreds of amino acids; 4 kcal/g; contain nitrogen in addition to carbon, hydrogen, and oxygen

B. Classification
   1. Complete protein: contains all the essential amino acids; usually from animal food sources.
   2. Incomplete protein: lacks one or more essential amino acids; usually from plant food sources

C. Amino acids
   1. Essential amino acids: eight amino acids that cannot be synthesized in the body and must be taken in food.
   2. Nonessential amino acids: 12 amino acids that can be synthesized in the body.

D. Functions of proteins
   1. Necessary for growth and continuous replacement of cells throughout life
   2. Play a role in the immune processes
   3. Participate in regulating body processes such as fluid balance, muscle contraction, mineral balance, iron transport, buffer actions
   4. Provide energy if necessary

E. Dietary sources: meat, fish, eggs, milk, cheese, poultry, grains, nuts, legumes (soybeans, lentils, peanuts, peanut butter)

F. Deficiencies
   1. Conditions
      a. Kwashiorkor
      b. Hypoproteinemia
      c. Marasmus (protein-kilocalorie malnutrition)
   2. Manifestations
      a. Generalized weakness
      b. Weight loss
      c. Lowered resistance to infection
      d. Slow wound healing and prolonged recovery from illness
      e. Growth failure

f. Brain damage to fetus or infant
g. Edema due to decreased albumin in blood
h. Anemia in severe deficiency
i. Fatty infiltration of liver and liver damage
3. Risk factors
a. Chronically ill
b. Elderly on fixed incomes
c. Low-income families
d. Strict vegetarians

G. Indications for high-protein diet
1. Burns, massive wounds when tissue building desired
2. Mild to moderate liver disease for organ repair when liver is still functioning
3. Malabsorption syndromes such as cystic fibrosis
4. Undernutrition
5. Pregnancy to meet needs of mother and developing fetus
6. Pregnancy-induced hypertension to replace protein lost in urine
7. Nephrosis to replace protein lost in urine
8. Deficiencies

H. Indications for low-protein diet
1. Liver failure (liver does not metabolize protein causing nitrogen toxicity to brain)
2. Kidney failure (kidneys can no longer excrete nitrogenous waste products causing toxic nitrogen levels in the brain)

I. Nursing interventions for clients needing low-protein diet
1. Increase carbohydrates so energy needs will be met by carbohydrates, not by breakdown of proteins
2. Protein intake that is allowed will be complete proteins (animal sources)

Energy Metabolism

A. Measurement of energy expressed in terms of heat units called kilocalories (kcal): amount of heat required to raise 1 kg water by 1°C

B. Energy expenditure
1. Basal metabolism
a. Amount of energy expended to carry on the involuntary work of the body while at rest
b. Factors influencing basal metabolic rate (BMR): body surface area, sex, age, body temperature, hormones, pregnancy, fasting, malnutrition
2. Physical activity: amount of energy expended depends upon the type of activity, the length of time involved, and the weight of the person

C. Factors determining total energy needs
1. Amount necessary for BMR
2. Amount required for physical activity

3. Specific dynamic action of food ingested
4. Growth
5. Climate

Minerals

Inorganic compounds that yield no energy; essential structural components involved in many body processes (see Table 1-2).

Vitamins

Organic compounds necessary in small quantities for cellular functions of the body; do not give energy; necessary in many enzyme systems (see Table 1-3).

A. Fat-soluble vitamins (A, D, E, K): can be stored in body; toxic in large amounts.
B. Water-soluble vitamins (B_1 [thiamin]; B_2 [riboflavin]; B_6 [pyridoxine]; B_{12} [hydroxycobalamin]; C[ascorbic acid]; folacin; niacin): cannot be stored in body so must be ingested daily; dissolve in cooking water, toxicity unlikely.

Water

A. Distribution: present in all body tissues; accounts for 50–60% total body weight in adults and 70–75% in infants.
   1. Intracellular fluid: exists within the cells.
   2. Extracellular fluid: includes plasma fluid, interstitial fluid, lymph, and secretions.

B. Functions: the medium of all body fluids.
   1. Necessary for many biologic reactions
   2. Acts as a solvent.
   3. Transports nutrients to cells and eliminates waste.
   4. Body lubricant.
   5. Regulates body temperature.

C. Sources.
   1. Ingestion of water and other beverages
   2. Water content of food eaten
   3. Water resulting from food oxidation

D. Recommended daily intake
   1. Replacement of losses through the kidneys, lungs, skin, and bowel
   2. Thirst usually a good guide
   3. Approximately 48 oz/day of water from all sources is adequate; requirement is higher if physical activity is strenuous or if sweating is profuse.

Dietary Guides

A. Food Pyramid
   1. Foods are grouped by composition and nutrient value: grains; vegetable group; fruit group; meat, poultry, fish, dry beans, eggs and nut group; and milk, yogurt and cheese group.

TABLE 1-2 Minerals

Mineral	Functions	Deficiency Syndrome	Food Sources	Comments
Calcium	Development of bones and teeth Transmission of nerve impulses Muscle contraction Permeability of cell membrane Catalyze thrombin formation Maintenance of normal heart rhythm	Rickets, osteoporosis, osteomalacia, stunted growth, fragile bones, tetany, occurs when parathyroids removed	Milk, cheese, ice cream, broccoli, collard greens, kale, oysters, shrimp, salmon, clams, sardines	Needs vitamin D and parathormone for utilization. Acid, lactose, and vitamin D favor absorption.
Phosphorus	Development of bones and teeth Transfer of energy in cells (ATP) Cell permeability Buffer salts Component in phospholipids	Rickets, stunted growth, poor bone mineralization	Milk, cheese, meat, fish, poultry, eggs, legumes, nuts, whole-grain cereals	Factors that affect calcium absorption also affect phosphorus. Inverse relationship to calcium.

Magnesium	Constituent of bones and teeth Cation in intracellular fluid Muscle and nerve irritability Activate enzymes in carbohydrate metabolism	Tremor observed in severe alcoholism, diabetic acidosis, severe renal disease	Milk, cheese, meat, nuts, legumes, green leafy vegetables, whole-grain cereals	Absorption similar to calcium.
Sulfur	Constituent of keratin in hair, skin, and nails Detoxification reactions Constituent of thiamin, biotin, insulin, coenzyme A, melanin, glutathione	None	Protein foods, eggs, meat, fish, poultry, milk, cheese, nuts	Diet adequate in protein provides sufficient sulfur.
Iron	Constituent of hemoglobin, myoglobin, oxidative enzymes	Anemia	Liver, organ meats, meat, poultry, egg yolk, whole-grain cereals, legumes, dark green vegetables, dried fruit	Ascorbic acid enhances absorption.

Continued

Table 1-2 Continued

Mineral	Functions	Deficiency Syndrome	Food Sources	Comments
Iodine	Constituent of thyroxine Regulate rate of energy metabolism	Simple goiter, creatinism, myxedema	Iodized salt, seafood	Allergies to iodine-rich foods may indicate allergy to iodine dyes used in diagnostic tests.
Sodium	Principle cation of extracellular fluid Osmotic pressure Water balance Regulate nerve irritability and muscle contraction Pump for active transport of glucose	Rare, seen in persons with Addison's disease	Table salt, protein foods, processed foods, baking soda	Diet usually provides excess. Increase in clients with cystic fibrosis and persons taking lithium. Decrease intake in clients with hypertension, congestive heart failure, renal failure, and edema.
Potassium	Principal cation of extracellular fluid Osmotic pressure	Muscle weakness, arrhythmias Deficiency may occur with diabetic acidosis	Oranges, bananas, dried fruits, melons, apricots, most fruits and vegetables, whole-grain cereals	Readily absorbed. Increase intake in clients taking thiazide and loop diuretics.

	Water balance Acid-base balance Regular heart rhythm Nerve irritability and muscle contraction	Deficiency may occur with thiazide and loop diuretics		Decrease intake for clients in renal failure.
Chlorine	Chief anion of extracellular fluid Constituent of gastric juice Acid-base balance Activate salivary amylase	Seen only after prolonged vomiting	Table salt, processed meats	Rapidly absorbed.

TABLE 1-3 Vitamins

Vitamin	Functions	Deficiency Syndrome	Food Sources	Comments
Fat Soluble				
Vitamin A (retinol)	Maintenance of mucous membranes Visual acuity in dim light, growth and bone development	Night blindness, xerophthalmia, keratinization of epithelium, poor bone and tooth development	Fish liver oils, liver, butter, cream, whole milk, egg yolk, dark green vegetables, yellow vegetables, yellow fruits, fortified margarine	Bile necessary for absorption. Large amounts are toxic.
Vitamin D (cholecalciferol)	Increase absorption of calcium and phosphorus Bone mineralization	Rickets, osteomalacia, enlarged joints, muscle spasms, delayed dentition	Fish liver oils, fortified milk	Synthesized in skin by activity of ultraviolet light. Large amounts are toxic.
Vitamin E (tocopherol)	Reduces oxidation of vitamin A, phospholipids, and polyunsaturated fatty acids	Hemolysis of red blood cells, deficiency not likely	Vegetable oils, wheat germ, nuts, legumes, green leafy vegetables	Not toxic.

Vitamin K (phylloquinone)	Formation of prothrombin and other clotting proteins	Prolonged clotting time, hemorrhagic disease in newborn and liver disease	Green leafy vegetables, cabbage, liver, alfalfa	Bile necessary for absorption; injectable form may be given in gallbladder and liver disease. Large amounts are toxic.
Water Soluble				
Vitamin B_1 (thiamine)	Involved in carbohydrate metabolism Thiamine pyrophosphate (TPP)	Beriberi, mental depression, polyneuritis, cardiac failure	Enriched cereals, whole grains, meat, organ meats, pork, fish, poultry, legumes, nuts	Very little storage.
Vitamin B_2 (riboflavin)	Coenzyme for transfer and removal of hydrogen Flavin adenine dinucleotide (FAD)	Cheilosis, photophobia, burning and itching of eyes, sore tongue and mouth	Milk, eggs, organ meats, green leafy vegetables	Limited storage.
Vitamin B_6 (pyridoxine, pyridoxal, pyridoxamine)	Coenzyme for transamination, transsulfuration, and decarboxylation	Convulsions, dermatitis, nervous irritability	Meat, poultry, fish, vegetables, potatoes	Converts glycogen to glucose. Given with isoniazid (INH) to prevent INH side effect of peripheral neuropathy.

Continued

Table 1-3 Continued

Vitamin	Functions	Deficiency Syndrome	Food Sources	Comments
Vitamin B_{12} (hydroxy-cobalamin)	Formation of mature red blood cells Synthesis of DNA and RNA	Pernicious anemia, neurologic degeneration, macrocytic anemia	Animal foods only	Intrinsic factor is necessary for absorption.
Vitamin C (ascorbic acid)	Synthesis of collagen Formation of intercellular cement Facilitation of iron absorption	Scurvy, bleeding gums, poor wound healing, cutaneous hemorrhage, capillary fragility	Citrus fruits, tomatoes, melon, raw cabbage, broccoli, strawberries	Most easily destroyed vitamin. Very little storage in body.
Folacin (folic acid)	Maturation of red blood cells, interrelated with vitamin B_{12}	Megaloblastic anemia, tropical sprue	Organ meats, muscle meats, poultry, fish, eggs, green leafy vegetables	Ascorbic acid necessary for utilization.
Niacin (nicotinamide)	Coenzyme to accept and transfer hydrogen, coenzyme for glycolysis	Pellagra, dermatitis, neurologic degeneration, glossitis, diarrhea	Meat, poultry, fish, whole grains, enriched breads, nuts, legumes	Amino acid tryptophan is a precursor.

2. Greater emphasis on fruits and vegetables with less emphasis on meats and fats than with basic four.
3. Recommends using fats and sweets sparingly.

B. Recommended daily allowances: established by the Food and Nutrition Board of the National Academy of Science; recommended nutrient intake is provided for infants, children, men, women, pregnant and lactating women; recommendations are stated for protein, kcal, and most vitamins and minerals.

C. Food composition tables: helpful in calculating the nutritive value of the daily diet; list nutrient content of foods.

D. Height and weight charts: ideal or desirable body weight for both men and women at specified heights with a small, medium, or large frame.

E. Exchange lists for meal planning
1. Foods are separated into six exchange lists.
2. Specific foods on each list are approximately equal in carbohydrate, protein, fat, and kcal content.
3. Individual foods on the same list may be exchanged for each other at the same meals.
4. Food lists are helpful in planning diets for weight control or diabetes.

Nutritional Assessment

Health History

A. Presenting problem
1. Weight changes
   a. Usual body weight 20% above or below normal standards.
   b. Recent loss or gain of 10% of usual body weight.
2. Appetite changes: may increase or decrease from usual.
3. Food intolerances: allergies, fluids, fat, salt, seafood
4. Difficulty swallowing
5. Dyspepsia or indigestion
6. Bowel dysfunction: record frequency, consistency, color of stools.
   a. Constipation
   b. Diarrhea

B. Lifestyle: eating behaviors such as fast foods, "junk foods," and skipping meals; cultural/religious concerns (vegetarian, kosher foods, exclusion of certain food groups); alcohol, socioeconomic status, living conditions (alone or with family).

C. Use of medications: vitamin supplements, antacids, antidiarrheals, laxatives, diuretics, antihypertensives, immunosuppressants, oral contraceptives, antibiotics, antidepressants, digitalis, anti-inflammatory agents, catabolic steroids.

D. Medical history: gastrointestinal diseases; endocrine diseases; hyperlipidemia; coronary artery disease; malabsorption syndrome; circulatory problems or heart failure; cancer; radiation therapy; chronic lung, renal, or liver disease; food allergies; recent major surgery; eating disorders; obesity.

E. Family history: obesity, allergies, cardiovascular diseases, diabetes, thyroid disease.
F. Dietary history: evaluation of the nutritional adequacy of diet
   1. 24-hour recall
   2. Food diary for a given number of days

Physical Examination

A. Assess for alertness and responsiveness
B. Record weight in relation to height, body build, and age
C. Inspect posture, muscle tone, skeleton for deformities
D. Elicit reflexes
E. Auscultate heart rate, rhythm; blood pressure
F. Inspect hair, skin, nails, oral mucosa, tongue, teeth
G. Inspect for swelling of legs or feet
H. Anthropometric measurements: indicators of available stores in muscle and fat compartments of body
   1. Height/weight ratio (Body Mass Index [BMI])
   2. Midarm muscle circumference
   3. Skinfold thickness (triceps, biceps, subscapular, abdominal, hip, pectoral, or calf)

Laboratory/Diagnostic Tests

A. Blood studies: serum albumin, iron-binding capacity, hemoglobin, hematocrit, lymphocyte count, blood sugar, total cholesterol, high-density lipids, low-density lipids, triglycerides, serum electrolytes
B. Urine studies, urinalysis, glucose, ketones, albumin, 24-hour creatinine
C. Nitrogen balance studies
D. Feces, hair
E. Intradermal delayed hypersensitivity testing

Analysis

Nursing diagnoses for the client with a nutritional dysfunction may include:
A. Imbalanced nutrition: less than body requirements
B. Imbalanced nutrition: more than body requirements
C. Risk for imbalanced nutrition: more than body requirements
D. Impaired oral mucous membrane
E. Self-care deficit, feeding
F. Disturbed sensory perceptions
G. Risk for impaired skin integrity
H. Impaired swallowing
I. Impaired tissue integrity
J. Activity intolerance
K. Disturbed body image
L. Constipation

M. Diarrhea
N. Deficient fluid volume
O. Excess fluid volume
P. Delayed growth and development
Q. Risk for infection
R. Deficient knowledge
S. Noncompliance

Planning and Implementation

Goals

A. Normal weight will be achieved and maintained.
B. Integrity of oral cavity will be maintained.
C. Client will feed self or receive help with feeding.
D. Normal skin integrity will be achieved/maintained.
E. Client will not aspirate.
F. Normal tissue integrity will be achieved/maintained.
G. Client will be able to exercise normally.
H. Client will maintain/develop satisfactory self-image.
I. Normal bowel functioning will be maintained.
J. Fluid and electrolyte balance will be achieved/maintained.
K. Client will have normal growth and development patterns.
L. Client will not develop infection.
M. Client will demonstrate knowledge of special dietary needs/prescriptions.
N. Client will comply with special diet.

Interventions

Care of the Client on a Special Diet

A. General information: therapeutic diets involve modifications of nutritional components necessitated by a client's disease state or nutritional status or to prepare a client for a procedure.
B. Nursing care in relation to special diets
   1. Assess client's mental, emotional, physical, and economic status; appropriateness of diet to client's condition; and ability to understand diet and comply with it.
   2. Maintain appropriate diet and teach client.
   3. Changing diet means changing lifelong patterns.
   4. Teach client importance of adhering to special diets that are long term.

Weight Control Diets

A. Underweight: 10% or more below individual's ideal weight
   1. Causes: failure to ingest enough kcal, excess energy expenditure, irregular eating habits, GI disturbances, mouth sores, cancer,

endocrine disorders, emotional disturbances, lack of education, economic problems.

2. Treatment: diet counseling, correction of underlying disease, nutritional supplements, behavioral therapy, social service referral.

B. Overweight: 10% or more above individual's ideal weight

C. Obesity: 20% or more above individual's ideal weight

1. Causes: overeating, underactivity, genetic factors, fat cell theory, alteration in hypothalamic function, endocrine disorders, emotional disturbances.
2. Treatment: diet counseling, nutritionally balanced diet, behavior modification, increased physical activity, medical treatment of any underlying disease, appropriate referrals.

D. Nursing care

1. Explain dietary instructions.
   a. Reducing fats and "empty calories" reduces caloric intake without sacrificing nutritional intake
   b. Increasing exercise increases metabolism
2. Caution against fad diets that may be nutritionally inadequate.
3. Encourage support groups if indicated.

Diabetic Diet

A. Prescribed for clients with diabetes mellitus.

B. Purposes include: attain or maintain ideal body weight, ensure normal growth, maintain plasma glucose levels as close to normal as possible.

C. Principles

1. Distribution of kcal: protein 12–20%; carbohydrates 55–60%; fats (unsaturated) 20–25%.
2. Daily distribution of kcal: equally divided among breakfast, lunch, supper, snacks.
3. Use foods high in fiber and complex carbohydrates.
4. Avoid simple sugars, jams, honey, syrup, frosting.

D. Teach client to utilize exchange lists.

E. New recommendations include low-fat, high fiber diet.

Protein-Modified Diets

A. Gluten-free diet

1. Purpose is to eliminate gluten (a protein) from the diet.
2. Indicated in malabsorption syndromes such as sprue and celiac disease.
3. Eliminate all barley, rye, oats, and wheat (BROW).
4. Avoid: cream sauces, breaded foods, cakes, breads, muffins.
5. Allow corn, rice, and soy flour.
6. Teach client to read labels of prepared foods.

B. PKU (Phenylketonuria) diet

1. Purpose is to control intake of phenylalanine, an amino acid that cannot be metabolized.

2. Diet will be prescribed until at least age 6 to prevent brain damage and mental retardation.
3. Avoid: breads, meat, fish, poultry, cheeses, legumes, nuts, eggs.
4. Give Lofenalac formula.
5. Teach family to use low-protein flour for baking.
6. Sugar substitutes such as Nutrasweet contain phenylalanine and must not be used.

C. Low-purine diet
   1. Indicated for gout, uric acid kidney stones, and uric acid retention.
   2. Purpose is to decrease the amount of purine, a precursor to uric acid.
   3. Teach client to avoid: organ meats, other meats, fowl, fish and lobster, lentils, dried peas and beans, nuts, oatmeal, whole wheat.
   4. Eggs are not high in purine.

Fat-Restricted Diets

Purpose is to restrict amount of fats ingested for clients with chronic pancreatitis, malabsorption syndromes, gallbladder disease, cystic fibrosis, and hyperlipidemia, and to control weight.

Consistency Modifications

A. Clear liquid diet
   1. Purpose is to rest GI tract and maintain fluid balance.
   2. Indications include difficulty chewing or swallowing; before certain diagnostic tests to reduce fecal material; immediate postoperative period (until bowel sounds have returned) to maintain electrolyte balance; and nausea, vomiting, and diarrhea.
   3. Foods allowed: "see-through foods" include water, tea, broth, jello, apple juice, clear carbonated beverages, and frozen ice pops.
   4. Not nutritionally adequate.

B. Full liquid diet
   1. Used as a transition diet between clear liquid and soft diet; usually short term.
   2. Foods allowed: clear liquids, milk and milk products, all fruit juices, cooked and strained cereals.
   3. Can be nutritionally adequate.

C. Soft diet
   1. Used as a transition diet between full liquid and regular diet.
   2. Indications include postoperatively, mild GI disturbances, chewing difficulties from lack of teeth or oral surgery.
   3. Foods allowed: foods low in fiber, connective tissue and fat (full liquid diet, pureed vegetables, eggs cooked any way except fried, tender meat, potatoes, cooked fruit).
   4. Nutritionally adequate.

D. Bland diet
   1. Promotes healing of the gastric mucosa and is chemically and mechanically nonstimulating.
   2. Foods allowed: soft diet without spices.

E. Low-residue diet
   1. Residue is the indigestible substances left in digestive tract after food has been digested.
   2. Indications include colon, rectal, or perineal surgery to reduce pressure on the operative site; prior to examination of the lower bowel to enhance visualization; internal radiation for cancer of the cervix; Crohn's disease or regional enteritis; ulcerative colitis to reduce irritation of the large bowel; and diarrhea.
   3. Teach client to avoid foods high in fiber, foods having skins and seeds, and milk and milk products.

Evaluation

A. Client's weight is within normal limits.
B. No lesions in oral cavity.
C. Client feeds self or receives needed assistance with feeding.
D. Skin and tissue integrity is maintained.
E. Client demonstrates ability to exercise.
F. Client makes positive statements about self-image.
G. Client's bowel functioning is normal.
H. Serum electrolytes are within normal limits.
I. Client will exhibit growth and development patterns appropriate for age.
J. Client shows no evidence of infection.
K. Client states reason for special diet.
L. Client describes foods allowed and not allowed on prescribed diet.
M. Client adheres to prescribed diet.

Enteral Nutrition

Preferred method for nutritional support for the malnourished client whose GI system is intact.

Oral Feeding

A. Always the first choice.
B. Oral formula supplements may be used between meals to provide added kcal and nutrients.
   1. Offer small quantities several times a day.
   2. Vary flavors, avoid taste fatigue.
   3. Chill and serve over ice.

Tube Feeding

A. Used for clients who have a functioning GI tract but cannot ingest food orally

1. Feeding tubes
   a. Short term: nasogastric tube
   b. Long term: esophagostomy, gastrostomy, or enterostomy tube
2. Formulas: nutritionally adequate, tolerated by client, easily prepared, easily digested, usual concentration 1 kcal/ml
3. Feeding schedules
   a. Intermittent: usually 4–6 times/day, volumes up to 400 ml, by slow gravity drip over 30–60 minutes
   b. Continuous: usually administered by pump through a duodenal or proximal jejunostomy feeding tube
4. Nursing responsibilities
   a. Administer formulas at room temperature (refrigerate unused portion).
   b. Gradually increase rate and concentration until desired amount is attained if there are no signs of intolerance (e.g., gastric residual greater than 120 ml, nausea, vomiting, diarrhea, distention, diaphoresis, increased pulse, glycosuria, aspiration).
   c. Check tube placement and elevate head of bed.
   d. Monitor I&O, serum electrolytes, fractional urines, serum glucose, daily weights; keep a stool record as well as an ongoing assessment of tolerance.

Parenteral Nutrition

Nutrients are infused directly into a vein for clients who are unable to eat or digest food through the GI tract, who refuse to eat, or who have inadequate oral intake.

Total Parenteral Nutrition (TPN)

A. Involves the infusion of nutrients through a central vein catheter. A central vein is needed because its larger caliber and higher blood flow will quickly dilute the hypertonic hyperalimentation solution to isotonic concentrations.

B. Hyperalimentation solutions
   1. Hypertonic glucose of 20–70%, amino acids, water, vitamins, and minerals with lipid emulsions given in a separate solution.
   2. Three-in-one solutions
      a. Lipids mixed with dextrose and amino acids in pharmacy.
      b. Comes in a three liter container and administered over 24 hours.

C. Nursing responsibilities
   1. For details of nursing care of the client with a central venous line.
   2. Inspect solution before hanging.
      a. Check for correct solution and additives against physician's order.

NURSING ALERT

To prevent hypoglycemic states, have dextrose 10% and water available as an alternate solution if a new TPN solution cannot be obtained.

   - **b.** Check expiration date.
   - **c.** Observe fluid for cloudiness or floating particulate matter.
- **3.** Control flow rate of solution.
   - **a.** Verify order and monitor flow rate.
   - **b.** Administration via pump is required.
   - **c.** Tubing with in-line filter is required.
   - **d.** Never attempt to speed up or slow down infusion rate.
      - **1)** speeding up infusion causes large amounts of glucose to enter body, causing hyperosmolar state.
      - **2)** slowing down infusion can cause hypoglycemic state, as it takes time for the pancreas to adjust to reduced glucose level.
- **4.** Monitor fluid balance.
- **5.** Assess client for signs and symptoms of infection (fever, chills, elevated WBC count).
- **6.** Obtain fractional urines or Accu-checks every 6 hours.
- **7.** Administer sliding scale insulin for hyperglycemia, as ordered.
- **8.** Provide psychological support.
- **9.** Encourage exercise regimen.

IV Lipid Emulsions

- **A.** May be given through a central vein or peripherally in order to prevent essential fatty acid deficiency in long-term TPN clients, or to provide supplemental kcal IV.
- **B.** Nursing care
   - **1.** Protect the stability of the emulsion.
      - **a.** Administer in its own separate IV bottle and IV tubing, and piggyback the emulsion into the Y connector closest to the catheter insertion. Follow hospital policy and manufacturer's recommendations for specific products.
      - **b.** Inspect solution for evidence of separation of oil, frothiness, inconsistency, particulate matter; discard solution if any of these signs of instability occur.
      - **c.** Do *not* shake the bottle; this might cause aggregation of fat globules.
      - **d.** Discard partially used bottles.
   - **2.** Control the infusion rate accurately and safely.

NURSING ALERT

When infusing fat emulsion and TPN, always infuse the fat emulsion through the correct size IV filter: 0.22 m for dextrose/amino acids; 1.2 m for three-in-one solutions.

   a. If using gravity method, lipid emulsion must hang higher than hyperalimentation to prevent backflow.
   b. Pump is preferred but may not be possible due to viscous nature of emulsion.
3. Prevent and assess for adverse reactions.
   a. Administer slowly according to package insert over first 30 minutes; if no adverse reactions, increase rate to complete infusion over the specified number of hours.
   b. Obtain baseline vital signs; repeat after first 30 minutes, and then every 1–2 hours until completion.
   c. Acute reactions may include: fever, chills, dyspnea, nausea, vomiting, headache, lethargy, syncope, chest or back pain, hypercoagulability, thrombocytopenia.
4. Evaluate tolerance and client response.

Peripheral Vein Parenteral Nutrition (PPN)

A. Can be used for short-term support, when the central vein is not available, and as a supplemental means of obtaining nutrients. Client must be able to tolerate a relatively high fluid volume.
B. Solution contains the same components as central vein therapy, but lower concentrations (less than 20% glucose).
C. Care is the same as for the client receiving hyperalimentation centrally.
D. Phlebitis and thrombosis are common and IV sites will need frequent changing.

■ INFECTION

Infection is an invasion of the body by pathogenic organisms that multiply and produce injurious effects. Communicable disease is an infectious disease that may be transmitted from one person to another.

Chain of Events

A. *Causative agent:* invading organism (e.g., bacteria, virus)
B. *Reservoir:* environment in which the invading organism lives and multiplies

C. *Portal of exit:* mode of escape from reservoir (e.g., respiratory tract, GI tract)
D. *Mode of transmission:* method by which invading organism is transported to new host (e.g., direct contact, air, food)
E. *Portal of entry:* means by which organism enters new host (e.g., respiratory tract, broken skin)
F. *Susceptible host:* susceptibility determined by factors such as number of invading organisms, duration of exposure, age, state of health, nutritional status.

Nursing Responsibilities in Prevention of Spread of Infection

A. Maintain an environment that is clean, dry, and well ventilated.
B. Use proper handwashing before and after client contact and after contact with contaminated material.
C. Disinfect and handle wastes and contaminated materials properly.
D. Prevent transmission of infectious droplets.
   1. Teach clients to cover mouth and nose when sneezing or coughing.
   2. Place contaminated tissues and articles in paper bag before disposing.
E. Institute proper isolation techniques as required by specific disease
F. Use surgical aseptic technique when appropriate: caring for open wounds, irrigating, or entering sterile cavities.
G. Practice universal precautions when caring for all clients regardless of their diagnosis in order to minimize contact with blood and body fluids and prevent the transmission of specific infections such as hepatitis B and human immunodeficiency virus (HIV).
   1. Hands must always be washed before and after contact with clients even when gloves have been used.
   2. If hands come in contact with blood, body fluids, or human tissue they should be immediately washed with soap and water.
   3. Gloves should be worn before touching blood or body fluids, mucous membranes, or nonintact skin.
   4. Gloves should be changed between each client contact and as soon as possible if torn.
   5. Wear masks and protective eyewear during procedures that are likely to generate splashes of blood or other body fluids.
   6. Wear gowns during procedures that are likely to generate splashes of blood or other body fluids and when cleaning spills from incontinent clients or changing soiled linen.
   7. Disposable masks should be used when performing CPR.
   8. Dispose of used needles properly. They should be promptly placed in a puncture-resistant container. They *should not* be recapped, bent, broken, or removed from syringes.

PAIN

Pain is an unpleasant sensation, entirely subjective, that produces discomfort, distress, or suffering.

Gate Control Theory

A. Substantia gelatinosa in the dorsal horn of the spinal cord acts as a gate mechanism that can close to keep pain impulses from reaching the brain, or can open to allow pain impulses to ascend to the brain.

B. Most pain impulses are conducted over small-diameter nerve fibers; if predominant nerve message is pain, the gate opens and allows pain impulses to reach the brain.

C. The gate can be closed by conflicting impulses from the skin conducted over large-diameter nerve fibers, by impulses from the reticular formation in the brainstem, or by impulses from the entire cerebral cortex or thalamus.

Acute Pain and Chronic Pain

A. Acute pain
1. Short duration; may last from split second to about 6 months.
2. Serves the purpose of warning the client that damage or injury has occurred in the body that requires treatment.
3. Subsides as healing occurs.
4. Usually associated with autonomic nervous system symptoms, e.g., increased pulse and blood pressure, sweating, pallor.

B. Chronic pain
1. Prolonged duration; lasts for 6 months or longer.
2. Serves no useful purpose.
3. Persists long after injury has healed.
4. Rarely accompanied by autonomic nervous system activity.

Assessment of Pain

See Table 1-4.

General Nursing Interventions

A. Establish nurse-client relationship.
1. Let the client know that you believe that his pain is real.
2. Respect the client's attitudes and behavioral responses to pain using a standardized pain scale appropriate to age and condition.
3. Document effectiveness of interventions in a timely manner.

B. Assess characteristics of pain and evaluate client's response to interventions.

C. Promote rest and relaxation.
1. Prevent fatigue.

TABLE 1-4 Pain Assessment

Influencing factors • Past experience with pain • Age (tolerance generally increases with age) • Culture and religious beliefs • Level of anxiety • Physical state (fatigue or chronic illness may decrease tolerance)
Characteristics of pain • Location • Quality • Intensity • Timing and duration • Precipitating factors • Aggravating factors • Alleviating factors • Interference with activities of daily living • Patterns of response

 2. Teach relaxation techniques, e.g., slow, rhythmic breathing, guided imagery.

D. Institute comfort measures.
 1. Positioning: support body parts.
 2. Decrease noxious stimuli such as noise or bright lights.

E. Provide cutaneous stimulation: massage, pressure, baths, vibration, heat, cold packs; increased input of large-diameter fibers closes gate.

F. Relieve anxiety and fears.
 1. Spend time with client.
 2. Offer reassurance, explanations.

G. Provide distraction and diversion, e.g., music, puzzles.

H. Administer pain medication as needed.
 1. Administer pain medication in early stages before pain becomes severe.
 2. Administer pain medication prior to procedure that produces discomfort.
 3. If pain is present most of the day, a preventative approach may be used, e.g., an around-the-clock schedule may be ordered in place of a prn schedule.
 4. Document effectiveness of intervention.

I. Teach client about pain and pain control measures, e.g., relaxation techniques, cutaneous stimulation.

DELEGATION TIP

Pain Assessment

It is the RN's responsibility to evaluate the patient's response to the pain-reduction interventions. Inform ancillary personnel or other care givers about the medications the patient is receiving if adverse effects are anticipated or are being monitored.

Specific Medical and Surgical Therapies for Pain

Nonnarcotic Analgesics

A. Salicylates

   1. Examples: Acetylsalicylic acid (ASA, aspirin (Ecotrin), choline magnesium trisalicylate (Trilisate), diflunisal (Dolobid), salsalate (Disalcid)

   2. Mechanism of action

      a. Analgesic action: produced by action on the hypothalamus and inhibition of prostaglandin synthesis

      b. Antipyretic action: acts on hypothalamus to produce peripheral vasodilation, which causes sweating and heat loss (diflunisal [Dolobid] has minimal antipyretic effect)

      c. Anti-inflammatory action: caused by inhibition of prostaglandin formation

      d. Antiplatelet activity: inhibits platelet aggregation (Trilisate, Dolobid, and Disalcid have no effect on platelet aggregation)

   3. Uses

      a. Relief of mild to moderate pain

      b. Reduction of elevated body temperature

      c. Symptomatic treatment of numerous inflammatory disorders

   4. Side effects

      a. Allergic reaction: varies from rash to anaphylaxis

      b. Anemia, decreased platelet aggregation, prolonged bleeding time (not with Trilisate, Dolobid, or Disalcid)

      c. Nausea, vomiting, gastritis, occult GI bleeding

      d. Renal failure with high doses

      e. Toxicity: tinnitus, visual changes, alterations in mental status

   5. Nursing interventions

      a. Give with food, milk, or antacid to decrease GI irritation; contraindicated in clients with ulcer disease.

      b. Check auditory and visual status periodically.

      c. Instruct client to watch for any signs of bleeding.

      d. Monitor renal function tests in clients receiving high doses or those in ASA toxicity.

B. Acetaminophen (Datril, Tylenol).
C. Nonsteroidal anti-inflammatory drugs (NSAIDs: ibuprofen [Motrin], indomethacin [Indocin], piroxicam [Feldene])
    1. Nursing interventions
        a. Administer with food or milk to prevent GI upset.
        b. Teach client to observe for and report signs of bleeding.
        c. Caution client that drowsiness and dizziness may occur and may impair ability to perform mechanical tasks.

Adjuvants

A. Includes several classes of drugs that may either:
    1. Potentiate the effects of narcotic or nonnarcotic analgesics, e.g., hydroxyzine (Vistaril, Atarax)
    2. Have independent analgesic properties in certain situations, e.g., tricyclic antidepressants such as amitriptyline (Elavil) for neuropathic pain
    3. Help control signs and symptoms associated with pain, e.g., anxiety, depression, nausea, and insomnia

Patient-Controlled Analgesia (PCA)

A. Type of intravenous pump that allows the client to administer narcotic analgesic (e.g., morphine) on demand within preset dose and frequency limits.
B. Goal is to achieve more constant level of analgesia as compared to prn IM injections; also, in general, causes less sedation and lower risk of respiratory depression.
C. Used most often for postoperative pain management; also used for intractable pain in terminal illness.
D. PCA pump may be used solely on PCA mode or may be combined with a continuous basal mode where client is receiving continuous infusion of narcotic in addition to self-administered bolus injections.
E. The dose of the analgesic bolus and the time interval between boluses (lockout period) is preset on the pump by the RN according to physician's orders.
F. Nursing Interventions
    1. Instruct client in use of PCA pump
        a. Demonstrate how to push control button.
        b. Explain concept of client-controlled analgesia.
    2. Assess client's level of consciousness, respiratory rate, and degree of pain relief frequently.
    3. Keep control button within client reach.

CLIENT TEACHING CHECKLIST

1. Explain purpose of PCA.
2. Teach how to report pain on a scale of 0–10.
3. Explain how to use the PCA button to administer a bolus of analgesic.
4. Explain that "Lockout" is an internal protection against overdosing.

Intraspinal Narcotic Infusion

A. Involves intraspinal infusion of narcotics or local anesthetic agents for relief of acute or chronic pain.

B. Medication is infused through catheter placed in the subarachnoid (intrathecal) or epidural space in the thoracic or lumbar area.

C. Repeated injections of narcotics produce analgesia without many of the side effects associated with systemic narcotics (e.g., sedation).

D. Indications

  1. Temporary intraspinal narcotic therapy is used most frequently for postoperative pain.

  2. For chronic pain, e.g., management of chronic cancer pain, the catheter may be tunneled under the skin and implanted subcutaneously in the abdomen; an implantable infusion device may be used to provide continuous narcotic infusion.

E. Nursing Interventions

  1. Monitor client closely for respiratory depression especially during initiation of treatment. (May be reversed with naloxone [Narcan]).

  2. Assess for other side effects:

    a. Urinary retention: Foley catheter may be used in post-op client until infusion is discontinued

    b. Pruritus: may be treated with antihistamine or medication rate reduction.

    c. Nausea and vomiting

  3. Check insertion site frequently for signs of infection.

Electrical Stimulation Techniques for Pain Control

A. *Transcutaneous electrical nerve stimulator (TENS)*

  1. Noninvasive alternative to traditional methods of pain relief

  2. Used in treating acute pain (e.g., post-op pain) and chronic pain (e.g., chronic low back pain)

  3. Consists of impulse generator connected by wires to electrodes on skin; produces tingling, buzzing sensation in the area.

  4. Mechanism based on gate-control theory: electrical impulse stimulates large diameter nerve fibers to "close the gate."

5. Nursing responsibilities
   a. Do not place electrodes over incision site, broken skin, carotid sinus, eyes, laryngeal or pharyngeal muscles.
   b. Do not use in client with cardiac pacemaker.
   c. Provide skin care.
      1) remove electrodes once a day; wash area with soap and water and air dry.
      2) wipe area with skin prep pad before reapplying electrode.
      3) assess area for signs of redness; reposition electrodes if redness persists for more than 30 minutes.

B. *Dorsal column stimulator*
   1. Used in selected clients for whom conventional methods of pain relief have not been effective.
   2. Electrode is surgically placed over the dorsal column of the spinal cord via laminectomy; connected by wires to a transmitter that may be worn externally or be implanted subcutaneously.

Neurosurgical Procedures for Pain Control

A. Performed for persistent intractable pain of high intensity
B. Involves surgical destruction of nerve pathways to block transmission of pain
C. Types
   1. *Neurectomy:* interruption of cranial or peripheral nerves by incision or injection
   2. *Rhizotomy:* interruption of posterior nerve root close to the spinal cord
      a. Laminectomy is necessary.
      b. Results in permanent loss of sensation and position sense in affected parts.
   3. *Chordotomy:* interruption of pain-conducting pathways within the spinal cord
      a. Laminectomy usually required.
      b. May be done by percutaneous needle insertion.
      c. Interrupts conduction of pain and temperature sense in affected parts.
   4. *Sympathectomy:* interruption of afferent pathways in the sympathetic division of the autonomic nervous system; used to control pain from causalgia and peripheral vascular disease.
D. Nursing responsibilities
   1. Provide pre- and post-op care for a laminectomy.
   2. Assess extremities for sensation (e.g., touch, pain, temperature, pressure, position sense) and movement.
   3. Provide safety measures to protect client from injury and carefully monitor skin for signs of damage or pressure.
   4. Teach client ways to compensate for loss of sensation in affected parts.
      a. Visually inspect skin for signs of injury or pressure.

   b. Check temperature of bath water.
   c. Avoid use of hot water bottles, heating pads.
   d. Avoid extremes of temperature.

Acupuncture

A. A Chinese technique of pain control by insertion of fine needles at various points on the body
B. Based on Eastern philosophy where insertion of needles is thought to block energy flow and restore the body's harmony
C. Mechanism of action: two theories
   1. Trigger points: the needles stimulate hypersensitive areas in muscle that produce local and referred pain. Extinction of the trigger point alleviates the referred pain.
   2. Endorphin system: needle insertion activates production of endorphins (body's natural opiates).
D. Acupressure: a less invasive variation; uses finger pressure and massage

Hypnosis

A. Has been used in dental procedures, labor and delivery, pain control in cancer.
B. Mechanism is thought to be related to positive suggestions that alter client's perception of pain.

Behavioral Techniques

A. Types
   1. *Operant conditioning:* based on decreasing positive reinforcement for pain behaviors
   2. *Biofeedback:* teaches clients to control physiologic responses to pain (e.g., muscle tension, heart rate, blood pressure) and to replace them with a state of relaxation.
B. Work best in conjunction with other types of pain management and stress reduction techniques.

FLUIDS AND ELECTROLYTES

Basic Principles

Fluids

A. Water constitutes over 50% of individual's weight; largest single component.
B. Body water divided into two compartments
   1. Intracellular: within cells
   2. Extracellular: outside cells, further divided into interstitial and intravascular fluid
C. Fluids in two compartments move among cells, tissue spaces, and plasma.

Electrolytes

- **A.** Salts or minerals in extracellular or intracellular body fluids
- **B.** If positively charged, called *cations*; if negatively charged, called *anions*
- **C.** Common electrolytes and normal blood values
  1. Sodium (Na)—135-148 mEq/liter
  2. Potassium (K)—3.5-5 mEq/liter
  3. Calcium (Ca)—4.5-5.3 mEq/liter, 9-11 mg/dl
  4. Magnesium (Mg)—1.3-2.1 mEq/liter
  5. Chloride (Cl)—98-106 mEq/liter

Movement of Fluids and Electrolytes

- **A.** Diffusion: movement of particles from an area of greater concentration to an area of lesser concentration as part of random activity
- **B.** Active transport: movement across cell membranes requiring energy from an outside source
- **C.** Osmosis: movement of water through a semipermeable membrane

Fluid and Electrolyte Imbalances

See Table 1-5.

- **A.** *Hypovolemia:* extracellular fluid volume deficit
- **B.** *Hypervolemia:* extracellular fluid volume excess
- **C.** *Water excess:* hypo-osmolar imbalances; water intoxication or solute deficit
- **D.** *Water deficit:* hyperosmolar imbalances; water depletion or solute excess
- **E.** *Hyperkalemia:* potassium excess, serum potassium above 5.5 mEq/liter
- **F.** *Hypokalemia:* potassium deficit, serum potassium below 3.5 mEq/liter
- **G.** *Hypernatremia:* sodium excess, serum sodium level above 145 mEq/liter
- **H.** *Hyponatremia:* sodium deficit, serum sodium level below 135 mEq/liter
- **I.** *Hypercalcemia:* calcium excess, serum calcium level above 5.8 mEq/liter
- **J.** *Hypocalcemia:* calcium deficit, serum calcium level below 4.5 mEq/liter
- **K.** *Hypermagnesemia:* magnesium excess, serum magnesium level above 3 mEq/liter
- **L.** *Hypomagnesemia:* magnesium deficit, serum magnesium level below 1.5 mEq/liter

■ ACID-BASE BALANCE

Basic Principles

- **A.** Normal pH of the body is 7.35-7.45.
- **B.** Buffer or control systems maintain normal pH. Kidneys excrete acids and reabsorb bicarbonate while the respiratory system gives off carbon dioxide in acidic states. In alkalotic states, the kidneys excrete bicarbonate and the respiratory system retains carbonic acid.

TABLE 1-5 Fluid and Electrolyte Imbalances

Imbalance	Causes	Assessment Findings	Nursing Interventions
Hypovolemia (extracellular fluid volume deficit)	Hemorrhage, diarrhea, vomiting, kidney disease, diaphoresis, burns, fever, draining fistulas, sequestration of fluids (peritonitis, edema associated with burns)	Nausea and vomiting, weakness, weight loss, anorexia, longitudinal wrinkles of the tongue, dry skin and mucous membranes, decreased fullness of neck veins, postural hypotension, oliguria to anuria, shock	Measure I&O. Weigh daily. Monitor closely and regulate isotonic IV infusion. Monitor blood pressure (determine lying down, sitting, and standing). Report urine output less than 30 ml/hr. Carefully assess skin and mucous membranes. Monitor for signs of shock.
Hypervolemia (extracellular fluid volume excess)	Excess or too rapid administration of any isotonic solution; side effect of corticosteroid administration; cardiac, liver, or renal disease; cerebral damage; stress	Weight gain, pitting edema, dyspnea, cough, diaphoresis, frothy or pink-tinged sputum, edema of the eyelids, distended neck veins, elevated blood pressure, moist rales (crackles)	Weigh daily. Measure I&O. Regulate IV fluids/administration of diuretics strictly and monitor carefully. Monitor abdominal girth. Assess for pitting edema. Restrict sodium and water intake.

Continued

Table 1-5 **Continued**

Imbalance	Causes	Assessment Findings	Nursing Interventions
Water excess syndromes	Excessive intake of water, inability to excrete water due to kidney or brain damage, excessive administration of electrolyte- free solutions, poor salt intake, use of diuretics, irrigation of nasogastric tube with plain water, administration of excessive amount of ice chips to a vomiting client or one with a nasogastric tube	Polyuria (in absence of renal disease), oliguria (with renal disease), twitching, hyper-irritability, disorientation, coma, convulsions, abdominal cramps	Measure I&O. Weigh daily. Restrict oral and IV intake. Replace fluid losses with isotonic solutions. Use normal saline solution for nasogastric tube irrigation.
Water deficit syndromes	Increased water output due to watery diarrhea, diabetic acidosis, excess TPN; dysphagia; impaired thirst mechanism; coma; general debility; diaphoresis; excess protein intake without sufficient water intake	Thirst, poor skin turgor, dry skin and mucous membranes, dry furrowed tongue, sunken eyeballs, weight loss, elevated temperature, apprehension, oliguria to anuria	Measure I&O. Weigh daily. Assess skin frequently. Ensure that clients with a high solute intake receive adequate water. Assess vital signs frequently, particularly temperature. Monitor TPN infusions

			accurately.
Hyperkalemia	Renal insufficiency, adrenocortical insufficiency, cellulose damage (burns), infection, acidotic states, rapid infusion of IV solutions with potassium, overzealous administration of potassium-conserving diuretics	Thready, slow pulse; shallow breathing; nausea and vomiting; diarrhea; intestinal colic, irritability; muscle weakness, numbness, flaccid paralysis; tingling; difficulty with phonation, respiration	Administer Kayexalate as ordered. Administer/monitor IV infusion of glucose and insulin. Control infection. Provide adequate calories and carbohydrates. Discontinue IV or oral sources of potassium.
Hypokalemia	Anorexia, alcoholism, gastric and intestinal suction, GI surgery, vomiting, diarrhea, laxative abuse, thiazide diuretics, steroid therapy, stress, alkalotic states	Thready, rapid, weak pulse; faint heart sounds; decreased blood pressure; skeletal muscle weakness; decreased or absent reflexes; shallow respirations; malaise; apathy; lethargy; loss of orientation; anorexia, vomiting, weight loss, gaseous intestinal distention	Be especially cautious if administering drugs that are not potassium sparing. Administer potassium supplements to replace losses. Monitor acid-base balance. Monitor pulse, blood pressure, and ECG.

Continued

Table 1-5 Continued

Imbalance	Causes	Assessment Findings	Nursing Interventions
Hypernatremia	Excessive/rapid IV administration of normal saline solution, inadequate water intake, kidney disease	Dry, sticky mucous membranes; flushed skin; rough, dry tongue; firm skin turgor; intense thirst; edema; oliguria to anuria	Weigh daily. Assess degree of edema frequently. Measure I&O. Assess skin frequently and institute nursing measures to prevent breakdown. Encourage sodium-restricted diet.
Hyponatremia	Decreased sodium intake, increased sodium excretion through diaphoresis or GI suctioning, adrenal insufficiency	Nausea and vomiting; abdominal cramps; weight loss; cold, clammy skin; decreased skin turgor; fingerprinting over the sternum; shrunken tongue; apprehension; headache; convulsions; confusion; weakness; fatigue; postural hypotension; rapid, thready pulse	Provide foods high in sodium. Administer normal saline solution IV. Assess blood pressure frequently (measure lying down, sitting, and standing).
Hypercalcemia	Hyperparathyroidism, immobility, increased vitamin D intake, osteoporosis and osteomalacia (early stages)	Nausea and vomiting, anorexia, constipation, headache, confusion, lethargy, stupor, decreased muscle tone, deep bone and/or flank pain	Encourage mobilization. Limit vitamin D and calcium intake. Administer diuretics. Protect from injury.

Hypocalcemia	Acute pancreatitis, diarrhea, hypoparathyroidism, lack of vitamin D in diet, long-term steroid therapy	Painful tonic muscle spasms, facial spasms, fatigue, laryngospasm, positive Trousseau's and Chvostek's signs, convulsions, dyspnea	Administer oral calcium lactate or IV calcium chloride or gluconate. Provide safety by padding side rails. Administer dietary sources of calcium. Provide quiet environment.
Hypermagnesemia	Renal insufficiency, dehydration, excessive use of magnesium-containing antacids or laxatives	Lethargy, somnolence, confusion, nausea and vomiting, muscle weakness, depressed reflexes, decreased pulse and respirations	Withhold magnesium-containing drugs/foods. Increase fluid intake (unless contraindicated).
Hypomagnesemia	Low intake of magnesium in diet, prolonged diarrhea, massive diuresis, hypoparathyroidism	Paresthesias, confusion, hallucinations, convulsions, ataxia, tremors, hyperactive deep reflexes, muscle spasm, flushing of the face, diaphoresis	Provide good dietary sources of magnesium.

TABLE 1-6 Acid-Base Imbalances

Imbalance	Causes	Assessment Findings	Nursing Interventions
Metabolic acidosis	Diabetic ketoacidosis, uremia, starvation, diarrhea, severe infections, renal tubular acidosis	Headache, nausea and vomiting, weakness, lethargy, disorientation, tremors, convulsions, coma	Administer sodium bicarbonate as ordered and monitor for signs of excess. Monitor for signs of hyperkalemia. Provide alkaline mouthwash (baking soda and water) to neutralize acids. Lubricate lips to prevent dryness from hyperventilation. Measure I&O. Institute seizure precautions. Monitor arterial blood gases and electrolytes.
Metabolic alkalosis	Severe vomiting, nasogastric suctioning, diuretic therapy, excessive ingestion of sodium bicarbonate, biliary drainage	Nausea and vomiting, diarrhea, numbness and tingling of extremities, tetany, bradycardia, decreased respirations	Replace fluid and electrolyte losses (potassium and chloride). Institute seizure precautions. Measure I&O. Assess for signs of hypokalemia. Monitor arterial blood gases and electrolytes.
Respiratory acidosis	COPD, barbiturate or sedative overdose, acute airway	Headache, weakness, visual disturbances, rapid respirations, confusion,	Position in semi-Fowler's. Maintain patent airway. Turn, cough, and

	obstruction, weakness of respiratory muscles	drowsiness, tachycardia, coma	deep breathe. Perform postural drainage. Administer fluids to help liquefy secretions (unless contraindicated). Administer low-concentration oxygen therapy. Monitor arterial blood gases and electrolytes. Administer prophylactic antibiotics as ordered.
Respiratory alkalosis	Hyperventilation, mechanical overventilation, encephalitis	Numbness and tingling of mouth and extremities, inability to concentrate, rapid respirations, dry mouth, coma	Offer reassurance. Encourage breathing into a paper bag or voluntary breath holding. Ensure adequate rest. Provide sedation as ordered. Monitor mechanical ventilation, arterial blood gases, and electrolytes.

Acid-Base Imbalances

See Table 1-6.

A. *Metabolic acidosis:* a primary deficit in the concentration of base bicarbonate in the extracellular fluid; decreased pH and bicarbonate, decreased pCO_2 (if respiratory compensation)

B. *Metabolic alkalosis:* a primary excess of base bicarbonate in the extracellular fluid; elevated pH and bicarbonate, elevated pCO_2 (if respiratory compensation)

C. *Respiratory acidosis:* a primary excess of carbonic acid in the extracellular fluid; decreased pH, elevated pCO_2 and bicarbonate (if renal compensation)

D. *Respiratory alkalosis:* a primary deficit of carbonic acid in the extracellular fluid; elevated pH, decreased $pCO_2$and bicarbonate (if renal compensation)

INTRAVENOUS THERAPY

Purposes

A. Maintenance of fluid and electrolyte balance
B. Replacement of fluid and electrolyte loss
C. Provision of nutrients
D. Provision of a route for medications

Nursing Interventions

A. Select correct solution after checking physician's order.
B. Note clarity of solution.
C. Calculate flow rate. Time-tape bag to assist in monitoring flow rate.
D. Assess infusion rate and site at least hourly.
E. Use infusion pump if administering medications (e.g., aminophylline, heparin, insulin).
F. Maintain I&O record.
G. Provide tubing change and IV site change according to hospital policy. Intravenous Nurses Society standards recommend IV site and tubing change every 48 hours.
H. Discontinue IV if complications occur.

Complications of Intravenous Therapy

See Table 1-7.

Central Lines

Uses

A. Administration of TPN
B. Measurement of central venous pressure (CVP)
C. IV therapy when suitable peripheral veins are not available
D. Long-term antibiotic therapy
E. Chemotherapy

Types

A. Nontunneled catheters: inserted into subclavian vein for short-term access
   1. Subclavian catheters: single lumen
   2. Multilumen catheters: double, triple, or quadruple lumens for simultaneous infusion of fluids or for blood drawing with fluid infusion.

TABLE 1-7 Complications of IV Therapy

Complication	Nursing Manifestation	Interventions
Infiltration	Blanching of skin, swelling, pain at site; cool to touch; decreased infusion rate	Discontinue IV. Restart in a new site. May apply warm compresses to increase fluid absorption.
Phlebitis	Redness, heat, and swelling at site; possible pain and red line along course of vein	Discontinue IV. Restart in new site. Apply warm compresses to site.
Pyrogenic reaction	Fever, chills, general malaise, nausea, vomiting, headache, backache	Discontinue infusion immediately. Monitor vital signs and notify physician. Retain IV equipment for culture/lab study.
Air embolism	Dyspnea, cyanosis, hypotension, tachycardia, loss of consciousness	Stop infusion immediately. Turn client on left side with his head down. Administer oxygen. Notify physician.
Circulatory overload.	Apprehension, shortness of breath, coughing, frothy sputum, crackles, engorged neck veins, increased blood pressure and pulse	Slow down IV rate. Monitor vital signs. Notify physician.

B. Tunneled catheters: long, silicone catheter threaded through subcutaneous layer to prevent infection with long-term use; catheter tip is located in the superior vena cava.

1. Hickman/Broviac catheters: single- or double-lumen catheters with external presentation; need to be flushed daily with a heparinized saline solution and must be clamped when not in use; repair kit available.
2. Groshong catheters: similar to Hickman/Broviac; difference is in valve at closed distal end of catheter that opens when used and remains closed at other times, preventing blood back-up into catheter; no clamping is necessary; flushing is done daily with saline in a vigorous manner.

3. Implantable ports: totally internal device consists of subcutaneous self-sealing injection port and a tunneled catheter; flushing is done with a heparinized saline solution every 28 days; access must be with a special noncoring needle.
4. Peripherally inserted central lines (PICC): short-term long lines that can be inserted by qualified nurses; inserted via a vessel in the antecubital fossa (median or cephalic); flushing is with a heparinized saline solution.

Care of the Client with a Central Venous Line

A. Assist physician with placement; catheters should initially be flushed with saline. Have fluids or cap and flush available (heparin or saline).

B. Confirm placement in superior vena cava by X-ray prior to catheter use.

C. Institute nursing measures to prevent infection (particularly important with TPN since high concentration of glucose encourages growth of bacteria).

1. Change dressings
   a. Usually 3 times/week and as needed (e.g., when loose or wet) but agency policies may vary
   b. Use sterile technique and apply sterile occlusive dressing.
2. Monitor for signs of infection: redness, drainage, odor at site, or elevated temperature.
3. Do not piggyback anything into a TPN infusion line except intralipids.

D. Monitor for infiltration: check for swelling of neck, face, and shoulder, and pain in upper arm.

E. Prevent catheter occlusion.

1. Keep infusion continuous.
2. Use infusion pump.
3. Check for kinks in tubing.
4. Evaluate for catheter migration or dislodgment.

F. Prevent air embolism.

1. Tighten and tape all tubing connections to prevent accidental disconnection.
2. Clamp catheter (except Groshong) and instruct client to perform Valsalva maneuver when changing or detaching tubing.
3. Check tubing for cracks or perforations.

G. Maintain proper infusion rate.

1. Monitor rate closely to prevent clotting, fluid depletion, or fluid overload.
2. Never attempt to speed up or slow down infusion.

H. With a multilumen catheter, flush ports not being used to prevent clotting (per agency's protocol).

I. With Hickman/Broviac catheters, Groshongs, PICCs, and implanted port provide other specific care according to agency protocol.
J. If clotting occurs, try to aspirate or add a declotting agent according to agency protocol. Do not irrigate. Do not use force to flush.
   1. Streptokinase requires 1 hour waiting time to achieve results.
   2. Urokinase requires 10 minutes waiting time to achieve results.
K. When drawing blood specimens, discard initial sample of 5–10 ml prior to drawing required volume for specimens. Flush with saline prior to flushing with heparinized saline solution or continuing fluids.

SHOCK

An abnormal physiologic state where an imbalance between the amount of circulating blood volume and the size of the vascular bed results in circulatory failure and oxygen and nutrient deprivation of tissues. See Table 1-8 for classification of shock.

Body's Response to Shock

A. Hyperventilation leading to respiratory alkalosis
B. Vasoconstriction: shunts blood to heart and brain
C. Tachycardia
D. Fluid shifts: intracellular to extracellular shift to maintain circulating blood volume
E. Impaired metabolism: tissue anoxia leads to anaerobic metabolism causing increased capillary permeability and lactic acid buildup, resulting in metabolic acidosis
F. Impaired organ function
   1. Kidney: decreased perfusion can result in renal failure.
   2. Lung: shock lung (adult respiratory distress syndrome ARDS)

Assessment Findings

A. Skin
   1. Cool, pale, moist in hypovolemic and cardiogenic shock
   2. Warm, dry, pink in septic and neurogenic shock
B. Pulse
   1. Tachycardia, due to increased sympathetic stimulation
   2. Weak and thready
C. Blood pressure
   1. Early stages: may be normal due to compensatory mechanisms
   2. Later stages: systolic and diastolic blood pressure drops
D. Respirations: rapid and shallow, due to tissue anoxia and excessive amounts of CO_2 (from metabolic acidosis)

TABLE 1-8 Classification of Shock

Type	Characteristics	Causes
Hypovolemic	Decreased circulating blood volume	Blood loss Plasma loss (e.g., burns) Fluid loss (e.g., excessive vomiting or diarrhea)
Cardiogenic	Failure of the heart to pump properly	Myocardial infarction Congestive heart failure Cardiac arrhythmias Pericardial tamponade Tension pneumothorax
Septic	Factors favoring septic shock • development of antibiotic-resistant organisms • invasive procedures such as urinary tract instrumentation • immunosuppression and old age • trauma: presence of blood in peritoneal cavity greatly increases likelihood of peritonitis	Release of bacterial toxins that act directly on the blood vessels producing massive vasodilation and pooling of blood; results most frequently from gram-negative septicemia.
Neurogenic	Failure of arteriolar resistance, leading to massive vasodilation and pooling of blood	Interruption of sympathetic impulses from • exposure to unpleasant circumstances • extreme pain • spinal cord injury • high spinal anesthesia • vasomotor depression • head injury
Anaphylactic	Massive vasodilation resulting from allergic reaction causing release of histamine and related substances	Allergic reaction to • insect venom or snake venom • medications • dyes used in radiologic studies

E. Level of consciousness: restlessness and apprehension, progressing to coma
F. Urinary output: decreases due to impaired renal perfusion
G. Temperature: decreases in severe shock (except septic shock).

Nursing Interventions

A. Maintain patent airway and adequate ventilation.
   1. Establish and maintain airway.
   2. Administer oxygen as ordered.
   3. Monitor respiratory status, blood gases.
   4. Start resuscitative procedures as necessary.
B. Promote restoration of blood volume; administer fluid and blood replacement as ordered.
   1. Crystalloid solutions: Ringer's lactate, normal saline
   2. Colloid solutions: albumin, plasmanate, dextran
   3. Blood products: whole blood, packed red blood cells, fresh frozen plasma
C. Administer drugs as ordered (see Table 1-9).
D. Minimize factors contributing to shock.
   1. Elevate lower extremities to 45° to promote venous return to heart, thereby improving cardiac output.
   2. Avoid Trendelenburg's position: increases respiratory impairment.
   3. Promote rest by using energy-conservation measures and maintaining as quiet an environment as possible.
   4. Relieve pain by cautious use of narcotics.
      a. Since narcotics interfere with vasoconstriction, give only if absolutely necessary, IV and in small doses.
      b. If given IM or subcutaneously, vasoconstriction may cause incomplete absorption; when circulation improves, client may get overdose.
   5. Keep client warm.
E. Maintain continuous assessment of the client.
   1. Check vital signs frequently.
   2. Monitor urine output: report urine output of less than 30 ml/hour.
   3. Observe color and temperature of skin.
   4. Monitor CVP.
   5. Monitor ECG.
   6. Check lab studies: CBC, electrolytes, BUN, creatinine, blood gases.
   7. Monitor other parameters such as arterial blood pressures, cardiac output, pulmonary artery pressures, pulmonary artery wedge pressures.
F. Provide psychologic support: reassure client to relieve apprehension, and keep family advised.

TABLE 1-9 Drugs Used to Treat Shock

Generic (Trade) Name	Action
Dopamine (Intropin)	*Low dosage:* Dilates renal, mesenteric, and splanchnic vessels, which in turn increases perfusion of kidneys and urine output. *High dosage:* Increases cardiac contractility; causes vasoconstriction (often given with nitroprusside [Nipride]).
Dobutamine (Dobutrex)	Increases myocardial contractility; vasodilator.
Isoproterenol (Isuprel)	Increases myocardial contractility; decreases peripheral resistance by dilating peripheral vascular bed; usefulness is limited by the tachycardia it produces.
Norepinephrine (Levophed)	Improves cardiac contractility and cardiac output; potent vasoconstrictor.
Sodium nitroprusside (Nipride)	Vasodilator; decreases peripheral resistance and workload of heart, thereby increasing cardiac output; used in cardiogenic shock and hypertensive emergencies.
Digitalis preparations	Improve cardiac performance.
Corticosteroids	Used especially in septic shock; help to protect cell membranes and decrease the inflammatory response to stress.
Antibiotics	Used in treating infectious processes related to septic shock.

Note: Vasopressors such as Levophed can cause almost complete occlusion of arterioles, causing a decrease of blood flow to larger tissue areas. Therefore, if blood pressure is adequate, a vasodilator such as Nipride could probably be given as well, to modify the vasoconstrictor effects.

MULTIPLE TRAUMA

Assessment and Emergency Care

Airway

A. Assess, establish, and maintain an adequate airway.
  1. Do not hyperextend the neck in a client with suspected cervical spine injury.
  2. Use jaw thrust instead.

B. Administer artificial resuscitation if necessary.

C. Observe for chest trauma such as open sucking wounds or flail chest.

D. Administer high-flow oxygen 85–100% to achieve maximum cellular oxygenation. Monitor for CO_2 retention in clients with COPD.

E. Draw blood samples for ABGs.

Hemorrhage and Shock

A. Deep wounds with pulsating blood flow
  1. Apply firm pressure over the wound with a sterile dressing.
  2. If wound is on a limb, elevate the extremity.
  3. Apply pressure with three fingers over appropriate pressure point.
  4. Once bleeding is controlled, apply a pressure dressing.
  5. Tourniquets should be used only when all other methods have failed.

B. Venous bleeding: apply direct pressure to bleeding site.

C. Never remove any foreign object, such as a knife, from the client; immobilize the object with packing.

D. Assess for and treat shock.

E. Administer tetanus booster as ordered.

Neurologic Injuries

A. Establish a baseline level of consciousness and reassess frequently.

B. Inspect the scalp, head, face, and neck for abrasions, hematomas, and lacerations.

C. Gently palpate the head for any injuries.

D. Inspect the nose and ears for leakage of cerebrospinal fluid.

E. Evaluate pupillary size, shape, equality, and reaction to light.

F. Assess for sensation and motor abilities.

G. Observe for signs of increased intracranial pressure.

H. For additional details of care see Head Injury and Spinal Cord Injury.

Abdominal Injuries

A. Keep client NPO.

B. Assist with insertion of nasogastric tube (for assessment of stomach bleeding and aspiration of stomach contents, which prevents vomiting).

C. Inspect abdomen for injuries.
D. Auscultate bowel sounds.
E. Do not palpate the abdomen (could aggravate possible internal injuries).
F. Prepare client for peritoneal lavage if indicated.
G. Insert Foley catheter.
   1. Measure urine output every 15 minutes.
   2. Assess for hematuria.

Musculoskeletal Injuries

A. Observe for sign of fracture: pain, swelling, tenderness, ecchymosis, crepitation (grating sound), loss of function, exposed bone fragments.
B. Cover open fracture with sterile dressing to prevent infection.
C. Immobilize any suspected fractures by splinting the joint above and below the injury.
D. Perform neurovascular check of area distal to fracture: assess for color, temperature, capillary refill, sensation, movement, pulses.

REVIEW QUESTIONS

1. A 27-year-old adult is admitted for treatment of Crohn's disease. Which information is most significant when the nurse assesses nutritional health?

   1. Anthropometric measurements.
   2. Bleeding gums.
   3. Dry skin.
   4. Facial rubor.

2. Total parenteral nutrition (TPN) is ordered for an adult client. Which nutrient is not likely to be in the solution?

   1. Dextrose 10%.
   2. Trace minerals.
   3. Electrolytes.
   4. Amino acids.

3. The nurse caring for an adult client who is receiving TPN will need to monitor for which of the following metabolic complications?

   1. Hypoglycemia and hypercalcemia.
   2. Hyperglycemia and hypokalemia.
   3. Hyperglycemia and hyperkalemia.
   4. Hyperkalemia and hypercalcemia.

4. Acetylsalicylic acid is being administered to an adult client. The nurse understands that the most common mechanism of action for nonnarcotic analgesics is their ability to
   1. inhibit prostaglandin synthesis.
   2. alter pain perception in the cerebellum.
   3. directly affect the central nervous system.
   4. target the pain-producing effect of kinins.
5. An adult has been taking acetylsalicylic acid (ASA) 650 mg four times a day for chronic back pain. The nurse assessing this client knows that a common side effect of high doses of ASA is
   1. liver failure.
   2. paralytic ileus.
   3. gastrointestinal bleeding.
   4. retinal detachment.
6. Ibuprofen (Motrin) is prescribed for an adult with chronic pain. The nurse must teach the client to observe which dietary precaution while taking ibuprofen?
   1. Eat a high-fiber diet.
   2. Drink citrus juices daily.
   3. Take the medication with milk.
   4. Omit spinach and other green leafy vegetables from the client's diet.
7. A 48-year-old woman has just returned to her room after having had a hysterectomy. She has patient-controlled analgesia (PCA). To reduce anxiety regarding receiving adequate pain relief, the client was most likely told that
   1. PCA is almost always effective.
   2. comfort will be assessed frequently.
   3. additional IM medication will be available.
   4. most therapies are better than frequent IM injections.
8. Preoperative teaching for an adult who is to have client controlled analgesia following surgery includes telling the client:
   1. "You will not be drowsy."
   2. "You will experience no pain."
   3. "Pain control will be adequate."
   4. "You will not have incisional pain but you may have muscle pain."

9. The client's family expresses concern that the client could overdose with a PCA. What protective mechanism prevents drug overdose with a PCA?
   1. The nurse controls the amount administered with each dose.
   2. Extensive client teaching precedes its use.
   3. The client can stop drug administration but not initiate it.
   4. After a bolus is administered, there is a mandatory waiting period before another dose is given.
10. The nurse is the first professional to arrive at the scene of a multivehicle accident. An adult was riding a motorcycle. Upon impact, he fell off the bike and it fell back on his legs. Priority care for the client should be directed toward
    1. assessing blood loss.
    2. monitoring respiratory status.
    3. obtaining vital signs.
    4. organizing lay people on the scene.
11. The nurse is at the scene of a multivehicle accident. A young man was injured when his motorcycle was hit by a car. He fell off the bike and then it fell back on his legs. He is bleeding profusely from a 4-inch gash on his left leg. Which of the following is the best approach for the nurse to take to stop the bleeding?
    1. Apply direct pressure to the wound.
    2. Move the motorcycle off his legs.
    3. Raise the extremity.
    4. Wrap a tourniquet above the wound.
12. The nurse is caring for a client who is receiving IV fluids. Which observation the nurse makes best indicates the IV has infiltrated?
    1. Pain at the site.
    2. A change in flow rate.
    3. Coldness around the insertion site.
    4. Redness around the insertion site.
13. The nurse is caring for a client whose arterial blood gases indicate metabolic acidosis. The nurse knows that, of the following, the least likely to cause metabolic acidosis is
    1. cardiac arrest.
    2. diabetic ketoacidosis.
    3. hypokalemia.
    4. renal failure.

14. An adult client is admitted with metabolic acidosis. Which set of arterial blood gases should the nurse expect to find in a client with metabolic acidosis?

1. pH 7.28; PCO_2 - 55; HCO - 26.
2. pH 7.50; PCO_2 - 40; HCO_3 - 31.
3. pH 7.48; PCO_2 - 30;HCO_3 - 22.
4. pH 7.30; PCO_2 - 36; HCO_3 - 18.

15. A 93-year-old adult is hospitalized for the treatment of gastroenteritis complicated by dehydration and hyponatremia. The nurse expects that an early symptom of hyponatremia exhibited by the client was

1. ataxia.
2. hunger.
3. thirst.
4. weakness.

16. An adult has just been brought in by ambulance after a motor vehicle accident and has moderate anxiety. When assessing the client, the nurse would expect which of the following from sympathetic nervous system stimulation?

1. A rapid pulse and increased respiratory rate.
2. Decreased physiologic functioning.
3. Rigid posture and altered perceptual focus.
4. Increased awareness and attending.

17. An adult has received an injection of immunoglobulin. The nurse knows that the client will develop which of the following types of immunity?

1. Active natural immunity.
2. Active artificial immunity.
3. Passive natural immunity.
4. Passive artificial immunity.

18. The nurse knows which of the following is true about immunity?

1. Antibody-mediated defense occurs through the T-cell system.
2. Cellular immunity is mediated by antibodies produced by the B-cells.
3. Antibodies are produced by the B-cells.
4. Humoral or circulating immunity is lost with AIDS.

19. An adult is on a clear liquid diet. The nurse can offer

1. milk.
2. Jello.

3. freshly squeezed orange juice.
4. ice cream.

20. An adult is being taught about a healthy diet. The nurse explains that the food pyramid can guide the client
    1. by indicating exactly how many servings of each group to eat.
    2. on how many calories the client should have.
    3. in making daily food choices.
    4. to divide food into four basic groups.
21. Before administering a tube feeding the nurse knows to perform which of the following assessments?
    1. The gastrointestinal (GI) tract, including bowel sounds, last BM, and distention.
    2. The client's neurologic status, especially gag reflex.
    3. The amount of air in the stomach.
    4. That the formula is used directly from the refrigerator.
22. The nurse knows which of the following indicates protein deficiency?
    1. Negative nitrogen balance.
    2. Koilonychia (spoon-shaped nails).
    3. Magenta tongue.
    4. Bleeding gums.
23. The nurse knows that a client understands a low residue diet when he selects which of the following from a menu?
    1. Rice and lean chicken.
    2. Eggs and bacon.
    3. Pasta with vegetables.
    4. Tuna casserole.
24. An adult is receiving total parenteral nutrition (TPN). The nurse knows which of the following assessments is essential?
    1. Evaluation of the peripheral intravenous (IV) site.
    2. Confirmation that the tube is in the stomach.
    3. Assessment of the GI tract, including bowel sounds.
    4. Fluid and electrolyte monitoring.
25. The nurse knows which of the following statements about TPN and peripheral parenteral nutrition (PPN) is true?

1. TPN is usually indicated for clients needing short-term (less than three weeks) nutritional support, while PPN is for long-term maintenance.
2. A client needing more than 3000 calories would receive PPN, whereas TPN is given to those requiring less than 3000 calories.
3. TPN is often given to those with fluid restrictions, whereas PPN is used for those without constraints on their fluid intake.
4. TPN is given to those who need to augment oral feedings, whereas PPN is used for those who are nothing by mouth (NPO).

26. When administering TPN, the nurse makes sure the

1. IV site is kept aseptic while infusing the solution.
2. feeding is poured into a pouch and then infused.
3. solution is only hung for a maximum of 8 hours at a time.
4. new formula is added to the partially used solution so the line does not run dry.

27. An adult has been treated for pulmonary tuberculosis (TB) and is being discharged home with his wife and two young children. His wife asks how TB is passed from one person to another so she can prevent any one else from catching it. The nurse responds,

1. "You should wear gloves when handling his linen and bedding, because you can get TB by touching the germs."
2. "You should keep the windows and doors closed so as not to spread the droplets."
3. "He must be careful to cough into a handkerchief that is washed in hot water or discarded."
4. "Make sure to boil all milk before drinking or using it."

28. The nurse is evaluating a certified nursing assistant (CNA). Which of the following CNAs understands universal precautions? The CNA who

1. wears gloves during all client contact.
2. cleans blood spills with soap and water.
3. pours bulk blood and other secretions down a drain connected to a sanitary sewer.
4. carries blood sample to the lab in an open basket.

29. An adult is on long-term aspirin therapy and is experiencing tinnitus. The nurse best interprets this to mean

1. the aspirin is working correctly.
2. the client ingested more medicine than was recommended.

3. the client has an upper GI bleed.
4. the client is experiencing a mild overdosage.

30. An adult is receiving a nonsteroidal anti-inflammatory drug (NSAID). The nurse is to assess for side effects. Which of the following would the nurse observe if the client is experiencing no side effects?
    1. The client is somnolent and hard to arouse.
    2. The client is having dark, tarry stools.
    3. There is no complaint of nausea or vomiting.
    4. The pain is still a 6 on a scale of 1–10.

31. An adult is to receive an intramuscular (IM) injection of morphine for post-op pain. Which of the following is necessary for the nurse to assess prior to giving a narcotic analgesic?
    1. The client's level of alertness and respiratory rate.
    2. The last time the client ate or drank something.
    3. The client's bowel habits and last bowel movement.
    4. The client's history of addictions.

32. An adult is to receive narcotic analgesic via a client-controlled analgesia (PCA). The nurse is evaluating the client's understanding of the procedure. Which of the following statements by the client indicates that she understands PCA?
    1. "When I press this button the machine will always give me more medicine."
    2. "I will press the button whenever I begin to experience pain."
    3. "I should press this button every hour so the pain doesn't come back."
    4. "With this machine I will experience no more pain."

33. An adult suffered second and third degree burns over 20% of his body two days ago. The nurse knows that the best way to assess fluid balance is to
    1. maintain strict records of intake and output.
    2. weigh the client daily.
    3. monitor skin turgor.
    4. check for edema.

34. A 78-year-old male has been working on his lawn for two days, although the temperature has been above 90° F. He has been on thiazide diuretics for hypertension. His lab values are: K 3.7 mEq/L, Na 129 mEq/L, Ca 4.9 mEq/L, and Cl 95 mEq/L. When planning for his care the nurse would

1. make sure he drinks eight glasses of water a day.
2. monitor for fatigue, muscle weakness, restlessness, and flushed skin.
3. look for signs of hyperchloremia.
4. observe for neurologic changes.

35. An adult who has gastroenteritis and is on digitalis has lab values of: K 3.2 mEq/L, Na 136 mEq/L, Ca 4.8 mEq/L, and Cl 98 mEq/L. The nurse puts which of the following on the client's plan of care?

1. Monitor for hyperkalemia.
2. Avoid foods rich in potassium.
3. Observe for digitalis toxicity.
4. Observe for Trousseau's and Chvostek's signs.

36. A client on hemodialysis is complaining of muscle weakness and numbness in his legs. His lab results are: Na 136 mEq/L, K 5.9 mEq/L, Cl 100 mEq/L, Ca 4.5 mEq/L. The nurse knows the client is suffering from

1. hyperkalemia.
2. hypernatremia.
3. hypocalcemia.
4. hypochloremia.

37. A woman has breast cancer that has metastasized to her bones. She is complaining of increased thirst, polyuria, and decreased muscle tone in her legs. Her lab values are: Na 139 mEq/L, K 4.0 mEq/L, Cl 103 mEq/L, and Ca 4.0 mEq/L. The nurse's best interpretation of the data is

1. hypocalcemia.
2. hypercalcemia.
3. hyperkalemia.
4. hypochloremia.

38. An adult who is anxious and hyperventilating has blood gases of: pH 7.47, $PaCO_2$ 33. What is the best initial action for the nurse to take?

1. Try to have the client breathe slower or into a paper bag.
2. Monitor the client's fluid balance.
3. Give O_2 via nasal cannula.
4. Administer sodium bicarbonate.

39. An adult has had gastroenteritis with vomiting for three days. He has taken baking soda without relief. His blood gases are as follows: pH 7.49, $PaCO_2$ 45, and HCO_3 30. The nurse would expect which of the following to be included in the plan of care?

1. Have the client drink at least eight glasses of water in the first day.
2. Administer $NaHCO_3$ IV as per physician's orders.
3. Continue sodium bicarbonate for nausea.
4. Monitor electrolytes for hypokalemia and hypocalcemia.

40. An adult's blood gas results are: pH 7.31, $PaCO_2$ 49, and HCO_3 24. The nurse interprets this as
    1. respiratory acidosis.
    2. respiratory alkalosis.
    3. metabolic acidosis.
    4. metabolic alkalosis.
41. An adult who has diabetes has infectious diarrhea. His arterial blood gases are: pH 7.30, $PaCO_2$ 35, and HCO_3 of 19. The nurse would monitor the client for which of the following?
    1. Trousseau's sign.
    2. Hypokalemia.
    3. Hypoglycemia.
    4. Respiratory changes.
42. An adult has an IV line in his right forearm infusing D5 1/2NS with 20 mEq of potassium at 75 ml/h. The nurse evaluating the client with no adverse reactions would expect to find which of the following?
    1. The area around the needle insertion is cool, blanched, and swollen.
    2. Redness and warmth at the needle site.
    3. An empty drip chamber and tubing.
    4. No blood in the IV tubing.
43. An adult has a central venous line. Which of the following should the nurse include in the care plan?
    1. Frequent monitoring of blood values including complete blood count (CBC) and electrolytes.
    2. Regular serial chest X-rays to ensure proper placement of the central line.
    3. Continuous infusion of a solution at a keep vein open rate.
    4. Any signs of infection, air embolus, and leakage or puncture.
44. An adult has a Hickman-type central venous catheter and needs to have blood drawn from it. Which of the following is the nurse going to do first?
    1. Use sterile technique to assemble the supplies needed.
    2. Aspirate and discard the first 5 ml of the blood.

3. Flush the catheter with normal saline according to hospital policy.
4. Remove the cap on the catheter and replace it with a new one.

45. An adult has a central line in his right subclavian vein. The nurse is to change the tubing. Which of the following should be done?
    1. Use the old solution with the new tubing.
    2. Connect the new tubing to the hub prior to running any fluid through the tubing.
    3. Close the roller clamp on the new tubing after priming it.
    4. Irrigate the hub prior to inserting the new tubing.

46. An adult suffered a diving accident and is being brought in by an ambulance intubated and on a backboard with a cervical collar. What is the first action the nurse would take on arrival in the hospital?
    1. Take the client's vital signs.
    2. Insert a large bore IV line.
    3. Check the lungs for equal breath sounds bilaterally.
    4. Perform a neurologic check using the Glasgow scale.

47. An adult has been shot. His vital signs are blood pressure (BP) 90/60, pulse (P) 120 weak and thready, respirations (R) 20. During the initial assessment, he is placed in a modified Trendelenburg position. If the position change has the desired effect the nurse would expect
    1. an increase in the client's blood pressure.
    2. an increase in the client's heart rate.
    3. an increase in the client's respiratory rate.
    4. a faster capillary refill time in the toes.

48. An adult has been stung by a bee and is in anaphylactic shock. An epinephrine (adrenaline) injection has been given. The nurse would expect which of the following if the injection has been effective?
    1. The client's breathing will become easier.
    2. The client's blood pressure will decrease.
    3. There will be an increase in angioedema.
    4. There will be a decrease in the client's level of consciousness.

49. An adult has been in a motor vehicle accident. She has a 4-in laceration on her forehead that is bleeding profusely. Her left ankle has an obvious deformity and is splinted. Her vital signs are BP 100/60, P 110, and R 16. What is the first action the nurse should take?
    1. Start an IV line.
    2. Place a Foley catheter.

3. Get an ECG.
4. Check her neurologic status.

50. An adult is brought in by ambulance after a motor vehicle accident. He is unconscious, on a backboard with his neck immobilized. He is bleeding profusely from a large gash on his right thigh. What is the first action the nurse should take?

1. Stop the bleeding.
2. Check his airway.
3. Take his vital signs.
4. Find out what happened from eyewitnesses.

ANSWERS AND RATIONALES

1. 1. Anthropometric measurements are the prime parameters used to evaluate fat and muscle stores in the body.

2. 1. The concentration of dextrose in TPN solutions is usually at least 30%.

3. 2. Metabolic complications from administration of TPN include hyperglycemia, hypoglycemia, hypocalcemia, hypokalemia, hypomagnesemia, hyponatremia, and hypophosphatemia. Hyperglycemia is the most common complication of TPN.

4. 1. Nonnarcotic analgesics inhibit prostaglandin synthesis. Prostaglandins increase the sensitivity of peripheral pain receptors to endogenous pain-producing substances.

5. 3. High doses of aspirin are associated with GI bleeding.

6. 3. NSAIDs such as ibuprofen are very irritating to the GI tract and should always be taken with milk or food to minimize the possibility of bleeding.

7. 2. Pain is an individual experience. It is important to reassure the client that assessments will be made frequently and that drug dosages will be adjusted according to the amount of pain the client perceives.

8. 3. Clients should be told that they will be able to control their pain.

9. 4. Immediately after a bolus dose of medication is administered the device enters a mandatory lockout mode where no other boluses of medication can be delivered.

10. 2. In the presence of multiple traumas, maintenance of a patent airway must always be the priority in the sequence of care delivery.

11. 1. Direct pressure to the wound will aid in the development of a blood clot, which is the first step in wound healing and will prevent hemorrhage.

12. 3. Coldness, pallor, and swelling around the insertion site are the best indicators that the fluid has infiltrated into subcutaneous tissue.

13. 3. Untreated hypokalemia will eventually lead to metabolic alkalosis. Potassium shifts from the serum into the cells in exchange for H+ ions. The absence of H+ ions causes a base excess, thus metabolic alkalosis.

14. 4. The pH is below the normal range of 7.35–7.45. The PCO_2 is within the normal range of 35–45, and the HCO_3 is below the normal limits of 21–28. These values indicate a metabolic problem because the PCO_2 is within normal limits. It is the low HCO_3 that is causing acidosis.

15. 3. Thirst is the body's attempt to restore blood volume depletion that occurs in hyponatremia.

16. 1. The sympathetic nervous system during moderate anxiety will increase the pulse and respirations.

17. 4. Passive artificial immunity occurs when antibodies are produced by another person or animal and injected into the recipient.

18. 3. Antibodies or immunoglobulins are produced by the B-cells and are part of the body's plasma proteins.

19. 2. Plain gelatins can be given on a clear liquid diet, as well as tea, coffee, ginger ale, or 7-Up.

20. 3. The pyramid helps to guide the client in choosing a variety of foods to obtain the nutrients needed. It also aids in eating more of some groups (bread, cereal, rice, and pasta) and less of others (fats, oils, and sweets).

21. 1. The GI tract should be assessed before each feeding to ensure functioning and minimal problems.

22. 1. A negative nitrogen balance indicates that protein catabolism exceeds protein anabolism. A positive nitrogen balance indicates intake exceeds output.

23. 1. A low residue diet includes rice, lean meats, and eggs.

24. 4. Clients receiving TPN can experience electrolyte imbalances, hypo- or hyperglycemia, as well as difficulties with fluid balance.

25. 3. TPN can provide a greater concentration of calories than PPN. Therefore, TPN is given to those with fluid restrictions.

26. 1. The IV site must be kept aseptic. It is a central line and the TPN with its high concentration of glucose provides an ideal medium for pathogens.

27. 3. TB is spread through residue of evaporated droplets and may remain in the air for long periods of time. Thus care should be given when coughing or sneezing.

28. 3. Bulk blood and other secretions like suctioned fluids are carefully poured down a drain connected to a sanitary sewer.?

29. 4. Tinnitus is a classic sign of aspirin overdosages, either from too much ingestion or limited excretion.

30. 3. NSAIDs often cause nausea or vomiting. This can be alleviated by taking the medicine with food, milk, or antacids.

31. 1. A decreasing level of alertness can signal early respiratory depression and a significant drop in the respiratory rate is a warning sign. Both should be taken prior to giving the medication for baseline purposes.

32. 2. PCA allows the client to administer more analgesic before the pain becomes severe, thus allowing better pain control.

33. 2. This is the best way to assess fluid balance, especially acute changes in those with large losses or acutely ill.

34. 4. Neurologic changes can occur from hyponatremia. They include confusion, disorientation, lethargy, seizures, and coma.

35. 3. Hypokalemia enhances digitalis toxicity and must be observed for carefully.

36. 1. Potassium is normally 3.5–5.5 mEq/L. Clients with renal failure are prone to hyperkalemia.

37. 1. The client's calcium is low. The normal values are 4.5–5.5 mEq/L. Hypocalcemia is common among those with bone cancer.

38. 1. The client is in respiratory alkalosis and needs to increase the carbon dioxide. The easiest way to do this is to try and calm the client and/or have him breathe in and out of a paper bag, thus inhaling the exhaled carbon dioxide.

39. 4. Hypokalemia and hypocalcemia are both common with metabolic alkalosis as a result of cellular buffering.

40. 1. A low pH indicates acidosis, whereas the high $PaCO_2$ indicates the problem is respiratory rather than metabolic.

41. 4. The client is in metabolic acidosis and the body will try to compensate through the respiratory system (with deep breaths), although it cannot completely correct the problem.

42. 4. Although blood return indicates the catheter is in a vein, it should not be in the tubing. If present, the nurse should find the reason and attempt to correct it.

43. 4. All of these are potential problems for those with a central line, which the nurse needs to be observant for.

44. 2. The first 5 ml are drawn off and discarded. Lab values can be altered by the solution remaining in the catheter from the infusion or flush.

45. 3. The roller clamp should be closed after priming, otherwise the fluid will continue to flow. Open the roller clamp after inserting the tubing into the hub.

46. 3. The airway is provided by the endotracheal tube. The nurse should assess breathing, the next step in the ABCs.

47. 1. The Trendelenburg position increases the blood return from the legs, thereby raising the blood pressure.

48. 1. The epinephrine would help to ease the client's respiratory distress.

49. 1. Her vital signs indicate that she is probably going into shock. Fluids are the first action to do after assessing ABCs.

50. 2. Airway is the first step of ABCs.

2

Aging

GENERAL INFORMATION

Aging is a normal developmental process occurring throughout the human life span that causes a mild progressive decline in body system functioning. The older client is generally regarded as one who is 65 years of age or older.

CHAPTER OUTLINE

Biologic Theories of Aging

A. Immune system theory
   1. The two primary immune organs, the thymus and bone marrow, are affected by the aging process, which contributes to a decline in T-cell production and stem cellefficiency.
   2. Increase of infections, autoimmune disease, and cancer with aging.

B. Cross-linking theory
   1. Cross-linking is a chemical reaction that binds glucose to protein, which causes abnormal division of DNA, interfering with normal cell functioning and intracellular transport over a lifetime.
   2. Eventually causes tissue and organ failure.

C. Free radical theory
   1. Molecules that are highly reactive as a result of oxygen metabolism in the body.
   2. Over time, cause physical decline by damaging proteins, enzymes, and DNA.
   3. Beta-carotene and vitamins C and E are naturally occurring antioxidants that counteract the free radicals.

D. Stress theory (wear and tear)
   1. The body, like any machine, will eventually "wear out" secondary to repetitive usage, damage, and stress.
   2. While this theory is seen as having some merit, individuals react differently to stress (positive and negative), causing controversy over the concept.

E. Genetics theory
   1. Preprogrammed life expectancy. Cells can only divide a specific number of times.
   2. Life expectancies among family members is similar, i.e., if the parents died over the age of 80, the children are more likely to live to that age.

F. Neuroendocrine theories
   1. Anterior pituitary hormones are thought to contribute to the aging process.
   2. An imbalance of certain chemicals in the brain may contribute to altered cell division within the body.

Age-Related Changes

See Table 2-1.

Psychosocial Changes in the Older Adult

A. A successful aging process includes physical, psychological, social, and cultural factors.
   1. Some cultures have a great respect for older persons.
   2. In the United States, much value is placed on youth.
   3. Be aware of ageism (discrimination against the older adult simply because of age).

B. Developmental tasks for the older adult
   1. Ego integrity vs. despair (Erikson)
      a. With ego integrity, the person's life is felt to have meaning and accomplishment.
      b. With despair, there are feelings of worthlessness for a life not well lived.
   2. Other possible developmental tasks
      a. Successfully adjusting to retirement.
      b. Making safe and satisfactory living arrangements.
      c. Adjusting to reduced income.
      d. Keeping socially active.
      e. Maintaining contact with friends and family.
      f. Making safe decisions about driving a car.
      g. Adjusting to death of spouse/significant other.
      h. Adjusting to idea of one's own death.

TABLE 2-1 Age-Related Changes

System	Change	Nursing Interventions
Special Senses		
Vision	Presbyopia: decreased ability to focus on near objects (often requiring reading glasses) Decreased lacrimal secretions—chronic dry eye, scratchiness Pupils: smaller—decreased peripheral vision and ability to adapt to the dark; increased sensitivity to glare Lens: larger, more rigid, and discolored (yellow opacity)—decreased depth perception and ability to focus Colors distorted, especially blue/green Red/orange more pleasing	Provide increased illumination without glare. Provide safe environment by orienting client to surroundings and removing potential hazards. Use sunglasses outdoors. Use large-print books. Avoid night driving.
Hearing	Presbycusis: decreased ability to hear pitch or level of sound (first high, then low and background) Tinnitus—"ringing in the ear"; results from decreased blood supply to neurosensory receptors in ear; problems distinguishing horns/sirens	Look directly at the client when speaking and speak clearly and slowly; low-pitched voice heard best. Decrease background noise.
Taste/Smell	Olfactory fibers atrophy—decreased sense of smell, decreased appetite/ability to enjoy foods	Provide attractive meals in comfortable social setting. Vary taste, textures, and colors of foods. Be alert for difficulty chewing or swallowing when selecting foods.
Touch	Sensory nerve receptors less acute—requires stronger stimuli, increased pain tolerance, skin tears, more	Protect skin from injury. Lower bath water temperature to 100–105° F. Provide for safety

	difficult to distinguish hot, cold, or pressure Fine discrimination abilities impaired, especially hands and feet	around hot liquids at mealtimes.
Nervous	Overall intellect remains the same Fewer neurons and reduced blood flow to brain—some short-term memory loss and learning ability slowed Myelin sheath degenerates—decreased reaction time, reduced deep tendon reflexes, and increased time to respond to stimuli Change in sleep patterns	Promote independence in daily activities. Allow ample time for completion of tasks. Offer back rub or warm milk at bedtime. Provide recreational and diversional activities. Maintain environmental stability, minimize frequency of transfers.
Integumentary	Sweat glands diminish—decreased thermoregulation Collagen and subcutaneous fat decreases (subcutaneous medications absorb more slowly)—wrinkles, poor turgor (poor estimate of hydration) Hair follicles decrease/produce less melanin—baldness/gray hair Vascular supply to nailbeds reduced—dull, brittle nails—hard to cut! Delayed wound healing	Provide adequate warmth. Maintain adequate hydration. Avoid overexposure to the sun. Provide adequate heat and humidity in environment. Keep skin clean, dry, lubricated, and pressure free. Decrease frequency of baths.
Musculoskeletal	Muscle fibers decrease and muscles atrophy—decreased strength and endurance Bone density decreases—osteoporosis, increased fractures	Encourage exercise program. Promote optimum physical activity within level of ability. Maintain optimum nutrition, especially intake

Continued

TABLE 2-1 Continued

System	Change	Nursing Interventions
	Ligaments and tendons lose elasticity—decreased ROM in joints Intervertebral disks narrow—increased spine curves, balance diminishes (center of gravity)	of protein, calcium, and vitamins. Encourage use of appropriate adaptive or assistive devices to enhance mobility.
Cardiovascular	Increased peripheral resistance/increased blood pressure, especially systolic Baroreceptors less sensitive—decreased sensitivity to change in positions (orthostatic hypotension) Decreased venous valve competency—increased dependent edema Mitral/aortic valves thicker and more rigid—more murmurs without disease Decreased stroke volume and cardiac output Decreased pacemaker cells—possible dysrhythmias	Assess symptoms and make appropriate modifications in care. Teach client to change positions slowly to avoid falls. Minimize edema and fatigue with rest periods and elevation of legs. Teach energy conservation methods in daily activities.
Respiratory	Muscles weaken and atrophy, rib cage calcifies, barrel-shaped chest—increased energy to expand lungs, harder to cough and deep breathe Less tidal volume and increased residual volume secondary to cell fibrosis Alveoli decrease and thicken—less sensitive to hypoxia and hypercapnia Atrophy of cilia—slowed cough reflex, increased risk of infection	Manipulate environment to enhance ventilation. Position client to promote optimum ventilation. Encourage exercises and prescribed pulmonary exercises. Encourage annual influenza vaccines and one-time pneumococcal vaccine.

Gastrointestinal	Decreased smooth muscle tone, difficulty in swallowing (minor) and decreased peristalsis—decreased esophageal motility, increased heartburn and constipation Decrease in digestive enzymes—altered absorption of fats, protein, B_{12}, folic acid, calcium, iron, medications Decreased saliva, loss of teeth Decreased sphincter tone—impactions, incontinence	Assess condition of teeth and mouth, fit and comfort of dentures, and ability to chew. Encourage fluids and foods high in fiber. Encourage optimal activity. Promote independence and privacy in use of bathroom. Keep stool record and observe for constipation.
Renal	Decreased GFR secondary to decreased kidney size and number of nephrons and decreased renal blood flow—ability to concentrate/dilute urine decreased, decreased excretion of medications Decreased bladder capacity and weakened bladder and pelvic muscles—frequency, urgency, nocturia, incontinence, retention, infections Prostate enlargement/obstruction (retention), dribbling, overflow incontinence	Assess voiding patterns. Provide adequate fluids. Establish a bladder program to promote continence (assist to bathroom or offer bedpan every 2-3 hours). Avoid catheterization unless comatose, skin breakdown, or bladder outlet obstruction.
Reproductive		
Female	Diminished vaginal secretions secondary to decreased estrogen—painful intercourse, infections	Promote good perineal care, treat with prescribed creams (e.g., estrogen). Use vaginal lubricant as needed.
Male	Slower erections and ejaculations secondary to sclerosis of penile veins and arteries—decrease in sexual activity	Provide encouragement and discuss modifications of sexual expression as necessary; rest before and after sexual activity.

Psychologic/Social Theories of Aging

A. Activity theory
   1. Maintaining a level of active involvement in life helps the older adult stay psychologically and socially healthy.
   2. As life roles or physical capacity are lost, the older adult will substitute new roles or intellectual activities.

B. Continuity or developmental theory
   1. Adjustment to old age is impacted by individual personality, and the older adult will exhibit similar choices and decisions to younger years.
   2. This theory allows for great variation in successful aging, as individual habits and preferences are unique.

C. Disengagement theory
   1. Gradual mutual withdrawal between the individual and society as the aging process continues.
   2. While this theory was a major milestone in aging research, it is now felt to be flawed, as many older adults remain engaged in psychosocial aspects of life.

■ PATTERNS OF HEALTH AND DISEASE IN THE OLDER ADULT

A. Diseases that occur to varying degrees in most older adults
   1. Cataracts
   2. Arteriosclerosis
   3. Benign prostatic hypertrophy (males)

B. Diseases with increased incidence with advancing age
   1. Neoplastic disease
   2. Diabetes mellitus
   3. Dementia disorders

C. Diseases that have more serious consequences in the elderly and make homeostasis more difficult to maintain
   1. Pneumonia
   2. Influenza
   3. Trauma

D. Chronic disease very common
   1. Seventy-nine percent of noninstitutionalized persons over age 70 have at least one chronic disease.
   2. Most common chronic diseases: arthritis, hypertension, heart disease.
   3. Most hospital visits for persons over 65 are for chronic diseases.

E. Functional disability (inability to perform activities of daily living [ADL])
   1. Thirty-two percent of persons over 65 have some limitation of functions.

TABLE 2-2 Chronic Disease vs. Acute Disease

Characteristic	Chronic Diseases	Acute Diseases
Cause	Multiple causes; often related to lifestyle	Specific etiologies
Onset	Slow, insidious	Rapid
Duration	Indeterminate; remissions and exacerbations	Short
Understanding of disease	Often difficult because of indeterminate course, remissions, and exacerbations	Simpler because symptoms more overt
Outcomes	Somewhat predictable but often debilitating and associated with long periods of illness Management of condition Lifestyle changes required Individual with disease must assume control of disease	Symptoms resolve with cure of disease Outcomes usually favorable; cures Health care provider directs care and cure

2. Twenty-five percent of persons over 65 require help with at least one ADL or IADL (instrumental activities of daily living; e.g., shopping, paying bills).

F. Chronic vs. acute diseases
See Table 2-2.

ASSESSMENT

Health History and Gerontologic Focus

A. Assessment of the older adult client is complex
1. Allow sufficient time to conduct a thorough health history interview.
2. Depending on the client's stability, the interview may take more than one session.

B. Presenting problem
1. Assess client systematically depending upon the presenting problem.
2. Typical presentations of disease may change with age (i.e., client may not exhibit chest pain with a myocardial infarction).
3. The problem is likely to have multiple contributing factors and affect the client's functional abilities.

C. Mental status and mental health
   1. It is important to obtain a baseline for orientation, memory, level of alertness, and decision-making capabilities.
   2. Assess the client for quality of life issues, mood, affect, and anxiety.

D. Lifestyle and function
   1. Often, there is little correlation between diseases and functional abilities.
   2. The functional assessment provides a clearer picture of physical, psychologic, and social health.
   3. Use the client's own baseline from previous assessments to determine any changes in function.
   4. Have the client demonstrate function wherever possible (i.e., observe gait and balance, drinking a glass of water, dressing self).

E. Medication usage
   1. Ask for information about all types of medications that the client is taking, including prescription medications, nonprescription medications (especially analgesics and laxatives), vitamin supplements, and herbal medications.
   2. Be sure the client understands the purpose, dosage, side effects, and any special considerations or interactions for all medications.
   3. Discuss the client's abilities to obtain medications (i.e., renewing prescriptions, paying for medications).
   4. Polypharmacy is often present. Average older adult takes 11 prescription medications per day.

F. Nutrition and hydration
   1. Obtain food/fluid intake profile (either 24 hours or 3 days).
   2. Determine any difficulties ingesting food/fluids (chewing, salivation, swallowing, manual dexterity, tremors).
   3. Any foods the client is unable to eat (dairy products, sodium, sugar) or foods the client should eat (potassium- or calcium-rich foods/fluids).
   4. Taking in adequate amounts of water daily to stay hydrated?
   5. Ability to afford/purchase/prepare food?

G. Past medical history
   1. Inquire about all chronic diseases and conditions. Be aware that the client may not even consider certain conditions treatable and therefore does not mention them, e.g., urinary incontinence or pain from arthritis.
   2. Obtain information about previous illnesses, hospitalizations, and surgeries.

Physical Examination

A. Assess body systems as indicated.

B. Note physical changes in the older adult (see Table 2-1).

Laboratory/Diagnostic Tests

A. Laboratory tests as indicated according to symptoms of individual client.
B. Interpret lab test results with aging changes in mind.

ANALYSIS

Nursing diagnoses for older adult clients may include:

A. Activity intolerance
B. Bowel incontinence, constipation, diarrhea
C. Acute or chronic pain
D. Anxiety or death anxiety
E. Deficient fluid volume
F. Risk for infection
G. Impaired memory
H. Impaired physical mobility
I. Impaired oral mucous membrane
J. Imbalanced nutrition: less or more than body requirements
K. Ineffective airway clearance or breathing pattern, or impaired gas exchange
L. Self-care deficits: feeding, bathing/hygiene, dressing/grooming, toileting
M. Disturbed body image or ineffective role performance
N. Disturbed sensory perception
O. Sexual dysfunction
P. Impaired skin integrity
Q. Disturbed sleep pattern
R. Disturbed thought processes
S. Ineffective tissue perfusion
T. Impaired urinary elimination
U. Deficient diversional activity
V. Wandering
W. Impaired social interaction
X. Risk for other-directed violence
Y. Risk for falls or injury
Z. Relocation stress syndrome
AA. Impaired home maintenance

PLANNING AND IMPLEMENTATION

Goals

Client will maintain:

A. Maximum functional independence
B. Normal bowel and bladder elimination patterns
C. Sufficient communication skills
D. Positive self-concept
E. Freedom from injury and infection

CLIENT TEACHING CHECKLIST

Ask the client if anyone has reviewed the dosage schedule with them, especially if the schedule has changed. The physician or pharmacist may do this.

F. Optimal cognitive functioning
G. Adequate nutritional status and fluid balance
H. A restful sleep pattern
I. Social contacts and interpersonal needs
J. Treatment regimens as prescribed

INTERVENTIONS

Pharmacotherapy in the Older Adult

A. General information

1. Decreased body weight, dehydration, alterations in fat to muscle ratio, and slowed organ functioning may cause accumulation of a drug in the body due to higher concentrations in the tissues and slowed metabolism and excretion of the drug.
2. Multiple chronic diseases affecting older adults may also cause changes in the metabolism and excretion of medications.
3. Medication errors among older community-dwelling adults are estimated to be 25–50%.
4. Drug-drug interactions are increased secondary to older adults often having more than one prescribing health care provider.

B. Nursing care

1. Conduct a "brown bag" evaluation to assess all prescription, over-the-counter, and herbal medications the client may be taking.
2. Assess the client's understanding of the reasons for the drug therapy.
3. Assess the client's vision, memory, judgment, reading level, and motivation to determine ability to self-medicate.
4. Provide instructions in large-print, premeasured syringes, memory aids, and daily drug dose containers to enhance self-medicating abilities.
5. Check with the pharmacist for any drug-drug interactions if unsure.
6. Before beginning a medication, obtain baseline vital signs, mental status, vision, and bowel/bladder function.
7. Drug-induced side effects may present as confusion, incontinence, falls, or immobility.
8. Assess the client's ability to pay for the prescriptions.
9. If the client requires assistance in taking medications, teach family members. Proper techniques for administering oral medications

include: position head forward with neck slightly flexed to facilitate swallowing and avoid risk of aspiration.

10. If client has swallowing difficulties, obtain liquid forms of oral medications wherever possible.
11. Assess client for effectiveness of medications and any adverse reactions.

EVALUATION

A. Client performs self-care activities or caregiver provides assistance as needed.
B. Client is continent of bowel and bladder; voids in adequate amounts and has regular bowel movements.
C. Client is able to successfully communicate needs and concerns.
D. Client makes positive statements about self.
E. Client/caregiver modifies environment to support safety.
F. Client is alert, calm, and oriented, if possible.
G. Skin is intact without pressure ulcers.
H. Client eats a nutritionally balanced diet and maintains a stable weight.
I. Client maintains friends, social interactions, and sexual function.
J. Client describes and adheres to treatment plan.

CONDITIONS

Senile Dementia, Alzheimer's Disease

A. General information
   1. In dementia, the elderly client is alert with a progressive decline in memory and cognition accompanied by personality and behavioral changes.
   2. Alzheimer's disease accounts for 60–75% of all dementias and is the number one reason for institutionalization of the elderly.
   3. Other types of dementias include:
      a. Vascular—small infarctions in the brain result in dementia. Risk factors include hyperlipidemia, hypertension, and smoking.
      b. Frontoparietal—atrophy of neurons in the frontal lobes of the brain. Early symptoms are behavioral rather than cognitive abnormalities. (Pick's disease is most common.)
B. Medical management
   1. Rule out other conditions that might be causing symptoms. A definitive diagnosis of Alzheimer's disease can only be made upon autopsy.
   2. Medications for treatment include tacrine (Cognex), donepezil (Aricept), rivastigmine (Exelon), or galantamine (Reminyl).

a. Used in mild to moderate stages of the disease: 25% of clients show symptom improvement, and 80% of clients show a delay in decline of cognition.
b. Nursing considerations: Monitor for bradycardia and GI side effects, including anorexia and weight loss.

3. Treatment goals are to minimize behavioral symptoms, i.e., agitation, and maximize quality of life.

C. Assessment findings
1. Early in the disease process, may become depressed or anxious. Increased risk of suicide at this time.
2. Early, mild impairment (Stage 1).
 a. May last 2–4 years.
 b. Mild short-term memory loss—forgets people's names, location of objects, current date.
 c. Social withdrawal; decreased interest in usual activities/ hobbies.
 d. Mood swings, irritability; insight is diminished.
3. Middle, moderate impairment (Stage 2).
 a. May last several years.
 b. Memory and math calculation faulty. Decreased abilities to perform ADLs.
 c. Disoriented to time and place.
 d. Can no longer drive.
 e. Needs assistance with complex ADLs, e.g., clothing selection and dressing (zippers/buttons).
 f. Personality and behavioral changes. Exhibits agitation, restlessness, and wandering.
 g. Incontinence begins.
4. Late, severe impairment (Stage 3).
 a. Assistance with all ADLs.
 b. Nonverbal or communication is incoherent.
 c. Becomes nonambulatory.
 d. Requires total support in all activities.
 e. Incontinent of bowel and bladder.
 f. Indifference to food.
 g. Agitation and aggression seen in this stage.

D. Nursing interventions
1. Provide a safe environment, e.g., bed in lowest position; check on client frequently; avoid restraints (increases agitation); use night-lights.
2. Provide structured environment and simple routines, e.g., lowered noise levels; appropriate lighting; confined area for wandering.
3. Enlist caregiver's assistance in assessing routine and establishing plan of care.
4. Use touch and a calm, relaxed manner in approaching the client.
5. Facilitate effective communication.

NURSING ALERT

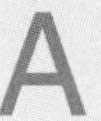 safe and secure environment is a high priority in caring for the client with Alzheimer's disease.

CLIENT TEACHING CHECKLIST

Encourage caregivers to monitor the client's fluid and food intake to detect imbalances. Limit the amount of food on plate to avoid having the client to make decisions.

   - **a.** Face the client and speak clearly using simple words and short sentences.
   - **b.** Keep directions simple and choices to a minimum; e.g., "Do you want to eat chicken or fish?"
   - **c.** Allow ample time for responses.

6. Encourage orientation with use of calendars and clocks; constantly reorienting the client is frustrating to all; consider validation therapy.
7. Have family bring items that stimulate memory, e.g., photographs and personal belongings, to the room.
8. Encourage mobility and provide opportunities for exercise, including walking and range of motion.
9. Avoid isolating the client; provide some stimulation such as soft music or television.
10. Provide nutritious, high-fiber foods and adequate fluids to maintain weight and hydration. Finger foods are a good choice.
11. Promote bowel and bladder continence by toileting at regular intervals.
12. Provide a simple bedtime routine that facilitates sleep, and encourage daytime activities to avoid excess napping.

ELDER MISTREATMENT

A. General information

1. Elder mistreatment can take the form of abuse or neglect.
2. Abuse may be actual injury inflicted or verbal insults, the use of physical or chemical restraints, financial abuse of money or assets, withholding food/fluids/medications, sexual abuse, or abandonment.

CLIENT TEACHING CHECKLIST

- Teach the client's family about environmental safety.
- Stress the importance of diet.
- Encourage the family to allow the client as much independence as possible.
- Refer the family to support groups such as the Alzheimer's Association.

3. The most common type of neglect is self-neglect in which the older adult is unable or unwilling to provide for him/herself. The responsible caregiver may also neglect by not providing necessary services or care.
4. An average of 5% of the older population experience elder mistreatment.

B. Assessment findings
1. Identify individuals at risk.
   a. Women over 75 years old who live with relatives and are physically, socially, and/or financially dependent.
   b. Persons whose primary caregivers express resentment, anger, or frustration with the older adult.
2. Clues to mistreatment
   a. Signs and symptoms may include poor hygiene and grooming, failure to thrive (malnutrition), oversedation, depression, and/or fearfulness.
   b. Skin provides objective evidence. Look for bruises, burns, lacerations, or pressure ulcers.
3. When assessing for mistreatment, the nurse should consider:
   a. Is the person in immediate danger of bodily harm?
   b. Is the person competent to make decisions regarding his/her care?
   c. What is the degree and significance of the person's functional impairments?
   d. What specific services might help to meet the unmet needs?
   e. Who in the family is involved and to what extent?
   f. Are the client and family willing to accept interventions?

C. Nursing interventions
1. Report suspected mistreatment to adult protective services.
2. Obtain client's consent for treatment.
3. Document nursing assessments of client's physical and emotional status.

REVIEW QUESTIONS

1. An 87-year-old woman has come to the medical clinic for her annual physical examination. The nurse assessing her knows that pulmonary function in elderly clients often shows
   1. reduction in vital capacity.
   2. a decrease in residual volume.
   3. an increase in functional alveoli.
   4. blood gases that reflect mild acidosis.
2. A normal sign of aging in the renal system is
   1. intermittent incontinence.
   2. concentrated urine.
   3. microscopic hematuria.
   4. a decreased glomerular filtration rate.
3. An older female client reports that she has been using more salt in her foods than she used to. The nurse understands that this is most likely because she
   1. has a decreased number of taste buds.
   2. is confused because of advanced age.
   3. needs more sodium to ensure renal function.
   4. is attempting to compensate for lost fluids.
4. Which assessment finding in the elderly is caused by decreased vessel elasticity and increased peripheral resistance?
   1. Confusion and disorientation.
   2. An irregular peripheral pulse rate.
   3. An increase in blood pressure.
   4. Wide QRS complexes on the ECG.
5. Which notation on the nursing care plan reflects inappropriate care of the older client with a hearing problem?
   1. Face the client, speaking slowly and clearly.
   2. Examine the ears for cerumen accumulation.
   3. Assess proper function of hearing aid daily.
   4. Speak loudly when talking to the client.
6. A 74-year-old, widowed client is hospitalized for cataract surgery. During his admission interview, he repeatedly talks about how he wishes he was

as strong and energetic as he was when he was younger. In planning care for this client, the nurse should include which of the following?

1. Use of the intervention reminiscence.
2. Confrontation of the client about being so grim.
3. Changing the topic whenever he brings it up.
4. Incorporation of a humorous view of the normal loss of strength.

7. A 74-year-old woman is hospitalized for dehydration. During the admission interview, she admits to the nurse that she is depressed. The nurse would expect this client to exhibit which of the following symptoms?

1. Increased energy level.
2. Increased anxiety.
3. Increased autonomy.
4. Increased socialization.

8. Knowing the difference between normal age-related changes and pathologic findings, which finding should the nurse identify as pathologic in a 74-year-old client?

1. Increase in residual lung volume.
2. Decrease in sphincter control of the bladder.
3. Increase in diastolic blood pressure.
4. Decreased response to touch, heat, and pain.

9. A sexually active 63-year-old client complains of painful intercourse secondary to vaginal dryness. Which information is most important for the nurse to include in a teaching plan for this client?

1. Ask the client for a list of all medications, including over-the-counter drugs, that she has taken in the past month in order to determine a possible etiology for the dryness.
2. Teach the client alternative methods of intimacy in the form of touch.
3. Instruct the client to use an artificial water-based lubricant in the vagina to decrease the discomfort of intercourse.
4. Prepare the client for a vascular work-up since the dryness is often related to vascular deficiencies.

10. An older, medically controlled manic-depressive and asthmatic man has been under the care of his primary physician for many years. Recently, a cardiologist prescribed cardiac medications for congestive heart failure. He complains to the home care nurse that he is nauseated. It would be justifiable for the nurse to reach which of the following conclusions as to the cause of the client's nausea?

1. The reaction between the new medication regime and the foods caused the nausea.
2. The problem of polypharmacy may exist as the client symptomatology may be a result of multiple drug interactions.
3. The nausea could be psychosomatic and related to the client's depression over having to take new medications.
4. The client may be taking too much of his new medications, which may contribute to his symptoms.

11. An older client has several medications ordered and has difficulty swallowing them. What strategy should the nurse use to administer these medications?

1. Hide the medication by placing them in meat.
2. Crush the medication and mix them with soft foods.
3. Substitute injectable medications.
4. Dissolve medications in liquid.

12. Which of the following measures is necessary to incorporate into a plan of care for a client who is diagnosed with senile dementia?

1. Because these clients are easily bored, they need to be challenged with new activities.
2. Environmental stimuli need to be eliminated.
3. Communicate in simple words, short sentences, and a calm tone of voice.
4. Schedule more demanding activities later in the day.

13. A 76-year-old man who is a resident in an extended care facility is in the late stages of Alzheimer's disease. He tells his nurse that he has sore back muscles from all the construction work he has been doing all day. Which response by the nurse is most appropriate?

1. "You know you don't work in construction anymore."
2. "What type of motion did you do to precipitate this soreness?"
3. "You're 76 years old and you've been here all day. You don't work in construction anymore."
4. "Would you like me to rub your back for you?"

14. An 86-year-old male with senile dementia has been physically abused and neglected for the past two years by his live-in caregiver. He has since moved and is living with his son and daughter-in-law. Which response by the client's son would cause the nurse great concern?

1. "How can we obtain reliable help to assist us in taking care of Dad? We can't do it alone."
2. "Dad used to beat us kids all the time. I wonder if he remembered that when it happened to him?"
3. "I'm not sure how to deal with Dad's constant repetition of words."
4. "I plan to ask my sister and brother to help my wife and me with Dad on the weekends."

15. An alert and oriented 84-year-old client is receiving home care services following a cerebrovascular accident (CVA) that has left her with right-sided hemiparesis. She lives with her middle-aged daughter and son-in-law. The nurse suspects she is being physically abused by her daughter. To elicit information effectively, the nurse should do which of the following?
   1. Directly ask the client if she has been physically struck or hurt by anyone.
   2. Wait until enough trust has been developed to enable the client to approach the nurse first.
   3. Confront the daughter with the suspicions.
   4. Interview the son-in-law to gain his perspective of the situation.

ANSWERS AND RATIONALES

1. 1. Residual volume increases with age, probably related to the loss of elastic forces in the lung.
2. 4. The glomerular filtration rate is decreased dramatically in the elderly due to changes in the renal tubules.
3. 1. The taste buds begin to atrophy at age 40, and insensitivity to taste qualities occurs after age 60. Studies related to diminished taste indicate that there are changes in the salt threshold for some elderly individuals.
4. 3. The blood pressure increases in response to the thickening of vessels and less distensible arteries and veins. There is also impedance to blood flow and increased systemic vascular resistance, contributing to hypertension.
5. 4. Raising the voice to speak loudly only increases the emission of higher frequency sounds, which the elderly client with presbycussis (a progressive bilateral perceptive loss of hearing in the older individual that occurs with the aging process) will have difficulty hearing.

6. 1. Assisting the older adult in reminiscing, or engaging in a "life review" process, is one way to assist the individual to accomplish his/her developmental tasks. One such task, adjusting to decreasing physical strength, needs to be met to establish and preserve ego integrity.

7. 2. Many psychosocial symptoms occur with depression, including feelings of hopelessness, helplessness, and increased anxiety, which contributes to despair rather than ego integrity.

8. 3. A modest increase in systolic blood pressure, not diastolic blood pressure, is an expected age-related change due to an increase in vascular resistance and vessel rigidity. An increase in diastolic blood pressure, however, is not an expected age-related change. It is pathologic and needs to be monitored.

9. 3. The decrease in vaginal secretions, which contributes to vaginal dryness and subsequent painful intercourse, is a normal age-related change. Using a lubricant will decrease or eliminate this discomfort.

10. 2. Polypharmacy is the prescription, use, or administration of five or more medications. If not coordinated, different physicians, each focusing on a specific disease process, contribute to polypharmacy. The background data indicate such may be the case.

11. 2. Medications, crushed and mixed with soft foods, are easier to digest for persons who have difficulty swallowing.

12. 3. Keep communications simple and concrete. Close-ended questions are more beneficial than open-ended questions, which may require complex answers that serve only to confuse the client. Even if the client isn't able to fully comprehend communications, a calm tone of voice may alleviate any stress.

13. 4. In the late stages of Alzheimer's disease, it is better to go along with the client's reality rather than confront him with logic and reasoning. Asking close-ended, simple questions that relate to his reality is nonthreatening and calming. Note that the nurse responds in a way that is congruent with his main concern, which is his sore back.

14. 2. This statement is a cause for concern. Victims 2 of abuse may alternate between generations. Abusive patterns are highly likely to be passed from parents to children. When children grow up and move into positions where they are caring for their aged parents (role reversal), the abusive behavior can surface.

15. 1. Direct questioning, in an open and accepting manner, is important. Abused elders are often reluctant to report abuse and will not volunteer the information on their own. Clients need to feel free to indicate the existence of an activity about which they may feel embarrassment and shame.

3

Perioperative Nursing

■ OVERVIEW

CHAPTER OUTLINE

Effects of Surgery on the Client

Physical Effects

A. Stress response (neuroendocrine response) is activated.
B. Resistance to infection is lowered due to surgical incision.
C. Vascular system is disturbed due to severing of blood vessels and blood loss.
D. Organ function may be altered due to manipulation.

Psychologic Effects

Common fears: pain, anesthesia, loss of control, disfigurement, separation from loved ones, alterations in roles or lifestyle

Factors Influencing Surgical Risk

A. *Age:* very young and elderly are at increased risk.
B. *Nutrition:* malnutrition and obesity increase risk of complications.
C. *Fluid and electrolyte balance:* dehydration, hypovolemia, and electrolyte imbalances can pose problems during surgery.
D. *General health status:* infection, cardiovascular disease, pulmonary problems, liver dysfunction, renal insufficiency, or metabolic disorders create increased risk.
E. *Medications*
1. Anticoagulants (including aspirin and NSAIDS) predispose to hemorrhage; discontinue 2 weeks before surgery.
2. Tranquilizers (e.g., phenothiazines) may cause hypotension and potentiate shock.
3. Antibiotics: aminoglycosides may intensify neuromuscular blockade of anesthesia with resultant respiratory paralysis.
4. Diuretics: may cause electrolyte imbalances.
5. Antihypertensives: can cause hypotension and contribute to shock.
6. Long-term steroid therapy: causes adrenocortical suppression; may need increased dosage during perioperative period.

F. *Type of surgery planned:* major surgery (e.g., thoracotomy) poses greater risk than minor surgery (e.g., dental extraction).
G. *Psychologic status of client:* excessive fear or anxiety may have adverse effect on surgery.

PREOPERATIVE PERIOD

Psychologic Support

A. Assess client's fears, anxieties, support systems, and patterns of coping.
B. Establish trusting relationship with client and significant others.
C. Explain routine procedures, encourage verbalization of fears, and allow client to ask questions.
D. Demonstrate confidence in surgeon and staff.
E. Provide for spiritual care if appropriate.

Preoperative Teaching

A. Frequently done on an outclient basis.
B. Assess client's level of understanding of surgical procedure and its implications.
C. Answer questions, clarify and reinforce explanations given by surgeon.
D. Explain routine pre- and post-op procedures and any special equipment to be used.
E. Teach coughing and deep-breathing exercises, splinting of incision, turning side to side in bed, and leg exercises; explain their importance in preventing complications; provide opportunity for return demonstration.
F. Assure client that pain medication will be available post-op.

Physical Preparation

A. Obtain history of past medical conditions, surgical procedures, allergies, dietary restrictions, and medications.
B. Perform baseline head-to-toe assessment, including vital signs, height, and weight.
C. Ensure that diagnostic procedures are performed as ordered: common tests are.
  1. CBC (complete blood count)
  2. Electrolytes
  3. PT/PTT (prothrombin time; partial thromboplastin time)
  4. Urinalysis
  5. ECG (electrocardiogram)
  6. Type and crossmatch
  7. Chest X-ray

D. Prepare client's skin.
  1. Shower with antibacterial soap to cleanse skin if ordered; client may do this at home the night before surgery if outclient admission.

2. Skin prep if ordered: shave or clip hairs and cleanse appropriate areas to reduce bacteria on skin and minimize chance of infection.

E. Administer enema if ordered (usually for surgery on GI tract, gynecologic surgery).

F. Promote adequate rest and sleep.

1. Provide back rub, clean linens.
2. Administer bedtime sedation.

G. Instruct client to remain NPO after midnight to prevent vomiting and aspiration during surgery.

Legal Responsibilities

A. Surgeon obtains operative permit (*informed consent*).

1. Surgical procedure, alternatives, possible complications, disfigurements, or removal of body parts are explained.
2. It is part of the nurse's role as client advocate to confirm that the client understands information given.

B. Informed consent is necessary for each operation performed, however minor. It is also necessary for major diagnostic procedures, e.g., bronchoscopy, thoracentesis, etc., where a major body cavity is entered.

C. Adult client (over 18 years of age) signs own permit unless unconscious or mentally incompetent.

1. If unable to sign, relative (spouse or next of kin) or guardian will sign.
2. In an emergency, permission via telephone or telegram is acceptable; have a second listener on phone when telephone permission being given.
3. Consents are not needed for emergency care if all four of the following criteria are met.
   - **a.** There is an immediate threat to life.
   - **b.** Experts agree that it is an emergency.
   - **c.** Client is unable to consent.
   - **d.** A legally authorized person cannot be reached.

D. Minors (under 18) must have consent signed by an adult (i.e., parent or legal guardian). An emancipated minor (married, college student living away from home, in military service, any pregnant female or any who has given birth) may sign own consent.

E. Witness to informed consent may be nurse, another physician, clerk, or other authorized person.

F. If nurse witnesses informed consent, specify whether witnessing explanation of surgery or just signature of client.

Preparation Immediately before Surgery

A. Obtain baseline vital signs; report elevated temperature or blood pressure.

B. Provide oral hygiene and remove dentures.

C. Remove client's clothing and dress in clean gown.

NURSING ALERT

Avoid incorrect surgical site errors by:

- Asking the client to mark the surgical site
- Orally verifying the surgery just before the start of the procedure
- Confirming correct person, surgical site, and correct procedure.

D. Remove nail polish, cosmetics, hair pins, contact lenses, prostheses, and any body jewelry.
E. Instruct client to empty bladder.
F. Check identification band.
G. Administer pre-op medications as ordered.
   1. Narcotic analgesics (meperidine [Demerol], morphine sulfate) relax client, reduce anxiety, and enhance effectiveness of general anesthesia.
   2. Sedatives (secobarbital sodium [Seconal]), sodium pentobarbital [Nembutal] decrease anxiety and promote relaxation and sleep.
   3. Anticholinergics (atropine sulfate, scopolamine [Hyoscine]) and glycopyrrolate (Robinul) decrease tracheobronchial secretions to minimize danger of aspirating secretions in lungs, decrease vagal response to inhibit undesirable effects of general anesthesia (bradycardia).
   4. Droperidol, fentanyl or a combination may be ordered; should not be given with sedatives because of danger of respiratory depression; also helpful in control of postoperative nausea and vomiting.
H. Elevate side rails and provide quiet environment.
I. Prepare client's chart for OR, including operative permit and complete pre-op check list.

INTRAOPERATIVE PERIOD

Anesthesia

General Anesthesia

A. General information
   1. Drug-induced depression of CNS; produces decreased muscle reflex activity and loss of consciousness.
   2. Balanced anesthesia: combination of several anesthetic drugs to provide smooth induction, appropriate depth and duration of anesthesia, sufficient muscle relaxation, and minimal complications.
B. Stages of general anesthesia: induction, excitement, surgical anesthesia, and danger stage (see Table 3-1).

TABLE 3-1 Stages of Anesthesia

Stage	From	To	Client Status
Stage I (induction)	Beginning administration of anesthetic agent	Loss of consciousness	May appear euphoric, drowsy, dizzy.
Stage II (delirium or excitement)	Loss of consciousness	Relaxation	Breathing irregular; may appear excited; very susceptible to external stimuli.
Stage III (surgical anesthesia)	Relaxation	Loss of reflexes and depression of vital functions	Regular breathing pattern; corneal reflexes absent; pupillary constriction.
Stage IV (danger stage)	Vital functions depressed	Respiratory arrest; possible cardiac arrest	No respirations; absent or minimal heartbeat; dilated pupils.

C. Agents for general anesthesia.

1. Inhalation agents may be gas or liquid.
2. IV anesthetics: used as induction agents because they produce rapid, smooth induction; may be used alone in short procedures such as endoscopies.
   a. Common IV anesthetics: methohexital (Brevital), sodium thiopental (Pentathol), midazolam hydrochloride (Versed)
   b. Disadvantages: poor relaxation; respiratory and myocardial depression in high doses; bronchospasm, laryngospasm; hypotension, respiratory depression
3. Dissociative agents: produce state of profound analgesia, amnesia, and lack of awareness without loss of consciousness; used alone in short surgical and diagnostic procedures or for induction prior to administration of more potent general anesthetics.
   a. Agent: ketamine (Ketalar)
   b. Side effects: tachycardia, hypertension, respiratory depression, hallucinations, delirium
   c. Precautions: decrease verbal, tactile, and visual stimulation during recovery period

4. Neuroleptics: produce state of neuroleptic analgesia characterized by reduced motor activity, decreased anxiety, and analgesia without loss of consciousness; used alone for short surgical and diagnostic procedures, as premedication or in combination with other anesthetics for longer anesthesia.
   a. Agent: fentanyl citrate with droperidol (Innovar)
   b. Side effects: hypotension, bradycardia, respiratory depression, skeletal muscle rigidity, twitching
   c. Precautions: reduce narcotic doses by ½ to ⅓ for at least 8 hours postanesthesia as ordered to prevent respiratory depression.

D. Adjuncts to general anesthesia: neuromuscular blocking agents: used with general anesthetics to enhance skeletal muscle relaxation.
   1. Agents: pancuronium (Pavulon), succinylcholine (Anectine), tubocurarine, atracurium besylate (Tracrium), vecuronium bromide (Norcuron)
   2. Precaution: monitor client's respirations for at least 1 hour after drug's effect has worn off.

Regional Anesthesia

A. General information (see also Table 3-2)
   1. Produces loss of painful sensation in one area of the body; does not produce loss of consciousness
   2. Uses: biopsies, excision of moles and cysts, endoscopies, surgery on extremities; childbirth
   3. Agents: lidocaine (Xylocaine), procaine (Novocain), tetracaine (Pontocaine)

Conscious Sedation

A. General information
   1. Intravenous conscious sedation is induced by pharmacologic agents.
   2. Sedative and analgesic medications are used to achieve an altered state of consciousness with minimal risk, relief of anxiety, an amnestic state, and pain relief from noxious stimuli.
   3. These agents may include a combination of a benzodiazepine (midazolam, diazepam) and a narcotic (fentanyl, morphine).
   4. This provides a safe and effective option for clients undergoing minor surgical and diagnostic procedures such as, but not limited to, endoscopic procedures, breast biopsy, dental surgery, and plastic surgery.
   5. Conscious sedation is extremely safe when administered by qualified providers.
      a. Certified registered nurse anesthetists (CRNAs), anesthesiologists, dentists, oral surgeons, and other physicians are qualified providers of conscious sedation.

TABLE 3-2 Regional Anesthesia

Types	Method
Topical	Cream, spray, drops, or ointment applied externally, directly to area to be anesthetized.
Local infiltration block	Injected into subcutaneous tissue of surgical area.
Field block	Area surrounding the surgical site injected with anesthetic.
Nerve block	Injection into a nerve plexus to anesthetize part of body.
Spinal	Anesthetic introduced into subarachnoid space of spinal cord producing anesthesia below level of diaphragm.
Epidural	Anesthetic injected extradurally to produce anesthesia below level of diaphragm; used in obstetrics.
Caudal	Variation of epidural block; produces anesthesia of perineum and occasionally lower abdomen; commonly used in obstetrics.
Saddle block	Similar to spinal, but anesthetized area is more limited; commonly used in obstetrics.

b. Specifically trained registered nurses may assist in the administration of conscious sedation.

6. Verbal communication with the client can be maintained throughout the procedure.

7. This will provide reassurance to a cooperative client and help monitor intact neurological status.

8. Supplemental oxygen should always be given to a client receiving conscious sedation.

9. Constant vigilance in monitoring of cardiorespiratory status (heart rate and rhythm, blood pressure, respiratory rate, and pulse oximetry) is crucial.

10. The provider who monitors the client receiving conscious sedation should have no other responsibilities during the procedure and should never abandon that client for any reason.

NURSING ALERT

Older clients are at greater risk for postoperative delirium.

POSTOPERATIVE PERIOD

Postoperative Care

Recovery Room (Immediate Postoperative Care)

A. Assess for and maintain patent airway.
   1. Position unconscious or semiconscious client on side (unless contraindicated) or on back with head to side and chin extended forward.
   2. Check for presence/absence of gag reflex.
   3. Maintain artificial airway in place until gag and swallow reflex have returned.

B. Administer oxygen as ordered.

C. Assess rate, depth, and quality of respirations.

D. Check vital signs every 15 minutes until stable, then every 30 minutes.

E. Note level of consciousness; reorient client to time, place, and situation.

F. Assess color and temperature of skin, color of nailbeds, and lips.

G. Monitor IV infusions: condition of site, type, and amount of fluid being infused and flow rate.

H. Check all drainage tubes and connect to suction or gravity drainage as ordered; note color, amount, and odor of drainage.

I. Assess dressings for intactness, drainage, hemorrhage.

J. Monitor and maintain client's temperature; may need extra blankets.

K. Encourage client to cough and deep breathe after airway is removed.

L. If spinal anesthesia used, maintain flat position and check for sensation and movement in lower extremities.

Care on Surgical Floor

A. Monitor respiratory status and promote optimal functioning.
   1. Encourage client to cough (if not contraindicated) and deep breathe every 1–2 hours.
   2. Instruct client to splint incision while coughing.
   3. Assist client to turn in bed every 2 hours.
   4. Encourage early ambulation.
   5. Encourage use of incentive spirometer every 2 hours: causes sustained, maximal inspiration that inflates the alveoli.
   6. Assess respiratory status and auscultate lungs every 4 hours; be alert for any signs of respiratory complications.

DELEGATION TIP

The assessment and management of the postoperative client require your knowledge and critical teaching skills. Other caregivers may record vital signs, provide basic comfort and hygiene, and empty, measure, and record drainage after the RN's initial assessment.

B. Monitor cardiovascular status and avoid post-op complications.
  1. Encourage leg exercises every 2 hours while in bed.
  2. Encourage early ambulation.
  3. Apply antiembolism stockings as ordered.
  4. Assess vital signs, color and temperature of skin every 4 hours.

C. Promote adequate fluid and electrolyte balance.
  1. Monitor IV and ensure adequate intake.
  2. Measure I&O.
  3. Irrigate NG tube properly, using normal saline solution.
  4. Observe for signs of fluid and electrolyte imbalances.

D. Promote optimum nutrition.
  1. Maintain IV infusion as ordered.
  2. Assess for return of peristalsis (presence of bowel sounds and flatus).
  3. Add progressively to diet as ordered and note tolerance.

E. Monitor and promote return of urinary function.
  1. Measure I&O.
  2. Assess client's ability to void.
  3. Report to surgeon if client has not voided within 8 hours after surgery.
  4. Check for bladder distention.
  5. Use measures to promote urination (e.g., assist male to sit on side of bed, pour warm water over female's perineum).

F. Promote bowel elimination.
  1. Encourage ambulation.
  2. Provide adequate food and fluid intake when tolerated.
  3. Keep stool record and note any difficulties with bowel elimination.

G. Administer post-op analgesics as ordered; provide additional comfort measures.

H. Encourage optimal activity, turning in bed every 2 hours, early ambulation if allowed (generally client will be out of bed within 24 hours; have client dangle legs before getting out of bed).

I. Provide wound care.
  1. Check dressings frequently to ensure they are clean, dry, and intact.
  2. Observe aseptic technique when changing dressings.
  3. Encourage diet high in protein and vitamin C.
  4. Report any signs of infection: redness, drainage, odor, fever.

CLIENT TEACHING CHECKLIST

- Provide the client with the physician's telephone number.
- Explain the signs and symptoms of infection to the client and family.
- Explain name, dose, schedule, and purpose of medications. Provide drug information leaflets.
- Explain exact activity restrictions.
- Explain dietary progression.
- Provide instruction sheet with written information that is clear and specific.

J. Provide adequate psychologic support to client/significant others.
K. Provide appropriate discharge teaching: dietary restrictions, medication regimen, activity limitations, wound care, and possible complications.

Postoperative Complications

Respiratory System

Common post-op complications of respiratory tract are atelectasis and pneumonia.

A. Predisposing factors.
  1. Type of surgery (e.g., thoracic or high abdomen surgery)
  2. Previous history of respiratory problems
  3. Age: greater risk over age 40
  4. Obesity
  5. Smoking
  6. Respiratory depression caused by narcotics
  7. Severe post-op pain
  8. Prolonged post-op immobility

B. Prevention: see Care on Surgical Floor.

Cardiovascular System

Common post-op complications of the cardiovascular system are deep vein thrombosis, pulmonary embolism, and shock.

A. Predisposing factors to deep venous thrombosis (DVT).
  1. Lower abdominal surgery or septic diseases (e.g., peritonitis)
  2. Injury to vein by tight leg straps during surgery
  3. Previous history of venous problems
  4. Increased blood coagulability due to dehydration, fluid loss

   5. Venous stasis in the extremity due to decreased movement during surgery
   6. Prolonged post-op immobilization
B. Predisposing factors to pulmonary embolism: may occur as a complication of DVT.
C. Most common causes of shock during post-op period
   1. Hemorrhage
   2. Sepsis
   3. Myocardial infarction and cardiac arrest
   4. Drug reactions
   5. Transfusion reactions
   6. Pulmonary embolism
   7. Adrenal failure
D. Prevention of DVT, pulmonary embolism, and shock.

Genitourinary System

Post-op complications of the genitourinary system often include urinary retention and urinary tract infection.

A. Predisposing factors to urinary retention include
   1. Anxiety
   2. Pain
   3. Lack of privacy
   4. Narcotics and certain anesthetics that diminish client's sense of a full bladder
B. Prevention and nursing interventions for urinary retention.
C. Post-op urinary tract infections are most commonly caused by catheterization; prevention consists of using strict sterile technique when inserting a catheter, and appropriate catheter care (every 8 hours or according to agency protocol).

Gastrointestinal System

An important GI post-op complication is paralytic ileus (paralysis of intestinal peristalsis).

A. Predisposing factors.
   1. Temporary: anesthesia, manipulation of bowel during abdominal surgery
   2. Prolonged: electrolyte imbalance, wound infection, pneumonia
B. Assessment findings
   1. Absent bowel sounds
   2. No passage of flatus
   3. Abdominal distention

NURSING ALERT

Wound dehiscence and evisceration usually occur 6–8 days after surgery.

C. Nursing interventions.
   1. Assist with insertion of nasogastric or intestinal tube with application of suction as ordered.
   2. Keep client NPO.
   3. Maintain IV therapy as ordered.
   4. Assess for bowel sounds every 4 hours; check for abdominal distention, passage of flatus.
   5. Encourage ambulation if appropriate.

Wound Complications

A. Wound infection
   1. Predisposing factors
      a. Obesity
      b. Diabetes mellitus
      c. Malnutrition
      d. Elderly clients
      e. Steroids and immunosuppressive agents
      f. Lowered resistance to infection, as found in clients with cancer
   2. Assessment findings: redness, tenderness, drainage, heat in incisional area; fever; usually occurs 3-5 days after surgery.
   3. Prevention: see Care on Surgical Floor.
   4. Nursing interventions
      a. Obtain culture and sensitivity of wound drainage (*S. aureus* most frequently cultured).
      b. Perform cleansing and irrigation of wound as ordered.
      c. Administer antibiotic therapy as ordered.

B. Wound dehiscence and evisceration.
   1. Dehiscence: opening of wound edges
   2. Evisceration: protrusion of loops of bowel through incision; usually accompanied by sudden escape of profuse, pink serous drainage
   3. Predisposing factors to wound dehiscence and evisceration
      a. Wound infection
      b. Faulty wound closure
      c. Severe abdominal stretching (e.g., coughing, retching)
   4. Nursing interventions for wound dehiscence
      a. Apply Steri-Strips to incision.
      b. Notify physician.
      c. Promote wound healing.

5. Nursing interventions for wound evisceration
   a. Place client in supine position.
   b. Cover protruding intestinal loops with moist normal saline soaks.
   c. Notify physician.
   d. Check vital signs.
   e. Observe for signs of shock.
   f. Start IV line.
   g. Prepare client for OR for surgical closure of wound.

REVIEW QUESTIONS

1. An adult man is in the postanesthesia care unit (PACU) following a hemicolectomy. While in the PACU, the nurse will monitor his vital signs
   1. continuously.
   2. every 5 minutes.
   3. every 15 minutes.
   4. on a prn basis.
2. An adult who has had general anesthesia for major surgery is in the PACU. One of the signs that may indicate that his artificial airway should be removed is
   1. gagging.
   2. restlessness.
   3. an increase in pain.
   4. clear lungs on auscultation.
3. An adult is 6 days post abdominal surgery. Which sign alerts the nurse to wound evisceration?
   1. Acute bleeding.
   2. Pink serous drainage.
   3. Purple drainage.
   4. Severe pain.
4. An adult client's wound has eviscerated. The nurse assesses his respiratory status because
   1. dehiscence elevates the diaphragm.
   2. coughing increases the risk of evisceration.

3. respiratory arrest commonly accompanies wound dehiscence.
4. splinting the wound will compromise respiratory status.

5. An adult client has acute leukemia and is scheduled for a Hickman catheter insertion under local anesthesia. A MAJOR advantage of regional anesthesia is that the client
    1. retains all reflexes.
    2. remains conscious.
    3. has retroactive amnesia.
    4. is in the OR for a short period of time.

6. An adult male is scheduled for surgery and the nurse is assessing for risk factors. Which of the following are the greatest risk factors?
    1. He is 5 ft 4 in tall and weighs 125 lb.
    2. He expresses a fear of pain in the post-op period.
    3. He is 5 ft 4 in tall, weighs 360 lb, and is diabetic.
    4. He expresses a fear of the unknown.

7. The nurse in an outclient department is interviewing an adult one week prior to her scheduled elective surgery. In planning for the surgery, which of the following should the nurse include in her teaching?
    1. The client will be able to return home alone following the surgery.
    2. Limitations of oral intake the day of the procedure.
    3. The laboratory studies ordered do not need to be done until after the surgery.
    4. The client should not take any of her routine medications the morning of the surgery.

8. The nurse enters a woman's room to administer 10 mg Valium PO, the ordered pre-op medication for her hysterectomy. During the conversation, the client tells the nurse that she and her husband are planning to have another child in the coming year. The best action for the nurse to take is which of the following?
    1. Do not administer the pre-op medication, notify the nursing supervisor and the physician.
    2. Go ahead and administer the medication as ordered.
    3. Check to see if the client has signed a surgical consent.
    4. Send the client to the operating room (OR) without the medication.

9. The nurse administers 10 mg intramuscular (IM) morphine as a pre-op medication, and then discovers that there is no signed operative permit. The best action for the nurse to take is to

1. send the client to surgery as scheduled.
2. notify the nursing supervisor, the OR, and the physician.
3. cancel the surgery immediately.
4. obtain the needed consent.

10. An adult received atropine sulfate (Atropine) as a pre-op medication 30 minutes ago and is now complaining of dry mouth and her pulse rate is higher than before the medication was administered. The nurse's best interpretation of these findings is that

1. the client is having an allergic reaction to the drug.
2. the client needs a higher dose of this drug.
3. this is a normal side effect of Atropine.
4. the client is anxious about the upcoming surgery.

11. An adult who has chronic obstructive pulmonary disease (COPD) is scheduled for surgery and the physician has recommended an epidural anesthetic. The nurse should know that general anesthesia was not recommended for this client because

1. there is too high a risk for pressures sores developing.
2. there is less effect on the respiratory system with epidural anesthesia.
3. central nervous system control of vascular constriction would be affected with general anesthesia.
4. there is too high a risk of lacerations to the mouth, bruising of lips, and damage to teeth.

12. An adult had a bunion removed under an epidural block. In the immediate post-op period, the nurse plans to assess the client for side effects of the epidural block that include which of the following?

1. Headache.
2. Hypotension, bradycardia, nausea, and vomiting.
3. Hypertension, muscular rigidity, fever, and tachypnea.
4. Urinary retention.

13. An adult received droperidol and fentanyl (Innovar) during surgery. In planning postoperative care, the nurse will need to monitor for which of the following during the immediate post-op period?

1. Restlessness and anxiety.
2. Delirium.
3. Dysrhythmias.
4. Respiratory depression.

14. An adult has just arrived on the general surgery unit from the postanesthesia care unit (PACU). Which of the following needs to be the initial intervention the nurse takes?
    1. Assess the surgical site, noting the amount and character of drainage.
    2. Assess for amount of urinary output and the presence of any distention.
    3. Allow the family to visit with the client to decrease the anxiety of the client.
    4. Take vital signs, assessing first for a patent airway and the quality of respirations.
15. An adult is receiving morphine via a PCA pump after her surgery. The best method for the nurse to use to evaluate her level of pain is to ask the client
    1. to rate her pain on a scale of 1–10.
    2. if the morphine is working for her.
    3. if she is feeling any pain.
    4. if she needs her morphine level increased.
16. A 58-year-old smoker underwent major abdominal surgery two days ago. During the respiratory assessment, the nurse notes he is taking shallow breaths and breath sounds are decreased in the bases. The best interpretation of these findings is that the client is experiencing post-op
    1. pneumonia.
    2. atelectasis.
    3. hemorrhage.
    4. thromboembolism.
17. To prevent thromboembolism in the post-op client the nurse should include which of the following in the plan of care?
    1. Place a pillow under the knees and restrict fluids.
    2. Use strict aseptic technique including handwashing and sterile dressing technique.
    3. Assess bowel sounds in all four quadrants on every shift and avoid early ambulation.
    4. Assess for Homan's signs on every shift, encourage early ambulation, and maintain adequate hydration.
18. It is 10:00 P.M and the nurse notes that an adult male who returned from the PACU at 2:00 P.M has not voided. The client has an out of bed order, but has not been up yet. The best action for the nurse to take is
    1. insert a Foley catheter into the client.
    2. straight-catheterize the client.

3. assist the client to stand at the side of his bed and attempt to void into a urinal.
4. encourage the client to lie on his left side in bed and attempt to void into a urinal.

19. When assessing a post-op client, the nurse notes a nasogastric tube to low constant suction, the absence of a bowel movement since surgery, and no bowel sounds. The most appropriate plan of care based on these findings is to
    1. increase the client's mobility and ensure he is receiving adequate pain relief.
    2. increase coughing, turning, and deep breathing exercises.
    3. discontinue the nasogastric tube as the client does not need it any more.
    4. assess for bladder pain and distention.

20. On the second post-op day following an inguinal herniorrhaphy, the nurse assessing a client's wound would expect to find
    1. a small amount of serous drainage, edges approximated, and a pink color.
    2. a large amount of sanguineous drainage and edges pink in color.
    3. no drainage, the edges brown and coming apart.
    4. a Penrose drain putting out large amounts of serosanguineous drainage.

ANSWERS AND RATIONALES

1. 3. While in the postanesthesia care unit (PACU) the client's vital signs are assessed every 15 minutes.
2. 1. The return of the gag reflex usually indicates that the client is able to manage his own secretions and maintain a patent airway.
3. 2. A sudden gush of serosanguinous drainage that looks like "pink lemonade" is usually the major symptom of wound dehiscence.
4. 2. Coughing increases intra-abdominal pressure, which could force loops of bowel out through the open wound.
5. 2. The client receiving regional anesthesia has nerve impulses blocked but does not lose consciousness.
6. 3. Obesity and diabetes are major risk factors with the potential for complications related to anesthesia.

7. 2. Instructions should be given to the client regarding limitations of oral intake to avoid nausea and vomiting from the anesthesia.
8. 1. No client should be administered the pre-op medication until the informed consent has been obtained. Informed consent means that the client understands the information about the surgery. Even if the consent form is signed, the nurse should withhold sedating medication. This client clearly does not understand the planned procedure.
9. 2. If a narcotic, sedative, or tranquilizing drug has been administered before signing of the consent, the drug's effects must be allowed to wear off before consent can be given.
10. 3. These are normal side effects of an anticholinergic drug; adverse side effects would include ECG changes, constipation, and urinary retention.
11. 2. Epidural anesthesia does not cause respiratory depression, but general anesthesia can, especially in a client with COPD.
12. 2. These are all symptoms of sympathetic nervous system blockade, so the client should be closely monitored for these.
13. 4. Depression of respiratory rate has been reported and tends to last longer than the analgesic effect when Innovar is used during surgery.
14. 4. A specific assessment priority is the evaluation of a patent airway and respiratory and circulatory adequacy.
15. 1. The client should obtain relief from pain, and using a scale to assess this is a more objective measure.
16. 2. Atelectasis occurs commonly after abdominal surgery, especially in smokers. This occurs when mucus blocks the bronchioles and causes decreased breath sounds and shallow breathing.
17. 4. Thromboembolism can be related to dehydration and immobility. These measures help prevent hypovolemia and subsequent sludging of cells. A positive Homan's sign is often associated with thromboembolism.
18. 3. Nursing interventions to facilitate voiding include ambulation and normal positioning for voiding. The normal voiding position for the male is standing.
19. 1. Paralytic ileus can be related to immobility and inadequate pain medication as well as bowel manipulation and the anesthetic used during surgery.
20. 1. An inguinal herniorrhaphy should have only minimal serous drainage (straw colored) during the post-op period.

4

Oncologic Nursing

PATHOPHYSIOLOGY AND ETIOLOGY OF CANCER

CHAPTER OUTLINE

Evolution of Cancer Cells

A. All cells constantly change through growth, degeneration, repair, and adaptation. Normal cells must divide and multiply to meet the needs of the organism as a whole, and this cycle of cell growth and destruction is an integral part of life processes. The activities of the normal cells in the human body are all coordinated to meet the needs of the organism as a whole, but when the regulatory control mechanisms of normal cells fail, and growth continues in excess of the body's needs, neoplasia results.

B. The term *neoplasia* refers to both benign and malignant growths, but malignant cells behave very differently from normal cells and have special features characteristic of the cancer process.

C. Since the growth control mechanism of normal cells is not entirely understood, it is not clear what allows the uncontrolled growth, therefore no definitive cure has been found.

Characteristics of Malignant Cells

Differentiation

A. Cancer cells are mutated stem cells that have undergone structural changes so that they are unable to perform the normal functions of specialized tissue (un- or dedifferentiation).

B. They may function in a disorderly way or cease normal function completely, only functioning for their own survival and growth.

C. The most undifferentiated cells are also called anaplastic.

Rate of Growth

A. Cancer cells have uncontrolled growth or cell division.

B. Rate at which a tumor grows involves both increased cell division and increased survival time of cells.

C. Malignant cells do not form orderly layers, but pile on top of each other to eventually form tumors.

Spread (Invasion and Metastasis)

A. Cancer cells are less adhesive than normal cells, more easily dissociated from their location.
B. Lack of adhesion and loss of contact inhibition make it possible for a cancer to spread to distant parts of the body (metastasis).
C. Malignant tumors are not encapsulated and expand into surrounding tissue (invasion).

Etiology (Carcinogenesis)

Actual cause of cancer is unknown but there are a number of theories; it is currently thought that there are probably multiple etiologies.

Environmental Factors

A. Majority (over 80%) of human cancers related to environmental carcinogens
B. Types
  1. Physical
    a. Radiation: X-rays, radium, nuclear explosion or waste, ultraviolet
    b. Trauma or chronic irritation
  2. Chemical
    a. Nitrites and food additives, polycyclic hydrocarbons, dyes, alkylating agents
    b. Drugs: arsenicals, stilbestrol, urethane
    c. Cigarette smoke
    d. Hormones

Genetics

A. Some cancers show familial pattern.
B. May be caused by inherited genetic defects.

Viral Theory

A. Viruses have been shown to be the cause of certain tumors in animals.
B. Oncoviruses (RNA-type viruses) thought to be culprit.
C. Viruses (HTLV-I, Epstein-Barr, Human Papilloma Virus) linked to human tumors.

Immunologic Factors

A. Failure of the immune system to respond to and eradicate cancer cells
B. Immunosuppressed individuals more susceptible to cancer

DIAGNOSIS OF CANCER

Classification and Staging

Tissue of Origin

A. *Carcinoma:* arises from surface, glandular, or parenchymal epithelium.
   1. *Squamous cell carcinoma:* surface epithelium
   2. *Adenocarcinoma:* glandular or parenchymal tissue
B. *Sarcoma:* arises from connective tissue.
C. *Leukemia, lymphoma, and multiple myeloma:* separate categories for each.

Stages of Tumor Growth

A. Several staging systems, important in selection of therapy
   1. TNM system: uses letters and numbers to designate the extent of the tumor.
      a. T: stands for primary growth; 1–4 with increasing size. T1S indicates carcinoma in situ.
      b. N: stands for lymph node involvement; 0–4 indicates progressively advancing nodal disease.
      c. M: stands for metastasis; 0 indicates no distant metastases, 1 indicates presence of metastases.
   2. Stages 0-IV: all cancers divided into five stages incorporating size, nodal involvement, and spread.
B. Cytologic diagnosis of cancer (e.g., Pap smear)
   1. Involves study of shed cells
   2. Classified by degree of cellular abnormality
      a. Normal
      b. Probably normal (slight changes)
      c. Doubtful (more severe changes)
      d. Probably cancer or precancerous
      e. Definitely cancer

Client Factors

Early detection of cancer is crucial in reducing morbidity and mortality. Clients need to be taught about

A. Seven warning signs of cancer (see Table 4-1).
B. Breast self-examination (BSE).
C. Importance of rectal exam for those over age 40
D. Hazards of smoking
E. Oral self-examination as well as annual exam of mouth and teeth
F. Hazards of excess sun exposure
G. Importance of Pap smear
H. Physical exam with lab work-up: every 3 years ages 20–40; yearly age 40 and over
I. Testicular self-examination (TSE)

TABLE 4-1 Seven Warning Signs of Cancer (Caution)

C — Change in bowel or bladder habits
A — A sore that doesn't heal
U — Unusual bleeding or discharge
T — Thickening or lump in breast (or elsewhere)
I — Indigestion or dysphagia
O — Obvious change in wart or mole
N — Nagging cough or hoarseness

1. *Testicular Cancer:* Most common cancer in young men between the ages of 15 and 34. Most testicular cancers are found by men themselves, by accident or when doing TSE.
2. *Testicular Self-Examination:* Ideally, should be performed monthly, after a warm shower or bath, when the skin of the scrotum is relaxed. Standing in front of a mirror, the man should gently roll each testicle between the thumb and fingers of both hands. The testes are smooth, oval-shaped, and rather firm.
3. *Warning Signs That Men Should Look For:*
   a. Painless swelling
   b. Feeling of heaviness
   c. Hard lump (size of a pea)
   d. Sudden collection of fluid in the scrotum
   e. Dull ache in the lower abdomen or in the groin
   f. Pain in a testicle or in the scrotum
   g. Enlargement or tenderness of the breasts.

TREATMENT OF CANCER

Chemotherapy

Principles

A. Based on ability of drug to kill cancer cells; normal cells may also be damaged, producing side effects discussed below. Effect is greatest on rapidly dividing cells, such as bone marrow cells, the GI tract, and hair.

B. Different drugs act on tumor cells in different stages of the cell growth cycle.

NURSING ALERT

When administering a chemotherapeutic agent intravenously, monitor the infusion site continuously for pain and burning or redness.

Types of Chemotherapeutic Drugs

A. Antimetabolites: foster cancer cell death by interfering with cellular metabolic process.
B. Alkylating agents: act with DNA to hinder cell growth and division.
C. Plant alkaloids: obtained from the periwinkle plant; makes the host's body a less favorable environment for the growth of cancer cells.
D. Antitumor antibiotics: affect RNA to make environment less favorable for cancer growth.
E. Steroids and sex hormones: alter the endocrine environment to make it less conducive to growth of cancer cells.

Major Side Effects and Nursing Interventions

A. GI System
- **1.** Nausea and vomiting
  - **a.** Administer antiemetics routinely every 4–6 hours as well as prophylactically before chemotherapy is initiated.
  - **b.** Withhold foods/fluids 4–6 hours before chemotherapy
  - **c.** Provide bland foods in small amounts after treatments.
- **2.** Diarrhea
  - **a.** Administer antidiarrheals.
  - **b.** Maintain good perineal care.
  - **c.** Give clear liquids as tolerated.
  - **d.** Monitor potassium, sodium, and chloride levels.
- **3.** Stomatitis
  - **a.** Provide and teach the client good oral hygiene, including avoidance of commercial mouthwashes.
  - **b.** Rinse with viscous lidocaine before meals to provide an analgesic effect.
  - **c.** Perform a cleansing rinse with plain water or dilute a water-soluble lubricant such as hydrogen peroxide after meals.
  - **d.** Apply water-soluble lubricant such as K-Y jelly to lubricate cracked lips.
  - **e.** Advise client to suck on Popsicles to provide moisture.

B. Hematologic System
- **1.** Thrombocytopenia
  - **a.** Teach client the importance of avoiding bumping or bruising the skin.
  - **b.** Protect client from physical injury.

   c. Avoid aspirin or aspirin products.
   d. Avoid giving IM injections.
   e. Monitor blood counts carefully.
   f. Assess for and teach signs of increased bleeding tendencies (epistaxis, petechiae, ecchymoses).
2. Leukopenia
   a. Use careful handwashing technique.
   b. Maintain reverse isolation if white blood cell count drops below $1000/mm^3$.
   c. Assess for signs of respiratory infection.
   d. Instruct client to avoid crowds/persons with known infection.
3. Anemia
   a. Provide for dequate rest periods.
   b. Monitor hemoglobin and hematocrit.
   c. Protect client from injury.
   d. Administer oxygen as necessary.

C. Integumentary System—Alopecia
1. Explain that hair loss is not permanent.
2. Offer support and encouragement.
3. Scalp tourniquets or scalp hypothermia via ice pack may be ordered to minimize hair loss with some agents.
4. Advise client to obtain a wig before initiating treatments.

D. Renal System
1. May cause direct damage to kidney by excretion of metabolites; encourage fluids and frequent voiding to prevent accumulation of metabolites in bladder.
2. Increased excretion of uric acid may damage kidneys.
3. Administer allopurinol (Zyloprim) as ordered to prevent uric acid formation; encourage fluids when administering allopurinol.

E. Reproductive System
1. Damage may occur to both men and women resulting in infertility and/or mutagenic damage to chromosomes.
2. Banking sperm often recommended for men before chemotherapy.
3. Clients and partners advised to use reliable methods of contraception during chemotherapy.

F. Neurologic System
1. Plant alkaloids (vincristine) cause neurologic damage with repeated doses.
2. Peripheral neuropathies, hearing loss, loss of deep tendon reflexes, and paralytic ileus may occur.

Radiation Therapy

Principles

A. Radiation therapy uses ionizing radiation to kill or limit the growth of cancer cells, may be internal or external.

B. It not only injures the cell membrane, but destroys or alters DNA so that the cells cannot reproduce.

C. Like chemotherapy, effect cannot be limited to cancer cells only; all exposed cells, including normal ones, will be injured, causing side effects discussed below. Localized effects are related to area of body being treated; generalized effects may be related to cellular breakdown products.

D. Types of energy emitted

1. Alpha: particles cannot pass through skin, rarely used
2. Beta: particles cannot pass through skin, somewhat more penetrating than alpha, generally emitted from radioactive isotopes, used for internal source
3. Gamma rays (electromagnetic or X-rays): penetrate deeper areas of body, most common form of external radiotherapy

Methods of Delivery

A. External radiation therapy: beams high-energy rays directly to the affected area.

B. Internal radiation therapy: radioactive material is injected or implanted in the client's body for a designated period of time.

1. Sealed implants: a radioisotope enclosed in a container so it does not circulate in the body; client's body fluids should not become contaminated with radiation.
2. Unsealed sources: a radioisotope that is not encased in a container and does circulate in the body and contaminate body fluids.

Factors Controlling Exposure

A. Half-life: time required for half of radioactive atoms to decay

1. Each radioisotope has a different half-life.
2. At the end of the half-life, the danger from exposure decreases.

B. Time: the shorter the duration, the less the exposure

C. Distance: the greater the distance from the radiation source the less the exposure

D. Shielding: all radiation can be blocked; rubber gloves stop alpha and usually beta rays; thick lead or concrete stops gamma rays

E. These factors affect health care worker's exposure as well as client's.

1. Health care worker at greater risk from internal than external sources
2. Film badge can measure the amount of exposure received
3. No pregnant nurses or visitors permitted near radiation source

Side Effects of Radiation Therapy and Nursing Interventions

A. Skin: itching, redness, burning, oozing, sloughing

1. Keep skin free from foreign substances.
2. Avoid use of medicated solutions, ointments, or powders that contain heavy metals such as zinc oxide.
3. Avoid pressure, trauma, infection to skin; use bed cradle.

NURSING ALERT

If the client is receiving internal radiation, excreted body fluids may be radioactive; double flush toilets after use.

CLIENT TEACHING CHECKLIST

In case of thrombocytopenia

- Monitor excreted stool and fluids for bleeding.
- Use an electric razor only for shaving.
- Avoid contact sports.
- Avoid aspirin and aspirin-containing products.
- Use soft toothbrushes and don't floss.

4. Wash affected areas with plain water and pat dry; avoid soap.
5. Use cornstarch, olive oil for itching; avoid talcum powder.
6. If sloughing occurs, use a sterile dressing with micropore tape.
7. Teach client to avoid exposing skin to heat, cold, or sunlight and to avoid constricting or irritating clothing.

B. Anorexia, nausea, and vomiting
1. Arrange mealtimes so they do not directly precede or follow therapy.
2. Encourage bland foods.
3. Provide small, attractive meals.
4. Avoid extremes of temperature.
5. Administer antiemetics as ordered before meals.

C. Diarrhea
1. Encourage low-residue, bland, high-protein foods.
2. Administer antidiarrheal drugs as ordered.
3. Provide good perineal care.
4. Monitor electrolytes, particularly sodium, potassium, and chloride.

D. Anemia, leukopenia, and thrombocytopenia
1. Isolate from those with known infections.
2. Provide frequent rest periods.
3. Encourage high-protein diet.
4. Instruct client to avoid injury.
5. Assess for bleeding.
6. Monitor CBC, leukocytes, and platelets.

Bone Marrow Transplant

A. General information
- **1.** Treatment alternative for a variety of diseases
  - **a.** Malignancies including several types of leukemias
  - **b.** Blood disorders including severe aplastic anemia, thalassemia
  - **c.** Solid tumors such as breast cancer and brain tumors; treatment for these diseases frequently causes bone marrow destruction; autologous bone marrow transplant may be indicated (Bone marrow harvested before chemotherapy or radiation destroys it and infused after therapy completed)
  - **d.** Other conditions including malignant infantile osteopetrosis, some inherited metabolic disorders
- **2.** Types
  - **a.** Autologous: client transplant with own harvested marrow
  - **b.** Syngeneic: transplant between identical twins
  - **c.** Allogeneic: transplant from a genetically nonidentical donor
    - **1)** most common transplant type
    - **2)** sibling most common donor
- **3.** Procedure
  - **a.** Donor suitability determined through tissue antigen typing; includes human leukocyte antigen (HLA) and mixed leukocyte culture (MLC) typing.
  - **b.** Donor bone marrow is aspirated from multiple sites along the iliac crests under general anesthesia.
  - **c.** Donor marrow is infused IV into the recipient.
- **4.** Early evidence of engraftment seen during the second week post-transplant; hematologic reconstitution takes 4–6 weeks; immunologic reconstitution takes months.
- **5.** Hospitalization of 2 or 3 months required.
- **6.** Prognosis is highly variable depending on indication for use.

B. Complications
- **1.** Failure of engraftment
- **2.** Infection: highest risk in first 3–4 weeks
- **3.** Pneumonia: nonbacterial or interstitial pneumonias are principal cause of death during first 3 months post-transplant
- **4.** *Graft vs. host disease (GVHD):* principal complication; caused by an immunologic reaction of engrafted lymphoid cells against the tissues of the recipient
  - **a.** Acute GVHD: develops within first 100 days post-transplant and affects skin, gut, liver, marrow, and lymphoid tissue
  - **b.** Chronic GVHD: develops 100–400 days post-transplant; manifested by multiorgan involvement
- **5.** Recurrent malignancy
- **6.** Late complications such as cataracts, endocrine abnormalities

C. Nursing care: pretransplant
   1. Recipient immunosuppression attained with total body irradiation (TBI) and chemotherapy to eradicate existing disease and create space in host marrow to allow transplanted cells to grow.
   2. Provide protected environment
      a. Client should be in a laminar airflow room or on strict reverse isolation; surveillance cultures done twice a week.
      b. Objects must be sterilized before being brought into the room.
      c. When working with children introduce new people where they can be seen, but outside child's room so child can see what they look like without isolation garb.
   3. Monitor central lines frequently; check patency and observe for signs of infection (fever, redness around site).
   4. Provide care for the client receiving chemotherapy and radiation therapy to induce immunosuppression.
      a. Administer chemotherapy as ordered, assist with radiation therapy if required.
      b. Monitor side effects and keep client as comfortable as possible.
      c. Monitor carefully for potential infection.
      d. Client will become very ill; prepare client and family.

D. Nursing care: post-transplant
   1. Prevent infection.
      a. Maintain protective environment.
      b. Administer antibiotics as ordered.
      c. Assess all mucous membranes, wounds, catheter sites for swelling, redness, tenderness, pain.
      d. Monitor vital signs frequently (every 1–4 hours as needed).
      e. Collect specimens for cultures as needed and twice a week.
      f. Change IV set-ups every 24 hours.
   2. Provide mouth care for stomatitis and mucositis (severe mucositis develops about 5 days after irradiation).
      a. Note tissue sloughing, bleeding, changes in color.
      b. Provide mouth rinses, viscous lidocaine, and antibiotic rinses.
      c. Do not use lemon and glycerin swabs.
      d. Administer parenteral narcotics as ordered if necessary to control pain.
      e. Provide care every 2 hours or as needed.
   3. Provide skin care: skin breakdown may result from profuse diarrhea from the TBI.
   4. Monitor carefully for bleeding.
      a. Check for occult blood in emesis and stools.
      b. Observe for easy bruising, petechiae on skin, mucous membranes.
      c. Monitor changes in vital signs.
      d. Check platelet count daily.
      e. Replace blood products as ordered (all blood products should be irradiated).

DELEGATION TIP

Instruct assistive personnel regarding the importance of recording accurate I&O and daily weight to assess hydration and promote nutrition.

5. Maintain fluid and electrolyte balance and promote nutrition.
   a. Measure I&O carefully.
   b. Provide adequate fluid, protein, and caloric intake.
   c. Weigh daily.
   d. Administer fluid replacement as ordered.
   e. Monitor hydration status: check skin turgor, moisture of mucous membranes, urine output.
   f. Check electrolytes daily.
   g. Check urine for glucose, ketones, protein.
   h. Administer antidiarrheal agents as needed.
6. Provide client teaching and discharge planning concerning
   a. Home environment (e.g., cleaning, pets, visitors)
   b. Diet modifications
   c. Medication regimen: schedule, dosages, effects, and side effects
   d. Communicable diseases and immunizations
   e. Daily hygiene and skin care
   f. Fever
   g. Activity

REVIEW QUESTIONS

1. A woman is undergoing chemotherapy treatment for uterine cancer. She asks the nurse how chemotherapeutic drugs work. The most accurate explanation would include which statement?
   1. They affect all rapidly dividing cells.
   2. Molecular structure of the DNA segment is altered.
   3. Chemotherapy stimulates cancer cells to divide.
   4. The cancer cells are sensitive to drug toxins.
2. An adult experiences severe vomiting from cancer chemotherapy drugs. Which acid-base imbalance should the nurse anticipate?
   1. Ketoacidosis.
   2. Metabolic acidosis.

3. Metabolic alkalosis.
4. Respiratory alkalosis.

3. A woman loses most of her hair as a result of cancer chemotherapy. The nurse understands that which of the following is true about chemotherapy-induced alopecia?
   1. New hair will be gray.
   2. Avoid the use of wigs.
   3. The hair loss is temporary.
   4. Pre-chemo hair texture will return.

4. An adult is diagnosed with Hodgkin's disease Stage 1A. He is being treated with radiation therapy. To minimize skin damage from radiation therapy, the nursing care plan should include which of the following?
   1. Avoid washing with water.
   2. Apply a heating pad to the site.
   3. Cover the area with an airtight dressing.
   4. Avoid applying creams and powders to the area.

5. An adult develops a second-degree or second-level skin reaction from radiation therapy. When evaluating his symptoms, the nurse can expect to find all of the following except
   1. scaly skin.
   2. an itchy feeling.
   3. dry desquamation.
   4. reddening of the skin.

6. An adult client is receiving radiation therapy. The nurse is teaching the client about signs of radiation-induced thrombocytopenia, which include
   1. fatigue.
   2. shortness of breath.
   3. elevated temperature.
   4. a tendency to bruise easily.

7. The nurse is caring for a client who is receiving radiation therapy. Which activity by the client indicates he does NOT understand the side effects of radiation therapy?
   1. Using an electric razor.
   2. Eating a high-protein diet.
   3. Taking his children to see Santa at the mall.
   4. Calling the doctor for a temperature of 101°F (38.3°C).

8. A man says to the nurse, "I don't understand how my wife could have come down with cancer. She doesn't smoke or drink. How do people get cancer?" Which of the following should be included in the nurse's response? Select the one or all that apply.

   ______ Bacteria.

   ______ Viruses.

   ______ Dietary factors.

   ______ Genetic factors.

9. A woman has breast cancer. Her physician has just told her that her cancer has been staged as "T2, N1, M0," and the client asks the nurse what this means. The nurse's answer is based on the understanding that

   1. the primary tumor is 2 cm in diameter, she has one positive lymph node, and no metastasis.
   2. there are two primary tumors, one involved lymph node chain, and no metastasis.
   3. the primary tumor is between 2 cm and 5 cm in size, she has metastasis to one movable lymph node, and no distant metastasis.
   4. there is carcinoma in situ, no regional lymph node metastasis, and the presence of distant metastasis cannot be assessed.

10. The nurse at a senior citizen center is teaching a class on the early warning signals of cancer. Which of the following will be a part of the teaching plan for this class?

    1. Reduction in the amount of dietary fat.
    2. Stop cigarette smoking.
    3. Avoid overexposure to the sun.
    4. Practice monthly breast self-exam (BSE).

11. Which statement tells the nurse that a man needs further information about testicular self-examination (TSE)?

    1. "The best time to perform TSE is immediately before sexual intercourse."
    2. "It's normal to find one testis lower than the other."
    3. "I should have my doctor examine any lumps I find, even though they might be benign."
    4. "That cord-like thing that I feel on the top and back of the testicle is not something to be worried about."

12. Which of the following actions is vital for the nurse to perform when assessing a client receiving chemotherapy?

1. Checking complete vital signs every 8 hours.
2. Taking rectal temperatures every 4 hours to check for infection.
3. Testing emesis for blood.
4. Avoiding fresh fruits and vegetables if absolute white blood count (WBC) is less than 1000/mm^3.

13. An adult asks the nurse how the chemotherapy that she is receiving for her lung cancer works. The nurse's best response is based on the knowledge that chemotherapeutic drugs
    1. block the sodium-potassium pump in the cell wall and cause cellular death due to an excess of intracellular potassium.
    2. prevent the entry of oxygen into the cell and cause cellular death due to cellular anoxia.
    3. shrink the size of the existing tumor, which causes the release of antitumor metabolites that are toxic to further tumor cell growth.
    4. destroy enough of the tumor so that the body's immune system can eradicate the remaining cells.
14. An adult, diagnosed with multiple myeloma, is receiving cyclophosphamide (Cytoxan). The nurse must include which of the following interventions in the nursing care plan of this client?
    1. High-flow oxygen delivery to combat interstitial pneumonitis, which routinely develops with cyclophosphamide therapy.
    2. Encouraging the client to empty his bladder every 2 to 3 hours to prevent development of hemorrhagic cystitis.
    3. Application of an ice cap to reduce or prevent alopecia.
    4. Antiemetic therapy for 7–10 days after cyclophosphamide administration, or until blood studies show nadir is reached.
15. An adult is receiving cancer chemotherapy and demonstrates alteration in her oral mucous membranes. Which of the following should be included in her plan of care?
    1. Brushing teeth and flossing after every meal and at bedtime.
    2. Using normal saline mouth rinses every 2 hours while awake.
    3. No use of dentures until mucous membranes have healed.
    4. Bland, mechanical, soft diet until mucous membranes have healed.
16. Ten days ago, a client received chemotherapy for his non-Hodgkin's lymphoma, stage IV. Drugs administered through his vascular access device ("Port-a-cath") included doxorubicin, cyclophosphamide, vincristine, and prednisone (CHOP protocol). This morning, his blood work is as follows: WBC: 1500/mm^3; hemoglobin (Hgb): 7.6 gm/dl; RBC

3,000,000/mm^3; hematocrit (Hct) 22.3%; platelets 20,000/mm^3. The nurse knows that the client's plan of care will include which of the following interventions?

1. Insertion of two extra IV lines for blood administration.
2. Cutting fingernails and toenails to prevent scratching that could lead to bleeding or infection.
3. Providing the client with a low residue diet.
4. Using a soft toothbrush and avoiding dental floss.

17. An adult who is receiving external radiation therapy for Hodgkin's disease makes all of the following statements to her nurse. Which statement tells the nurse that the client needs further teaching about the care she requires because of her radiation therapy?

1. "I will check my mouth frequently for signs of irritation."
2. "I know that if I get tired easily, it may be from the radiation and doesn't necessarily mean my Hodgkin's disease is getting worse."
3. "I will use a good quality lotion on my skin to keep the radiation from burning it."
4. "I may lose some of my hair during radiation and foods may not taste right."

18. A client asks the nurse to explain how the radiation therapy she will be receiving for her neck cancer is effective. The nurse's best response is based on the knowledge that

1. radiation causes breakage in the strands of the DNA helix, which leads to cell death.
2. radiation is antagonistic to glucose, which cells need for energy and replication; radiation prevents glucose from entering cells, leading to cell death.
3. cell walls are broken down by gamma rays during radiation therapy, leading to cell death.
4. oxygen cannot enter cells that have been irradiated, so the cell converts to anaerobic metabolism that causes its death.

19. The nurse manager on the oncology unit is assessing the knowledge level of the staff in regard to safety requirements for the client receiving internal radiation therapy. Which observation by the nurse manager indicates that further instruction is necessary?

1. The physical therapist is ambulating the client in the hall.
2. The nurse uses rubber gloves when emptying the bedpan.
3. The dietitian provides a low residue diet for the client.

4. The housekeeping staff calls for Radiation Safety personnel to inspect the room before the client is discharged.

20. A woman is receiving internal radiation therapy for cancer of the cervix. Which statement indicates to the nurse that the client understands precautions necessary during her treatment?

1. "I should get out of bed and walk around in my room at least every other hour."
2. "My seven-year-old twins should not come to visit me while I'm receiving treatment."
3. "I will try not to cough, because the force might make me expel the applicator."
4. "I know that my primary nurse has to wear one of those badges like the people in the X-ray department wear, but they aren't necessary for anyone else who comes in here."

21. An adult is receiving internal radiation therapy for cancer of the cervix. Her radiation source, a rod, becomes dislodged. The nurse's best first action is to

1. notify the Radiation Safety personnel at once and wait further information.
2. use long-handled forceps to remove the rod and place in a lead-lined container.
3. apply two sets of rubber gloves and pick up the rod; place it in a white plastic "biohazard" bucket and call Radiation Safety personnel for a special pick-up.
4. use long-handled forceps to pick up rod; clean with normal saline, and reinsert into client's vagina, stopping when the rod meets resistance. This indicates that it is against the cervix.

22. In caring for the client receiving external radiation therapy, the nurse assesses for which of the following side effects?

1. Extravasation injury at the IV site used for contrast media injection.
2. Generalized or local edema.
3. Infection and bleeding.
4. Allergic reactions, particularly anaphylaxis.

ANSWERS AND RATIONALES

1. 1. There are numerous mechanisms of action for cancer chemotherapeutic drugs, but most affect rapidly dividing cells. The drugs interfere with cell division and prevent rapid division of cells.

2. 3. Severe vomiting results in a loss of hydrochloric acid and acids from extracellular fluids, leading to metabolic alkalosis.

3. 3. Alopecia from chemotherapy is only temporary.

4. 4. Creams and powders, many of which contain heavy metals, will further irritate skin sensitized by radiation therapy and reduce the effectiveness of therapy by blocking radiation.

5. 4. Reddening of the skin will not be seen in a second-level or second-degree reaction. A second-degree skin reaction would be evidenced by scaly skin, an itchy feeling, and dry desquamation.

6. 4. Clients with decreased platelet count (thrombocytopenia) bleed easily. Thrombocytes are clotting cells.

7. 3. People being treated with radiation therapy should avoid crowds because of the increased risk of infection. Crowds at Christmastime can be very large and children are frequent carriers of infection.

8. Bacteria should be marked. *Helicobacter pylori*, which causes stomach ulcers, has been linked to stomach cancer.

Viruses should be marked. Viruses are thought to insinuate themselves into the genetic structure of cells, thereby altering future generations of that cell. Epstein-Barr is strongly implicated in the development of Burkitt's lymphoma. Some types of human papilloma virus, which causes genital warts, cause cancer of the cervix.

Dietary factors should be marked. Approximately 40–60% of all environmental cancers are thought to have links to dietary factors such as fats, alcohol, foods containing nitrates/nitrites, and salt-cured and smoked meats.

Genetic factors should be marked. Genetics are involved in cancer cell development. Damage to the DNA in certain populations of cells may lead to mutant cells being transmitted to future generations. Examples of cancers associated with familial inheritance include breast, colon, and rectal cancers.

9. 3. In the TNM staging classification system, T refers to the primary tumor, and T2 is between 2 cm and 5 cm without extension to chest wall or skin. The N refers to regional lymph node involvement, with N1 indicating spread to an ipsilateral movable node. N0 indicates no regional lymph node spread; N2 indicates metastasis to an ipsilateral axillary node fixed to another node or other structure. M refers to distant metastasis, with MX indicating that metastasis cannot be assessed, M0 that there is no distant spread, and M1 that there is spread present.

10. 4. Only this answer, practicing breast self-exam, will yield a "warning signal of cancer" (i.e., a breast lump). Be certain that your response answers the question, not just that it contains factual information.

11. 1. The man is mistaken (and needs more teaching) if he says that testicular self-exam should be performed immediately prior to sexual intercourse. The best time to do TSE is when the scrotum is relaxed, such as after a warm bath or shower.

12. 3. Because of the bleeding disorders common in clients receiving chemotherapy, all body secretions, including emesis, should be assessed for obvious and occult blood.

13. 4. Each time the tumor is exposed to the chemotherapeutic drug, a certain percentage of cells are killed. (The exact percentage is determined by the drug dosage used.) Because a percentage of tumor is killed, a part of tumor will remain (there is no percentage—except for zero—which yields zero) after therapy. It is up to the body's immune system to destroy the remaining tumor, which an intact immune system may be able to do if the tumor is made small enough.

14. 2. If the metabolites of cyclophosphamide are allowed to accumulate in the bladder, the subsequent irritation of the bladder wall capillaries will cause hemorrhagic cystitis. This condition is preventable; if it develops, one of its serious sequelae is bladder fibrosis. In addition to monitoring BUN and creatinine prior to administration, the nurse must promote hydration of at least 3 liters a day and frequent voiding.

15. 2. The client will use normal saline mouth rinses every 2 hours while awake and every 6 hours at night to aid in the removal of thick secretions, debris, and bacteria.

16. 4. By using a soft toothbrush and avoiding dental floss, the client promotes a healthy oral cavity without risking bleeding or disruption of skin integrity, which could lead to infection.

17. 3. It is important to protect skin from irritation, and lotions, creams, powders, and ointments can all contribute to skin problems. Clients are advised to consult their radiation oncologists for troublesome skin problems and should be advised that after treatment, reepithelialization will occur.

18. 1. There are two types of ionizing radiation: electromagnetic rays and particulate radiation. Either of these can cause tissue disruption, the most harmful of which is the alteration in the structure of the cell's DNA molecules; this will lead to cell death.

19. 1. The client will be restricted to her room to minimize exposure of staff, visitors, and other clients to the radiation source.

20. 2. Visitors younger than 18 years of age, and pregnant visitors, are not allowed during internal radiation therapy.

21. 2. Long-handled forceps and a lead-lined container (sometimes called a "lead pig") must be kept in the room of any client receiving internal radiation therapy for this very occurrence.

22. 3. If bone marrow-producing sites are included in the field being irradiated, anemia, leukopenia (low white blood cells), and thrombocytopenia (low platelets) may occur; these may lead to infection and/or bleeding.

5

The Neurosensory System

■ OVERVIEW OF ANATOMY AND PHYSIOLOGY

The Nervous System

The functional unit of the nervous system is the nerve cell, or neuron. The nervous system consists of the central nervous system (CNS), which includes the brain and spinal cord, and the peripheral nervous system (PNS), which includes the cranial nerves and the spinal nerves. The autonomic nervous system (ANS) is a subdivision of the PNS that automatically controls body functions such as breathing and heartbeat. It is further divided into the sympathetic and parasympathetic nervous systems. The special senses of vision and hearing are also covered in this section.

CHAPTER OUTLINE

Neuron

A. Primary component of the nervous system; composed of cell body (gray matter), axon, and dendrites

B. *Axon:* elongated process or fiber extending from the cell body; transmits impulses (messages) away from the cell body to dendrites or directly to the cell bodies of other neurons; neuron usually has only one axon.

C. *Dendrites:* short, branching fibers that receive impulses and conduct them toward the nerve cell body. Neurons may have many dendrites.

D. *Synapse:* junction between neurons where an impulse is transmitted

E. *Neurotransmitters:* chemical agents (e.g., acetylcholine, norepinephrine) involved in the transmission of impulse across synapse

F. *Myelin sheath:* a wrapping of myelin (a whitish, fatty material) that protects and insulates nerve fibers and enhances the speed of impulse conduction

1. Both axons and dendrites may or may not have a myelin sheath (myelinated/unmyelinated)
2. Most axons leaving the CNS are heavily myelinated by *Schwann cells*

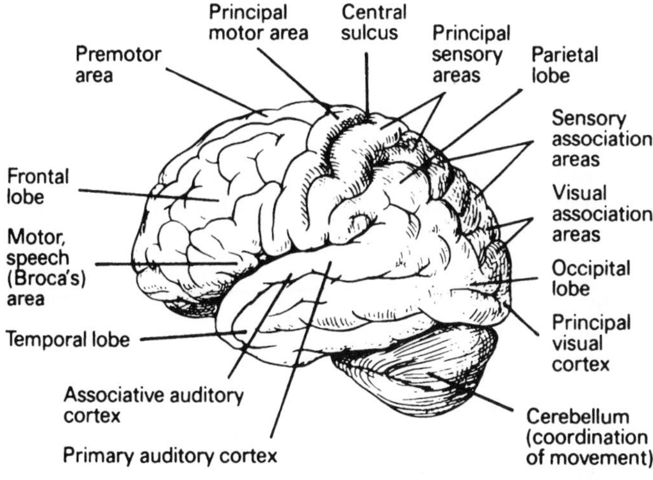

FIGURE 5-1 Side view of the brain, showing principal functional areas

Functional Classification

A. *Afferent (sensory) neurons:* transmit impulses from peripheral receptors to the CNS

B. *Efferent (motor) neurons:* conduct impulses from CNS to muscles and glands

C. *Internuncial neurons (interneurons):* connecting links between afferent and efferent neurons

Central Nervous System: Brain and Spinal Cord

Brain

A. *Cerebrum:* outermost area (cerebral cortex) is gray matter; deeper area is composed of white matter

  1. Two hemispheres: right and left

  2. Each hemisphere divided into four lobes; many of the functional areas of the cerebrum have been located in these lobes (see Figure 5-1).

    a. *Frontal lobe*

      1) personality, behavior

      2) higher intellectual functioning

      3) precentral gyrus: motor function

      4) Broca's area: specialized motor speech area

    b. *Parietal lobe*

      1) postcentral gyrus: registers general sensation (e.g., touch, pressure)

      2) integrates sensory information

    c. *Temporal lobe*

      1) hearing, taste, smell

2) Wernicke's area: sensory speech area (understanding/formulation of language)

d. *Occipital lobe:* vision

3. *Corpus callosum:* large fiber tract that connects the two cerebral hemispheres
4. *Basal ganglia:* islands of gray matter within white matter of cerebrum
   a. Regulate and integrate motor activity originating in the cerebral cortex
   b. Part of extrapyramidal system

B. *Diencephalon:* connecting part of the brain, between the cerebrum and the brain stem.Contains several small structures; the thalamus and hypothalamus are most important.

1. *Thalamus*
   a. Relay station for discrimination of sensory signals (e.g., pain, temperature, touch).
   b. Controls primitive emotional responses (e.g., rage, fear).
2. *Hypothalamus*
   a. Found immediately beneath the thalamus.
   b. Plays major role in regulation of vital functions such as blood pressure, sleep, food and water intake, and body temperature.
   c. Acts as control center for pituitary gland and affects both divisions of the autonomic nervous system.

C. *Brain stem*

1. Contains midbrain, pons, and medulla oblongata.
2. Extends from the cerebral hemispheres to the foramen magnum at the base of the skull.
3. Contains nuclei of the cranial nerves and the long ascending and descending tracts connecting the cerebrum and the spinal cord.
4. Contains vital centers of respiratory, vasomotor, and cardiac functions.

D. *Cerebellum:* coordinates muscle tone and movements and maintains position in space (equilibrium).

Spinal Cord

A. Serves as a connecting link between the brain and the periphery.

B. Extends from foramen magnum to second lumbar vertebra.

C. H-shaped gray matter in the center (cell bodies) surrounded by white matter (nerve tracts and fibers).

D. *Gray matter*

1. Anterior horns: contain cell bodies giving rise to efferent (motor) fibers
2. Posterior horns: contain cell bodies connecting with afferent (sensory) fibers from dorsal root ganglion
3. Lateral horns: in thoracic region, contain cells giving rise to autonomic fibers of sympathetic nervous system

E. *White matter*
  1. Ascending tracts (sensory pathways)
    a. Posterior columns: carry impulses concerned with touch, pressure, vibration, and position sense.
    b. Spinocerebellar: carry impulses concerned with muscle tension and position sense to cerebellum.
    c. Lateral spinothalamic: carry impulses resulting in pain and temperature sensations.
    d. Anterior spinothalamic: carry impulses concerned with crude touch and pressure.
  2. Descending tracts (motor pathways)
    a. Corticospinal (pyramidal, upper motor neuron): conduct motor impulses from motor cortex to anterior horn cells (cross in the medulla).
    b. Extrapyramidal: help to maintain muscle tone and to control body movement, especially gross automatic movements such as walking.

F. *Reflex arc*
  1. Reflex consists of an involuntary response to a stimulus occurring over a neural pathway called a reflex arc.
  2. Not relayed to and from brain; takes place at cord levels.
  3. Components
    a. Sensory receptor: receives/reacts to a stimulus.
    b. Afferent pathway: transmits impulses to spinal cord.
    c. Interneuron: synapses with a motor neuron (anterior horn cell).
    d. Efferent pathway: transmits impulses from motor neuron to effector.
    e. Effector: muscle or organ that responds to stimulus.

Supporting Structures

A. Skull
  1. Rigid; numerous bones fused together.
  2. Protects and supports the brain.

B. Spinal column
  1. Consists of 7 cervical, 12 thoracic, and 5 lumbar vertebrae, as well as sacrum and coccyx.
  2. Supports the head and protects the spinal cord.

C. Meninges
  1. Membranes between the skull and brain and the vertebral column and spinal cord.
  2. Layers
    a. *Dura mater:* outermost layer, tough, leathery
    b. *Arachnoid mater:* middle layer, weblike
    c. *Pia mater:* innermost layer, delicate, clings to surface of brain
  3. Area between arachnoid and pia mater is called *subarachnoid space.*

D. Ventricles
   1. Four fluid-filled cavities connecting with one another and the spinal canal.
   2. Produce and circulate cerebrospinal fluid.
E. *Cerebrospinal fluid (CSF)*
   1. Surrounds brain and spinal cord.
   2. Offers protection by functioning as a shock absorber.
   3. Allows fluid shifts from the cranial cavity to the spinal cavity.
   4. Carries nutrients to and waste products away from nerve cells.
F. Vascular supply
   1. Two *internal carotid arteries* **anteriorly**
   2. Two *vertebral arteries* **leading to basilar artery posteriorly**
   3. These arteries communicate at the base of the brain through the *circle of Willis.*
   4. Anterior, middle, and posterior cerebral arteries are the main arteries for distributing blood to each hemisphere of the brain.
   5. Brain stem and cerebellum are supplied by branches of the vertebral and basilar arteries.
   6. Venous blood drains into dural sinuses and then into internal jugular veins.
G. *Blood-brain barrier:* protective barrier preventing harmful agents from entering the capillaries of the CNS; protects brain and spinal cord.

Peripheral Nervous System

Spinal Nerves

A. 31 pairs: carry impulses to and from spinal cord.
B. Each segment of the spinal cord contains a pair of spinal nerves (one for each side of the body).
C. Each nerve is attached to the spinal cord by two roots.
   1. Dorsal (posterior) root: contains afferent (sensory) nerve whose cell body is in the dorsal root ganglion.
   2. Ventral (anterior) root: contains efferent (motor) nerve whose nerve fibers originate in the anterior horn cell of the spinal cord (lower motor neuron).

Cranial Nerves

A. 12 pairs: carry impulses to and from brain (see Table 5-1).
B. May have sensory, motor, or mixed functions.

Autonomic Nervous System

A. Part of the peripheral nervous system
B. Includes those peripheral nerves (both cranial and spinal) that regulate functions occurring automatically in the body; ANS regulates smooth muscle, cardiac muscle, and glands.

TABLE 5-1 Cranial Nerves

Name and Number	Function
Olfactory: cranial nerve I	Sensory: carries impulses for sense of smell
Optic: cranial nerve II	Sensory: carries impulses for vision
Oculomotor: cranial nerve III	Motor: muscles for pupillary constriction, elevation of upper eyelid; 4 out of 6 extraocular movements
Trochlear: cranial nerve IV	Motor: muscles for downward, inward movement of eye
Trigeminal: cranial nerve V	Mixed: impulses from face, surface of eyes (corneal reflex); muscles controlling mastication
Abducens: cranial nerve VI	Motor: muscles for lateral deviation of eye
Facial: cranial nerve VII	Mixed: impulses for taste from anterior tongue; muscles for facial movement
Acoustic: cranial nerve VIII	Sensory: impulses for hearing (cochlear division) and balance (vestibular division)
Glossopharyngeal: cranial nerve IX	Mixed: impulses for sensation to posterior tongue and pharynx; muscles for movement of pharynx (elevation) and swallowing
Vagus: cranial nerve X	Mixed: impulses for sensation to lower pharynx and larynx; muscles for movement of soft palate, pharynx, and larynx
Spinal accessory: cranial nerve XI	Motor: movement of sternomastoid muscles and upper part of trapezius muscles
Hypoglossal: cranial nerve XII	Motor: movement of tongue

C. Components
   1. *Sympathetic nervous system:* generally accelerates some body functions in response to stress
   2. *Parasympathetic nervous system:* controls normal body functioning
D. Effects of ANS activity: see Table 5-2.

Vision

External Structures of Eye

A. Eyelids (palpebrae) and eyelashes: protect the eye from foreign particles
B. *Conjunctiva*
   1. Palpebral conjunctiva: pink; lines inner surface of eyelids.
   2. Bulbar conjunctiva: white with small blood vessels, covers anterior sclera.
C. *Lacrimal apparatus* (lacrimal gland and its ducts and passages): produces tears to lubricate the eye and moisten the cornea; tears drain into the nasolacrimal duct, which empties into nasal cavity.
D. Movement of the eye is controlled by six extraocular muscles.

Internal Structures of Eye

A. Three layers of the eyeball
   1. Outer layer
      a. *Sclera:* tough, white connective tissue (''white of the eye''); located anteriorly and posteriorly
      b. *Cornea:* transparent tissue through which light enters the eye; located anteriorly
   2. Middle layer
      a. *Choroid:* highly vascular layer, nourishes retina; located posteriorly
      b. *Ciliary body:* anterior to choroid, secretes aqueous humor; muscles change shape of lens
      c. *Iris:* pigmented membrane behind cornea, gives color to eye; located anteriorly. ***Pupil*** **is a circular opening in the middle of the iris that constricts or dilates to regulate amount of light entering eye.**
   3. Inner layer: *retina*
      a. Light-sensitive layer composed of rods and cones (visual cells)
         1) Cones: specialized for fine discrimination and color vision
         2) Rods: more sensitive to light than cones, aid in peripheral vision
      b. *Optic disk:* area in retina for entrance of optic nerve, has no photoreceptors
B. *Lens:* transparent body that focuses image on retina
C. Fluids of the eye
   1. *Aqueous humor:* clear, watery fluid in anterior and posterior chambers in anterior part of eye; serves as refracting medium and provides nutrients to lens and cornea; contributes to maintenance of intraocular pressure.

TABLE 5-2 Effects of Autonomic Nervous System Activity

Effector	Sympathetic (Adrenergic) Effects	Parasympathetic (Cholinergic) Effects
Eye	Dilates pupil (mydriasis)	Constricts pupil (miosis)
Glands of head		
Lacrimal	No effect	Stimulates secretion
Salivary	Scanty thick, viscous secretions; dry mouth	Copious thin, watery secretions
Heart	Increases rate and force of contraction	Decreases rate
Blood vessels	Constricts smooth muscles of skin, abdominal blood vessels, and cutaneous blood vessels Dilates smooth muscle of bronchioles, blood vessels of heart, and skeletal muscles	No effect
Lungs	Bronchodilation	Bronchoconstriction
GI tract	Decreases motility Constricts sphincters Possibly inhibits secretions Inhibits activity of gallbladder and ducts Inhibits glycogenolysis in liver	Increases motility Relaxes sphincters Stimulates secretion Stimulates activity of gallbladder and ducts
Adrenal gland	Stimulates secretion of epinephrine and norepinephrine	No effects
Urinary tract	Relaxes detrusor muscle Contracts trigone sphincter (prevents voiding)	Contracts detrusor muscle Relaxes trigone sphincter (allows voiding)

2. *Vitreous humor:* clear, gelatinous material that fills posterior cavity of eye; maintains transparency and form of eye.

Visual Pathways

A. Retina (rods and cones) translates light waves into neural impulses that travel over the optic nerves.
B. Optic nerves for each eye meet at the optic chiasm.
   1. Fibers from median halves of the retinas cross here and travel to the opposite side of the brain.
   2. Fibers from lateral halves of retinas remain uncrossed.
C. Optic nerves continue from optic chiasm as optic tracts and travel to the cerebrum (occipital lobe), where visual impulses are perceived and interpreted.

Hearing

External Ear

A. Auricle (pinna): outer projection of ear composed of cartilage and covered by skin; collects sound waves.
B. *External auditory canal:* lined with skin; glands secrete cerumen (wax), providing protection; transmits sound waves to tympanic membrane.
C. *Tympanic membrane (eardrum):* at end of external canal; vibrates in response to sound and transmits vibrations to middle ear.

Middle Ear

A. *Ossicles*
   1. 3 small bones: *malleus (hammer)* attached to tympanic membrane, *incus (anvil)*, *stapes (stirrup)*
   2. Ossicles are set in motion by sound waves from tympanic membrane.
   3. Sound waves are conducted by vibration to the footplate of the stapes in the *oval window* (an opening between the middle ear and the inner ear).
B. *Eustachian tube:* connects nasopharynx and middle ear; brings air into middle ear, thus equalizing pressure on both sides of eardrum.

Inner Ear

A. *Cochlea*
   1. Contains *organ of Corti*, **the receptor end-organ for hearing**
   2. Transmits sound waves from the oval window and initiates nerve impulses carried by cranial nerve VIII (acoustic branch) to the brain (temporal lobe of cerebrum).
B. *Vestibular apparatus*
   1. Organ of balance
   2. Composed of three semicircular canals and the utricle.

ASSESSMENT

Health History

Nervous System

A. Presenting problem: symptoms may include behavior changes, memory loss, mood changes, nervousness or anxiety, headache, seizures, syncope, vertigo, loss of consciousness; problems with speech, vision, or smell; motor problems (paralysis, tremor); sensory problems (pain, paresthesias)

B. Lifestyle: drug and alcohol intake, exposure to toxins, recent travel, employment, stressors

C. Use of medications: prescribed and over-the-counter (OTC)

D. Past medical history

1. Perinatal exposure to toxic agents, X-rays; difficult labor and delivery
2. Childhood and adult: history of systemic diseases; seizures; loss of consciousness; head trauma

E. Family history: may uncover diseases with hereditary or congenital background

Eye

A. Presenting problem: symptoms may include blurred vision, decreased vision, or blind spots; pain, redness, excessive tearing; double vision (diplopia); drainage

B. Use of eyeglasses, contact lenses; date of last eye exam

C. Lifestyle: occupation (exposure to fumes, smoke, or eye irritant); use of safety glasses

D. Use of medications: cortisone preparations may contribute to formation of glaucoma and cataracts

E. Past medical history: systemic diseases; previous childhood or adult eye disorders, eye trauma

F. Family history: many eye disorders may be inherited

Ear

A. Presenting problem: symptoms may include hearing loss, tinnitus (ringing in ear), dizziness or vertigo, pain, drainage

B. Lifestyle: occupation (exposure to excessive noise levels), swimming habits

C. Use of medications: ototoxic drugs; aspirin (tinnitus)

D. Past medical history

1. Perinatal: rubella in first trimester of pregnancy
2. Childhood and adult: otitis media, perforated eardrum, measles, mumps, allergies, tonsillectomy, and adenoidectomy

E. Family history: hearing loss in family members

Physical Examination

Nervous System

A. Neurologic examination
   1. Mental status exam (cerebral function); see also Psychiatric-Mental Health Nursing.
      a. General appearance and behavior
      b. Level of consciousness; see Neuro Check.
      c. Intellectual function: memory (recent and remote), attention span, cognitive skills
      d. Emotional status
      e. Thought content
      f. Language/speech
         1) *expressive aphasia:* inability to speak
         2) *receptive aphasia:* inability to understand spoken words
         3) *dysarthria:* difficult speech due to impairment of muscles involved with production of speech
   2. Cranial nerves (see Table 5-1)
   3. Cerebellar function: posture, gait, balance, coordination
   4. Motor function: muscle size, tone, strength; abnormal or involuntary movements
   5. Sensory function: light touch, superficial pain, temperature, vibration, and position sense
   6. Reflexes
      a. Deep tendon: grade from 0 (no response) to 4 (hyperactive); 2 is normal
      b. Superficial
      c. Pathologic: *Babinski's reflex* (dorsiflexion of great toe with fanning of other toes) indicates damage to corticospinal tracts (see Figure 5-2)

B. Neuro check
   1. *Level of consciousness (LOC)*
      a. Orientation to time, place, and person
      b. Speech: clear, garbled, rambling
      c. Ability to follow commands
      d. If client does not respond to verbal stimuli, apply a painful stimulus (e.g., pressure on nailbeds, squeeze trapezius muscle); note response to pain
         1) appropriate: withdrawal, moaning
         2) inappropriate: nonpurposeful
      e. Abnormal posturing (may occur spontaneously or in response to stimulus)
         1) *decorticate posturing:* extension of legs, internal rotation and adduction of arms with flexion of elbows, wrists, and fingers (damage to corticospinal tracts; cerebral hemispheres)

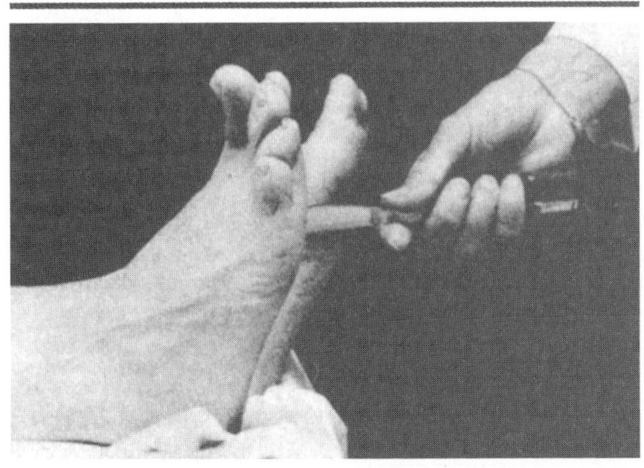

FIGURE 5-2 Pathologic Reflex (Babinski)

2) *decerebrate posturing:* back arched, rigid extension of all four extremities with hyperpronation of arms and plantar flexion of feet (damage to upper brain stem, midbrain, or pons)

2. *Glasgow coma scale* (see Figure 5-3)
   a. Objective evaluation of LOC, motor/verbal response; a standardized system for assessing the degree of neurologic impairment in critically ill clients.
   b. Cannot replace a complete neurologic check, but can be used as an aid in evaluation and to eliminate ambiguous terms such as stupor and lethargy.
   c. A score of 15 indicates client is awake and oriented; the lowest score, 3, is deep coma; a score of 7 or below is considered coma.
3. Pupillary reaction and eye movements
   a. Observe size, shape, and equality of pupils (note size in millimeters)
   b. Reaction to light: pupillary constriction
   c. Corneal reflex: blink reflex in response to light stroking of cornea
   d. Oculocephalic reflex (doll's eyes): present in unconscious client with intact brainstem
4. Motor function
   a. Movement of extremities (paralysis)
   b. Muscle strength
5. Vital signs: respiratory patterns (may help localize possible lesion)
   a. *Cheyne-Stokes respiration:* regular, rhythmic alternating between hyperventilation and apnea; may be caused by structural cerebral dysfunction or by metabolic problems, such as diabetic coma.
   b. *Central neurogenic hyperventilation:* sustained, rapid, regular respirations (rate of 25/minute) with normal blood oxygen levels; usually due to brain stem dysfunction.

Subscale	Response	Score
Best eye opening (E)	Spontaneous	4
	To voice	3
	To pain	2
	None	1
Best verbal response (V)	Oriented	5
	Confused conversation	4
	Inappropriate words	3
	Incomprehensible sounds	2
	None	1
Best motor response, upper limb (M)	Obeys commands	6
	Localizes to pain	5
	Flexor withdrawal (decorticate posturing)	4
	Abnormal flexion (decerebrate posturing)	3
	Extension	2
	Flaccid	1

FIGURE 5-3 Glasgow Coma Scale

c. *Apneustic breathing:* prolonged inspiratory phase, followed by a 2- to 3-second pause; usually indicates dysfunction of respiratory center in pons.
d. *Cluster breathing:* clusters of irregular breathing, irregularly followed by periods of apnea; usually caused by a lesion in upper medulla and lower pons.
e. *Ataxic breathing:* breathing pattern completely irregular; indicates damage to respiratory centers of the medulla.

Eye

A. Visual acuity: Snellen chart
B. Visual fields (peripheral vision)
   1. Confrontation method
   2. Perimetry: more precise method
C. External structures
   1. Position and alignment of eyes
   2. Eyebrows, eyelids, lacrimal apparatus, conjunctiva, sclera, cornea, iris, pupils (size, shape, equality, and reaction to light)
D. Extraocular movements; note paralysis, nystagmus (rapid, abnormal movement of the eyeball)
E. Corneal reflex

Ear

A. Inspection and palpation of auricle, preauricular area, and mastoid area
B. Hearing acuity
  1. Whispered voice or ticking watch tests: gross estimation
  2. Audiometry: more precise method
C. Tuning fork tests distinguish between sensorineural and conductive hearing loss.
  1. Conductive hearing loss: secondary to problem in external or middle ear; transmission of sound waves to inner ear impaired
  2. Sensorineural (perceptive) hearing loss: disease of inner ear or cranial nerve VIII (acoustic branch)
  3. *Weber's test:* handle of vibrating tuning fork placed on midline of client's skull, sound should be heard equally in midline or in both ears; in conductive hearing loss, sound is louder in poorer ear; in sensorineural hearing loss, sound is louder in better ear.
  4. *Rinne's test:* tuning fork placed on mastoid process (bone conduction) until sound no longer heard, then placed in front of the ear (air conduction); sound should be heard longer (almost twice as long) with air conduction than with bone conduction; bone conduction greater than air conduction indicates conductive hearing deficit.

Laboratory/Diagnostic Tests

Nervous System

A. Lumbar puncture (LP)
  1. A hollow spinal needle introduced into subarachnoid space of spinal canal between L_4/L_5 for diagnostic or therapeutic reasons
  2. Purposes
    a. Measures CSF pressure (normal opening pressure 60–150 mm H_2O)
    b. Obtain specimens for lab analysis (protein [normally not present], sugar [normally present], cytology, C&S)
    c. Check color of CSF (normally clear) and check for blood
    d. Inject air, dye, or drugs into the spinal canal
  3. Nursing care: pretest
    a. Have client empty bladder.
    b. Position client in lateral recumbent position with head and neck flexed onto the chest and knees pulled up.
    c. Explain the need to remain still during the procedure.
  4. Nursing care: posttest
    a. Ensure labeling of CSF specimens in proper sequence.
    b. Keep client flat for 12–24 hours as ordered.
    c. Force fluids.
    d. Check puncture site for bleeding, leakage of CSF.
    e. Assess sensation and movement in lower extremities.

f. Monitor vital signs.
g. Administer analgesics for headache as ordered.

B. X-rays of skull and spine
1. Used to detect atrophy, erosion, or fractures of bones; calcifications
2. Pretest nursing care: remove hairpins, glasses, hearing aids.

C. Computerized tomography (CT scan)
1. Skull/spinal cord are scanned in successive layers by a narrow beam of X-rays; computer uses information obtained to construct a picture of the internal structure of the brain; contrast medium may or may not be used.
2. Used to detect intracranial and spinal cord lesions and monitor effects of surgery or other therapy.
3. Nursing care
a. Explain appearance of scanner.
b. Instruct client to lie still during procedure.
c. Check for allergy to iodine if contrast material is used.
d. Remove hairpins, etc.

D. Magnetic resonance imaging (MRI)
1. Also known as nuclear magnetic resonance (NMR)
2. Computer-drawn, detailed pictures of structures of the body through use of large magnet, radio waves
3. Used to detect intracranial and spinal abnormalities associated with disorders such as cerebrovascular disease, tumors, abscesses, cerebral edema, hydrocephalus, multiple sclerosis
4. Nursing care
a. Instruct client to remove jewelry, hairpins, glasses, wigs (with metal clips), and other metallic objects.
b. Be aware that this test cannot be performed on anyone with orthopedic hardware, intrauterine devices, pacemaker, internal surgical clips, or other fixed metallic objects in the body.
c. Inform client of need to remain still while completely enclosed in scanner throughout the procedure, which lasts 45–60 minutes.
d. Teach relaxation techniques to assist client to remain still and to help prevent claustrophobia.
e. Warn client of normal audible humming and thumping noises from the scanner during test.
f. Have client void before test.
g. Sedate client if ordered.

E. Brain scan
1. Injection of radioactive isotope, followed by scanning of head; isotopes will accumulate in abnormal lesions and be recorded by the scanner.
2. Used to detect intracranial masses, vascular lesions, infarcts, hemorrhage
3. Nursing care: check for allergy to iodine.

F. Myelography

G. Cerebral angiography

1. Injection of radiopaque substance into the cerebral circulation via carotid, vertebral, femoral, or brachial artery followed by X-rays
2. Used to visualize cerebral vessels and detect tumors, aneurysms, occlusions, hematomas, or abscesses
3. Nursing care: pretest
   a. Explain that client may have warm, flushed feeling and salty taste in mouth during procedure.
   b. Check for allergy to iodine.
   c. Keep NPO after midnight or offer clear liquid breakfast only.
   d. Take baseline vital signs and neuro check.
   e. Administer sedation if ordered.
4. Nursing care: posttest
   a. Maintain pressure dressing over site if femoral or brachial artery used; apply ice as ordered.
   b. Maintain bed rest until next morning as ordered.
   c. Monitor vital signs and neuro checks frequently; report any changes immediately.
   d. Check site frequently for bleeding or hematoma; if carotid artery used, assess for swelling of neck, difficulty swallowing or breathing.
   e. Check pulse, color, and temperature of extremity distal to site used.
   f. Keep extremity extended and avoid flexion.

H. Echoencephalography: use of ultrasound to detect midline shift of intracranial contents due to brain tumors, hematomas.

I. Electroencephalography (EEG)

1. Graphic recording of electrical activity of the brain by several small electrodes placed on the scalp
2. Used to detect focus or foci of seizure activity and to quantitatively evaluate level of brain function (determine brain death)
3. Pretest nursing care: withhold sedatives, tranquilizers, stimulants for 2–3 days.
4. Posttest nursing care: remove electrode paste with acetone and shampoo hair.

Eye

A. Ophthalmoscopic exam

B. Refraction: detects refractive errors and provides information for prescription of eyeglasses and contact lenses

C. Perimetry: assesses peripheral vision, visual fields

D. Tonometry: measures intraocular pressure (normal: 12–20 mmHg)

Ear

A. Otoscopic exam

B. Audiometry: screening test for hearing loss and diagnostic test to determine degree and type of hearing loss

C. Vestibular function
   1. Caloric test
   2. Electronystagmography (ENG)

ANALYSIS

Nursing diagnoses for clients with disorders of the neurosensory system may include

A. Imbalanced nutrition: less than body requirements
B. Ineffective thermoregulation
C. Autonomic dysreflexia
D. Constipation
E. Bowel incontinence
F. Impaired urinary elimination
G. Urinary retention
H. Ineffective tissue perfusion: cerebral
I. Ineffective airway clearance
J. Ineffective breathing pattern
K. Risk for injury
L. Risk for aspiration
M. Risk for disuse syndrome
N. Risk for impaired skin integrity
O. Impaired verbal communication
P. Sexual dysfunction
Q. Impaired physical mobility
R. Feeding self-care deficit
S. Impaired swallowing
T. Bathing/hygiene self-care deficit
U. Dressing/grooming self-care deficit
V. Toileting self-care deficit
W. Disturbed sensory perception: visual, auditory, kinesthetic, gustatory, tactile, olfactory
X. Unilateral neglect
Y. Disturbed thought processes

PLANNING AND IMPLEMENTATION

Goals

A. Nutritional state will be optimal.
B. Normal body temperature will be maintained.
C. Complications will be recognized early and treated promptly.
D. Adequate bowel and bladder elimination will be maintained.
E. Cerebral perfusion will be improved.
F. Adequate respiratory function will be maintained.
G. Client will remain free from any injury resulting from neurosensory deficits.

DELEGATION TIP

You may delegate the preparation of external feeding to assistive personnel, but you must assess the client's abdomen, assess the feeding-tube placement, and instruct to place only a 4-hour supply of feeding in the reservoir bag.

H. Client's skin integrity will be maintained.
I. Client's ability to communicate will be improved.
J. Sexual health will return to optimal level.
K. Mobility will be restored to optimal level.
L. Maximum independence in self-care activities will be attained.
M. Sensory perception will be improved.
N. Optimal cognitive functioning will be attained.

Interventions

Care of the Unconscious Client

A. Maintain a clear, patent airway.
   1. Place client in a side-lying or three-quarters prone position to prevent tongue from obstructing airway.
   2. If tongue is obstructing, insert oral airway.
   3. Prepare for insertion of a cuffed endotracheal or tracheostomy tube as the client's condition requires.
   4. Suction as needed.
   5. Check respiratory rate, depth, and quality every 1–2 hours and as needed.
   6. Auscultate breath sounds for crackles (rales), rhonchi, or absent breath sounds every 4 hours and before and after suctioning.

B. Take vital signs and perform neuro checks at specified intervals as ordered; report any significant changes immediately.

C. Maintain fluid and electrolyte balance and ensure adequate nutrition.
   1. Administer IV fluids, nasogastric tube feedings as ordered.
   2. Maintain accurate I&O.
   3. Assess client's hydration status: skin turgor, check for dry mucous membranes.
   4. Provide mouth care to keep mucous membranes clean, moist, and intact.

D. Provide for client's safety.
   1. Keep side rails up at all times.
   2. Avoid restraints if at all possible.
   3. Observe client carefully for seizures and intervene to avoid precipitating factors: fever, hypoxia, electrolyte imbalance.

4. Protect client if seizure occurs.
5. Speak softly and use client's name during nursing care.
6. Touch client as gently as possible.
7. Protect client's eyes from corneal irritation.
   a. Check for corneal reflex.
   b. Instill artificial tears as ordered; patch eye.

E. Prevent complications of immobility.
1. Keep skin clean, dry, and pressure free.
2. Turn and reposition client every 2 hours.
3. Perform passive range-of-motion (ROM) exercises every 4 hours.
4. Use nursing measures to prevent deformities: footboard/high-topped sneakers to prevent footdrop, splint to prevent wrist drop.

F. Maintain adequate bladder and bowel elimination.
1. Urinary: indwelling catheter (may use external device in male)
2. Bowel: stool softeners and suppositories as ordered

Care of the Client with Increased Intracranial Pressure (ICP)

A. General information
1. An increase in intracranial bulk due to an increase in any of the major intracranial components: brain tissue, CSF, or blood.
2. Increased ICP may be caused by tumors, abscesses, hemorrhage, edema, hydrocephalus, inflammation.
3. Untreated increased ICP can lead to displacement of brain tissue (herniation).
4. Presents life-threatening situation because of pressure on vital structures in the brain stem, nerve tracts, and cranial nerves.

B. Assessment findings
1. Earliest sign: decrease in LOC; progresses from restlessness to confusion and disorientation to lethargy and coma
2. Changes in vital signs (may be a late sign)
   a. Systolic blood pressure rises while diastolic pressure remains the same (widening pulse presence)
   b. Pulse slows
   c. Abnormal respiratory patterns (e.g., Cheyne-Stokes respirations)
   d. Elevated temperature
3. Pupillary changes
   a. Ipsilateral (same side) dilation of pupil with sluggish reaction to light from compression of cranial nerve III
   b. Pupil eventually becomes fixed and dilated.
4. Motor abnormalities
   a. Contralateral (opposite side) hemiparesis from compression of corticospinal tracts
   b. Decorticate or decerebrate rigidity
5. Headache, projectile vomiting, papilledema (edema of the optic disc)

C. Nursing care
  1. Maintain patent airway and adequate ventilation.
    a. Prevention of hypoxia and hypercarbia (increased CO_2) important: hypoxia may cause brain swelling and hypercarbia causes cerebral vasodilation, which increases ICP.
    b. Before and after suctioning, hyperventilate the client with a resuscitator bag connected to 100% oxygen. Limit suctioning to 15 seconds.
    c. Assist with mechanical hyperventilation as indicated: produces hypocarbia (decreased CO_2) causing cerebral vasoconstriction and decreased ICP.
  2. Monitor vital sign and neuro checks frequently to detect rises in ICP.
  3. Maintain fluid balance: fluid restriction to 1200–1500 ml/day may be ordered.
  4. Position client with head of bed elevated to 30–45° and neck in neutral position unless contraindicated (improves venous drainage from brain).
  5. Prevent further increases in ICP.
    a. Maintain quiet, comfortable environment.
    b. Avoid use of restraints.
    c. Prevent straining at stool; administer stool softeners and mild laxatives as ordered.
    d. Prevent vomiting; administer antiemetics as ordered.
    e. Prevent excessive coughing.
    f. Avoid clustering nursing care activities together.
  6. Prevent complications of immobility.
  7. Administer medications as ordered.
    a. Hyperosmotic agents (mannitol [Osmitrol]) to reduce cerebral edema; monitor urine output every hour (should increase).
    b. Corticosteroids (dexamethasone [Decadron]); anti-inflammatory effect reduces cerebral edema
    c. Diuretics (furosemide [Lasix]) to reduce cerebral edema.
    d. Anticonvulsants (phenytoin [Dilantin]) to prevent seizures.
    e. Analgesics for headache as needed
      1) small doses of codeine
      2) stronger opiates may be contraindicated since they potentiate respiratory depression, alter LOC, and cause pupillary changes.
  8. Assist with ICP monitoring when indicated.
    a. ICP monitoring records the pressure exerted within the cranial cavity by the brain, cerebral blood, and CSF.
    b. Types of monitoring devices
      1) Intraventricular catheter: inserted in lateral ventricle to give direct measurement of ICP; also allows for drainage of CSF if needed

2) Subarachnoid screw (bolt): inserted through skull and dura mater into subarachnoid space
3) Epidural sensor: least invasive method; placed in space between skull and dura mater for indirect measurement of ICP

c. Monitor ICP pressure readings frequently and prevent complications.
   1) Normal ICP reading is 0–15 mmHg; a sustained increase above 15 mmHg is considered abnormal.
   2) Use strict aseptic technique when handling any part of the monitoring system.
   3) Check insertion site for signs of infection; monitor temperature.
   4) Assess system for CSF leakage, loose connections, air bubbles in lines, and occluded tubing.

9. Provide intensive nursing care for client treated with barbiturate therapy or administration of paralyzing agents.
   a. Intravenous administration of barbiturates may be ordered to induce coma artificially in the client who has not responded to conventional treatment.
   b. Paralytic agents such as vecuronium bromide (Norcuron) may be administered to paralyze the client.
   c. Reduces cellular metabolic demands that may protect the brain from further injury.
   d. Constant monitoring of the client's ICP, arterial blood pressures, pulmonary pressures, arterial blood gases, serum barbiturate levels, and ECG is necessary.
   e. EEG monitoring as necessary.
   f. Provide appropriate nursing care for the client on a ventilator.
10. Observe for hyperthermia secondary to hypothalamus damage.

Care of the Client with Hyperthermia

A. General information
   1. Abnormal elevation of body temperation to 41°C (106°F) or above
   2. Caused by dysfunction of hypothalamus (temperature regulating center) from edema, head injury, hemorrhage, CVA, brain tumor, or intracranial surgery
   3. Hyperthermia increases cerebral metabolism; predisposes to seizures; may cause neurologic damage if prolonged

B. Nursing care
   1. Remove blankets and excess clothing if temperature rises above 38.4°C (101°F).
   2. Maintain room temperature at 21.1°C (70°F).

3. Administer antipyretic drugs (acetaminophen [Tylenol]) orally or rectally every 4 hours as ordered.
4. Increase fluid intake to 3000 ml/day unless contraindicated (in increased ICP).
5. Monitor vital signs, especially temperature, every 2–4 hours (more often if hypothermia is used).
6. Monitor urine output and urine specific gravity and assess for signs of dehydration.
7. Observe for seizure activity and protect client if seizures occur.
8. Change linen frequently if client is diaphoretic (sweating profusely).
9. Apply methods for inducing hypothermia as ordered: cool or tepid sponge baths, fans, hypothermia blanket.
10. Provide special care for the client with a hypothermia blanket.
    a. Reduce temperature gradually to prevent shivering and serious dysrhythmias; chlorpromazine (Thorazine) may be given for shivering.
    b. Provide frequent skin care to prevent breakdown.
        1) check every hour for signs of tissue damage or frostbite.
        2) apply lotion to skin to prevent drying.
        3) turn every 2 hours if not contraindicated because of increased intracranial pressure.
    c. Monitor core body temperature.

Care of the Client with Diminished Eyesight

A. Always speak and identify yourself upon entering the room to prevent startling the client.
B. Orient the client to his surroundings.
    1. Walk the client around the room and have him touch the objects in the room, e.g., table, chair.
    2. Keep personal belongings and objects in the room in the same place in order to increase client's independence and sense of security.
    3. Explain noises or other activities going on in the room.
C. Provide safety measures.
    1. Keep call bell nearby.
    2. Keep at least one side rail up.
    3. Keep the room orderly and free of clutter.
D. Assist the client in walking by having him take your arm; walk a half step in front of the client.
E. Offer explanations to the client and tell him what to expect next.
F. Provide mental stimulation and prevent sensory deprivation by providing frequent contacts with the staff, visitors, use of radio, TV, etc.

Communicating with the Client with Impaired Hearing

A. Attract the client's attention by raising an arm or hand.
B. Face the client directly when speaking.
C. Do not obscure the client's view of your mouth in any way.
D. Initially state the topic or subject of your conversation to give the client clues as to what you are going to say.
E. Speak slowly and distinctly, but do not overaccentuate words.
F. Speak in a normal tone of voice; do not shout.
G. Verify that the client has understood you, if necessary.

Irrigation of the Ear

A. Introduction of fluid into external auditory canal for cleansing purposes; may be used to apply antiseptic solutions.
B. Nursing care
   1. Explain procedure to the client.
   2. Prepare supplies needed: irrigating solution (about 500 ml normal saline at body temperature), irrigating syringe, basin, towel, cotton-tipped applicators, cotton balls.
   3. Assist client to a sitting or lying position with head tilted toward the affected ear.
   4. Straighten ear canal by pulling auricle upward and backward (down and backward on a child under 3 years).
   5. Insert tip of syringe into auditory meatus and direct the solution gently upward toward the top of the canal.
   6. Collect returning fluid in basin.
   7. Dry the outer ear with cotton balls.
   8. Instruct client to lie on affected side to encourage drainage of solution.
   9. Record the procedure and results.

EVALUATION

A. Client maintains normal weight; no evidence of malnutrition.
B. Client's temperature is maintained within normal limits.
C. Dysreflexia will be prevented or recognized early and treated promptly.
D. Client has regular bowel movements.
E. Client has adequate patterns of urinary elimination.
F. Neuro checks are within normal limits.
G. Client maintains patent airway and has effective respiratory patterns.
H. Client remains free from injuries.
I. Client remains free from aspiration and complications of immobility.
J. Client's skin remains clear and intact.
K. Client communicates effectively, responds appropriately to others.
L. Client experiences satisfying sexual activity/expression.
M. No contractures or limitations in motor function have occurred or loss of mobility has been kept to a minimum.

N. Client attains independence in self-care activities; uses assistive devices as necessary.

O. Sensory dysfunction is corrected or compensated for.

P. Client is oriented to time, place, and person; memory is intact; able to evaluate reality.

DISORDERS OF THE NERVOUS SYSTEM

Headache

A. General information
- **1.** Diffuse pain in different parts of the head
- **2.** Types
  - **a.** Functional
    - **1)** tension (muscle contraction): associated with tension or anxiety
    - **2)** migraine: recurrent throbbing headache
      - **a)** often starts in adolescence
      - **b)** affects women more than men
      - **c)** vascular origin: vasoconstriction or spasm of cerebral blood vessels (producing an aura) then vasodilation
    - **3)** cluster: similar to migraine (vascular origin); recur several times a day over a period of weeks followed by remission lasting for weeks or months
  - **b.** Organic: secondary to intracranial or systemic disease (e.g., brain tumor, sinus disease)

B. Assessment findings
- **1.** Tension headache: pain usually bilateral, often occurring in the back of the neck and extending diffusely over top of head
- **2.** Migraine headache: severe, throbbing pain, often in temporal or supraorbital area, lasting several hours to days; may be an aura (e.g., visual disturbance) preceding the pain; nausea and vomiting; pallor; sweating; irritability
- **3.** Cluster headache: intense, throbbing pain, usually affecting only one side of face and head; abrupt onset, lasts 30–90 minutes; eye and nose water on side of pain; skin reddens
- **4.** Diagnostic tests may be used to rule out organic causes.

C. Nursing interventions
- **1.** Carefully assess details regarding the headache.
- **2.** Provide quiet, dark environment.
- **3.** Administer medications as ordered.
  - **a.** Symptomatic during acute attack
    - **1)** nonnarcotic analgesics (aspirin, acetaminophen [Tylenol])
    - **2)** Fiorinal (analgesic-sedative/tranquilizer combination)
    - **3)** for migraines, ergotamine tartrate (Gynergen) or ergotamine with caffeine (Cafergot); vasoconstrictors given during aura may prevent the headache

4) Midrin (vasoconstrictor and sedative)
5) Sumatriptan (Imitrex) causes vasoconstriction in cerebral arteries; given via cutaneous injection.

b. Prophylactic to prevent migraine attacks
1) methysergide maleate (Sansert): after 6 months' use, drug should be discontinued for a 2-month period before resuming
2) propranolol (Inderal) and amytriptyline (Elavil): have also been used in migraine prevention

4. Provide additional nursing interventions for pain.
5. Provide client teaching and discharge planning concerning
   a. Identification of factors including diet that appear to precipitate attacks
   b. Examination of lifestyle, identification of stressors, and development of more positive coping behaviors
   c. Importance of daily exercise and relaxation periods
   d. Relaxation techniques
   e. Use and side effects of prescribed medications
   f. Alternative ways of handling the pain of headache: meditation, relaxation, self-hypnosis, yoga

Meningitis

A. General information
   1. Inflammation of the meninges of the brain and spinal cord
   2. Caused by bacteria, viruses, or other microorganisms
   3. May reach CNS
      a. Via the blood, CSF, lymph
      b. By direct extension from adjacent cranial structures (nasal sinuses, mastoid bone, ear, skull fracture)
      c. By oral or nasopharyngeal route
   4. Most common organisms: meningococcus, pneumococcus, *H. influenzae*, **streptococcus**

B. Assessment findings
   1. Headache, photophobia, malaise, irritability
   2. Chills and fever
   3. Signs of meningeal irritation
      a. Nuchal rigidity: stiff neck
      b. *Kernig's sign:* contraction or pain in the hamstring muscle when attempting to extend the leg when the hip is flexed
      c. Opisthotonos: head and heels bent backward and body arched forward
      d. *Brudzinski's sign:* flexion at the hip and knee in response to forward flexion of the neck
   4. Vomiting
   5. Possible seizures and decreasing LOC

6. Diagnostic test: lumbar puncture (measurement and analysis of CSF shows increased pressure, elevated WBC and protein, decreased glucose and culture positive for specific microorganism)

C. Nursing interventions
   1. Administer large doses of antibiotics IV as ordered.
   2. Enforce respiratory isolation for 24 hours after initiation of antibiotic therapy for some types of meningitis (consult hospital's infection control manual for specific directions).
   3. Provide nursing care for increased ICP, seizures, and hyperthermia if they occur.
   4. Provide nursing care for delirious or unconscious client as needed.
   5. Provide bed rest; keep room quiet and dark if client has headache or photophobia.
   6. Administer analgesics for headache as ordered.
   7. Maintain fluid and electrolyte balance.
   8. Prevent complications of immobility.
   9. Monitor vital signs and neuro checks frequently.
   10. Provide client teaching and discharge planning concerning
       a. Importance of good diet: high protein, high calorie with small, frequent feedings
       b. Rehabilitation program for residual deficits.

Encephalitis

A. General information
   1. Inflammation of the brain caused by a virus, e.g., herpes simplex (type I) or arbovirus (transmitted by mosquito or tick)
   2. May occur as a sequela of other diseases such as measles, mumps, chickenpox.

B. Assessment findings
   1. Headache
   2. Fever, chills, vomiting
   3. Signs of meningeal irritation
   4. Possibly seizures
   5. Alterations in LOC

C. Nursing interventions
   1. Monitor vital signs and neuro checks frequently.
   2. Provide nursing measures for increased ICP, seizures, hyperthermia if they occur.
   3. Provide nursing care for confused or unconscious client as needed.
   4. Provide client teaching and discharge planning: same as for meningitis.

Brain Abscess

A. General information
   1. Collection of free or encapsulated pus within the brain tissue

NURSING ALERT

Signs of brain herniation include

- Decreased level of consciousness
- Change in pupil size
- Rapid change in respiration
- Deteriorating motor response

2. Usually follows an infectious process elsewhere in the body (ear, sinuses, mastoid bone)

B. Assessment findings
  1. Headache, malaise, anorexia
  2. Vomiting
  3. Signs of increased ICP
  4. Focal neurologic deficits (hemiparesis, seizures)

C. Nursing interventions
  1. Administer large doses of antibiotics as ordered.
  2. Monitor vital signs and neuro checks.
  3. Provide symptomatic and supportive care.
  4. Prepare client for surgery if indicated.

Brain Tumors

A. General information
  1. Tumor within the cranial cavity; may be benign or malignant
  2. Types
    a. Primary: originates in brain tissue (e.g., glioma, meningioma)
    b. Secondary: metastasizes from tumor elsewhere in the body (e.g., lung, breast)

B. Medical management
  1. Craniotomy: to remove the tumor when possible
  2. Radiation therapy and chemotherapy: may follow surgery; also for inaccessible tumors and metastatic tumors
  3. Drug therapy: hyperosmotic agents, corticosteroids, diuretics to manage increased ICP

C. Assessment findings
  1. Headache: worse in the morning and with straining and stooping
  2. Vomiting
  3. Papilledema
  4. Seizures (focal or generalized)
  5. Changes in mental status

6. Focal neurologic deficits (e.g., aphasia, hemiparesis, sensory problems)
7. Diagnostic tests
   a. Skull X-ray, CT scan, MRI, brain scan: reveal presence of tumor
   b. Abnormal EEG
   c. Brain biopsy

D. Nursing interventions
   1. Monitor vital signs and neuro checks; observe for signs and symptoms of increased ICP.
   2. Administer medications as ordered.
      a. Drugs to decrease ICP, e.g., dextromethasone (Decadron)
      b. Anticonvulsants, e.g., phenytoin (Dilantin)
      c. Analgesics for headache, e.g., acetaminophen (Tylenol)
   3. Provide supportive care for any neurologic deficit (see Cerebrovascular Accident).
   4. Prepare client for surgery.
   5. Provide care for effects of radiation therapy or chemotherapy.
   6. Provide psychologic support to client/significant others.
   7. Provide client teaching and discharge planning concerning
      a. Use and side effects of prescribed medications.
      b. Rehabilitation program for residual deficits.

Cerebrovascular Accident (CVA)

A. General information
   1. Destruction (infarction) of brain cells caused by a reduction in cerebral blood flow and oxygen
   2. Affects men more than women; incidence increases with age
   3. Caused by thrombosis, embolism, hemorrhage
   4. Risk factors
      a. Hypertension, diabetes mellitus, arteriosclerosis/atherosclerosis, cardiac disease (valvular disease/replacement, chronic atrial fibrillation, myocardial infarction)
      b. Lifestyle: obesity, smoking, inactivity, stress, use of oral contraceptives
   5. Pathophysiology
      a. Interruption of cerebral blood flow for 5 minutes or more causes death of neurons in affected area with irreversible loss of function
      b. Modifying factors
         1) cerebral edema: develops around affected area causing further impairment
         2) vasospasm: constriction of cerebral blood vessel may occur, causing further decrease in blood flow
         3) collateral circulation: may help to maintain cerebral blood flow when there is compromise of main blood supply

6. Stages of development
    a. *Transient ischemic attack (TIA)*
        1) warning sign of impending CVA
        2) brief period of neurologic deficit: visual loss, hemiparesis, slurred speech, aphasia, vertigo
        3) may last less than 30 seconds, but no more than 24 hours with complete resolution of symptoms
    b. *Stroke in evolution*: progressive development of stroke symptoms over a period of hours to days
    c. *Completed stroke*: neurologic deficit remains unchanged for a 2- to 3-day period.

B. Assessment findings
1. Headache
2. Generalized signs: vomiting, seizures, confusion, disorientation, decreased LOC, nuchal rigidity, fever, hypertension, slow bounding pulse, Cheyne-Stokes respirations
3. Focal signs (related to site of infarction): hemiplegia, sensory loss, aphasia, homonymous hemianopsia
4. Diagnostic tests
    a. CT and brain scan: reveal lesion
    b. EEG: abnormal changes
    c. Cerebral arteriography: may show occlusion or malformation of blood vessels

C. Nursing interventions: acute stage
1. Maintain patent airway and adequate ventilation.
2. Monitor vital signs and neuro checks and observe for signs of increased ICP, shock, hyperthermia, and seizures.
3. Provide complete bed rest as ordered.
4. Maintain fluid and electrolyte balance and ensure adequate nutrition.
    a. IV therapy for the first few days
    b. Nasogastric tube feedings if client unable to swallow
    c. Fluid restriction as ordered to decrease cerebral edema
5. Maintain proper positioning and body alignment.
    a. Head of bed may be elevated 30–45° to decrease ICP
    b. Turn and reposition every 2 hours (only 20 minutes on the affected side)
    c. Passive ROM exercises every 4 hours.
6. Promote optimum skin integrity: turn client and apply lotion every 2 hours.
7. Maintain adequate elimination.
    a. Offer bedpan or urinal every 2 hours, catheterize only if absolutely necessary.
    b. Administer stool softeners and suppositories as ordered to prevent constipation and fecal impaction.
8. Provide a quiet, restful environment.

9. Establish a means of communicating with the client.
10. Administer medications as ordered.
    a. Hyperosmotic agents, corticosteroids to decrease cerebral edema
    b. Anticonvulsants to prevent or treat seizures
    c. Thrombolytics given to dissolve clot (hemorrhage must be ruled out)
        1) tissue plasminogen activator (tPA, Alteplase)
        2) streptokinase, urokinase
        3) must be given within 2 hours of episode
    d. Anticoagulants for stroke in evolution or embolic stroke (hemorrhage must be ruled out)
        1) heparin
        2) warfarin (Coumadin) for long-term therapy
        3) aspirin and dipyridamole (Persantine) to inhibit platelet aggregation in treating TIAs
    e. Antihypertensives if indicated for elevated blood pressure

D. Nursing interventions: rehabilitation
1. *Hemiplegia:* results from injury to cells in the cerebral motor cortex or to corticospinal tracts (causes contralateral hemiplegia since tracts cross in medulla)
    a. Turn every 2 hours (20 minutes only on affected side).
    b. Use proper positioning and repositioning to prevent deformities (foot drop, external rotation of hip, flexion of fingers, wrist drop, abduction of shoulder and arm).
    c. Support paralyzed arm on pillow or use sling while out of bed to prevent subluxation of shoulder.
    d. Elevate extremities to prevent dependent edema.
    e. Provide active and passive ROM exercises every 4 hours.
2. Susceptibility to hazards
    a. Keep side rails up at all times.
    b. Institute safety measures.
    c. Inspect body parts frequently for signs of injury.
3. *Dysphagia* (difficulty swallowing)
    a. Check gag reflex before feeding client.
    b. Maintain a calm, unhurried approach.
    c. Place client in upright position.
    d. Place food in unaffected side of mouth.
    e. Offer soft foods.
    f. Give mouth care before and after meals.
4. *Homonymous hemianopsia:* loss of right or left half of each visual field
    a. Approach client on unaffected side.
    b. Place personal belongings, food, etc., on unaffected side.
    c. Gradually teach client to compensate by scanning, i.e., turning the head to see things on affected side.

5. Emotional lability: mood swings, frustration
   a. Create a quiet, restful environment with a reduction in excessive sensory stimuli.
   b. Maintain a calm, nonthreatening manner.
   c. Explain to family that the client's behavior is not purposeful.
6. *Aphasia:* most common in right hemiplegics; may be receptive/ expressive
   a. Receptive aphasia
      1) give simple, slow directions.
      2) give one command at a time; gradually shift topics.
      3) use nonverbal techniques of communication (e.g., pantomime, demonstration).
   b. Expressive aphasia
      1) listen and watch very carefully when the client attempts to speak.
      2) anticipate client's needs to decrease frustration and feelings of helplessness.
      3) allow sufficient time for client to answer.
7. *Sensory/perceptual deficits:* more common in left hemiplegics; characterized by impulsiveness, unawareness of disabilities, visual neglect (neglect of affected side and visual space on affected side)
   a. Assist with self-care.
   b. Provide safety measures.
   c. Initially arrange objects in environment on unaffected side.
   d. Gradually teach client to take care of the affected side and to turn frequently and look at affected side.
8. *Apraxia:* loss of ability to perform purposeful, skilled acts
   a. Guide client through intended movement (e.g., take object such as washcloth and guide client through movement of washing).
   b. Keep repeating the movement.
9. Generalizations about clients with left hemiplegia versus right hemiplegia and nursing care
   a. Left hemiplegia
      1) Perceptual, sensory deficits; quick and impulsive behavior
      2) Use safety measures, verbal cues, simplicity in all areas of care
   b. Right hemiplegia
      1) Speech-language deficits; slow and cautious behavior
      2) Use pantomime and demonstration

Cerebral Aneurysm

A. General information
   1. Dilation of the walls of a cerebral artery, resulting in a sac-like outpouching of vessel
   2. Caused by congenital weakness in the vessel, trauma, arteriosclerosis, hypertension

3. Pathophysiology
   a. Aneurysm compresses nearby cranial nerves or brain substance, producing dysfunction.
   b. Aneurysm may rupture, causing subarachnoid hemorrhage or intracerebral hemorrhage.
   c. Initially a clot forms at the site of rupture, but fibrinolysis (dissolution of the clot) tends to occur within 7–10 days and may cause rebleeding.

B. Assessment findings
   1. Severe headache and pain in the eyes
   2. Diplopia, tinnitus, dizziness
   3. Nuchal rigidity, ptosis, decreasing LOC, hemiparesis, seizures

C. Nursing interventions
   1. Maintain a patent airway and adequate ventilation.
      a. Instruct client to take deep breaths but to avoid coughing.
      b. Suction only with a specific order.
   2. Monitor vital signs and neuro checks and observe for signs of vasospasm, increased ICP, hypertension, seizures, and hyperthermia.
   3. Enforce strict bed rest and provide complete care.
   4. Keep head of bed flat or elevated to 20–30° as ordered.
   5. Maintain a quiet, darkened environment.
   6. Avoid taking temperature rectally and instruct client to avoid sneezing, coughing, and straining at stool.
   7. Enforce fluid restriction as ordered; maintain accurate I&O.
   8. Administer medications as ordered.
      a. Antihypertensive agents to maintain normotensive levels
      b. Corticosteroids to prevent increased ICP
      c. Anticonvulsants to prevent seizures
      d. Stool softeners to prevent straining
      e. Aminocaproic acid (Amicar) to decrease fibrinolysis of the clot (administered IV)
   9. Prevent complications of immobility.
   10. Institute seizure precautions.
   11. Provide nursing care for the unconscious client if needed.
   12. Prepare the client for surgery if indicated.

Parkinson's Disease

A. General information
   1. A progressive disorder with degeneration of the nerve cells in the basal ganglia resulting in generalized decline in muscular function; disorder of the extrapyramidal system
   2. Usually occurs in the older population
   3. Cause unknown; predominantly idiopathic, but sometimes disorder is postencephalitic, toxic, arteriosclerotic, traumatic, or drug induced

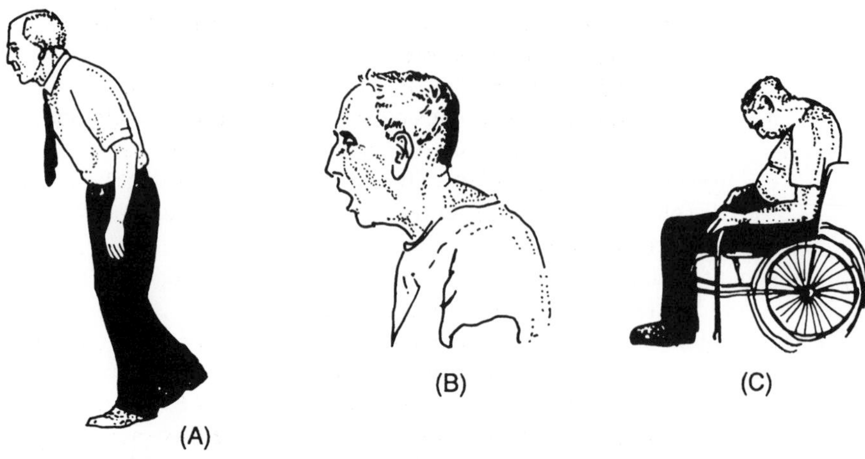

FIGURE 5-4 The shuffling gait and early postural changes of Parkinson's disease shown in (A). (B) and (C) show an advanced stage of the disease with head held forward, mouth open, and inability to stand.

(reserpine, methyldopa [Aldomet], haloperidol [Haldol], phenothiazines)

4. Pathophysiology
   a. Disorder causes degeneration of the dopamine-producing neurons in the substantia nigra in the midbrain.
   b. Dopamine influences purposeful movement.
   c. Depletion of dopamine results in degeneration of the basal ganglia.

B. Assessment findings
   1. Tremor: mainly of the upper limbs, "pill-rolling," resting tremor; most common initial symptom
   2. Rigidity: cogwheel type
   3. Bradykinesia: slowness of movement
   4. Fatigue
   5. Stooped posture; shuffling, propulsive gait (see Figure 5-4)
   6. Difficulty rising from sitting position
   7. Masklike face with decreased blinking of eyes
   8. Quiet, monotone speech
   9. Emotional lability, depression
   10. Increased salivation, drooling
   11. Cramped, small handwriting
   12. Autonomic symptoms: excessive sweating, seborrhea, lacrimation, constipation; decreased sexual capacity

C. Nursing interventions
   1. Administer medications as ordered
      a. Levodopa (L-dopa)

1) increases level of dopamine in the brain; relieves tremor, rigidity, and bradykinesia.
2) side effects: anorexia; nausea and vomiting; postural hypotension; mental changes such as confusion, agitation, and hallucinations; cardiac arrhythmias; dyskinesias.
3) contraindications: narrow-angle glaucoma; clients taking MAO inhibitors, reserpine, guanethidine, methyldopa, antipsychotics; acute psychoses.
4) avoid multiple vitamin preparations containing vitamin B_6 (pyridoxine) and foods high in vitamin B_6.
5) be aware of any worsening of symptoms with prolonged high-dose therapy: ''on-off'' syndrome.
6) administer with food or snack to decrease GI irritation.
7) inform client that urine and sweat may be darkened.

b. Carbidopa-levodopa (Sinemet): prevents breakdown of dopamine in the periphery and causes fewer side effects.

c. Amantadine (Symmetrel): used in mild cases or in combination with L-dopa to reduce rigidity, tremor, and bradykinesia.

d. Anticholinergic drugs: benztropine mesylate (Cogentin), procyclidine (Kemadrin), trihexyphenidyl (Artane)
1) inhibit action of acetylcholine
2) used in mild cases or in combination with L-dopa
3) relieve tremor and rigidity
4) side effects: dry mouth, blurred vision, constipation, urinary retention, confusion, hallucinations, tachycardia

e. Antihistamines: diphenhydramine (Benadryl)
1) decrease tremor and anxiety
2) side effect: drowsiness

f. Bromocriptine (Parlodel)
1) stimulates release of dopamine in the substantia nigra.
2) often employed when L-dopa loses effectiveness.

g. Eldepryl (Selegilene) a MAO inhibitor inhibits dopamine breakdown and slows progression of disease

h. Tricyclic antidepressants given to treat depression commonly seen in Parkinson's disease

2. Provide a safe environment.

a. Side rails on bed; rails and handlebars in toilet, bathtub, and hallways; no scatter rugs

b. Hard-back or spring-loaded chair to make getting up easier

3. Provide measures to increase mobility.

a. Physical therapy: active and passive ROM exercises; stretching exercises; warm baths

b. Assistive devices

c. If client ''freezes,'' suggest thinking of something to walk over.

CLIENT TEACHING CHECKLIST

To ensure safety at home instruct the client to:

- Wear sturdy, proper-fitting shoes
- Focus on standing upright
- Not have scatter rugs or obstacles in walkways or hallways in the home
- Install side rails in hallways
- Have a raised toilet seat installed

4. Encourage independence in self-care activities: alter clothing for ease in dressing; use assistive devices; do not rush client.
5. Improve communication abilities: instruct client to practice reading aloud, to listen to own voice, and enunciate each syllable clearly.
6. Refer for speech therapy when indicated.
7. Maintain adequate nutrition.
   a. Cut food into bite-sized pieces.
   b. Provide small, frequent feedings.
   c. Allow sufficient time for meals, use warming tray.
8. Avoid constipation and maintain adequate bowel elimination.
9. Provide psychologic support to client/significant others; depression is common due to changes in body image and self-concept.
10. Provide client teaching and discharge planning concerning
    a. Nature of the disease
    b. Use of prescribed medications and side effects
    c. Importance of daily exercise: walking, swimming, gardening as tolerated; balanced activity and rest
    d. Activities/methods to limit postural deformities: firm mattress with a small pillow; keep head and neck as erect as possible; use broad-based gait; raise feet while walking
    e. Promotion of active participation in self-care activities

Multiple Sclerosis (MS)

A. General information
   1. Chronic, intermittently progressive disease of the CNS, characterized by scattered patches of demyelination within the brain and spinal cord
   2. Incidence
      a. Affects women more than men
      b. Usually occurs from 20–40 years of age
      c. More frequent in cool or temperate climates

3. Cause unknown; may be a slow-growing virus or possibly of autoimmune origin
4. Signs and symptoms are varied and multiple, reflecting the location of demyelination within the CNS
5. Characterized by remissions and exacerbations

B. Assessment findings
1. Visual disturbances: blurred vision, scotomas (blind spots), diplopia
2. Impaired sensation: touch, pain, temperature, or position sense; paresthesias such as numbness, tingling
3. Euphoria or mood swings
4. Impaired motor function: weakness, paralysis, spasticity
5. Impaired cerebellar function: scanning speech, ataxic gait, nystagmus, dysarthria, intention tremor
6. Bladder: retention or incontinence
7. Constipation
8. Sexual impotence in the male
9. Diagnostic tests:
   a. CSF studies: increased protein and IgG (immunoglobulin)
   b. Visual evoked response (VER) determined by EEG: may be delayed
   c. CT scan: increased density of white matter
   d. MRI: shows areas of demyelination

C. Nursing interventions
1. Assess the client for specific deficits related to location of demyelinization.
2. Promote optimum mobility.
   a. Muscle-stretching and strengthening exercises
   b. Walking exercises to improve gait: use wide-based gait
   c. Assistive devices: canes, walker, rails, wheelchair as necessary
3. Administer medications as ordered.
   a. For acute exacerbations: corticosteroids (ACTH [IV], prednisone) to reduce edema at sites of demyelinization
   b. For spasticity: baclofen (Lioresal), dantrolene (Dantrium), diazepam (Valium)
   c. Beta interferon (Betaseron) to alter immune response
4. Encourage independence in self-care activities.
5. Prevent complications of immobility.
6. Institute bowel program.
7. Maintain urinary elimination.
   a. Urinary retention
      1) administer bethanecol chloride (Urecholine) as ordered.
      2) perform intermittent catheterization as ordered.
   b. Urinary incontinence
      1) establish voiding schedule.
      2) administer propantheline bromide (Pro-Banthine) if ordered.
   c. Force fluids to 3000 ml/day.

    d. Promote use of acid-ash foods like cranberry or grape juice.
8. Prevent injury related to sensory problems.
    a. Test bath water with thermometer.
    b. Avoid heating pads, hot-water bottles.
    c. Inspect body parts frequently for injury.
    d. Make frequent position changes.
9. Prepare client for plasma exchange (to remove antibodies) if indicated.
10. Provide psychologic support to client/significant others.
    a. Encourage positive attitude and assist client in setting realistic goals.
    b. Provide compassion in helping client adapt to changes in body image and self-concept.
    c. Do not encourage false hopes during remission.
    d. Refer to multiple sclerosis societies and community agencies.
11. Provide client teaching and discharge planning concerning
    a. General measures to ensure optimum health
        1) balance between activity and rest
        2) regular exercise such as walking, swimming, biking in mild cases
        3) use of energy conservation techniques
        4) well-balanced diet
        5) fresh air and sunshine
        6) avoiding fatigue, overheating or chilling, stress, infection
    b. Use of medications and side effects
    c. Alternative methods for sexual gratification; refer for sexual counseling if indicated.

Myasthenia Gravis

A. General information
    1. A neuromuscular disorder in which there is a disturbance in the transmission of impulses from nerve to muscle cells at the neuromuscular junction, causing extreme muscle weakness
    2. Incidence
        a. Highest between ages 15 and 35 for women, over 40 for men.
        b. Affects women more than men
    3. Cause: thought to be autoimmune disorder whereby antibodies destroy acetylcholine receptor sites on the postsynaptic membrane of the neuromuscular junction.
    4. Voluntary muscles are affected, especially those muscles innervated by the cranial nerves.

B. Medical management
    1. Drug therapy
        a. Anticholinesterase drugs: ambenonium (Mytelase), neostigmine (Prostigmin), pyridostigmine (Mestinon)

    1) block action of cholinesterase and increase levels of acetylcholine at the neuromuscular junction
    2) side effects: excessive salivation and sweating, abdominal cramps, nausea and vomiting, diarrhea, fasciculations (muscle twitching)
  - **b.** Corticosteroids: prednisone
    1) used if other drugs are not effective
    2) suppress autoimmune response

2. Surgery (thymectomy)
  - **a.** Surgical removal of the thymus gland (thought to be involved in the production of acetylcholine receptor antibodies)
  - **b.** May cause remission in some clients especially if performed early in the disease

3. Plasma exchange
  - **a.** Removes circulating acetylcholine receptor antibodies
  - **b.** Use in clients who do not respond to other types of therapy

C. Assessment findings
  - **1.** Diplopia, dysphagia
  - **2.** Extreme muscle weakness, increased with activity and reduced with rest
  - **3.** Ptosis, masklike facial expression
  - **4.** Weak voice, hoarseness
  - **5.** Diagnostic tests
    - **a.** Tensilon test: IV injection of Tensilon provides spontaneous relief of symptoms (lasts 5–10 minutes)
    - **b.** Electromyography (EMG): amplitude of evoked potentials decreases rapidly
    - **c.** Presence of antiacetylcholine receptor antibodies in the serum

D. Nursing interventions
  - **1.** Administer anticholinesterase drugs as ordered.
    - **a.** Give medication exactly on time.
    - **b.** Give with milk and crackers to decrease GI upset.
    - **c.** Monitor effectiveness of drugs: assess muscle strength and vital capacity before and after medication.
    - **d.** Avoid use of the following drugs: morphine and strong sedatives (respiratory depressant effect), quinine, curare, procainamide, neomycin, streptomycin, kanamycin and other aminoglycosides (skeletal muscle blocking effects).
    - **e.** Observe for side effects.
  - **2.** Promote optimal nutrition.
    - **a.** Mealtimes should coincide with the peak effects of the drugs: give medications 30 minutes before meals.
    - **b.** Check gag reflex and swallowing ability before feeding.
    - **c.** Provide a mechanical soft diet.

  - **d.** If the client has difficulty chewing and swallowing, do not leave alone at mealtimes; keep emergency airway and suction equipment nearby.

3. Monitor respiratory status frequently: rate, depth; vital capacity; ability to deep breathe and cough.
4. Assess muscle strength frequently; plan activity to take advantage of energy peaks and provide frequent rest periods.
5. Observe for signs of myasthenic or cholinergic crisis.
   - **a.** *Myasthenic crisis*
     - **1)** abrupt onset of severe, generalized muscle weakness with inability to swallow, speak, or maintain respirations
     - **2)** caused by undermedication, physical or emotional stress, infection
     - **3)** symptoms will improve temporarily with Tensilon test
   - **b.** *Cholinergic crisis*
     - **1)** symptoms similar to myasthenic crisis and, in addition, the side effects of anticholinesterase drugs (e.g., excessive salivation and sweating, abdominal cramps, nausea and vomiting, diarrhea, fasciculations)
     - **2)** caused by overmedication with the cholinergic (anticholinesterase) drugs
     - **3)** symptoms worsen with Tensilon test; keep atropine sulfate and emergency equipment on hand
   - **c.** Nursing care in crisis
     - **1)** maintain tracheostomy or endotracheal tube with mechanical ventilation as indicated.
     - **2)** monitor arterial blood gases and vital capacities.
     - **3)** administer medications as ordered.
       - **a)** *myasthenic crisis:* increase doses of anticholinesterase drugs as ordered.
       - **b)** *cholinergic crisis:* discontinue anticholinesterase drugs as ordered until the client recovers.
     - **4)** establish a method of communication.
     - **5)** provide support and reassurance.
6. Provide nursing care for the client with a thymectomy.
7. Provide client teaching and discharge planning concerning
   - **a.** Nature of the disease
   - **b.** Use of prescribed medications, their side effects and signs of toxicity
   - **c.** Importance of checking with physician before taking any new medications including OTC drugs
   - **d.** Importance of planning activities to take advantage of energy peaks and of scheduling frequent rest periods
   - **e.** Need to avoid fatigue, stress, people with upper-respiratory infections

f. Use of eye patch for diplopia (alternate eyes)
g. Need to wear Medic-Alert bracelet
h. Myasthenia Gravis Foundation and other community agencies

Head Injury

A. General information
1. Usually caused by car accidents, falls, assaults
2. Types
a. *Concussion:* severe blow to the head jostles brain, causing it to strike the skull; results in temporary neural dysfunction
b. *Contusion:* results from more severe blow that bruises the brain and disrupts neural function
c. Hemorrhage
1) *epidural hematoma:* accumulation of blood between the dura mater and skull; commonly results from laceration of middle meningeal artery during skull fracture; blood accumulates rapidly
2) *subdural hematoma:* accumulation of blood between the dura and arachnoid; venous bleeding that forms slowly; may be acute, subacute, or chronic
3) *subarachnoid hematoma:* bleeding in subarachnoid space
4) *intracerebral hematoma:* accumulation of blood within the cerebrum
d. Fractures: linear, depressed, comminuted, compound

B. Assessment findings (depend on type of injury)
1. Concussion: headache, transient loss of consciousness, retrograde or posttraumatic amnesia, nausea, dizziness, irritability
2. Contusion: neurologic deficits depend on the site and extent of damage; include decreased LOC, aphasia, hemiplegia, sensory deficits
3. Hemorrhages
a. Epidural hematoma: brief loss of consciousness followed by lucid interval; progresses to severe headache, vomiting, rapidly deteriorating LOC, possible seizures, ipsilateral pupillary dilation
b. Subdural hematoma: alterations in LOC, headache, focal neurologic deficits, personality changes, ipsilateral pupillary dilation
c. Intracerebral hematoma: headache, decreased LOC, hemiplegia, ipsilateral pupillary dilation
4. Fractures
a. Headache, pain over fracture site
b. Compound fractures: rhinorrhea (leakage of CSF from nose); otorrhea (leakage of CSF from ear)

5. Diagnostic tests
    a. Skull X-ray: reveals skull fracture or intracranial shift
    b. CT scan: reveals hemorrhage

C. Nursing interventions
1. Maintain a patent airway and adequate ventilation.
2. Monitor vital signs and neuro checks; observe for changes in neurologic status, signs of increased ICP, shock, seizures, and hyperthermia.
3. Observe for CSF leakage.
    a. Check discharge for positive Testape or Dextrostix reaction for glucose; bloody spot encircled by watery, pale ring "halo" on pillowcase or sheet.
    b. Never attempt to clean the ears or nose of a head-injured client or use nasal suction unless cleared by physician.
4. If a CSF leak is present
    a. Instruct client not to blow nose.
    b. Elevate head of bed 30° as ordered.
    c. Observe for signs of meningitis and administer antibiotics to prevent meningitis as ordered.
    d. Place a cotton ball in the ear to absorb otorrhea; replace frequently.
    e. Gently place a sterile gauze pad at the bottom of the nose for rhinorrhea; replace frequently.
5. Prevent complications of immobility.
6. Prepare the client for surgery if indicated.
    a. Depressed skull fracture: surgical removal or elevation of splintered bone; debridement and cleansing of area; repair of dural tear if present; cranioplasty (if necessitated for large cranial defect)
    b. Epidural or subdural hematoma: evacuation of the hematoma
7. Provide psychologic support to client/significant others.
8. Observe for hemiplegia, aphasia, and sensory problems, and plan care accordingly
9. Provide client teaching and discharge planning concerning rehabilitation for neurologic deficits; note availability of community agencies.

Intracranial Surgery

A. Types
1. *Craniotomy:* surgical opening of skull to gain access to intracranial structures; used to remove a tumor, evacuate blood clot, control hemorrhage, relieve increased ICP
2. *Craniectomy:* excision of a portion of the skull; sometimes used for decompression
3. *Cranioplasty:* repair of a cranial defect with a metal or plastic plate

B. Nursing interventions: preoperative

1. Routine pre-op care.

2. Provide emotional support; explain post-op procedures and that client's head will be shaved, there will be a large bandage on head, possibly temporary swelling and discoloration around the eye on the affected side, and possible headache.

3. Shampoo the scalp and check for signs of infection.

4. Shave hair.

5. Evaluate and record baseline vital signs and neuro checks.

6. Avoid enemas unless directed (straining increases ICP).

7. Give pre-op steroids as ordered to decrease brain swelling.

8. Insert Foley catheter as ordered.

C. Nursing interventions: postoperative

1. Provide nursing care for the unconscious client.

2. Maintain a patent airway and adequate ventilation.

a. Supratentorial incision: elevate head of bed 15–45° as ordered; position on back (if intubated or conscious) or on unaffected side; turn every 2 hours to facilitate breathing and venous return.

b. Infratentorial incision: keep head of bed flat or elevate 20–30° as ordered; do not flex head on chest; turn side to side every 2 hours using a turning sheet; check respirations closely and report any signs of respiratory distress.

c. Instruct the conscious client to breathe deeply but not to cough; avoid vigorous suctioning.

3. Check vital signs and neuro checks frequently; observe for decreasing LOC, increased ICP, seizures, hyperthermia.

4. Monitor fluid and electrolyte status.

a. Maintain accurate I&O.

b. Restrict fluids to 1500 ml/day or as ordered to decrease cerebral edema.

c. Avoid overly rapid infusions.

d. Watch for signs of diabetes insipidus (severe thirst, polyuria, dehydration) and inappropriate ADH secretion (decreased urine output, hunger, thirst, irritability, decreased LOC, muscle weakness).

e. For infratentorial surgery: may be NPO for 24 hours due to possible impaired swallowing and gag reflexes.

5. Assess dressings frequently and report any abnormalities.

a. Reinforce as needed with sterile dressings.

b. Check dressings for excessive drainage, CSF, infection, displacement and report to physician.

c. If surgical drain is in place, note color, amount, and odor of drainage.

6. Administer medications as ordered.

a. Corticosteroids: to decrease cerebral edema

b. Anticonvulsants: to prevent seizures

c. Stool softeners: to prevent straining
d. Mild analgesics
7. Apply ice to swollen eyelids; lubricate lids and areas around eyes with petrolatum jelly.
8. Refer client for rehabilitation for residual deficits.

Spinal Cord Injuries

A. General information
1. Occurs most commonly in young adult males between ages 15 and 25
2. Common traumatic causes: motor vehicle accidents, diving in shallow water, falls, industrial accidents, sports injuries, gunshot or stab wounds
3. Nontraumatic causes: tumors, hematomas, aneurysms, congenital defects (spina bifida)
4. Classified by extent, level, and mechanism of injury
a. Extent of injury
1) may affect the vertebral column: fracture, fracture/dislocation
2) may affect anterior or posterior ligaments, causing compression of spinal cord
3) may be to the spinal cord and its roots: concussion, contusion, compression or laceration by fracture/dislocation or penetrating missiles
b. Level of injury: cervical, thoracic, lumbar
c. Mechanisms of injury
1) hyperflexion
2) hyperextension
3) axial loading (force exerted straight up or down spinal column as in a diving accident)
4) penetrating wounds
5. Pathophysiology: hemorrhage and edema cause ischemia, leading to necrosis and destruction of the cord
B. Medical management: immobilization and maintenance of normal spinal alignment to promote fracture healing
1. Horizontal turning frames (Stryker frame)
2. Skeletal traction: to immobilize the fracture and maintain alignment of the cervical spine
a. *Cervical tongs (Crutchfield, Gardner- Wells, Vinke):* inserted through burr holes; traction is provided by a rope extended from the center of tongs over a pulley with weights attached at the end.
b. *Halo traction*
1) stainless steel halo ring fits around the head and is attached to the skull with four pins; halo is attached to plastic body cast or plastic vest
2) permits early mobilization, decreased period of hospitalization and reduces complications of immobility

3. Surgery: decompression laminectomy, spinal fusion
   a. Depends on type of injury and the preference of the surgeon
   b. Indications: unstable fracture, cord compression, progression of neurologic deficits

C. Assessment findings
   1. Spinal shock
      a. Occurs immediately after the injury as a result of the insult to the CNS
      b. Temporary condition lasting from several days to three months
      c. Characterized by absence of reflexes below the level of the lesion, flaccid paralysis, lack of temperature control in affected parts, hypotension with bradycardia, retention of urine and feces
   2. Symptoms depend on the level and the extent of the injury.
      a. Level of injury
         1) *quadriplegia:* cervical injuries (C_1–C_8) cause paralysis of all four extremities; respiratory paralysis occurs in lesions above C_6 due to lack of innervation to the diaphragm; (phrenic nerves at the C_4–C_5 level).
         2) *paraplegia:* thoraco/lumbar injuries (T_1–L_4) cause paralysis of the lower half of the body involving both legs
      b. Extent of injury
         1) complete cord transection
            a) loss of all voluntary movement and sensation below the level of the injury; reflex activity below the level of the lesion may return after spinal shock resolves.
            b) lesions in the conus medullaris or cauda equina result in permanent flaccid paralysis and areflexia.
         2) incomplete lesions: varying degrees of motor or sensory loss below the level of the lesion depending on which neurologic tracts are damaged and which are spared.
   3. Diagnostic test: spinal X-rays may reveal fracture.

D. Nursing interventions: emergency care
   1. Assess airway, breathing, circulation
      a. Do not move the client during assessment.
      b. If airway obstruction or inadequate ventilation exists: do not hyperextend neck to open airway, use jaw thrust instead.
   2. Perform a quick head-to-toe assessment: check for LOC, signs of trauma to the head or neck, leakage of clear fluid from ears or nose, signs of motor or sensory impairment.
   3. Immobilize the client in the position found until help arrives.
   4. Once emergency help arrives, assist in immobilizing the head and neck with a cervical collar and place the client on a spinal board; avoid any movement during transfer, especially flexion of the spinal column.

5. Have suction available to clear the airway and prevent aspiration if the client vomits; client may be turned slightly to the side if secured to a board.
6. Evaluate respiration and observe for weak or labored respirations.

E. Nursing interventions: acute care
   1. Maintain optimum respiratory function.
      a. Observe for weak or labored respirations; monitor arterial blood gases.
      b. Prevent pneumonia and atelectasis: turn every 2 hours; cough and deep breathe every hour; use incentive spirometry every 2 hours.
      c. Tracheostomy and mechanical ventilation may be necessary if respiratory insufficiency occurs.
   2. Maintain optimal cardiovascular function.
      a. Monitor vital signs; observe for bradycarida, arrhythmias, hypotension.
      b. Apply thigh-high elastic stockings or Ace bandages.
      c. Change position slowly and gradually elevate the head of the bed to prevent postural hypotension.
      d. Observe for signs of deep-vein thrombosis.
   3. Maintain fluid and electrolyte balance and nutrition.
      a. Nasogastric tube may be inserted until bowel sounds return.
      b. Maintain IV therapy as ordered; avoid overhydration (can aggravate cord edema).
      c. Check bowel sounds before feeding client (paralytic ileus is common).
      d. Progress slowly from clear liquid to regular diet.
      e. Provide diet high in protein, carbohydrates, calories.
   4. Maintain immobilization and spinal alignment always.
      a. Turn every hour on turning frame.
      b. Maintain cervical traction at all times if indicated.
   5. Prevent complications of immobility; use footboard/high-topped sneakers to prevent footdrop; provide splint for quadriplegic client to prevent wrist drop.
   6. Maintain urinary elimination.
      a. Provide intermittent catheterization or maintain indwelling catheter as ordered.
      b. Increase fluids to 3000 ml/day.
      c. Provide acid-ash foods/fluids to acidify urine and prevent infection.
   7. Maintain bowel elimination: administer stool softeners and suppositories to prevent impaction as ordered.
   8. Monitor temperature control.
      a. Check temperature every 4 hours.
      b. Regulate environment closely.
      c. Avoid excessive covering or exposure.

9. Observe for and prevent infection.
   a. Observe tongs or pin site for redness, drainage.
   b. Provide tong- or pin-site care. Cleanse with antiseptic solution according to agency policy.
   c. Observe for signs of respiratory or urinary infection.
10. Observe for and prevent stress ulcers.
   a. Assess for epigastic or shoulder pain.
   b. If corticosteroids are ordered, give with food or antacids; administer H_2 blocker as ordered.
   c. Check nasogastric tube contents and stools for blood.

F. Nursing interventions: chronic care
1. *Neurogenic bladder*
   a. Reflex or upper motor neuron bladder; reflex activity of the bladder may occur after spinal shock resolves; the bladder is unable to store urine very long and empties involuntarily
   b. Nonreflexive or lower motor neuron bladder: reflex arc is disrupted and no reflex activity of the bladder occurs, resulting in urine retention with overflow
   c. Management of reflex bladder
      1) intermittent catheterization every 4 hours and gradually progress to every 6 hours.
      2) regulate fluid intake to 1800–2000 ml/day.
      3) bladder taps or stimulating trigger points to cause reflex emptying of the bladder.
   d. Management of nonreflexive bladder
      1) intermittent catheterization every 6 hours.
      2) Credé maneuver or rectal stretch.
      3) regulate intake to 1800–2000 ml/day to prevent overdistention of bladder.
   e. Management depends on lifestyle, age, sex, home care, and availability of caregiver.
2. *Spasticity*
   a. Return of reflex activity may occur after spinal shock resolves; severe spasticity may be detrimental
   b. Drug therapy: baclofen (Lioresal), dantrolene (Dantrium), diazepam (Valium)
   c. Physical therapy: stretching exercises, warm tub baths, whirlpool
   d. Surgery: chordotomy
3. *Autonomic dysreflexia*
   a. Rise in blood pressure, sometimes to fatal levels
   b. Occurs in clients with cord lesions above T_6 and most commonly in clients with cervical injuries
   c. Reflex response to stimulation of the sympathetic nervous system
   d. Stimulus may be overdistended bladder or bowel, decubitus ulcer, chilling, pressure from bedclothes

NURSING ALERT

If the stimulus for autonomic dysreflexia is not completely removed, the dysreflexia may reoccur. Use caution if the source is bladder distention. Slowly remove urine at a rate of approximately 500 ml every 15 minutes. Assess for blood pressure fluctuations.

   e. Symptoms: severe headache, hypertension, bradycardia, sweating, goose bumps, nasal congestion, blurred vision, convulsions
   f. Interventions
      1) raise client to sitting position to decrease BP.
      2) check for source of stimulus (bladder, bowel, skin).
      3) remove offending stimulus (e.g., catheterize client, digitally remove impacted feces, reposition client).
      4) monitor blood pressure.
      5) administer antihypertensives (e.g., hydralazine HCl [Apresoline]) as ordered.

G. Nursing interventions: general rehabilitative care
   1. Provide psychologic support to client/significant others.
      a. Support during grieving process.
      b. Assist client to adjust to effects of injury.
      c. Encourage independence.
      d. Involve the client in decision making.
   2. Provide sexual counseling.
      a. Work with the client and partner.
      b. Explore alternative methods of sexual gratification.
   3. Initiate rehabilitation program.
      a. Physical therapy
      b. Vocational rehabilitation
      c. Psychologic counseling
      d. Use of braces, electronic wheelchair, and other assistance devices to maximize independence

Specific Disorders of the Peripheral Nervous System

Trigeminal Neuralgia (Tic Douloureux)

A. General information
   1. Disorder of cranial nerve V causing disabling and recurring attacks of severe pain along the sensory distribution of one or more branches of the trigeminal nerve
   2. Incidence increased in elderly women
   3. Cause unknown

B. Medical management
  1. Anticonvulsant drugs: carbamazepine (Tegretol), phenytoin (Dilantin)
  2. Nerve block: injection of alcohol or phenol into one or more branches of the trigeminal nerve; temporary effect, lasts 6–18 months
  3. Surgery
    a. Peripheral: avulsion of peripheral branches of trigeminal nerve
    b. Intracranial
      1) retrogasserian rhizotomy: total severance of the sensory root of the trigeminal nerve intracranially; results in permanent anesthesia, numbness, heaviness, and stiffness in affected part; loss of corneal reflex
      2) microsurgery: uses more precise cutting and may preserve facial sensation and corneal reflex
      3) percutaneous radio-frequency trigeminal gangliolysis: current surgical procedure of choice; thermally destroys the trigeminal nerve in the area of the ganglion; provides permanent pain relief with preservation of sense of touch, proprioception, and corneal reflex; done under local anesthesia
      4) microvascular decompression of trigeminal nerve: decompresses the trigeminal nerve; craniotomy necessary; provides permanent pain relief while preserving facial sensation

C. Assessment findings
  1. Sudden paroxysms of extremely severe shooting pain in one side of the face
  2. Attacks may be triggered by a cold breeze, foods/fluids of extreme temperature, toothbrushing, chewing, talking, or touching the face
  3. During attack: twitching, grimacing, and frequent blinking/tearing of the eye
  4. Poor eating and hygiene habits
  5. Withdrawal from interactions with others
  6. Diagnostic tests: X-rays of the skull, teeth, and sinuses may identify dental or sinus infection as an aggravating factor.

D. Nursing interventions
  1. Assess characteristics of the pain including triggering factors, trigger points, and pain management techniques.
  2. Administer medications as ordered; monitor response.
  3. Maintain room at an even, moderate temperature, free from drafts.
  4. Provide small, frequent feedings of lukewarm, semiliquid, or soft foods that are easily chewed.
  5. Provide the client with a soft washcloth and lukewarm water and perform hygiene during periods when pain is decreased.
  6. Prepare the client for surgery if indicated.
  7. Provide client teaching and discharge planning concerning

a. Need to avoid outdoor activities during cold, windy, or rainy weather
b. Importance of good nutrition and hygiene
c. Use of medications, side effects, and signs of toxicity
d. Specific instructions following surgery for residual effects of anesthesia and loss of corneal reflex
  1) protective eye care
  2) chew on unaffected side only
  3) avoid hot fluids/foods
  4) mouth care after meals to remove particles
  5) good oral hygiene; visit dentist every 6 months
  6) protect the face during extremes of temperature

Bell's Palsy

A. General information
  1. Disorder of cranial nerve VII resulting in the loss of ability to move the muscles on one side of the face
  2. Cause unknown; may be viral or autoimmune
  3. Complete recovery in 3–5 weeks in majority of clients
B. Assessment findings
  1. Loss of taste over anterior two-thirds of tongue on affected side
  2. Complete paralysis of one side of face
  3. Loss of expression, displacement of mouth toward unaffected side, and inability to close eyelid (all on affected side)
  4. Pain behind the ear
C. Nursing interventions
  1. Assess facial nerve function regularly (see Table 5-1).
  2. Administer medications as ordered.
    a. Corticosteroids: to decrease edema and pain
    b. Mild analgesics as necessary
  3. Provide soft diet with supplementary feedings as indicated.
  4. Instruct to chew on unaffected side, avoid hot fluids/foods, and perform mouth care after each meal.
  5. Provide special eye care to protect the cornea.
    a. Dark glasses (cosmetic and protective reasons) or eyeshield
    b. Artificial tears to prevent drying of the cornea
    c. Ointment and eye patch at night to keep eyelid closed
  6. Provide support and reassurance.

Guillain-Barré Syndrome

A. General information
  1. Symmetrical, bilateral, peripheral polyneuritis characterized by ascending paralysis
  2. Can occur at any age; affects women and men equally

3. Cause unknown; may be an autoimmune process
4. Precipitating factors: antecedent viral infection, immunization
5. Progression of disease is highly individual; 90% of clients stop progression in 4 weeks; recovery is usually from 3–6 months; may have residual deficits

B. Medical management
1. Mechanical ventilation if respiratory problems present
2. Plasmapheresis to reduce circulating antibodies
3. Continuous ECG monitoring to detect alteration in heart rate and rhythm
4. Propranolol to prevent tachycardia
5. Atropine may be given to prevent episodes of bradycardia during endotracheal suctioning and physical therapy

C. Assessment findings
1. Mild sensory changes; in some clients severe misinterpretation of sensory stimuli resulting in extreme discomfort
2. Clumsiness: usually first symptom
3. Progressive motor weakness in more than one limb (classically is ascending and symmetrical)
4. Cranial nerve involvement (dysphagia)
5. Ventilatory insufficiency if paralysis ascends to respiratory muscles
6. Absence of deep tendon reflexes
7. Autonomic dysfunction
8. Diagnostic tests
   a. CSF studies: increased protein
   b. EMG: slowed nerve conduction

D. Nursing interventions
1. Maintain adequate ventilation.
   a. Monitor rate and depth of respirations; serial vital capacities.
   b. Observe for ventilatory insufficiency.
   c. Maintain mechanical ventilation as needed; keep airway free of secretions and prevent pneumonia.
2. Check individual muscle groups every 2 hours in acute phase to check for progression of muscle weakness.
3. Assess cranial nerve function: check gag reflex and swallowing ability; ability to handle secretions; voice.
4. Monitor vital signs and observe for signs of autonomic dysfunction such as acute periods of hypertension fluctuating with hypotension, tachycardia, arrhythmias.
5. Administer corticosteroids to suppress immune reaction as ordered.
6. Administer antiarrhythmic agents as ordered.
7. Prevent complications of immobility.
8. Promote comfort (especially in clients with sensory changes): foot cradle, sheepskin, guided imagery, relaxation techniques.
9. Promote optimum nutrition.

  a. Check gag reflex before feeding.
  b. Start with pureed foods.
  c. Assess need for nasogastric tube feedings if unable to swallow.
10. Provide psychologic support and encouragement to client/significant others.
11. Refer for rehabilitation to regain strength and to treat any residual deficits.

Amyotrophic Lateral Sclerosis (Lou Gehrig's Disease)

A. General information
  1. Progressive motor neuron disease, which usually leads to death in 2–6 years
  2. Onset usually between ages 40 and 70; affects men more than women
  3. Cause unknown
  4. There is no cure or specific treatment; death usually occurs as a result of respiratory infection secondary to respiratory insufficiency
B. Assessment findings
  1. Progressive weakness and atrophy of the muscles of the arms, trunk, or legs
  2. Dysarthria, dysphagia
  3. Fasciculations
  4. Respiratory insufficiency
  5. Diagnostic tests: EMG and muscle biopsy can rule out other diseases
C. Nursing interventions
  1. Provide nursing measures for muscle weakness and dysphagia.
  2. Promote adequate ventilatory function.
  3. Prevent complications of immobility.
  4. Encourage diversional activities; spend time with the client.
  5. Provide compassion and intensive support to client/significant others.
  6. Provide or refer for physical therapy as indicated.
  7. Promote independence for as long as possible.

■ DISORDERS OF THE EYE

Cataracts

A. General information
  1. Opacity of the ocular lens
  2. Incidence increases with age
  3. May be caused by changes associated with aging (''senile'' cataract); may be congenital; or may develop secondary to trauma, radiation, infection, certain drugs (corticosteroids)
B. Assessment findings
  1. Blurred vision
  2. Progressive decrease in vision
  3. Glare in bright lights

4. Pupil may develop milky-white appearance
5. Diagnostic test: ophthalmoscopic exam confirms presence of cataract

C. Nursing interventions: prepare client for cataract surgery.

Cataract Surgery

A. General information
1. Performed when client can no longer remain independent because of reduced vision
2. Surgery performed on one eye at a time; usually in a same-day surgery unit
3. Local anesthesia and intravenous sedation usually used
4. Types
   a. *Extracapsular extraction:* lens capsule is excised and the lens is expressed; posterior capsule is left in place (may be used to support new artificial lens implant).
   b. *Phacoemulsification:* a type of extracapsular extraction; a hollow needle capable of ultrasonic vibration is inserted into lens, vibrations emulsify the lens, which is then aspirated.
   c. *Intracapsular extraction:* lens is totally removed within its capsule, may be delivered from eye by cryoextraction (lens is frozen with a metal probe and removed).
5. *Peripheral iridectomy* may be performed at the time of surgery; small hole cut in iris to prevent development of secondary glaucoma
6. *Intraocular lens implant* often performed at the time of surgery.

B. Nursing interventions: preoperative
1. Assess vision in the unaffected eye since the affected eye will be patched post-op.
2. Provide pre-op teaching regarding measures to prevent increased intraocular pressure post-op.
3. Administer medications as ordered.
   a. Topical mydriatics and cycloplegics to dilate the pupil
   b. Topical antibiotics to prevent infection
   c. Acetazolamide (Diamox) and osmotic agents (oral glycerin or IV mannitol) to decrease intraocular pressure to provide a soft eyeball for surgery

C. Nursing interventions: postoperative
1. Reorient the client to surroundings.
2. Provide safety measures: elevate side rails, provide call bell, assist with ambulation when fully recovered from anesthesia.
3. Prevent increased intraocular pressure and stress on the suture line.
   a. Elevate head of bed 30–40°.
   b. Have client lie on back or unaffected side.

c. Avoid having client cough, sneeze, bend over, or move head too rapidly.
d. Treat nausea with antiemetics as ordered to prevent vomiting.
e. Give stool softeners as ordered to prevent straining.
f. Observe for and report signs of increased intraocular pressure: severe eye pain, restlessness, increased pulse.

4. Protect eye from injury.
    a. Dressings are usually removed the day after surgery.
    b. Eyeglasses or eye shield used during the day.
    c. Always use eye shield during the night.
5. Administer medications as ordered.
    a. Topical mydriatics and cycloplegics to decrease spasm of ciliary body and relieve pain
    b. Topical antibiotics and corticosteroids
    c. Mild analgesics as needed
6. Provide client teaching and discharge planning concerning
    a. Technique of eyedrop administration
    b. Use of eye shield at night
    c. No bending, stooping, or lifting
    d. Report signs or symptoms of complications immediately to physician: severe eye pain, decreased vision, excessive drainage, swelling of eyelid.
    e. Cataract glasses/contact lenses
        1) if a lens implant has not been performed, the client will need glasses or contact lenses.
        2) temporary glasses are worn for 1–4 weeks, then permanent glasses fitted.
        3) cataract glasses magnify objects by $\frac{1}{3}$ and distort peripheral vision; have client practice manual coordination with assistance until new spatial relationships become familiar; have client practice walking, using stairs, reaching for articles.
        4) contact lenses cause less distortion of vision; prescribed at one month.

Glaucoma

A. General information
1. Characterized by increased intraocular pressure resulting in progressive loss of vision; may cause blindness if not recognized and treated
2. Risk factors: age over 40, diabetes, hypertension, heredity; history of previous eye surgery, trauma, or inflammation
3. Types
    a. *Chronic (open-angle) glaucoma:* most common form, due to obstruction of the outflow of aqueous humor, in trabecular meshwork or canal of Schlemm

b. *Acute (closed-angle) glaucoma:* due to forward displacement of the iris against the cornea, obstructing the outflow of the aqueous humor; occurs suddenly and is an emergency situation; if untreated, blindness will result

c. *Chronic (closed-angle) glaucoma:* similar to acute (closed-angle) glaucoma, with the potential for an acute attack

4. Early detection is very important; regular eye exams including tonometry for persons over age 40 is recommended.

B. Medical management

1. Chronic (open-angle) glaucoma
   - a. Drug therapy: one or a combination of the following
     - 1) miotic eyedrops (pilocarpine) to increase outflow of aqueous humor
     - 2) epinephrine eyedrops to decrease aqueous humor production and increase outflow
     - 3) acetazolamide (Diamox): carbonic anhydrase inhibitor to decrease aqueous humor production
     - 4) timolol maleate (Timoptic): topical beta-adrenergic blocker to decrease intraocular pressure
   - b. Surgery (if no improvement with drugs)
     - 1) filtering procedure (trabeculectomy, trephining) to create artificial openings for the outflow of aqueous humor
     - 2) laser trabeculoplasty: noninvasive procedure performed with argon laser that can be done on an outclient basis; produces similar results as trabeculectomy
2. Acute (closed-angle) glaucoma
   - a. Drug therapy (before surgery)
     - 1) miotic eyedrops (e.g., pilocarpine) to cause pupil to contract and draw iris away from cornea
     - 2) osmotic agents (e.g., glycerin [oral], mannitol [IV]) to decrease intraocular pressure
     - 3) narcotic analgesics for pain
   - b. Surgery
     - 1) peripheral iridectomy: portion of the iris is excised to facilitate outflow of aqueous humor
     - 2) argon laser beam surgery: noninvasive procedure using laser that produces same effect as iridectomy; done on an outclient basis
     - 3) iridectomy usually performed on second eye later since a large number of clients have an acute attack in the other eye
3. Chronic (closed-angle) glaucoma
   - a. Drug therapy: miotics (pilocarpine)
   - b. Surgery: bilateral peripheral iridectomy to prevent acute attacks

C. Assessment findings
   1. Chronic (open-angle) glaucoma: symptoms develop slowly; impaired peripheral vision (tunnel vision); loss of central vision if unarrested; mild discomfort in the eyes; halos around lights
   2. Acute (closed-angle) glaucoma: severe eye pain; blurred, cloudy vision; halos around lights; nausea and vomiting; steamy cornea; moderate pupillary dilation
   3. Chronic (closed-angle) glaucoma: transient blurred vision; slight eye pain; halos around lights
   4. Diagnostic tests
      a. Visual acuity: reduced
      b. Tonometry: reading of 24–32 mmHg suggests glaucoma; may be 50 mmHg or more in acute (closed-angle) glaucoma
      c. Ophthalmoscopic exam: reveals narrowing of small vessels of optic disk, cupping of optic disk
      d. Perimetry: reveals defects in visual fields
      e. Gonioscopy: examine angle of anterior chamber

D. Nursing interventions
   1. Administer medications as ordered.
   2. Provide quiet, dark environment.
   3. Maintain accurate I&O with the use of osmotic agents.
   4. Prepare the client for surgery if indicated.
   5. Provide post-op care.
   6. Provide client teaching and discharge planning concerning
      a. Self-administration of eyedrops
      b. Need to avoid stooping, heavy lifting, or pushing, emotional upsets, excessive fluid intake, constrictive clothing around the neck
      c. Need to avoid the use of antihistamines or sympathomimetic drugs (found in cold preparations) in closed-angle glaucoma since they may cause mydriasis
      d. Importance of follow-up care
      e. Need to wear Medic-Alert tag

Detached Retina

A. General information
   1. Detachment of the sensory retina from the pigment epithelium of the retina
   2. Caused by trauma, aging process, severe myopia, postcataract extraction, severe diabetic retinopathy
   3. Pathophysiology: tear in the retina allows vitreous humor to seep behind the sensory retina and separate it from the pigment epithelium

B. Medical management
   1. Bed rest with eyes patched and detached areas dependent to prevent further detachment

2. Surgery: necessary to repair detachment
   a. *Photocoagulation:* light beam (argon laser) through dilated pupil creates an inflammatory reaction and scarring to heal the area
   b. *Cryosurgery* or *diathermy:* application of extreme cold or heat to the external globe; inflammatory reaction causes scarring and healing of area
   c. *Scleral buckling:* shortening of sclera to force pigment epithelium close to retina

C. Assessment findings
   1. Flashes of light, floaters
   2. Visual field loss, veil-like curtain coming across field of vision
   3. Diagnostic test: ophthalmoscopic examination confirms diagnosis

D. Nursing interventions: preoperative
   1. Maintain bed rest as ordered with head of bed flat and detached area in a dependent position.
   2. Use bilateral eye patches as ordered; elevate side rails to prevent injury.
   3. Identify yourself when entering the room.
   4. Orient the client frequently to time, date, and surroundings; explain procedures.
   5. Provide diversional activities to provide sensory stimulation.

E. Nursing interventions: postoperative
   1. Check orders for positioning and activity level.
      a. May be on bed rest for 1–2 days.
      b. May need to position client so that detached area is in dependent position.
   2. Administer medications as ordered: topical mydriatics, analgesics as needed.
   3. Provide client teaching and discharge planning concerning
      a. Technique of eyedrop administration
      b. Use of eye shield at night
      c. No bending from waist; no heavy work or lifting for 6 weeks
      d. Restriction of reading for 3 weeks or more
      e. May watch television
      f. Need to check with physician regarding combing and shampooing hair and shaving
      g. Need to report complications such as recurrence of detachment

Eye Injuries/Emergency Care

A. Removal of loose foreign body from conjunctiva
   1. Foreign bodies, e.g., sand, dust, may cause pain and lacrimation.
   2. Instruct client to look upward.
   3. Evert lower lid to expose the conjunctival sac.

   4. Gently remove the particle with a cotton applicator dipped in sterile normal saline using a twisting motion.
   5. If particle is not found, examine the upper lid.
   6. Place cotton applicator stick or tongue blade horizontally on outer surface of upper lid; grasp under eyelashes with fingers of other hand and pull the upper lid outward and upward over the applicator stick.
   7. Gently remove the particle as above.

B. Penetrating injuries to the eye
   1. Examples: darts, scissors, flying metal.
   2. Do not attempt to remove object.
   3. Do not allow client to apply pressure to the eye.
   4. Cover eye lightly with sterile eye patch for embedded objects, e.g., metal; apply protective shield, e.g., paper cup, for impaled objects such as darts.
   5. Cover uninjured eye to prevent excessive movement of injured eye.
   6. Refer the client to an emergency room immediately.

C. Chemical burns
   1. Flush eye immediately with copious amounts of water for 15–20 minutes.
      a. Have client hold head under faucet to let water run over eye to thoroughly wash it out; may need to forcibly separate eyelids during flush
      b. If available, flush eye with syringe
   2. After flushing, refer client to an emergency room immediately.

DISORDERS OF THE EAR

Otosclerosis

A. General information
   1. Formation of new spongy bone in the labyrinth of the ear causing fixation of the stapes in the oval window; this prevents transmission of auditory vibration to the inner ear
   2. Found more often in females
   3. Cause unknown, but there is a familial tendency

B. Medical management: stapedectomy is the procedure of choice.

C. Assessment findings
   1. Progressive loss of hearing
   2. Tinnitus
   3. Diagnostic tests
      a. Audiometry: reveals conductive hearing loss
      b. Weber's and Rinne's tests: show bone conduction is greater than air conduction

D. Nursing interventions: see Stapedectomy.

Stapedectomy

A. General information
  1. Removal of diseased portion of stapes and replacement with a prosthesis to conduct vibrations from the middle ear to inner ear; usually performed under local anesthesia
  2. Used to treat otosclerosis

B. Nursing interventions: preoperative
  1. Provide general pre-op nursing care, including an explanation of post-op expectations.
  2. Explain to the client that hearing may improve during surgery and then decrease due to edema and packing.

C. Nursing interventions: postoperative
  1. Position the client according to the surgeon's orders (possibly with operative ear uppermost to prevent displacement of the graft).
  2. Have client deep breathe every 2 hours while in bed, but no coughing.
  3. Elevate side rails; assist the client with ambulation and move slowly (may have some vertigo).
  4. Administer medications as ordered: analgesics, antibiotics, antiemetics, anti-motion-sickness drugs.
  5. Check dressings frequently for excessive drainage or bleeding.
  6. Assess facial nerve function, i.e., ask client to wrinkle forehead, close eyelids, puff out cheeks, smile and show teeth; check for any asymmetry.
  7. Question client about pain, headache, vertigo, and unusual sensations in the ear; report existence to physician.
  8. Provide client teaching and discharge planning concerning
    a. Warnings against blowing nose or coughing; sneeze with the mouth open
    b. Need to keep ear dry in the shower; no shampooing until allowed
    c. No flying for 6 months, especially if an upper respiratory tract infection is present
    d. Placement of cotton ball in auditory meatus after packing is removed; change twice a day

Ménière's Disease

A. General information
  1. Disease of the inner ear resulting from dilation of the endolymphatic system and increased volume of endolymph; characterized by recurrent and usually progressive triad of symptoms: vertigo, tinnitus, and hearing loss

2. Incidence highest between ages 30 and 60
3. Cause unknown; theories include allergy, toxicity, localized ischemia, hemorrhage, viral infection, or edema

B. Medical management
1. Acute: atropine (decreases autonomic nervous system activity), diazepam (Valium), fentanyl, and droperidol (Innovar)
2. Chronic
   a. Drug therapy: vasodilators (nicotinic acid), diuretics, mild sedatives or tranquilizers (diazepam [Valium]), antihistamines (diphenhydramine [Benadryl], meclizine [Antivert])
   b. Low-sodium diet, restricted fluid intake, restrict caffeine and nicotine.
3. Surgery
   a. Surgical destruction of labyrinth causing loss of vestibular and cochlear function (if disease is unilateral)
   b. Intracranial division of vestibular portion of cranial nerve VIII
   c. Endolymphatic sac decompression or shunt to equalize pressure in endolymphatic space

C. Assessment findings
1. Sudden attacks of vertigo lasting hours or days; attacks occur several times a year
2. Nausea, tinnitus, progressive hearing loss
3. Vomiting, nystagmus
4. Diagnostic tests
   a. Audiometry: reveals sensorineural hearing loss
   b. Vestibular tests: reveal decreased function

D. Nursing interventions
1. Maintain bed rest in a quiet, darkened room in position of choice; elevate side rails as needed.
2. Only move the client for essential care (bath may not be essential).
3. Provide an emesis basin for vomiting.
4. Monitor IV therapy; maintain accurate I&O.
5. Assist with ambulation when the attack is over.
6. Administer medications as ordered.
7. Prepare the client for surgery as indicated (post-op care includes using above measures).
8. Provide client teaching and discharge planning concerning
   a. Use of medication and side effects
   b. Low-sodium diet and decreased fluid intake
   c. Importance of eliminating smoking

REVIEW QUESTIONS

1. An adult has a medical diagnosis of increased intracranial pressure and is being cared for on the neurology unit. The nursing care plan includes elevating the head of the bed and positioning the client's head in proper alignment. The nurse recognizes that these actions are effective because they act by
   1. making it easier for the client to breathe.
   2. preventing a Valsalva maneuver.
   3. promoting venous drainage.
   4. reducing pain.
2. A client begins to have Cheyne-Stokes respirations. This type of breathing pattern is best explained as
   1. completely irregular breathing pattern with random deep and shallow respirations.
   2. prolonged inspirations with inspiratory and/or expiratory pauses.
   3. rhythmic waxing and waning of both rate and depth of respiration with brief periods of interspersed apnea.
   4. sustained, regular, rapid respirations of increased depth.
3. Which of the following reduces cerebral edema by constricting cerebral veins?
   1. Dexamethasone (Decadron).
   2. Mechanical hyperventilation.
   3. Mannitol (Osmitrol).
   4. Ventriculostomy.
4. The nurse is caring for an adult client who was admitted unconscious. The initial assessment utilized the Glasgow Coma Scale. The nurse knows that of the following, which are included when assessing a client using the Glasgow Coma Scale? Select all that apply.
   1. ______ Eye opening.
   2. ______ Motor response.
   3. ______ Pupillary reaction
   4. ______ Verbal performance.
5. An adult's Glasgow Coma Scale score is indicative of coma. Her score is
   1. 0.
   2. 2.

3. 6.
4. 10.

6. When the nurse tested an unconscious client for noxious stimuli, the client responded with decorticate rigidity or posturing. This is best described as
   1. flexion of the upper and lower extremities into a fetal-like position.
   2. rigid extension of the upper and lower extremities and plantar flexion.
   3. complete flaccidity of both upper and lower extremities and hyperextension of the neck.
   4. flexion of the upper extremities, extension of the lower extremities, and plantar flexion.
7. An adult male is receiving cryotherapy for repair of a detached retina. When taking a history from him, which symptom should the nurse expect him to have?
   1. Diplopia.
   2. Severe eye pain.
   3. Sudden blindness.
   4. Bright flashes of light.
8. An adult who has a detached retina asks the nurse what may have contributed to the development of his detached retina. The nurse explains that the client at greatest risk for development of a retinal tear usually has
   1. hypertension.
   2. nearsightedness.
   3. cranial tumors.
   4. sinusitis.
9. The nurse is explaining cryotherapy to a client who has a detached retina. The nurse should explain that the MAJOR purpose of cryotherapy in the treatment of detached retina is to
   1. create a scar that promotes healing.
   2. disintegrate debris in the eye.
   3. freeze small blood vessels.
   4. halt secretions of the lacrimal duct.
10. An adult client has a stapedectomy. Which of the following is most important for the nurse to include in the post-op care plan?
    1. Checking the gag reflex.
    2. Encouraging independence.

3. Instructing the client not to blow her nose.
4. Positioning the client on the operative side.

11. The nurse is assessing reflexes on a client. A positive Babinski's reflex is
    1. extension of the elbow and contraction of the triceps tendon.
    2. supination and flexion of the forearm.
    3. dorsiflexion of the great toe with fanning of the other toes.
    4. flexion of the arm at the antecubital fossa and contraction of the biceps.

12. The nurse is assessing the optic nerve of a client. Which of the following is a correct method to evaluate cranial nerve (CN) II, the optic nerve?
    1. Inspect the pupils for reaction.
    2. Test extraocular movements.
    3. Use of a Snellen chart.
    4. Test for a corneal reflex.

13. Which of the following tests or tools could the nurse use to assess CN VIII, the acoustic nerve?
    1. Romberg.
    2. Rosenbaum chart.
    3. Inspection of pupils.
    4. Audiometry.

14. A nurse is obtaining a Glasgow Coma Score on a client. The score is as follows:
    Best eye opening 3
    Best motor response 6
    Best verbal response 4
    The nurse interprets these findings as the client
    1. opens eyes to speech, obeys verbal commands, and is confused.
    2. opens eyes to pain, decoricates to pain, and does not speak.
    3. opens eyes to pain, no motor response, and has inappropriate speech.
    4. opens eyes spontaneously, obeys verbal commands, and is oriented × 3.

15. A nurse is preparing a client for an MRI. Which of the following conditions would *exclude* a client from an MRI?
    1. Wearing jewelry.
    2. Cardiac pacemaker.
    3. Claustrophobia.
    4. Allergy to iodine.

16. A nurse is assessing a client who has returned from a cerebral arteriogram. The left carotid was the site punctured. Which of the following indicates complications?
    1. Difficulty in swallowing.
    2. Puncture site is dry and red.
    3. BP 120/82, HR 86, RR 22.
    4. No swelling or hematoma at the site.
17. A client with a closed head injury is confused, drowsy, and has unequal pupils. Which of the following nursing diagnosis is *most important* at this time?
    1. Altered level of cognitive function.
    2. High risk for injury.
    3. Altered cerebral tissue perfusion.
    4. Sensory perceptual alteration.
18. A client is admitted with a head injury. To monitor hypothalamic function, the nurse should monitor what parameters?
    1. Temperature and urinary output.
    2. Gastric aspirate and BP.
    3. Heart rate and pupillary responses.
    4. Respiratory rate and skin integrity.
19. Which of the following is the best way for the nurse to assist a blind client in ambulation?
    1. Allow client to take nurse's arm with the nurse walking slightly ahead of the client.
    2. Allow client to walk beside the nurse with the nurse's hand on the client's back.
    3. Allow client to walk down the hall with his or her hand along the wall.
    4. Push the client in a wheelchair.
20. Which of the following is the best way for the nurse to communicate with the hearing impaired client?
    1. Talk directly into the impaired ear.
    2. Speak directly and clearly facing the person.
    3. Shout into the good ear.
    4. Write out all communication.

21. A nurse is assessing a client who is unable to extend the legs without pain, has a temperature of 103° F, and on flexion of the neck also flexes the hip and knee. Based on this assessment, the nurse suspects the client has (a)
   1. meningitis.
   2. brain abscess.
   3. brain tumor.
   4. epilepsy.
22. A client has a fever of 103° F, nuchal rigidity, pain on extension of the legs, and opisthotonos. Based on these findings, the *most important* nursing diagnosis is
   1. acute pain.
   2. ineffective tissue perfusion
   3. anxiety.
   4. risk for injury.
23. A client presents with symptoms of increased intracranial pressure, papilledema, and headache. No history of trauma is found. Vital signs are: BP 110/60, HR 80, T 98.9° F, RR 24. Based on this assessment, the nurse suspects the client has a(n)
   1. brain tumor.
   2. meningitis.
   3. skull fracture.
   4. encephalitis.
24. What should the nurse include in the plan of care for a newly admitted client with an infratentorial craniotomy for a brain tumor?
   1. Keep the head of the bed elevated 30–45° and a large pillow under the client's head and shoulder.
   2. Keep the head of the bed flat with a small pillow under the nape of the neck.
   3. Assess vital signs and pupils every four hours.
   4. Flex neck every 2 hours to prevent stiffness.
25. The home health nurse observes an aide who is transferring a client with hemiplegia from a sitting position in the bed to the wheelchair. Which action by the aide requires correction? The aide transfers the client by
   1. grasping the client's arms to pull the client to a standing position.
   2. reminding the client to lean forward before rising.
   3. moving the client toward the unaffected side.
   4. bracing the affected knee and foot to assist the client to stand.

26. When comparing a cerebrovascular accident (CVA) to a transient ischemic attack (TIA), the nurse understands that a TIA is

1. permanent with long-term focal deficits.

2. intermittent with spontaneous resolution of the neurologic deficit.

3. intermittent with permanent motor and sensory deficits.

4. permanent with no long-term neurologic deficits.

27. The nurse is teaching a client with transient ischemic attacks about aspirin therapy. Which statement by the client indicates understanding of the reason for his aspirin therapy?

1. "I must take the aspirin regularly to prevent the headache that many people have with this disorder."

2. "If I take aspirin, I am less likely to develop bleeding in my brain."

3. "The aspirin will help to prevent me from having a stroke."

4. "Taking aspirin regularly will reduce my chances of having a heart attack."

28. A client with Parkinson's disease is receiving combination therapy with levodopa (L-dopa) and carbidopa (Sinemet). Which of the following manifestations indicates to the nurse that an adverse drug reaction is occurring?

1. Involuntary head movement.

2. Bradykinesia.

3. Shuffling gait.

4. Depression.

29. A nurse is teaching the family of a client with Parkinson's disease. Which of the following statements by the family reflects a need for more education?

1. "We can buy lots of soups for Dad."

2. "We are teaching Dad posture exercises."

3. "Dad is going to do his range of motion (ROM) exercises three times a day."

4. "The bath bars will be installed before Dad comes home."

30. A 36-year-old female reports double vision, visual loss, weakness, numbness of the hands, fatigue, tremors, and incontinence. On assessment, the nurse notes nystagmus, scanning speech, ataxia, and muscular weakness. Based on these findings, the nurse suspects the client has

1. Parkinson's disease.

2. myasthenia gravis (MG).

3. amyotrophic lateral sclerosis (ALS).
4. multiple sclerosis (MS).

31. Which nursing diagnosis is of the *highest priority* when caring for a client with myasthenia gravis (MG)?
    1. Pain.
    2. Risk for injury.
    3. Ineffective coping.
    4. Ineffective airway clearance.

32. The nurse has explained the use of neostigmine methylsulfate (Prostigmin) to a client with myasthenia gravis. Which comment by the client indicates the need for further instruction?
    1. "I need to take the medication regularly, even when I feel strong."
    2. "I should take the medication once daily at bedtime."
    3. "If I take too much medication, I can become weak and have breathing problems."
    4. "I may have difficulty swallowing my saliva if I take too much medication."

33. A nurse is assessing a client with a head injury. The client has clear drainage from the nose and ears. How can the nurse determine if the drainage is cerebrospinal fluid (CSF)?
    1. Measure the pH of the fluid.
    2. Measure the specific gravity of the fluid.
    3. Test for glucose.
    4. Test for chloride.

34. The nurse is caring for a confused client who sustained a head injury resulting in a subdural hematoma. The client's blood pressure is 100/60 mmHg and he is unresponsive. Select the most effective position for the client as the nurse transports him to the operating room.
    1. Semi-Fowler's.
    2. Trendelenburg.
    3. High-Fowler's.
    4. Supine.

35. A client who has been treated in the emergency room for a head injury is preparing for discharge. The nurse is teaching the family about the signs of complications that may occur within the first 24 hours and the appropriate action to take if a complication is suspected. Which statement by the client's spouse would require further teaching by the nurse?

1. "I'm not looking forward to checking on my husband all night long."
2. "If he can just get a long nap, I'm sure that my husband will be fine."
3. "I'll call the doctor immediately if my husband starts to vomit."
4. "If my husband has trouble talking, I'll bring him to the hospital."

36. A client is admitted postcraniotomy. Decadron 4 mg IV is ordered every 6 hours. The nurse understands the Decadron is ordered to
    1. stabilize the blood sugar.
    2. decrease cerebral edema.
    3. prevent seizures.
    4. maintain the integrity of the gastric mucosa.

37. A client is admitted with a C7 complete transection. In the *immediate* postinjury period, the nurse must plan for
    1. bladder and bowel training.
    2. possible ventilatory support.
    3. complications of autonomic dysreflexia.
    4. diaphragmatic pacing.

38. A client fell backward over a stair rail to the floor below and is not breathing. After calling for assistance, how should the nurse proceed?
    1. Initiate rescue breathing by performing a chin tilt maneuver and administering two breaths.
    2. After determining absence of breathing, administer 15 chest compressions at the rate of 60 per minute.
    3. Initiate rescue breathing by performing a jaw thrust maneuver and administering two breaths.
    4. After determining pulselessness, administer five chest compressions at the rate of 60 per minute.

39. A client with a cervical spine injury was placed in Halo traction yesterday. When the client complains of discomfort around the pins, what action should the nurse take?
    1. Carefully loosen the pins and notify the physician immediately.
    2. Cleanse the skin around the pin sites and dry the area thoroughly.
    3. Give the ordered analgesic and reassure the client that the pain is temporary.
    4. Loosen the pins immediately and maintain the head in a neutral position.

40. A client with a C6 spinal cord injury 2 months ago now complains of a pounding headache. The pulse is 64 and the blood pressure is 220/110 mmHg. Which of the following actions should the nurse take first?

1. Give the analgesic as ordered.
2. Check for fecal impaction.
3. Elevate the client's head and lower the legs.
4. Notify the physician.

41. The nurse is evaluating the ability of a client with trigeminal neuralgia to implement the treatment that has been suggested. Which of the following behaviors by the client will be most effective in controlling manifestations? The client

1. exercises the facial muscles at least twice daily.
2. puts the affected arm through full range of motion daily.
3. avoids extremes in temperature of food and drink.
4. uses proper body mechanics in sitting and bending.

42. A client with Bell's palsy asks the nurse why artificial tears were ordered by the physician. Select the best reply by the nurse.

1. "When your affected eye fails to make tears, the eye can become irritated and ulcerated."
2. "Because your eye remains closed, foreign matter can be trapped beneath the lid."
3. "Artificial tears will remove the purulent drainage from your eye, which speeds healing."
4. "Because you cannot blink the affected eye, it can become dry and irritated."

43. A nurse is caring for a client with Guillain-Barré syndrome. Which of the following strategies is of the *most importance* in the plan of care?

1. Range of motion exercises three to four times per day.
2. Frequent measurement of vital capacity.
3. Use of artificial tears.
4. Starting an enteral feeding.

44. The nurse has presented information about amyotrophic lateral sclerosis (ALS) to a newly diagnosed client. Which question by the client indicates that he understands the nature of the disease?

1. "How can I avoid infecting my family with the virus?"
2. "How can I execute a living will?"
3. "How can I prevent an exacerbation of the disease?"
4. "How many people achieve remission with chemotherapy?"

45. A client reports gradual painless blurring of vision. On assessment, the nurse notes a cloudy opaque lens. Based on this assessment, the nurse suspects the client has

1. glaucoma.

2. cataracts.

3. retinal detachment.

4. diabetic retinopathy.

46. Which of the following risk factors would the nurse assess for in a client with glaucoma?

1. Family history, increased intraocular pressure, and age of 45–65.

2. History of diabetes and age greater than 50.

3. Female gender, cigarette smoking, age greater than 65.

4. Myopia, history of diabetes, and sudden severe physical exertion.

47. The nurse has been planning for home care with the family of a client who will undergo extracapsular lens extraction with an intraocular lens implant. Because the client and family speak very little English, the nurse takes extra care to evaluate their understanding. Which behavior by the client and/or family shows progress in understanding post-op home care instructions?

1. Using a chart showing various sleeping positions, the client points to a person lying on the affected side.

2. The family demonstrates that the eye should be cleaned with a washcloth, soap, and water.

3. The client demonstrates medication instillation by carefully dropping the solution on the cornea.

4. The family shows the nurse the sunglasses they have purchased for the client to wear post-op.

48. A nurse is admitting a client who reports vision loss. To determine if a client has glaucoma or a detached retina, the nurse understands that a client with glaucoma will report

1. seeing floating spots.

2. eye pain.

3. seeing flashing lights.

4. sudden loss of vision.

49. Which of the following techniques should the nurse use to evaluate a client's understanding of self-care for chronic (primary) open-angle glaucoma?

1. The nurse measures the client's blood pressure at each visit.
2. The nurse measures hearing acuity at each visit.
3. The nurse observes the client's technique for monitoring blood glucose.
4. The nurse observes the client's administration of eye drops.

50. A client is admitted with a detached retina of the left eye. The nurse patches both eyes. What is the rationale for patching both eyes?

1. To prevent eye infections.
2. To decrease eye movement.
3. To prevent photophobia.
4. To prevent nystagmus.

51. A neighbor splashes chlorine bleach in her eyes and calls the nurse for immediate help. The *first* action the nurse should take is to

1. lift the upper lid over the lower lid of each eye.
2. close and patch both eyes with a loose bandage.
3. continuously flush the eyes with tap water for 20 minutes.
4. instill an over-the-counter anti-irritant solution, such as Visine.

52. A client reports bilateral hearing loss. On assessment of the ear, the nurse observes chalky white plaques on the eardrum and the eardrum appears pinkish orange in color. The Rinne test favors bone conduction. Based on this assessment, the nurse suspects the client has (a)

1. cholesteatoma.
2. actinic keratosis.
3. external otitis.
4. otosclerosis.

53. The nurse is teaching a post-op stapedectomy client. What should be included in the teaching?

1. Work can be resumed the next day.
2. Gently sneeze or cough with the mouth closed.
3. Blow the nose gently one side at a time.
4. Resume exercise in one week.

54. A client reports very loud, overpowering ringing in the ears, fluctuating hearing loss on the right side with severe vertigo accompanied by nausea and vomiting, and a feeling of fullness in the right ear. The nurse suspects the client has (a)

1. Ménière's disease.
2. acoustic neuroma.

3. otosclerosis.
4. cholesteatoma.

55. What is the *priority* nursing diagnosis for a client with very loud overpowering ringing in his ears, fluctuating hearing loss on the right side with severe vertigo accompanied by nausea and vomiting and a feeling of fullness in the right ear?
    1. Knowledge deficit related to the disease process.
    2. Anxiety.
    3. Impaired physical mobility.
    4. Pain.

ANSWERS AND RATIONALES

1. 3. It has been demonstrated that positioning the client with the head elevated to 30° decreases ICP by promoting venous drainage from the head by gravity. Pronounced angulation of the head can obstruct venous return and increase ICP.

2. 3. Cheynes-Stokes respirations are a pattern of breathing in which phases of hyperapnea regularly alternate with apnea. The pattern waxes (crescendo) and wanes (decrescendo).

3. 2. Mechanical hyperventilation to reduce CO_2 levels to 25 mmHg produces cerebral vasoconstriction and thereby decreases ICP.

4. *Eye opening* should be selected. The Glasgow Coma Scale is a practical scale that independently evaluates three features: eye opening, motor response in the upper limb, and verbal performance.

   Motor response should be selected. The Glasgow Coma Scale is a practical scale that independently evaluates three features: eye opening, motor response in the upper limb, and verbal performance.

   Verbal performance should be selected. The Glasgow Coma Scale is a practical scale that independently evaluates three features: eye opening, motor response in the upper limb, and verbal performance.

5. 4. A score of 7 or less defines coma. The lowest achievable score is 3, which indicates deep coma. Fifteen is a perfect score.

6. 4. Decorticate rigidity or posturing is best described as an abnormal flexor response in the arm with extension and plantar flexion in the lower extremities.

7. 4. Momentary bright flashes of light are a common symptom of retinal detachment.

8. 2. Myopia or nearsightedness is a predisposing factor in the development of a retinal tear.
9. 1. Cryotherapy is used to produce a chorioretinal adhesion or scar that allows the retina to return to its normal position.
10. 3. The client should be taught to avoid blowing the nose because this action could increase the pressure in the eustachian tube and dislodge the surgical graft.
11. 3. It is abnormal in an adult. It signifies an upper motor neuron lesion. The response describes the Babinski reflex.
12. 3. To correctly test cranial nerve II, the optic nerve, use a Snellen chart to assess visual acuity.
13. 4. An audiometry test tests different pitches and sounds.
14. 1. 3 points are given for opening eyes to speech, 6 points are given for obeying verbal commands related to motor response, and 4 points are given for best verbal response when client is confused.
15. 2. Pacemakers and cerebral aneurysm clips are the exclusions for an MRI.
16. 1. Difficulty swallowing occurs from a hematoma developing and pushing on the trachea.
17. 3. The client is manifesting symptoms of increased intracranial pressure.
18. 1. Increased intracranial pressure causes hypothalamic dysfunction creating hypo/hyperthermia, SIADH, and diabetes insipidus. The hypothalamus regulates body temperature, osmolality of body fluids, hunger, and satiety.
19. 1. This method allows the client to have a feeling of control.
20. 2. Facing the person and speaking clearly is the best way to communicate with the hearing impaired.
21. 1. These are some of the symptoms of meningitis.
22. 2. The ineffective tissue perfusion is related to the increased intracranial pressure and inflammatory process.
23. 1. These findings are consistent with a brain tumor.
24. 2. This is the correct position for an infratentorial approach.
25. 1. Pulling the client's paralyzed arm can result in shoulder subluxation and pain. The client's unaffected hand must be free to reach for the arm of the wheelchair.
26. 2. A TIA is a temporary loss of function due to cerebral ischemia.
27. 3. Platelet-inhibiting drugs such as aspirin are taken prophylactically to prevent cerebral infarction secondary to embolism and thrombosis.

28. 4. Depression, confusion, and hallucinations are adverse effects that can occur after prolonged use of L-dopa. A "drug holiday" under medical supervision may restore drug effectiveness.

29. 1. The client should have semisolid, thickened food. Soup is thin in texture and could be aspirated by the client.

30. 4. These are the symptoms of MS, which is more common in women ages 20–40.

31. 4. Clients with MG have respiratory muscle failure.

32. 2. The client is confused about the timing of medication administration. The anticholinesterase medication should be taken 30 minutes prior to meals to enhance the muscle strength needed for chewing and swallowing.

33. 3. Cerebrospinal fluid is positive for glucose.

34. 1. The client's head should be elevated about 30° to lower the intracranial pressure, which may be dangerously elevated in a subdural hematoma. The venous blood pressure begins to decline as intracranial pressure rises.

35. 2. The wife may not understand that she must interrupt the client's sleep to detect early signs of increased intracranial pressure caused by contusion or hematoma development.

36. 2. Cerebral edema is common after surgery. Decadron (a corticosteroid) is given to decrease the edema.

37. 2. Edema above the area of the lesion can cause respiratory depression and arrest.

38. 3. When initiating rescue breathing for a client with a suspected spinal injury, the jaw thrust maneuver is used with rescue breathing at the rate of 12 breaths per minute.

39. 3. Discomfort at the pin sites is expected for several days after application of the Halo device. The pain can be controlled with mild analgesic medication. The client can benefit from the reassurance that the pain will not continue for the weeks that the traction will be in place.

40. 3. The client is showing signs of autonomic dysreflexia. Placing the client in a sitting position will allow blood to pool in the legs, which should lower the blood pressure and prevent possible hypertensive hemorrhage.

41. 3. Extremes of temperature of food or drink can trigger paroxysms of severe facial pain along the pathways of the trigeminal nerve. Meals are better tolerated if served at room temperature.

42. 4. Bell's palsy may cause paralysis of the eyelid and loss of the blink reflex on the affected side. The eye may not close completely. These problems render the eye susceptible to drying and irritation from dust or other debris.

43. 2. Clients with Guillain-Barré have respiratory muscle weakness and respiratory failure.

44. 2. Clients with ALS often experience respiratory failure as the disease progresses and need to communicate their wishes regarding ventilator support. The nurse should explore the client's wishes and facilitate discussion within the family. Arranging for the client to sign a living will, if the client wishes to do so, is also a nursing responsibility.

45. 2. These are the assessment findings of cataracts.

46. 1. These are common risk factors for glaucoma.

47. 4. Sunglasses should be worn post-op for comfort and protection when outdoors.

48. 2. Eye pain is present with open- and narrow-angle glaucoma, but not with a detached retina.

49. 4. Glaucoma is usually treated with eye drops, such as betaxolol (Timoptic), a beta-adrenergic antagonist. The eye can be damaged when eye drops are used incorrectly.

50. 2. Eye movements can increase the amount of detachment.

51. 3. Immediate irrigation with copious amounts of water or normal saline solution may reduce alkaline burns of the cornea and conjunctiva. Any delay in initiating the irrigation can result in serious damage to eye structures.

52. 4. These are classic signs of otosclerosis.

53. 3. The client should blow the nose gently one side at a time to prevent pressure changes in the ear.

54. 1. These are classic signs of Ménière's disease.

55. 1. This client most likely has Ménière's disease. In Ménière's disease, client education is paramount. The client needs to be taught that with the increased volume of hydrolymph, excessive fluid intake increases the volume even more and exacerbates the disease. They should also be taught not to ambulate or make extreme movements during the acute attacks.

6

The Cardiovascular System

OVERVIEW OF ANATOMY AND PHYSIOLOGY

The cardiovascular system consists of the heart, arteries, veins, and capillaries. The major functions are circulation of blood, delivery of oxygen and other nutrients to the tissues of the body, and removal of carbon dioxide and other products of cellular metabolism.

CHAPTER OUTLINE

Heart

The heart is a muscular pump that propels blood into the arterial system and receives blood from the venous system.

Heart Wall

A. *Pericardium:* composed of fibrous (outermost layer) and serous pericardium (parietal and visceral); a sac that functions to protect the heart from friction.
B. *Epicardium:* covers surface of heart, becomes continuous with visceral layer of serous pericardium.
C. *Myocardium:* middle, muscular layer.
D. *Endocardium:* thin, inner membranous layer lining the chambers of the heart.
E. *Papillary muscles:* arise from the endocardial and myocardial surface of the ventricles and attach to the chordae tendinae.
F. *Chordae tendinae:* attach to the tricuspid and mitral valves and prevent eversion during systole.

Chambers

A. *Atria:* two chambers, function as receiving chambers, lie above the ventricles
   1. Right atrium: receives systemic venous blood through the superior vena cava, inferior vena cava, and coronary sinus.

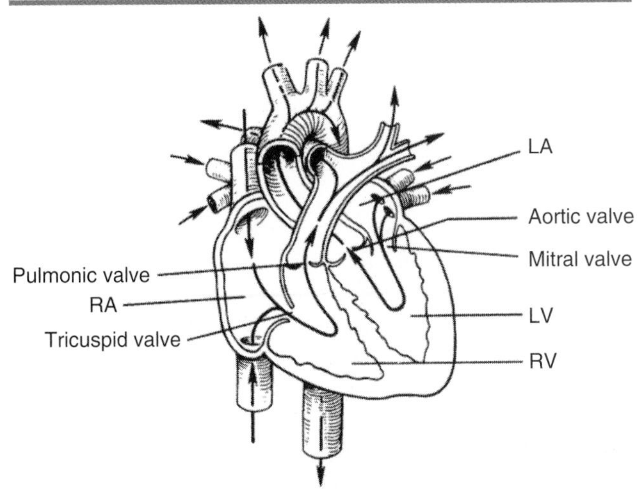

FIGURE 6-1 The valves of the heart; arrows indicate the direction of blood flow.

2. Left atrium: receives oxygenated blood returning to the heart from the lungs through the pulmonary veins.

B. *Ventricles:* two thick-walled chambers; major responsibility for forcing blood out of the heart; lie below the atria.

1. Right ventricle: contracts and propels deoxygenated blood into the pulmonary circulation via the pulmonary artery.
2. Left ventricle: propels blood into the systemic circulation via the aorta during ventricular systole.

Valves

See Figure 6-1.

A. Atrioventricular (AV) valves

1. *Mitral valve:* located between the left atrium and left ventricle; contains two leaflets attached to the chordae tendinae.
2. *Tricuspid valve:* located between the right atrium and right ventricle; contains three leaflets attached to the chordae tendinae.
3. Functions
   a. Permit unidirectional flow of blood from specific atrium to specific ventricle during ventricular diastole.
   b. Prevent reflux flow during ventricular systole.
   c. Valve leaflets open during ventricular diastole and close during ventricular systole; valve closure produces *first heart sound* (S_1).

B. Semilunar valves

1. *Pulmonary valve:* located between right ventricle and pulmonary artery
2. *Aortic valve:* located between left ventricle and aorta
3. Functions

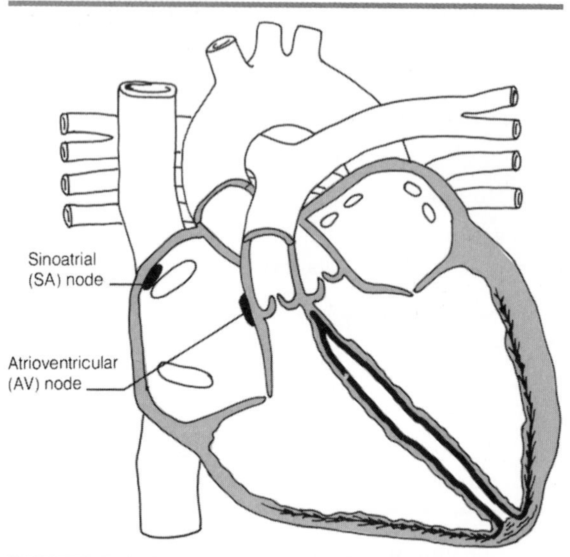

FIGURE 6-2
Conduction system of the heart

a. Permit unidirectional flow of blood from specific ventricle to arterial vessel during ventricular systole.
b. Prevent reflux blood flow during ventricular diastole.
c. Valves open when ventricles contract and close during ventricular diastole; valve closure produces *second heart sound* (S_2).

Conduction System

See Figure 6-2.

A. *Sinoatrial (SA) node:* the pacemaker of the heart; initiates the cardiac impulse, which spreads across the atria and into AV node.
B. *Atrioventricular (AV) node:* delays the impulse from the atria while the ventricles fill.
C. *Bundle of His:* arises from the AV node and conducts impulse to the bundle branch system.
   1. Right bundle branch: divided into anterior, lateral, and posterior; transmits impulses down the right side of the interventricular septum toward the right ventricular myocardium
   2. Left bundle branch: divided into anterior and posterior
      a. Anterior portion transmits impulses to the anterior endocardial surface of the left ventricle.
      b. Posterior portion transmits impulses over the posterior and inferior endocardial surfaces of the left ventricle.
D. *Purkinje fibers:* transmit impulses to the ventricles and provide for depolarization after ventricular contraction.

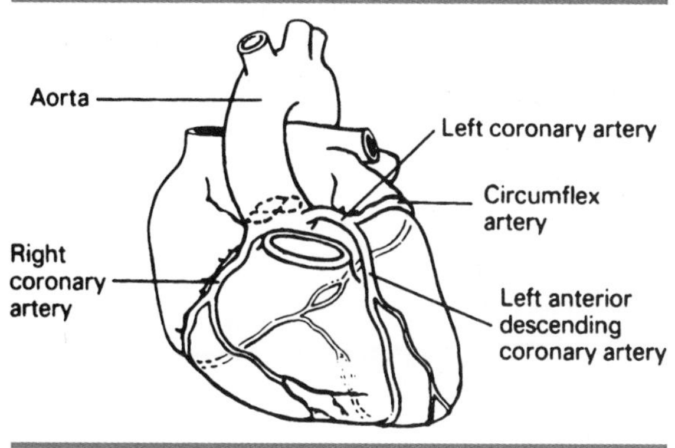

FIGURE 6-3 Coronary circulation

E. Electrical activity of heart can be visualized by attaching electrodes to the skin and recording activity by electrocardiograph.

Coronary Circulation

See Figure 6-3.

A. Coronary arteries: branch off at the base of the aorta and supply blood to the myocardium and the conduction system; two main coronary arteries are *right* and *left.*

B. Coronary veins: return blood from the myocardium back to the right atrium via the coronary sinus.

Vascular System

The major function of the blood vessels is to supply the tissues with blood, remove wastes, and carry unoxygenated blood back to the heart.

Types of Blood Vessels

A. *Arteries:* elastic-walled vessels that can stretch during systole and recoil during diastole; they carry blood away from the heart and distribute oxygenated blood throughout the body.

B. *Arterioles:* small arteries that distribute blood to the capillaries and function in controlling systemic vascular resistance and, therefore, arterial pressure.

C. *Capillaries:* the following exchanges occur in the capillaries

1. Oxygen and carbon dioxide
2. Solutes between the blood and tissues
3. Fluid volume transfer between the plasma and interstitial spaces

D. *Venules:* small veins that receive blood from the capillaries and function as collecting channels between the capillaries and veins.

E. *Veins:* low-pressure vessels with thin walls and less muscle than arteries; most contain valves that prevent retrograde blood flow; they carry deoxygenated blood back to the heart. When skeletal muscles surrounding veins contract, the veins are compressed, promoting movement of blood back to the heart.

ASSESSMENT

Health History

A. Presenting problem
   1. Nonspecific symptoms may include fatigue, shortness of breath, cough, dizziness, syncope, headache, palpitations, weight loss/gain, anorexia, difficulty sleeping.
   2. Specific signs and symptoms
      a. Chest pain: note character, quality, location, radiation, frequency, and whether it is associated with precipitating factors (exertion, eating, excitement).
      b. Dyspnea (shortness of breath): note kind and extent of precipitating activities.
      c. Orthopnea (form of dyspnea that develops when client lies down): determine how many pillows are used when sleeping; note any paroxysmal nocturnal dyspnea (PND) (client awakens suddenly in the night, breathing with difficulty).
      d. Palpitations (awareness of heartbeat, fluttering feeling): assess precipitating factors (anxiety, caffeine, nicotine, stress); ask client to tap out the rhythm.
      e. Edema (abnormal accumulation of fluid in tissues): note whether unilateral/bilateral, location, time of day when most apparent.
      f. Cyanosis (dusky, bluish coloration to the skin): note whether peripheral or central.

B. Lifestyle: occupation, hobbies, financial status, stressors, unusual life patterns, relaxation time, exercise, living conditions, smoking, sleep habits

C. Use of medications: OTC drugs, cardiac drugs, oral contraceptives, or estrogen replacement therapy

D. Personality profile: Type A, manic-depressive, anxieties

E. Nutrition: dietary habits; calorie, cholesterol, salt intake; alcohol consumption

F. Past medical history
   1. Heart murmurs, rheumatic fever, sexually transmitted diseases, angina, myocardial infarction (MI), hypertension, CVA, alcoholism, obesity, hyperlipidemia, varicose veins, claudication
   2. Pregnancies, contraceptive use

G. Family history: heart disease (congenital, acute, chronic); risk factors (diabetes, hypertension, obesity)

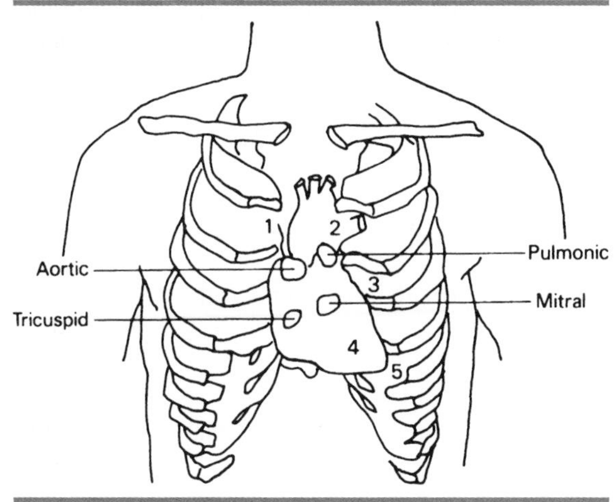

FIGURE 6-4 Heart valves and areas of auscultation: (1) aortic area; (2) pulmonic area; (3) Erb's point; (4) tricuspid area; (5) mitral area

Physical Examination

A. Skin and mucous membranes: note color/texture, temperature, hair distribution on extremities, atrophy or edema, venous pattern, petechiae, lesions, ulcerations or gangrene; examine nails.

B. Peripheral pulses: palpate and rate all arterial pulses (temporal, carotid, brachial, radial, femoral, popliteal, dorsalis pedis, and posterior tibial) on scale of: 0 = absent, 1 = palpable, 2 = normal, 3 = full, 4 = full and bounding.

C. Assess for arterial insufficiency and venous impairment.

D. Measure and record blood pressure.

E. Inspect and palpate the neck vessels.

1. Jugular veins: note location, characteristics; measure jugular venous pressure.
2. Carotid arteries: note location, characteristics

F. Precordium

1. Inspect and palpate sternoclavicular, aortic, pulmonic, Erb's point, tricuspid, apical, epigastric sites.
2. Note point of maximum impulse (PMI), pulsations, thrills.

G. Auscultate aortic, pulmonic, Erb's point, tricuspid, mitral or apical, xiphoid areas; note heart rate and rhythm (see Figure 6-4).

1. Normal heart sounds (S_1 and S_2): note location, intensity, splitting.
2. Abnormal heart sounds (S_3, S_4): note location, occurrence in cardiac cycle
3. Murmurs: note location, occurrence in cardiac cycle
4. Friction rubs

Laboratory/Diagnostic Tests

A. Blood chemistry and electrolyte analysis
   1. Serial cardiac enzymes (protein assays) will be evaluated with symptoms of acute coronary syndrome, chest pain/ischemia with and without infection, congestive heart failure, area post cardiac surgical intervention, and post chest trauma.
      a. Nonspecific enzymes, elevated in myocardial injury and with other systems:
         1) creatine kinase (CK); normally 50–325 mU/ml
         2) myoglobin
         3) LDH
         4) AST (SGOT); normally 7–40 U/ml
      b. Specific cardiac isoenzymes, elevated in myocardial injury:
         1) creatine kinase-MB (CKMB); normally 0%
         2) LDH_1 and LDH_2
         3) troponin I or cardiac troponin T (currently used in place of LDH isoenzymes)
      c. Specific enzymes, elevations correlated with vascular inflammation, irritability of atherosclerotic plaque, and future coronary risk:
         1) ischemic modified albumin (IMA)
         2) serum lipids (HDLs, LDLs, VDRLs)
         3) C-reactive protein (CRP)
         4) lipoprotein phospholipase A2 (PLAQ test)
      d. Specific cardiac proteins, elevated in congestive heart failure:
         1) B-type natriuretic peptide and N-terminal proB-type natriuretic peptide (BNP)

B. Hematologic studies
   1. CBC (see Hematologic system for values)
   2. Coagulation time: 5–15 min.; increased levels indicate bleeding tendency, used to monitor heparin therapy
   3. Prothrombin time (PT) 9.5–12 sec.; INR 1.0, increased levels indicate bleeding tendency, used to monitor warfarin therapy
   4. Activated partial thromboplastin time (APTT) 20–45 sec., increased levels indicate bleeding tendency, used to monitor heparin therapy
   5. Erythrocyte sedimentation rate (ESR) <20 mm/hr; increased level indicate inflammatory process

C. Urine studies: routine urinalysis

D. Electrocardiogram (ECG or EKG)
   1. Noninvasive test that produces a graphic record of the electrical activity of the heart. In addition to determining cardiac rhythm, pattern variations may reveal pathologic processes (MI and ischemia, electrolyte and acid-base imbalance, chamber enlargement, block of the right or left bundle branch).

2. Portable recorder (Holter monitor) provides continuous recording of ECG for up to 24 hours; client keeps a diary noting presence of symptoms or any unusual activities.

E. Stress tests may show heart disease when resting ECG does not. Stress test types:
   1. Exercise: treadmill or bicycle
   2. Chemical: Persantine, Dobutamine

F. Cardiac nuclear scan: Radionucleotide imaging to identify ischemic/ infracted tissue.

G. *Phonocardiogram:* noninvasive device to amplify and record heart sounds and murmurs.

H. *Echocardiogram:* noninvasive recording of the cardiac structures using ultrasound.

I. *Cardiac catheterization:* invasive, but often definitive test for diagnosis of cardiac disease.
   1. A catheter is inserted into the right or left side of the heart to obtain information.
      a. Right-sided catheterization: the catheter is inserted into an antecubital vein and advanced into the vena cava, right atrium, and right ventricle with further insertion into the pulmonary artery.
      b. Left-sided catheterization: performed by inserting the catheter into a brachial or femoral artery; the catheter is passed retrograde up the aorta and into the left ventricle.
   2. Purpose: to measure intracardiac pressures and oxygen levels in various parts of the heart; with injection of a dye, it allows visualization of the heart chambers, blood vessels, and course of blood flow (*angiography*).
   3. Nursing care: pretest
      a. Confirm that informed consent has been signed.
      b. Ask about allergies, particularly to iodine, if dye being used.
      c. Keep client NPO for 8–12 hours prior to test.
      d. Record height and weight, take baseline vital signs, and monitor peripheral pulses.
      e. Inform client that a feeling of warmth and fluttering sensation as catheter is passed is common.
   4. Nursing care: posttest
      a. Assess circulation to the extremity used for catheter insertion.
      b. Check peripheral pulses, color, sensation of affected extremity every 15 minutes for 4 hours.
      c. If protocol requires, keep affected extremity straight for approximately 8 hours.
      d. Observe catheter insertion site for swelling and bleeding; a sandbag or pressure dressing may be placed over insertion site.
      e. Assess vital signs and report significant changes from baseline.

J. *Aortography*

1. Injection of radiopaque contrast medium into the aorta to visualize the aorta, valve leaflets, and major vessels on a movie film.
2. Purpose: to determine and diagnose aortic valve incompetence, aneurysms of the ascending aorta, abnormalities of major branches of the aorta.
3. Nursing care: pretest
   - **a.** Confirm that informed consent has been signed.
   - **b.** Inform client that a dye will be injected and to report any dyspnea, numbness, or tingling.
4. Nursing care: posttest
   - **a.** Assess the puncture site frequently for bleeding or inflammation.
   - **b.** Assess peripheral pulses distal to the injection site every hour for 4–8 hours posttest.

K. *Coronary arteriography*

1. Visualization of coronary arteries by injection of radiopaque contrast dye and recording on a movie film.
2. Purpose: evaluation of heart disease and angina, location of areas of infarction and extent of lesions, ruling out coronary artery disease in clients with myocardial disease.
3. Nursing care: same as for Aortography (above).

ANALYSIS

Nursing diagnoses for the client with a cardiovascular dysfunction may include

A. Excess fluid volume
B. Decreased cardiac output
C. Ineffective tissue perfusion
D. Impairment of skin integrity
E. Activity intolerance
F. Pain
G. Ineffective individual coping
H. Fear
I. Anxiety

PLANNING AND IMPLEMENTATION

Goals

A. Fluid imbalance will be resolved, edema minimized.
B. Cardiac output will be improved.
C. Cardiopulmonary and peripheral tissue perfusion will be improved.
D. Adequate skin integrity will be maintained.
E. Activity tolerance will progressively increase.
F. Pain in the chest or in the affected extremity will be diminished.
G. Client will use effective coping techniques.
H. Client's level of fear and anxiety will be decreased.

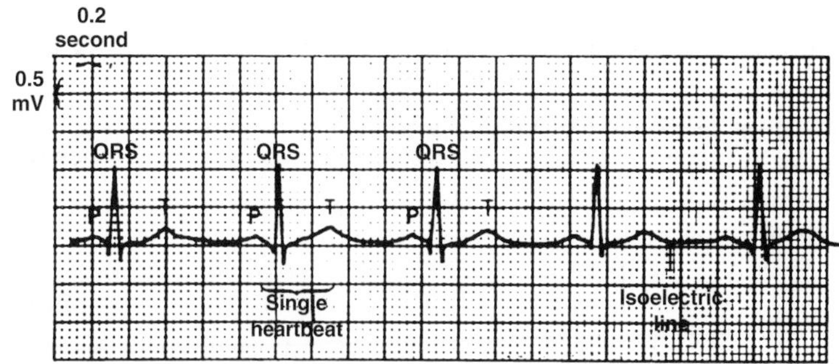

FIGURE 6-5 A typical ECG; all beats appear as a similar pattern, equally spaced, and have three major units: P wave, QRS complex, and T wave.

Interventions

Cardiac Monitoring

A. The cardiac monitor provides continuous information regarding the cardiac rhythm and rate (ECG). Constant surveillance and understanding of the basic electrocardiographic system is imperative to avoid/treat arrhythmias (see Figure 6-5).

1. ECG strip: each small square represents 0.04 second, each large square 0.2 second.
2. P wave: produced by atrial depolarization; indicates SA node function.
3. P-R interval
   - **a.** Indicates atrioventricular conduction time or the time it takes an impulse to travel from the atria down and through the AV node
   - **b.** Measured from beginning of P wave to beginning of QRS complex
   - **c.** Normal: 0.12–0.20 second.
4. QRS complex
   - **a.** Indicates ventricular depolarization
   - **b.** Measured from onset of Q wave to end of S wave
   - **c.** Normal: 0.06–0.10 seconds
5. ST segment
   - **a.** Indicates time interval between complete depolarization of ventricles and repolarization of ventricles
   - **b.** Measured after QRS complex to beginning of T wave
6. T wave
   - **a.** Represents ventricular repolarization
   - **b.** Follows ST segment

Hemodynamic Monitoring (Swan-Ganz Catheter)

A. A pulmonary artery (PA) catheter with a balloon tip that is advanced through the superior vena cava into the right atrium, right ventricle, and pulmonary artery. When it is wedged it is in the distal arterial branch of the pulmonary artery.

B. Purposes

1. Proximal port: measures right atrial pressure
2. Distal port
   a. Measures pulmonary artery (PA) pressure (reflects left and right heart pressures) and pulmonary capillary wedge pressure (PCWP) (reflects left atrial and left ventricular end diastolic pressure)
   b. Normal values: PA systolic 15–30 mmHg and diastolic 4–12 mmHg; PCWP 6–12 mmHg
3. Balloon port: inflated with 1–1.5 cc air to obtain PCWP
4. Thermistor lumen: used to measure cardiac output if ordered

C. Nursing care

1. A sterile dry dressing should be applied to site and changed every 24 hours; inspect site daily and report signs of infection.
2. If catheter is inserted via an extremity, immobilize extremity to prevent catheter dislodgment or trauma.
3. Observe catheter site for leakage.
4. Ensure that balloon is deflated with a syringe attached, except when PCWP is read.
5. Continuously monitor PA systolic and diastolic pressures and report significant variations.
6. Maintain client in same position for each reading.
7. Maintain pressure bag at 300 mmHg.
8. Record PA systolic and diastolic readings at least every hour and PCWP as ordered, noting position of client.

Central Venous Pressure (CVP)

A. Obtained by inserting a catheter into the external jugular, antecubital, or femoral vein and threading it into the vena cava. The catheter is attached to an IV infusion and H_2O manometer by a three-way stopcock or electronic transducer.

B. Purposes

1. Reveals right atrial pressure, reflecting alterations in the right ventricular pressure
2. Provides information concerning blood volume and adequacy of central venous return
3. Provides an IV route for drawing blood samples, administering fluids or medication, and possibly inserting a pacing catheter

C. Normal range is 4–10 cm H_2O or 2–6 mmHg; elevation indicates hypervolemia, decreased level indicates hypovolemia.

D. Nursing care

1. Ensure client is relaxed.

2. Maintain zero point of manometer always at level of right atrium (midaxillary line).
3. Determine patency of catheter by opening IV infusion line.
4. Turn stopcock to allow IV solution to run into manometer to a level of 10–20 cm above expected pressure reading.
5. Turn stopcock to allow IV solution to flow from manometer into catheter; fluid level in manometer fluctuates with respiration.
6. Stop ventilatory assistance during measurement of CVP.
7. After CVP reading, return stopcock to IV infusion position.
8. Record CVP reading and position of client.
9. Electronic transducer
   a. Ensure client is relaxed.
   b. Make sure transducer is zeroed and calibrated.
   c. If CVP line is in use, turn stopcock to allow pressure measurement from transducer, which will temporarily stop infusion.
   d. Ensure that infusion is reinitiated upon completion of reading.
   e. Record CVP.

EVALUATION

A. Resolution of peripheral edema and neck vein distention; weight stable; lungs clear.
B. Capillary refill is less than 3 seconds; balanced I&O with urine output at least 30 ml/hour; hemodynamic measurements within normal range; usual mental status.
C. Stable vital signs; skin warm and dry; peripheral pulses present, equal, and strong; absence of edema; increased tolerance to activity; usual mentation; absence of pain.
D. Client's skin warm and dry, shows absence of redness and irritation; healing of lesions.
E. Progressive increase in tolerance for activity with heart rate and blood pressure stable; absence of pain.
F. Client expresses relief from pain; relaxed facial expression; stable vital signs; progressive increase in activity tolerance.
G. Demonstrates the use of effective coping skills and problem-solving techniques.
H. Verbalizes awareness of feelings of fear and anxiety. Client reports fear/anxiety as reduced/controlled.

DISORDERS OF THE CARDIOVASCULAR SYSTEM

The Heart

Coronary Artery Disease (CAD)

A. General information

NURSING ALERT

The average duration of original pain is less than 15 minutes and not greater than 30 minutes.

1. CAD refers to a variety of pathologic conditions that cause narrowing or obstruction of the coronary arteries, resulting in decreased blood supply to the myocardium.
2. *Atherosclerosis* (deposits of cholesterol and lipids within the walls of the artery) is the major causative factor.
3. Occurs most often between ages 30 and 50; men affected more often than women; nonwhites have higher mortality rates.
4. May manifest as angina pectoris or MI.
5. Risk factors: family history of CAD, elevated serum lipoproteins, cigarette smoking, diabetes mellitus, hypertension, obesity, sedentary and/or stressful/competitive lifestyle, elevated serum uric acid levels.

B. Medical management, assessment findings, and nursing interventions: see Angina Pectoris (below) and Myocardial Infarction.

Angina Pectoris

A. General information
1. Transient, paroxysmal chest pain produced by insufficient blood flow to the myocardium resulting in myocardial ischemia
2. Risk factors: CAD, atherosclerosis, hypertension, diabetes mellitus, thromboangiitis obliterans, severe anemia, aortic insufficiency
3. Precipitating factors: physical exertion, consumption of a heavy meal, extremely cold weather, strong emotions, cigarette smoking, sexual activity

B. Medical management
1. Drug therapy: nitrates, beta-adrenergic blocking agents, and/or calcium-blocking agents, lipid reducing drugs if cholesterol elevated
2. Modification of diet and other risk factors
3. Surgery: coronary artery bypass surgery
4. Percutaneous transluminal coronary angioplasty (PTCA)

C. Assessment findings
1. Pain: substernal with possible radiation to the neck, jaw, back, and arms; relieved by rest
2. Palpitations, tachycardia
3. Dyspnea
4. Diaphoresis
5. Increased serum lipid levels

6. Diagnostic tests
   a. ECG may reveal ST segment depression and T-wave inversion during chest pain.
   b. Stress test may reveal an abnormal ECG during exercise.

D. Nursing interventions
1. Administer oxygen.
2. Give prompt pain relief with nitrates or narcotic analgesics as ordered.
3. Monitor vital signs, status of cardiopulmonary function.
4. Monitor ECG.
5. Place client in semi- to high-Fowler's position.
6. Provide emotional support.
7. Provide client teaching and discharge planning concerning
   a. Proper use of nitrates
      1) nitroglycerin tablets (sublingual)
         a) allow tablet to dissolve.
         b) relax for 15 minutes after taking tablet to prevent dizziness.
         c) if no relief with 1 tablet, take additional tablets at 5-minute intervals, but no more than 3 tablets within a 15-minute period.
         d) know that transient headache is a frequent side effect.
         e) keep bottle tightly capped and prevent exposure to air, light, heat.
         f) ensure tablets are within reach at all times.
         g) check shelf life, expiration date of tablets.
      2) nitroglycerin ointment (topical)
         a) rotate sites to prevent dermal inflammation.
         b) remove previously applied ointment.
         c) avoid massaging/rubbing as this increases absorption and interferes with the drug's sustained action.
   b. Ways to minimize precipitating events
      1) reduce stress and anxiety (relaxation techniques, guided imagery)
      2) avoid overexertion and smoking
      3) maintain low-cholesterol, low-saturated fat diet and eat small, frequent meals
      4) avoid extremes of temperature
      5) dress warmly in cold weather
   c. Gradual increase in activities and exercise
      1) participate in regular exercise program
      2) space exercise periods and allow for rest periods
8. Instruct client to notify physician immediately if pain occurs and persists, despite rest and medication administration.

Dysrhythmias

A dysrhythmia, often called an arrhythmia, is a disruption in the normal events of the cardiac cycle. It may take a variety of forms. Treatment varies depending on the type of dysrhythmia.

Sinus Tachycardia

A. General information
  1. A heart rate of over 100 beats/minute, originating in the SA node
  2. May be caused by fever, apprehension, physical activity, anemia, hyperthyroidism, drugs (epinephrine, theophylline), myocardial ischemia, caffeine

B. Assessment findings
  1. Rate: 100–160 beats/minute
  2. Rhythm: regular
  3. P wave: precedes each QRS complex with normal contour
  4. P-R interval: normal (0.08 second)
  5. QRS complex: normal (0.06 second)

C. Treatment: correction of underlying cause, elimination of stimulants; sedatives, propranolol (Inderal).

Premature Atrial Complex

A. General information
  1. Physical appearance: single ECG complex that occurs early
  2. Causes: nicotine, alcohol, anxiety, low potassium level, hypovolemia, myocardial ischemia

B. Assessment findings
  1. Ventricular and atrial rate dependent on underlying rhythm
  2. Rhythm; irregular due to premature complexes
  3. QRS shape; usually normal
  4. P wave: morphology may be the same, different, or absent
  5. P-R interval: may be shorter but within limits (0.12–.20 second)
  6. P-QRS: 1:1

Sinus Bradycardia

A. General information
  1. A slowed heart rate initiated by SA node
  2. Caused by excessive vagal or decreased sympathetic tone, MI, intracranial tumors, meningitis, myxedema, cardiac fibrosis; a normal variation of the heart rate in well-trained athletes

B. Assessment findings
  1. Rate: less than 60 beats/minute
  2. Rhythm: regular
  3. P wave: precedes each QRS with a normal contour

   4. P-R interval: normal
   5. QRS complex: normal
C. Treatment: usually not needed; if cardiac output is inadequate, atropine and isoproterenol (Isuprel) are usually prescribed; if drugs are not effective, a pacemaker may need to be inserted.

Atrial Tachycardia

A. General information
   1. A heart rate above 160–250, originates in the SA node
   2. May be drug induced (including substance abuse), caused by fever, severe blood loss, thyroid storm, electrolyte imbalances, severe hypoxia
B. Assessment findings
   1. Rate: 160–250 beats/minute
   2. Rhythm: regular
   3. P Wave: precedes each QRS complex with normal contour
   4. P-R interval: normal (0.08 second)
   5. QRS complex: normal (0.06 second)
C. Treatment: correction of underlying problem, beta-blockers, calcium channel blocker, amniodarone

Atrial Flutter

A. General information
   1. Atrial rate between 250 and 400, ventricular rate between 75 and 150
   2. May be idiopathic, associated with advanced age, valvular disease, HTN, cardiomyopathy, pulmonary disease, hyperthyroidism, moderate-to-heavy alcohol consumption
B. Assessment findings
   1. Rate: 250–400 beats/minute
   2. Rhythm: irregular
   3. P Wave: varies to QRS
   4. P-R interval: difficult to distinguish due to rate
   5. QRS complex: normal or abnormal
C. Treatment: correction of underlying problem, beta-blockers, calcium channel blocker, amniodarone, digitalis

Atrial Fibrillation

A. General information
   1. An arrhythmia in which ectopic foci in the atria cause rapid, irregular contractions of the heart
   2. Commonly seen in clients with rheumatic mitral stenosis, thyrotoxicosis, cardiomyopathy, hypertensive heart disease, pericarditis, and coronary heart disease

B. Assessment findings
   1. Rate
      a. Atrial: 350–600 beats/minute
      b. Ventricular: varies between 100–160 beats/minute
   2. Rhythm: atrial and ventricular regularly irregular
   3. P wave: no definite P wave; rapid undulations called fibrillatory (f) waves
   4. P-R interval: not measurable
   5. QRS complex: generally normal

C. Treatment: digitalis preparations, propranolol, verapamil in conjunction with digitalis; direct-current cardioversion

Premature Ventricular Contractions (PVCs)

A. General information
   1. Irritable impulses originate in the ventricles
   2. Caused by electrolyte imbalance (hypokalemia); digitalis drug therapy; myocardial disease; stimulants (caffeine, epinephrine, isoproterenol); hypoxia; congestive heart failure

B. Assessment findings
   1. Rate: varies according to number of PVCs
   2. Rhythm: irregular because of PVCs
   3. P wave: normal; however, often lost in QRS complex
   4. P-R interval: often not measurable
   5. QRS complex: wide and distorted in shape, greater than 0.12 second

C. Treatment
   1. IV push of lidocaine (50–100 mg) followed by IV drip of lidocaine at rate of 1–4 mg/minute
   2. Procainamide (Pronestyl), quinidine
   3. Treatment of underlying cause

Ventricular Tachycardia

A. General information
   1. A run of three or more consecutive PVCs; occurs from repetitive firing of an ectopic focus in the ventricles
   2. Caused by acute MI, CAD, digitalis intoxication, hypokalemia

B. Assessment findings
   1. Rate
      a. Atrial: 60–100 beats/minute
      b. Ventricular: 110–250 beats/minute
   2. Rhythm: atrial (regular), ventricular (occasionally irregular)
   3. P wave: often lost in QRS complex
   4. P-R interval: usually not measurable
   5. QRS complex: greater than 0.12 second, wide

C. Treatment
   1. IV push of lidocaine (1 mg/kg for a dose of 50–100 mg), then IV drip of lidocaine 1–4 mg/minute
   2. Procainamide via IV infusion of 2–6 mg/minute
   3. Direct-current cardioversion
   4. Bretylium, propranolol (Inderal)

Ventricular Fibrillation

A. General information
   1. Rapid and disorganized rhythm caused by quivering of the ventricles
   2. No atrial activity is seen
   3. May be caused by idiopathic sudden death, electrical shock
B. Assessment findings
   1. Ventricular rate: greater than 300
   2. Ventricular rhythm irregular, without specific pattern
   3. QRS shape and duration: irregular, undulating waves without recognizable QRS pattern
C. Treatment: counter-shock (defibrillation)

Myocardial Infarction (MI)

A. General information
   1. The death of myocardial cells from inadequate oxygenation, often caused by a sudden complete blockage of a coronary artery; characterized by localized formation of necrosis (tissue destruction) with subsequent healing by scar formation and fibrosis.
   2. Risk factors: atherosclerotic CAD, thrombus formation, hypertension, diabetes mellitus, hyperlipidemia, and genetic predisposition
B. Assessment findings
   1. Pain usually substernal with radiation to the neck, arm, jaw, or back; severe, crushing, viselike with sudden onset; *unrelieved by rest or nitrates*
   2. Nausea and vomiting
   3. Dyspnea
   4. Skin: cool, clammy, ashen
   5. Elevated temperature
   6. Initial increase in blood pressure and pulse, with gradual drop in blood pressure
   7. Restlessness
   8. Occasional findings: rales or crackles; presence of S_4; pericardial friction rub; split S_1, S_2
   9. Diagnostic tests
      a. Elevated WBC
      b. Elevated CPK and CPK-MB
      c. Elevated SGOT or AST

d. Elevated LDH, LDH_1, and LDH_2
e. Elevated troponin levels
f. ECG changes (specific changes dependent on location of myocardial damage and phase of the MI; inverted T wave and ST segment changes seen with myocardial ischemia
g. Increased ESR, elevated serum cholesterol

C. Nursing interventions
1. Establish a patent IV line
2. Provide pain relief; morphine sulfate IV (given IV because after an infarction there is poor peripheral perfusion and because serum enzymes would be affected by IM injections) as ordered.
3. Administer oxygen as ordered to relieve dyspnea and prevent arrhythmias.
4. Provide bed rest with semi-Fowler's position to decrease cardiac workload.
5. Monitor ECG and hemodynamic procedures.
6. Administer antiarrhythmias as ordered.
7. Perform complete lung/cardiovascular assessment.
8. Monitor urinary output and report output of less than 30 ml/hour; indicates decreased cardiac output.
9. Maintain full liquid diet with gradual increase to soft; low sodium.
10. Maintain quiet environment.
11. Administer stool softeners as ordered to facilitate bowel evacuation and prevent straining.
12. Relieve anxiety associated with coronary care unit (CCU) environment.
13. Administer anticoagulants, as ordered.
14. Administer thrombolytics (tissue-type plasminogen activator or t-pa and streptokinase) and monitor for side effects; bleeding.
15. Provide client teaching and discharge planning concerning
    a. Effects of MI, healing process, and treatment regimen
    b. Medication regimen including name, purpose, schedule, dosage, side effects
    c. Risk factors, with necessary lifestyle modifications
    d. Dietary restrictions: low sodium, low cholesterol, avoidance of caffeine
    e. Importance of participation in a progressive activity program
    f. Resumption of sexual activity according to physician's orders (usually 4–6 weeks)
    g. Need to report the following symptoms: increased persistent chest pain, dyspnea, weakness, fatigue, persistent palpitations, light-headedness
    h. Enrollment of client in a cardiac rehabilitation program

Percutaneous Transluminal Coronary Angioplasty

A. General information

1. Percutaneous transluminal coronary angioplasty (PTCA), with or without placement of a stent, can be performed as an alternative to coronary artery bypass graft surgery (CABG).
2. The aim of PTCA is to revascularize the myocardium, decrease angina, and increase survival.
3. PTCA is performed in the cardiac catheterization lab and is accomplished by insertion of a balloon-tipped catheter into the stenotic, diseased coronary artery. The balloon is inflated with a controlled pressure and thereby decreases the stenosis of the vessel.

B. Nursing interventions

Preoperative and postoperative care is similar to the care of the client undergoing cardiac catheterization.

Coronary Artery Bypass Surgery

A. General information

1. A coronary artery bypass graft is the surgery of choice for clients with severe CAD.
2. New supply of blood brought to diseased/occluded coronary artery by bypassing the obstruction with a graft that is attached to the aorta proximally and to the coronary artery distally.
3. Several bypasses can be performed depending on the location and extent of the blockage.
4. Procedure frequently requires use of extracorporeal circulation (heart-lung machine, cardiopulmonary bypass). Some clients may be candidates for off pump coronary artery bypass (OPCAB).

B. Nursing interventions: preoperative

1. Explain anatomy of the heart, function of coronary arteries, effects of CAD.
2. Explain events of the day of surgery: length of time in surgery, length of time until able to see family.
3. Orient to the critical and coronary care units and introduce to staff.
4. Explain equipment to be used (monitors, hemodynamic procedures, ventilator, endotracheal tube, drainage tubes).
5. Demonstrate activity and exercises (turning from side to side, dangling, sitting in a chair, ROM exercises for arms and legs, effective deep breathing, and coughing).
6. Reassure client that pain medication is available.

C. Nursing interventions: postoperative

1. Maintain patent airway.
2. Promote lung reexpansion.
   - **a.** Monitor drainage from chest/mediastinal tubes, and check patency of chest drainage system.
   - **b.** Assist client with turning, coughing, and deep breathing.

3. Monitor cardiac status.
   a. Monitor vital signs and cardiac rhythm and report significant changes, particularly temperature elevation.
   b. Perform peripheral pulse checks.
   c. Carry out hemodynamic monitoring.
   d. Administer anticoagulants as ordered and monitor hematologic test results carefully.
4. Maintain fluid and electrolyte balance.
   a. Maintain accurate I&O with hourly outputs; report if less than 30 ml/hour urine.
   b. Assess color, character, and specific gravity of urine.
   c. Daily weights.
   d. Assess lab values, particularly BUN, creatinine, sodium, and potassium levels.
5. Maintain adequate cerebral circulation: frequent neuro checks.
6. Provide pain relief.
   a. Administer narcotics cautiously and monitor effects.
   b. Assist with positioning for maximum comfort.
   c. Teach relaxation techniques.
7. Prevent abdominal distension.
   a. Monitor nasogastric drainage and maintain patency of system.
   b. Assess for bowel sounds every 2–4 hours.
   c. Measure abdominal girths if necessary.
8. Monitor for and prevent the following complications.
   a. Thrombophlebitis/pulmonary embolism
   b. Cardiac tamponade
   c. Arrhythmias
      1) maintain continuous ECG monitoring and report changes.
      2) assess electrolyte levels daily and report significant changes, particularly potassium.
      3) administer antiarrhythmics as ordered.
   d. Heart failure (see below)
9. Provide client teaching and discharge planning concerning
   a. Limitation with progressive increase in activities
      1) encourage daily walking with gradual increase in distance weekly
      2) avoid heavy lifting and activities that require continuous arm movements (vacuuming, playing golf, bowling)
      3) avoid driving a car until physician permits
   b. Sexual intercourse: can usually be resumed by third or fourth week post-op; avoid sexual positions in which the client would be supporting weight
   c. Medical regimen: ensure client/family are aware of drugs, dosages, proper times of administration, and side effects
   d. Meal planning with prescribed modifications (decreased sodium, cholesterol, and possibly carbohydrates)

e. Wound cleansing daily with mild soap and H_2O and report signs of infection
f. Symptoms to be reported: fever, dyspnea, chest pain with minimal exertion

Heart Failure (HF)

A. General information: inability of the heart to pump an adequate supply of blood to meet the metabolic needs of the body.
B. Types
   1. *Left-sided heart failure*
      a. Left ventricular damage causes blood to back up through the left atrium and into the pulmonary veins. Increased pressure causes transudation into the interstitial tissues of the lungs with resultant pulmonary congestion.
      b. Caused by left ventricular damage (usually due to an MI), hypertension, ischemic heart disease, aortic valve disease, mitral stenosis
      c. Assessment findings
         1) dyspnea, orthopnea, PND, tiredness, muscle weakness, cough
         2) tachycardia, PMI displaced laterally, possible S_3, bronchial wheezing, rales or crackles, cyanosis, pallor
         3) decreased pO_2, increased pCO_2
         4) diagnostic tests
            a) chest X-ray: shows cardiac hypertrophy
            b) PAP and PCWP usually increased; however, this is dependent on the degree of heart failure
         5) Echocardiography: shows increased size of cardiac chambers
   2. *Right-sided heart failure*
      a. Weakened right ventricle is unable to pump blood into the pulmonary system; systemic venous congestion occurs as pressure builds up.
      b. Caused by left-sided heart failure, right ventricular infarction, atherosclerotic heart disease, COPD, pulmonic stenosis, pulmonary embolism.
      c. Assessment findings
         1) anorexia, nausea, weight gain
         2) dependent pitting edema, jugular venous distension, bounding pulses, hepatomegaly, cool extremities, oliguria
         3) elevated CVP, decreased pO_2, increased ALT (SGPT)
         4) diagnostic tests
            a) chest X-ray: reveals cardiac hypertrophy
            b) echocardiography: indicates increased size of cardiac chambers

3. *High-output failure*
    a. Cardiac output is adequate but exceeded by the metabolic needs of the tissues; the exorbitant demands made on the heart eventually cause ventricular failure.
    b. Caused by hyperthyroidism, anemia, AV fistula, pregnancy

C. Medical management (all types)
1. Determination and elimination/control of underlying cause
2. Drug therapy: digitalis preparations, diuretics, vasodilators
3. Sodium-restricted diet to decrease fluid retention
4. If medical therapies unsuccessful, mechanical assist devices (intra-aortic balloon pump), cardiac transplantation, or mechanical hearts may be employed.

D. Nursing interventions
1. Monitor respiratory status and provide adequate ventilation (when HF progresses to pulmonary edema).
    a. Administer oxygen therapy.
    b. Maintain client in semi- or high-Fowler's position.
    c. Monitor ABGs.
    d. Assess for breath sounds, noting any changes.
2. Provide physical and emotional rest.
    a. Constantly assess level of anxiety.
    b. Maintain bed rest with limited activity.
    c. Maintain quiet, relaxed environment.
    d. Organize nursing care around rest periods.
3. Increase cardiac output.
    a. Administer digitalis as ordered and monitor effects.
    b. Monitor ECG and hemodynamic monitoring.
    c. Administer vasodilators as ordered.
    d. Monitor vital signs.
4. Reduce/eliminate edema.
    a. Administer diuretics as ordered.
    b. Daily weights.
    c. Maintain accurate I&O.
    d. Assess for peripheral edema.
    e. Measure abdominal girths daily.
    f. Monitor electrolyte levels.
    g. Monitor CVP and Swan-Ganz readings.
    h. Provide sodium-restricted diet as ordered.
    i. Provide meticulous skin care.
5. Provide client teaching and discharge planning concerning
    a. Need to monitor self daily for signs and symptoms of HF (pedal edema, weight gain of 1–2 kg in a 2-day period, dyspnea, loss of appetite, cough)
    b. Medication regimen including name, purpose, dosage, frequency, and side effects (digitalis, diuretics)

c. Prescribed dietary plan (low sodium; small, frequent meals)
d. Need to avoid fatigue and plan for rest periods

Pulmonary Edema

A. General information
   1. A medical emergency that occurs when the capillary pressure within the lungs becomes so great that fluid moves from the intravascular space into the alveoli, bronchi, and bronchioles. Death occurs by suffocation if this condition is untreated.
   2. Caused by left-sided heart failure, rapid administration of IV fluids.
B. Medical management
   1. Oxygen therapy
   2. Endotracheal/nasotracheal intubation (possible)
   3. Drug therapy
      a. Morphine sulfate to induce vasodilation and decrease anxiety; 5 mg IV, administer slowly
      b. Digitalis to improve cardiac output
      c. Diuretics (furosemide [Lasix] is drug of choice) to relieve fluid retention
      d. Aminophylline to relieve bronchospasm and increase cardiac output; 250–500 mg IV, administer slowly
      e. Vasodilators (nitroglycerin, isosorbide dinitrate) to dilate the vessels, thereby reducing amount of blood returned to the heart
   4. Rotating tourniquets or phlebotomy
C. Assessment findings
   1. Dyspnea
   2. Cough with large amounts of blood-tinged sputum
   3. Tachycardia, pallor, wheezing, rales or crackles, diaphoresis
   4. Restlessness, fear/anxiety
   5. Jugular vein distension
   6. Decreased pO_2, increased pCO_2, elevated CVP
D. Nursing interventions
   1. Assist with intubation (if necessary) and monitor mechanical ventilation.
   2. Administer oxygen by mask in high concentrations (40–60%) if not intubated.
   3. Place client in semi-Fowler's position or over bedside table to ease dyspnea.
   4. Administer medications as ordered.
   5. Assist with phlebotomy (removal of 300–500 ml of blood from a peripheral vein) if performed.
   6. CVP/hemodynamic monitoring.
   7. Provide client teaching and discharge planning concerning

a. Prescribed medications, including name, purpose, schedule, dosage, and side effects
b. Dietary restrictions: low sodium, low cholesterol
c. Importance of adhering to planned rest periods with gradual progressive increase in activities
d. Daily weights
e. Need to report the following symptoms to physician immediately: dyspnea, persistent productive cough, pedal edema, restlessness

Pacemakers

A. General information
1. A pacemaker is an electronic device that provides repetitive electrical stimulation to the cardiac musculature to control the heart rate.
2. Artificial pacing system consists of a battery-powered generator and a pacing wire that delivers the stimulus to the heart.

B. Indications for use
1. Adams-Stokes attack
2. Acute MI with Mobitz II AV block
3. Third-degree AV block with slow ventricular rate
4. Right bundle branch block
5. New left bundle branch block
6. Symptomatic sinus bradycardia
7. Sick sinus syndrome
8. Arrhythmias (during or after cardiac surgery)
9. Drug-resistant tachyarrhythmia

C. Modes of pacing
1. Fixed rate: pacemaker fires electrical stimuli at preset rate, regardless of the client's rate and rhythm.
2. Demand: pacemaker produces electrical stimuli only when the client's own heart rate drops below the preset rate per minute on the generator.

D. Types of pacemakers
1. Temporary
   a. Used in emergency situations and performed via an endocardial (transvenous) or transthoracic approach to the myocardium.
   b. Performed at bedside or using fluoroscopy.
2. Permanent
   a. Endocardial or transvenous procedure involves passing endocardial lead into right ventricle with subcutaneous implantation of pulse generator into right or left subclavian areas. Usually done under local anesthesia.
   b. Epicardial or myocardial method involves passing the electrode transthoracically to the myocardium where it is sutured in place. The pulse generator is implanted into the abdominal wall.

E. Nursing interventions

1. Assess pacemaker function
   a. Monitor heart rate, noting deviations from the preset rate.
   b. Observe the presence of pacemaker spikes on ECG tracing or cardiac monitor; spike before P wave with atrial pacemaker; spike before QRS complex with ventricular pacemaker
   c. Assess for signs of pacemaker malfunction, such as weakness, fainting, dizziness, or hypotension.
2. Maintain the integrity of the system
   a. Ensure that catheter terminals are attached securely to the pulse generator (temporary pacemaker)
   b. Attach pulse generator to client securely to prevent accidental dislodgment (temporary pacemaker)
3. Provide safety and comfort
   a. Provide safe environment by properly grounding all equipment in the room.
   b. Monitor electrolyte level periodically, particularly potassium.
4. Prevent infection
   a. Assess vital signs, particularly temperature changes.
   b. Assess catheter insertion site daily for signs of infection.
   c. Maintain sterile dressing over catheter insertion site.

F. Provide client teaching and discharge planning concerning

1. Fundamental concepts of cardiac physiology
2. Daily pulse check for one minute
3. Need to report immediately any sudden slowing or increase in pulse rate
4. Importance of adhering to weekly monitoring schedule during first month after implantation and when battery depletion is anticipated (depending on type of battery)
5. Wear loose-fitting clothing around the area of the pacemaker for comfort
6. Notify physician of any pain or redness over incision site
7. Avoid trauma to area of pulse generator
8. Avoid heavy contact sports
9. Carry an identification card/bracelet that indicates physician's name, type and model number of pacemaker, manufacturer's name, pacemaker rate
10. Display identification card and request scanning by hand scanner when going through weapons detector at airport
11. Remember that periodic hospitalization is necessary for battery changes/pacemaker unit replacement

Cardiac Arrest

A. General information: sudden, unexpected cessation of breathing and adequate circulation of blood by the heart

B. Medical management

1. Cardiopulmonary resuscitation (CPR); see below
2. Drug therapy
   a. Lidocaine, procainamide, verapamil for ventricular tachycardia
   b. Dopamine (Intropin), isoproterenol (Isuprel), norepinephrine (Levophed).
   c. Epinephrine to enhance myocardial automaticity, excitability, conductivity, and contractility
   d. Atropine sulfate to reduce vagus nerve's control over the heart, thus increasing the heart rate
   e. Sodium bicarbonate to correct respiratory and metabolic acidosis
   f. Calcium chloride: calcium ions help the heart beat more effectively by enhancing the myocardium's contractile force
3. Defibrillation (electrical countershock)

C. Assessment findings: unresponsiveness, cessation of respiration, pallor, cyanosis, absence of heart sounds/blood pressure/palpable pulses, dilation of pupils, ventricular fibrillation or asystole (if client on a monitor)

D. Nursing interventions: monitored arrest caused by ventricular fibrillation
1. CPR until defibrillation possible.
2. If defibrillation unsuccessful, continue CPR and assist with administration of and monitor effects of additional emergency drugs.
3. If defibrillation successful, monitor client status.

Cardiopulmonary Resuscitation (CPR)

A. General information: process of externally supporting the circulation and respiration of a person who has had a cardiac arrest

B. Nursing interventions: unwitnessed cardiac arrest
1. Assess LOC.
   a. Shake victim's shoulder and shout.
   b. If no response, summon help.
2. Position victim supine on a firm surface.
3. Open airway.
   a. Use head tilt, chin lift maneuver.
   b. Place ear over nose and mouth.
      1) look to see if chest is moving.
      2) listen for escape of air.
      3) feel for movement of air against face.
   c. If no respiration, proceed to #4.
4. Ventilate twice, allowing for deflation between breaths.
5. Assess circulation: in adults palpate for carotid pulse; if not present, proceed to #6.
6. Initiate external cardiac compressions
   a. Proper placement of hands: lower half of the sternum
   b. Depth of compressions: 1½–2 inches for adults
   c. 15 compressions (at rate of 80–100 per minute) with 2 ventilations

NURSING ALERT

Low grade fevers (99–102 °F) may indicate subacute endocarditis. High grade fevers (103–104 °F) may indicate acute infective endocarditis.

Endocarditis

A. General information
   1. Inflammation of the endocardium; platelets and fibrin deposit on the mitral and/or aortic valves causing deformity, insufficiency, or stenosis.
   2. Caused by bacterial infection: commonly *S. aureus, S. viridans*, B-hemolytic streptococcus, gonococcus
   3. Precipitating factors: rheumatic heart disease, open-heart surgery procedures, GU/Ob-Gyn instrumentation/surgery, dental extractions, invasive monitoring, septic thrombophlebitis
B. Medical management
   1. Drug therapy
      a. Antibiotics specific to sensitivity of organism cultured
      b. Penicillin G and streptomycin if organism not known
      c. Antipyretics
   2. Cardiac surgery to replace affected valve
C. Assessment findings
   1. Fever, malaise, fatigue, dyspnea and cough (if extensive valvular damage), acute upper quadrant pain (if splenic involvement), joint pain
   2. Petechiae, murmurs, edema (if extensive valvular damage), splenomegaly, hemiplegia and confusion (if cerebral infarction), hematuria (if renal infarction)
   3. Elevated WBC and ESR, decreased Hgb and Hct
   4. Diagnostic tests: positive blood culture for causative organism
D. Nursing interventions
   1. Administer antibiotics as ordered to control the infectious process.
   2. Control temperature elevation by administration of antipyretics.
   3. Assess for vascular complications.
   4. Provide client teaching and discharge planning concerning
      a. Types of procedures/treatments (e.g., tooth extractions, GU instrumentation) that increase the chances of recurrences
      b. Antibiotic therapy, including name, purpose, dose, frequency, side effects
      c. Signs and symptoms of recurrent endocarditis (persistent fever, fatigue, chills, anorexia, joint pain)
      d. Avoidance of individuals with known infections

Pericarditis

A. General information
   1. An inflammation of the visceral and parietal pericardium
   2. Caused by a bacterial, viral, or fungal infection; collagen diseases; trauma; acute MI; neoplasms; uremia; radiation therapy; drugs (procainamide, hydralazine, doxorubicin HCl [Adriamycin])

B. Medical management
   1. Determination and elimination/control of underlying cause
   2. Drug therapy
      a. Medication for pain relief
      b. Corticosteroids, salicylates (aspirin), and indomethacin (Indocin) to reduce inflammation
      c. Specific antibiotic therapy against the causative organism may be indicated.

C. Assessment findings
   1. Chest pain with deep inspiration (relieved by sitting up), cough, hemoptysis, malaise
   2. Tachycardia, fever, pleural friction rub, cyanosis or pallor, accentuated component of S_2, pulsus paradoxus, jugular vein distension
   3. Elevated WBC and ESR, normal or elevated AST (SGOT)
   4. Diagnostic tests
      a. Chest X-ray may show increased heart size if effusion occurs
      b. ECG changes: ST elevation (precordial leads and 2- or 3-limb heads), T wave inversion

D. Nursing interventions
   1. Ensure comfort: bed rest with semi- or high-Fowler's position.
   2. Monitor hemodynamic parameters carefully.
   3. Administer medications as ordered and monitor effects.
   4. Provide client teaching and discharge planning concerning
      a. Signs and symptoms of pericarditis indicative of a recurrence (chest pain that is intensified by inspiration and position changes, fever, cough)
      b. Medication regimen including name, purpose, dosage, frequency, side effects

Cardiac Tamponade

A. General information
   1. An accumulation of fluid/blood in the pericardium that prevents adequate ventricular filling; without emergency treatment client will die.
   2. Caused by blunt or penetrating chest trauma, malignant pericardial effusion; can be a complication of cardiac surgery.

B. Medical management: emergency treatment of choice is *pericardiocentesis* (insertion of a needle into the pericardial sac to aspirate fluid/blood and relieve the pressure on the heart)

C. Assessment findings
  1. Chest pain
  2. Hypotension, distended neck veins, tachycardia, muffled or distant heart sounds, paradoxical pulse, pericardial friction rub
  3. Elevated CVP, decreased Hgb and Hct if massive hemorrhage
  4. Diagnostic test: chest X-ray reveals enlarged heart and widened mediastinum.

D. Nursing interventions
  1. Administer oxygen therapy
  2. Monitor CVP/IVs closely
  3. Assist with pericardiocentesis
     a. Monitor ECG, blood pressure, and pulse.
     b. Assess aspirated fluid for color, consistency.
     c. Send specimen to lab immediately.

The Blood Vessels

Hypertension

A. General information
  1. According to the World Health Organization, hypertension is a persistent elevation of the systolic blood pressure above 140 mmHg and of the diastolic above 90 mmHg.
  2. Types
     a. Essential (primary, idiopathic): marked by loss of elastic tissue and arteriosclerotic changes in the aorta and larger vessels coupled with decreased caliber of the arterioles
     b. Benign: a moderate rise in blood pressure marked by a gradual onset and prolonged course
     c. Malignant: characterized by a rapid onset and short dramatic course with a diastolic blood pressure of more than 150 mmHg
     d. Secondary: elevation of the blood pressure as a result of another disease such as renal parenchymal disease, Cushing's disease, pheochromocytoma, primary aldosteronism, coarctation of the aorta
  3. Essential hypertension usually occurs between ages 35 and 50; more common in men over 35, women over 45; African-American men affected twice as often as white men/women
  4. Risk factors for essential hypertension include positive family history, obesity, stress, cigarette smoking, hypercholesteremia, increased sodium intake

B. Medical management
  1. Diet and weight reduction (restricted sodium, kcal, cholesterol)

2. Lifestyle changes: alcohol moderation, exercise regimen, cessation of smoking
3. Antihypertensive drug therapy

C. Assessment findings
1. Pain similar to anginal pain; pain in calves of legs after ambulation or exercise (*intermittent claudication*); severe occipital headaches, particularly in the morning; polyuria; nocturia; fatigue; dizziness; epistaxis; dyspnea on exertion
2. Blood pressure consistently above 140/90, retinal hemorrhages and exudates, edema of extremities (indicative of right-sided heart failure)
3. Rise in systolic blood pressure from supine to standing position (indicative of essential hypertension)
4. Diagnostic tests; elevated serum uric acid, sodium, cholesterol levels

D. Nursing interventions
1. Record baseline blood pressure in three positions (lying, sitting, standing) and in both arms.
2. Continuously assess blood pressure and report any variables that relate to changes in blood pressure (positioning, restlessness).
3. Administer antihypertensive agents as ordered; monitor closely and assess for side effects.
4. Monitor intake and hourly outputs.
5. Provide client teaching and discharge planning concerning
   a. Risk factor identification and development/implementation of methods to modify them
   b. Restricted sodium, kcal, cholesterol diet; include family in teaching
   c. Antihypertensive drug regimen (include family).
      1) names, actions, dosages, and side effects of prescribed medications
      2) take drugs at regular times and avoid omission of any doses
      3) never abruptly discontinue the drug therapy
      4) supplement diet with potassium-rich foods if taking potassium-wasting diuretics
      5) avoid hot baths, alcohol, or strenuous exercise within 3 hours of taking medications that cause vasodilation
   d. Development of a graduated exercise program
   e. Importance of routine follow-up care

Arteriosclerosis Obliterans

A. General information
1. A chronic occlusive arterial disease that may affect the abdominal aorta or the lower extremities. The obstruction to blood flow with resultant ischemia usually affects the femoral, popliteal, aortal, and iliac arteries.
2. Occurs most often in men ages 50–60
3. Caused by atherosclerosis

4. Risk factors: cigarette smoking, hyperlipidemia, hypertension, diabetes mellitus

B. Medical management

1. Drug therapy
   a. Vasodilators: papaverine, isoxsuprine HCl (Vasodilan), nylidrin HCl (Arlidin), nicotinyl alcohol (Roniacol), cyclandelate (Cyclospasmol), tolazoline HCl (Priscoline) to improve arterial circulation; effectiveness questionable
   b. Analgesics to relieve ischemic pain
   c. Anticoagulants to prevent thrombus formation
   d. Lipid-reducing drug: cholestyramine (Questran), colestipol HCl (Cholestid), dextrothyroxine sodium (Choloxin), clofibrate (Atromid-S), gemfibrozil (Lopid), niacin, lovastatin (Mevacor)
2. Surgery: bypass grafting, endarterectomy, balloon catheter dilation; lumbar sympathectomy (to increase blood flow), amputation may be necessary

C. Assessment findings

1. Pain, both intermittent claudication and rest pain, numbness or tingling of the toes
2. Pallor after 1–2 minutes of elevating feet, and dependent hyperemia/rubor; diminished or absent dorsalis pedis, posterior tibial and femoral pulses; trophic changes; shiny, taut skin with hair loss on lower legs
3. Diagnostic tests
   a. Oscillometry may reveal decrease in pulse volume
   b. Doppler ultrasound reveals decreased blood flow through affected vessels
   c. Angiography reveals location and extent of obstructive process
4. Elevated serum triglycerides; sodium

D. Nursing interventions

1. Encourage slow, progressive physical activity (out of bed at least 3–4 times/day, walking 2 times/day).
2. Administer medications as ordered.
3. Assist with Buerger-Allen exercises qid.
   a. Client lies with legs elevated above heart for 2–3 minutes
   b. Client sits on edge of bed with legs and feet dependent and exercises feet and toes—upward and downward, inward and outward—for 3 minutes
   c. Client lies flat with legs at heart level for 5 minutes
4. Assess for sensory function and trophic changes.
5. Protect client from injury.
6. Provide client teaching and discharge planning concerning
   a. Restricted kcal, low-saturated-fat diet; include family
   b. Importance of continuing with established exercise program
   c. Measures to reduce stress (relaxation techniques, biofeedback)

   d. Importance of avoiding smoking, constrictive clothing, standing in any position for a long time, injury
   e. Importance of foot care, immediately taking care of cuts, wounds, injuries
7. Prepare client for surgery if necessary.

Thromboangiitis Obliterans (Buerger's Disease)

A. General information
   1. Acute, inflammatory disorder affecting medium/smaller arteries and veins of the lower extremities. Occurs as focal, obstructive process; results in occlusion of a vessel with subsequent development of collateral circulation.
   2. Most often affects men ages 25–40.
   3. Disease is idiopathic; high incidence among smokers.
B. Medical management: see Arteriosclerosis Obliterans, above; only really effective treatment is cessation of smoking.
C. Assessment findings
   1. Intermittent claudication, sensitivity to cold (skin of extremity may at first be white, changing to blue, then red)
   2. Decreased or absent peripheral pulses (posterior tibial and dorsalis pedis), trophic changes, ulceration and gangrene (advanced)
   3. Diagnostic tests: same as in Arteriosclerosis Obliterans except no elevation in serum triglycerides
D. Nursing interventions
   1. Prepare client for surgery.
   2. Provide client teaching and discharge planning concerning
      a. Drug regimen (vasodilators, anticoagulants, analgesics) to include names, dosages, frequency, and side effects
      b. Need to avoid trauma to the affected extremity
      c. Need to maintain warmth, especially in cold weather
      d. Importance of stopping smoking.

Raynaud's Phenomenon

A. General information
   1. Intermittent episode of arterial spasms, most frequently involving the fingers
   2. Most often affects women between the teenage years and age 40
   3. Cause unknown
   4. Predisposing factors: collagen diseases (systemic lupus erythematosus, rheumatoid arthritis), trauma (e.g., from typing, piano playing, operating a chain saw)
B. Medical management: vasodilators, catecholamine-depleting antihypertensive drugs (reserpine, guanethidine monosulfate [Ismelin])
C. Assessment findings

1. Coldness, numbness, tingling in one or more digits; pain (usually precipitated by exposure to cold, emotional upsets, tobacco use)
2. Intermittent color changes (pallor, cyanosis, rubor); small ulcerations and gangrene at tips of digits (advanced)

D. Nursing interventions
1. Provide client teaching concerning
   - **a.** Importance of stopping smoking
   - **b.** Need to maintain warmth, especially in cold weather
   - **c.** Need to use gloves when handling cold objects/opening freezer or refrigerator door
   - **d.** Drug regimen

Aneurysms

An aneurysm is a sac formed by dilation of an artery secondary to weakness and stretching of the arterial wall. The dilation may involve one or all layers of the arterial wall.

Classification

A. *Fusiform:* uniform spindle shape involving the entire circumference of the artery

B. *Saccular:* outpouching on one side only, affecting only part of the arterial circumference

C. *Dissecting:* separation of the arterial wall layers to form a cavity that fills with blood

D. *False:* the vessel wall is disrupted, blood escapes into surrounding area but is held in place by surrounding tissue

Thoracic Aortic Aneurysm

A. General information
1. An aneurysm, usually fusiform or dissecting, in the descending, ascending, or transverse section of the thoracic aorta
2. Usually occurs in men ages 50–70
3. Caused by arteriosclerosis, infection, syphilis, hypertension

B. Medical management
1. Control of underlying hypertension
2. Surgery: resection of the aneurysm and replacement with a Teflon/Dacron graft; clients will need extracorporeal circulation (heart-lung machine).

C. Assessment findings
1. Often asymptomatic
2. Deep, diffuse chest pain; hoarseness; dysphagia; dyspnea
3. Pallor, diaphoresis, distended neck veins, edema of head and arms
4. Diagnostic tests

   a. Aortography shows exact location of the aneurysm
   b. X-rays: chest film reveals abnormal widening of aorta; abdominal film may show calcification within walls of aneurysm

D. Nursing interventions: see Cardiac Surgery.

Abdominal Aortic Aneurysm

A. General information
   1. Most aneurysms of this type are saccular or dissecting and develop just below the renal arteries but above the iliac bifurcation
   2. Occur most often in men over age 60
   3. Caused by atherosclerosis, hypertension, trauma, syphilis, other types of infectious processes

B. Medical management: surgical resection of the lesion and replacement with a graft (extracorporeal circulation not needed)

C. Assessment findings
   1. Severe mid- to low-abdominal pain, low-back pain
   2. Mass in the periumbilical area or slightly to the left of the midline with bruits heard over the mass
   3. Pulsating abdominal mass
   4. Diminished femoral pulses
   5. Diagnostic tests: same as for thoracic aneurysms

D. Nursing interventions: preoperative
   1. Prepare client for surgery: routine pre-op care.
   2. Assess rate, rhythm, character of the peripheral pulses and mark all distal pulses.

E. Nursing interventions: postoperative
   1. Provide routine post-op care.
   2. Monitor the following parameters
      a. Hourly circulation checks noting rate, rhythm, character of all pulses distal to the graft
      b. CVP/PAP/PCWP
      c. Hourly outputs through Foley catheter (report less than 30 ml/hour)
      d. Daily BUN/creatinine/electrolyte levels
      e. Presence of back pain (may indicate retroperitoneal hemorrhage)
      f. IV fluids
      g. Neuro status including LOC, pupil size and response to light, hand grasp, movement of extremities
      h. Heart rate and rhythm via monitor
   3. Maintain client flat in bed without sharp flexion of hip/knee (avoid pressure on femoral/popliteal arteries).
   4. Auscultate lungs and encourage turning, coughing, and deep breathing.
   5. Assess for signs and symptoms of paralytic ileus.

6. Prevent thrombophlebitis.
    a. Encourage client to dorsiflex foot while in bed.
    b. Use elastic stockings or sequential compression devices as ordered.
    c. Assess for signs and symptoms (see Thrombophlebitis discussion that follows).
7. Provide client teaching and discharge planning concerning
    a. Importance of changes in color/temperature of extremities
    b. Avoidance of prolonged sitting, standing, and smoking
    c. Need for a gradual progressive activity regimen
    d. Adherence to low-cholesterol, low-saturated-fat diet

Femoral-Popliteal Bypass Surgery

A. General information
    1. Most common type of surgery to correct arterial obstructions of the lower extremities
    2. Procedure involves bypassing the occluded vessel with a graft, such as Teflon, Dacron, or an autogenous artery or vein (saphenous).
B. Nursing interventions: preoperative
    1. Provide routine pre-op care.
    2. Monitor and correct potassium imbalances to prevent cardiac arrhythmias.
    3. Assess for focus of infection (infected tooth) or infectious processes (urinary tract infections).
    4. Mark distal peripheral pulses.
C. Nursing interventions: postoperative
    1. Provide routine post-op care.
    2. Assess the following
        a. Circulation, noting rate, rhythm, and quality of peripheral pulses distal to the graft; color; temperature; and sensation
        b. Signs and symptoms of thrombophlebitis (see discussion that follows)
        c. Neuro checks
        d. Hourly outputs
        e. CVP
        f. Wound drainage, noting amount, color, and characteristics
    3. Elevate legs above the level of the heart.
    4. Encourage turning, coughing, and deep breathing while splinting incision.

Venous Stasis Ulcers

A. General information
    1. Usually a complication of thrombophlebitis and varicose veins.

2. Ulcers result from incompetent valves in the veins, causing high pressure with rupture of small skin veins and venules.

B. Medical management
   1. Antibiotic therapy (specific to organism cultured); topical bacteriocidal solutions
   2. Skin grafting
   3. Enzymatic or surgical debridement

C. Assessment findings
   1. Pain in the limb in dependent position or during ambulation
   2. Skin of leathery texture, brownish pigment around ankles; positive pulses but edema makes palpation difficult.

D. Nursing interventions
   1. Provide bed rest, elevating extremity.
   2. Provide a balanced diet with added protein and vitamin supplements.
   3. Administer antibiotics as ordered to control infection.
   4. Promote healing by cleansing ulcer with prescribed agents.
   5. Provide client teaching and discharge planning concerning
      a. Importance of avoiding trauma to affected limb
      b. Skin care regimen
      c. Use of elastic support stockings (after ulcer is healed)
      d. Need for planned rest periods with elevation of the extremities
   6. Adherence to balanced diet with vitamin supplements.

Thrombophlebitis

A. General information
   1. Inflammation of the vessel wall with formation of a clot (thrombus); may affect superficial or deep veins.
   2. Most frequent veins affected are the saphenous, femoral, and popliteal.
   3. Can result in damage to the surrounding tissues, ischemia, and necrosis.
   4. Risk factors: obesity, HF, prolonged immobility, MI, pregnancy, oral contraceptives, trauma, sepsis, cigarette smoking, dehydration, severe anemias, venous cannulation, complication of surgery.

B. Medical management
   1. Anticoagulant therapy
      a. Heparin
         1) blocks conversion of prothrombin to thrombin and reduces formation or extension of thrombus
         2) side effects: spontaneous bleeding, injection site reactions, ecchymoses, tissue irritation and sloughing, reversible transient alopecia, cyanosis, pain in arms or legs, thrombocytopenia

b. Warfarin (Coumadin)
   1) blocks prothrombin synthesis by interfering with vitamin K synthesis
   2) side effects
      a) GI: anorexia, nausea and vomiting, diarrhea, stomatitis
      b) hypersensitivity: dermatitis, urticaria, pruritus, fever
      c) other: transient hair loss, burning sensation of feet, bleeding complications

2. Surgery
   a. Vein ligation and stripping
   b. *Venous thrombectomy:* removal of a clot in the iliofemoral region
   c. *Plication of the inferior vena cava:* insertion of an umbrella-like prosthesis into the lumen of the vena cava to filter incoming clots

C. Assessment findings
1. Pain in the affected extremity
2. Superficial vein: tenderness, redness, induration along course of the vein
3. Deep vein: swelling, venous distension of limb, tenderness over involved vein, positive Homan's sign, cyanosis
4. Elevated WBC and ESR
5. Diagnostic tests
   a. Venography (phlebography): increased uptake of radioactive material
   b. Doppler ultrasonography: impairment of blood flow ahead of thrombus
   c. Venous pressure measurements: high in affected limb until collateral circulation is developed

D. Nursing interventions
1. Provide bed rest, elevating involved extremity to increase venous return and decrease edema.
2. Apply continuous warm, moist soaks to decrease lymphatic congestion.
3. Administer anticoagulants as ordered
   a. Heparin
      1) monitor PTT; dosage should be adjusted to keep PTT between 1.5–2.5 times normal control level.
      2) use infusion pump to administer IV heparin.
      3) ensure proper injection technique.
         a) use 26- or 27-gauge syringe with ½ - ⅝ -inch needle, inject into fatty layer of abdomen above iliac crest.
         b) avoid injecting within 2 inches of umbilicus.
         c) insert needle at 45–90° to skin.
         d) do not withdraw plunger to assess blood return.
         e) apply gentle pressure after removal of needle, avoid massage.

4) assess for increased bleeding tendencies (hematuria; hematemesis; bleeding gums; petechiae of soft palate, conjunctiva, retina; ecchymoses, epistaxis, bloody sputum, melena) and instruct client to observe for and report these.
5) have antidote (protamine sulfate) available.
6) instruct client to avoid aspirin, antihistamines, and cough preparations containing glyceryl guaiacolate, and to obtain physician's permission before using other OTC drugs.

b. Warfarin (Coumadin)
1) assess PT daily; dosage should be adjusted to maintain PT at 1.5–2.5 times normal control level; INR of 2.
2) obtain careful medication history (there are many drug-drug interactions).
3) advise client to withhold dose and notify physician immediately if bleeding or signs of bleeding occur (see Heparin, above).
4) instruct client to use a soft toothbrush and to floss gently.
5) have antidote (vitamin K) available.
6) alert client to factors that may affect the anticoagulant response (high-fat diet or sudden increases in vitamin K-rich foods).
7) instruct client to wear Medic-Alert bracelet.

4. Assess vital signs every 4 hours.
5. Monitor for chest pain or shortness of breath (possible pulmonary embolism).
6. Measure thighs, calves, ankles, and instep every morning.
7. Provide client teaching and discharge planning concerning
a. Need to avoid standing, sitting for long periods; constrictive clothing; crossing legs at the knees; smoking; oral contraceptives
b. Importance of adequate hydration to prevent hypercoagulability
c. Use of elastic stockings when ambulatory
d. Importance of planned rest periods with elevation of the feet
e. Drug regimen
f. Plan for exercise/activity
1) begin with dorsiflexion of the feet while sitting or lying down
2) swim several times weekly
3) gradually increase walking distance
g. Importance of weight reduction if obese

Pulmonary Embolism

A. General information
1. Most pulmonary emboli arise as detached portions of venous thrombi formed in the deep veins of the legs, right side of the heart, or pelvic area.

CLIENT TEACHING CHECKLIST

Teach the client about the anticoagulation medication and the signs of bleeding. The client should watch for:

- Bloody stool
- Blood in urine
- Bleeding gums
- Bleeding hemorrhoids
- Large bruises
- Excessive menstrual flow

2. Distribution of emboli is related to blood flow; emboli involve the lower lobes of the lung because of higher blood flow.
3. Embolic obstruction to blood flow increases venous pressure in the pulmonary artery and pulmonary hypertension.
4. Risk factors: venous thrombosis, immobility, pre- and post-op states, trauma, pregnancy, HF, use of oral contraceptives, obesity

B. Medical management
   1. Drug therapy
      a. Anticoagulants
      b. Thrombolytics: streptokinase or urokinase
      c. Dextran 70 to decrease blood viscosity and aggregation of blood cells
      d. Narcotics for pain relief
      e. Vasopressors (in the presence of shock)
   2. Surgery: *embolectomy* (surgical removal of an embolus from the pulmonary arteries)

C. Assessment findings
   1. Chest pain (pleuritic), severe dyspnea, feeling of impending doom
   2. Tachypnea, tachycardia, anxiety, hemoptysis, shock symptoms (if massive)
   3. Decreased pCO_2; increased pH (due to hyperventilation)
   4. Increased temperature
   5. Intensified pulmonic S_2; rales or crackles
   6. Diagnostic tests
      a. Pulmonary angiography: reveals location/extent of embolism
      b. Lung scan reveals adequacy/inadequacy of pulmonary circulation

D. Nursing interventions
   1. Administer medications as ordered; monitor effects and side effects.
   2. Administer oxygen therapy to correct hypoxemia.

3. Assist with turning, coughing, deep breathing, and passive ROM exercises.
4. Provide adequate hydration to prevent hypercoagulability.
5. Offer support/reassurance to client/family.
6. Elevate head of bed to relieve dyspnea.
7. Provide client teaching and discharge planning: same as for thrombophlebitis.

Varicose Veins

A. General information
   1. Dilated veins that occur most often in the lower extremities and trunk. As the vessel dilates, the valves become stretched and incompetent with resultant venous pooling/edema
   2. Most common between ages 30 and 50
   3. Predisposing factor: congenital weakness of the veins, thrombophlebitis, pregnancy, obesity, heart disease
B. Medical management: vein ligation (involves ligating the saphenous vein where it joins the femoral vein and stripping the saphenous vein system from groin to ankle)
C. Assessment findings
   1. Pain after prolonged standing (relieved by elevation)
   2. Swollen, dilated, tortuous skin veins
   3. Diagnostic tests
      a. Trendelenburg test: varicose veins distend very quickly (less than 35 seconds)
      b. Doppler ultrasound: decreased or no blood flow heard after calf or thigh compression
D. Nursing interventions
   1. Elevate legs above heart level.
   2. Measure circumference of ankle and calf daily.
   3. Apply knee-length elastic stockings.
   4. Provide adequate rest.
   5. Prepare client for vein ligation, if necessary.
      a. Provide routine pre-op care; usually outpatient surgery.
      b. In addition to routine post-op care
         1) keep affected extremity elevated above the level of the heart to prevent edema.
         2) apply elastic bandages and stockings, which should be removed every 8 hours for short periods and reapplied.
         3) assist out of bed within 24 hours, ensuring that elastic stockings are applied.
         4) assess for increased bleeding, particularly in the groin area.
   6. Provide client teaching and discharge planning: same as for thrombophlebitis.

Amputation

A. General information
   1. Surgical procedure done for peripheral vascular disease if medical management is ineffective and the symptoms become worse.
   2. The level of amputation is determined by the extent of the disease process.
      a. Above knee (AK): performed between the lower third to the middle of the thigh
      b. Below knee (BK): usually done in middle third of leg, leaving a stump of 12.5–17.5 cm

B. Nursing interventions: preoperative
   1. Provide routine pre-op care.
   2. Offer support/encouragement and accept client's response of anger/grief.
   3. Discuss
      a. Rehabilitation program and use of prosthesis
      b. Upper extremity exercises such as push-ups in bed
      c. Crutch walking
      d. Amputation dressings/cast
      e. Phantom limb sensation as a normal occurrence

C. Nursing interventions: postoperative
   1. Provide routine post-op care.
   2. Prevent hip/knee contractures.
   3. Avoid letting client sit in chair with hips flexed for long periods of time.
   4. Have client assume prone position several times a day and position hip in extension (unless otherwise ordered).
   5. Avoid elevation of the stump after 12–24 hours.
   6. Observe stump dressing for signs of hemorrhage and mark outside of dressing so rate of bleeding can be assessed.
   7. Administer pain medication as ordered.
   8. Ensure that stump bandages fit tightly and are applied properly to enhance prosthesis fitting.
   9. Initiate active ROM exercises of all joints (when medically advised), crutch walking, and arm/shoulder exercises.
   10. Provide stump care.
      a. Inspect daily for signs of skin irritation.
      b. Wash thoroughly daily with warm water and bacteriostatic soap; rinse and dry thoroughly.
      c. Avoid use of irritating substances such as lotions, alcohol, powders.

REVIEW QUESTIONS

1. An adult is admitted to the coronary care unit to rule out a myocardial infarction. The client states, "I am not sure if it is just angina, and I cannot understand the difference between angina and heart attack pain." Which response is most appropriate for the nurse to make?
   1. Anginal pain usually lasts only 3–5 minutes.
   2. Anginal pain produces clenching of the fists over the chest while acute MI pain does not.
   3. Anginal pain requires morphine for relief.
   4. Anginal pain radiates to the left arm while acute MI pain does not.
2. An adult woman is admitted to the cardiac care unit with a myocardial infarction. The morning after admission she and her husband tell the nurse that she must be home tonight to care for the children when her husband goes to work. The problem identified at this point would be
   1. anxiety related to physical limitations.
   2. alteration in cardiac output.
   3. inability of client/family to understand disease process.
   4. safety needs related to inability to cope.
3. The nurse is caring for an adult admitted to the coronary care unit with a myocardial infarction. During the second night in the CCU, the client develops heart failure. A pulmonary artery catheter is inserted to monitor the client for left ventricular function because
   1. it provides information about pulmonary resistance.
   2. it measures myocardial oxygen consumption.
   3. it controls renal blood flow.
   4. it controls afterload.
4. The nurse is planning care for a client who is in heart failure. Which of the following goals are appropriate? Select all that apply.

   ____ An increase in cardiac output.

   ____ An elevation in renal blood flow.

   ____ A reduction in the heart's workload.

   ____ A decrease in myocardial contractility.
5. The nurse is caring for an adult who is being treated for a myocardial infarction. Oxygen is ordered. Administering oxygen to this client is related to which of the following client problems?
   1. Anxiety.

2. Chest pains.
3. Ineffective myocardial perfusion.
4. Alteration in heart rate, rhythm, or conduction.

6. The nurse reading an ECG rhythm strip notes that there are 8 QRS complexes in a 6-second strip. The heart rate is
   1. 48.
   2. 64.
   3. 80.
   4. 120.

7. A 57-year-old is being treated in the clinic for hypertension. His blood pressure is 170/92 and he is complaining of fatigue and lassitude. He has been taking propranolol (Inderal) 80 mg bid. The best indication that previous teaching about this drug has been successful is that he
   1. checks his pulse for bradycardia.
   2. makes an appointment as soon as he notices fatigue.
   3. stops the drug when he experiences chest pain.
   4. takes the drug with breakfast and dinner.

8. A 56-year-old obese man is recovering from a bowel resection for cancer of the colon. On his third post-op day he complains that the area around the calf of his leg is warm and tender. Suspecting he may have developed a thrombus, the nurse performs a thorough assessment. When assessing for common clinical manifestations of deep vein thrombosis, the nurse will observe the client for
   1. absence of a pulse distal to the clot.
   2. cyanosis distal to the clot.
   3. pain on dorsiflexion.
   4. reddened area around the clot.

9. A 68-year-old man has been treated over the years for chronic venous insufficiency. Today he came to the medical clinic complaining of severe pain in his legs. They were swollen and covered with deep, draining, foul-smelling ulcers. He is admitted to the hospital for aggressive treatment. The nurse reminds him that the underlying cause of his venous insufficiency is
   1. congestive heart failure.
   2. hypertrophied leg muscles.
   3. decreased hemoglobin levels.
   4. poor blood return to the heart.

10. A 65-year-old man is admitted with venous stasis ulcers and chronic venous insufficiency. A goal of care for this client is the control of swelling. The primary mechanism for achieving this is to

1. exercise vigorously.
2. restrict fluid intake.
3. promote gravity drainage.
4. eat a high-protein, low-salt diet.

11. A client is being assessed to rule out cardiovascular problems. The nurse understands that some of the common symptoms associated with cardiovascular disease are

1. shortness of breath, chest discomfort, palpitations.
2. dyspnea, chest discomfort, sputum production.
3. fatigue, weight changes, mood swings.
4. mood swings, headaches, fainting.

12. Which of the following assessment findings by the nurse is abnormal?

1. S_1 heard at the fourth-fifth left intercostals space in a 35-year-old man.
2. S_2 heard at the second-third left intercostals space in a 40-year-old female.
3. S_4 heard at the apex in an 80-year-old male.
4. S_3 heard at the apex in a 15-year-old female.

13. Which of the following instructions should the nurse give to a client prior to an exercise electrocardiogram?

1. Avoid coffee, tea, and alcohol the day of the test.
2. Smoking is permitted up to the time of the test.
3. Allow only 3 hours of sleep the night prior to the test.
4. Take all medications as prescribed prior to the test.

14. To prevent possible complication, which of the following questions should a nurse ask a client prior to a cardiac catheterization?

1. "Have you ever had a cardiac catheterization before?"
2. "Can you eat shellfish?"
3. "Do you understand the procedure?"
4. "Have you ever had a heart attack?"

15. Which of the following should the nurse include in the plan of care for a post-op coronary arteriogram client?

1. Assess pedal pulses.
2. Assess lung sounds.

3. Provide early ambulation.
4. Monitor vital signs every 8 hours.

16. A client has the following rhythm. The client has no pulse or blood pressure.

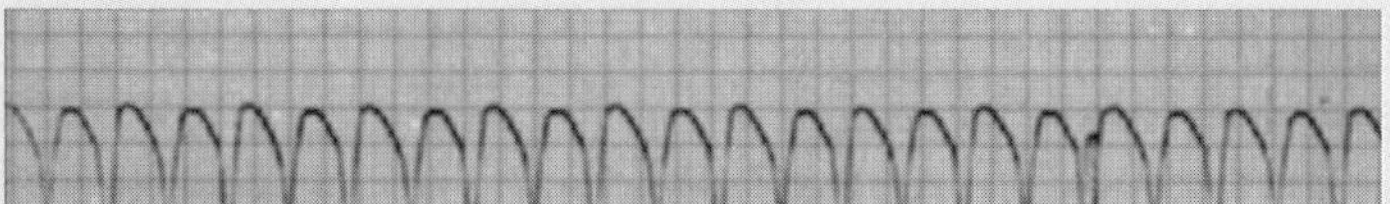

The nurse interprets the rhythm as
1. ventricular tachycardia.
2. ventricular fibrillation.
3. sinus tachycardia.
4. supraventricular tachycardia.

17. A client has the following rhythm. The client has no pulse or blood pressure.

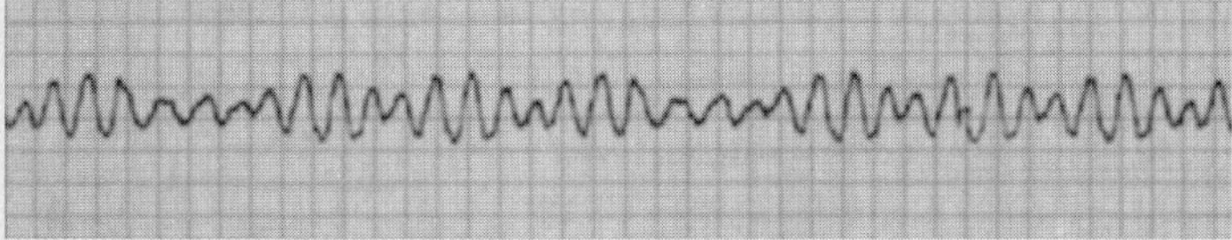

The nurse interprets the rhythm as
1. ventricular tachycardia.
2. ventricular fibrillation.
3. sinus tachycardia.
4. supraventricular tachycardia.

18. A client had a myocardial infarction yesterday. His cardiac monitor shows 6 to 8 PVCs per minute, with occasional couplets. The best action by the nurse at this time is to
1. monitor the client for development of ventricular tachycardia.
2. administer the ordered prn dose of lidocaine.
3. perform a precordial thump.
4. initiate manual chest compressions.

19. A client is admitted in cardiogenic shock. To *best* evaluate the heart's hemodynamic performance, the nurse anticipates the insertion of a(n)
1. intra-arterial line.
2. pulmonary artery catheter.
3. intra-aortic balloon pump (IABP).
4. central venous pressure line (CVP).

20. Which of the following statements by a client to the nurse indicates a risk factor for coronary artery disease?

1. "I exercise four times a week."
2. "No one in my family has heart problems."
3. "My cholesterol is 189."
4. "I smoke 1½ packs of cigarettes per day."

21. An adult female has a history of coronary artery disease and angina pectoris. After walking to the bathroom, she complains of aching substernal pain that radiates to her left shoulder. The nurse should

1. assist her to lie down and elevate her legs.
2. administer a prn dose of nitroglycerin sublingually.
3. use pillows to support and immobilize the left shoulder.
4. administer a prn dose of aspirin or acetaminophen (Tylenol).

22. A nitroglycerin transdermal patch was prescribed 6 weeks ago for an adult to treat angina pectoris. The nurse knows that the patch has been effective if

1. the client's serum cholesterol level has decreased.
2. the client's pressure is within normal limits.
3. the client reports no episodes of chest pain.
4. pulse oximetry shows the client's oxygen saturation is improved.

23. An adult has developed angina pectoris secondary to coronary artery disease. A low-fat, low cholesterol diet is prescribed for the client. The nurse should praise the client for a wise choice if which of the following was selected for an evening snack?

1. Cheese cubes and crackers.
2. Half tuna salad sandwich.
3. Yogurt with fresh strawberries.
4. Jello mold with fruit slices.

24. Lidocaine is mixed 2 g in 500 ml D_5W. The nurse prepared to start an infusion at 2 mg/h using a 60-drop tubing. Which of the following is the correct rate to start the infusion on a pump?

1. 15 ml.
2. 30 ml.
3. 45 ml.
4. 60 ml.

25. An adult male is transferred to the step-down unit on the third day after a myocardial infarction. Which of the following should the nurse include in his care plan at this time?

1. Enforcing complete bed rest.
2. Supervising short walks in the hallway.
3. Performing passive range of motion exercises.
4. Having him sit on the side of the bed and dangle his legs.

26. A 55-year-old man with a history of angina pectoris complains of chest pain radiating to the jaw. After taking three nitroglycerin gr 1/150 tablets he is still having the chest pain. His skin is cool and pale and he is diaphoretic and mildly short of breath. The best initial action for the nurse to take is to

1. auscultate heart and lung sounds.
2. administer another nitroglycerin tablet.
3. initiate telemetry monitoring.
4. assist him to a supine position.

27. An adult male is being discharged from the hospital following a myocardial infarction. The nurse knows that he understands the guidelines for resuming sexual activity if he states that

1. bedtime is the best time to have intercourse.
2. he should exercise for 10–15 minutes before intercourse, to "warm up."
3. he should take a nitroglycerin before intercourse to prevent chest pain.
4. it is best to avoid having intercourse when the stomach is empty.

28. An adult is scheduled for a percutaneous transluminal coronary angioplasty (PTCA). The client says to the nurse, "Can you tell me again what the doctor is going to do? I don't remember exactly what she told me." The most appropriate response by the nurse would be,

1. "A clot dissolving drug is administered through a catheter into the blocked section of your artery."
2. "A piece of vein from your leg is used to bypass the blocked section of your artery."
3. "A tiny rotating blade is used to scrape off the plaque that is blocking your artery."
4. "A balloon is placed next to the plaque blocking your artery, then the balloon is inflated to crush the plaque."

29. A man is being discharged following coronary artery bypass graft surgery (CABG). The nurse recognizes that he needs additional teaching if he makes which of the following statements?

1. "I'll be going to a support group to help me quit smoking."
2. "I need to use a golf cart instead of walking around the course."
3. "I should bake or broil my chicken instead of frying it."
4. "I've learned a breathing exercise to help me calm down if I get upset."

30. Which of the following assessment findings by the nurse indicates right ventricular failure in a client?

1. Pink frothy sputum.

2. Paroxysmal nocturnal dyspnea.

3. Jugular venous distention.

4. Crackles.

31. A nurse is assessing a client with fatigue, tachycardia, crackles, and pink frothy sputum. Which nursing diagnosis is of the *most* importance?

1. Impaired skin integrity.

2. Impaired gas exchange.

3. Potential for injury.

4. Anxiety.

32. An adult is admitted with an acute exacerbation of congestive heart failure. Vital signs are: T 99, P 115, R 32, BP 154/100. Ankles are edematous and crackles are auscultated at the bases of both lungs, 0.5 mg of digoxin (Lanoxin) IV and 40 mg of furosemide (Lasix) IV are administered immediately. The nurse recognizes that the medications are having a therapeutic effect if

1. the client's pulse rate decreases below 100.

2. the client has an increased urine specific gravity.

3. the client expectorates frothy sputum.

4. the client's lungs are clear to auscultation.

33. A client is admitted with pulmonary edema. The nurse is preparing to administer morphine sulfate. What beneficial effect does morphine have in pulmonary edema?

1. Decreases anxiety, work of breathing, and vasodilates.

2. Decreases respiratory rate.

3. Provides an analgesic and sedative effect.

4. Decreases anxiety and vasoconstricts.

34. An adult female is being discharged after having a ventricular demand pacemaker inserted. The nurse should include which of the following in the teaching plan for this client?

1. She should not use remote control devices (e.g., TV channel selector).

2. She must leave the room while a microwave oven is in operation.

3. She will need to avoid air travel.

4. She should not pass through metal detectors.

35. An adult has a ventricular demand pacemaker that is set at 72 beats per minute. The nurse knows that the client's pacemaker is functioning correctly if which of the following appears on the ECG?

1. Pacemaker spikes instead of QRS complexes.
2. Pacemaker spikes followed by QRS complexes.
3. Pacemaker spikes before each P wave.
4. Pacemaker spikes appearing only if the heart rate is over 72.

36. Which strategy by the nurse provides safety during a defibrillation attempt?

1. A verbal and visual check of "all clear."
2. No lubricant on the paddles.
3. Placing paddles lightly on the chest.
4. Standing in alignment with the bed while administering the shock.

37. An adult client has experienced a cardiac arrest and the nurse is performing CPR. The correct position of the nurse's hands on the client's chest is

1. over the upper half of the sternum.
2. two finger widths below the sternal notch.
3. two finger widths above the xiphoid process.
4. over the xiphoid process.

38. A client with a history of a myocardial infarction two days ago reports chest pain that is worse on inspiration but is relieved on sitting forward. Based on this finding, the nurse suspects the client is experiencing the pain of

1. endocarditis.
2. angina pectoris.
3. pericarditis.
4. recurrent myocardial infarction.

39. An adult has prazocin hydrochloride (Minipress) prescribed to treat hypertension. The nurse should instruct the client to

1. take the medication with meals.
2. take the first dose at bedtime.
3. report a pulse rate below 50 to the physician.
4. check the ankles daily for edema.

40. An adult has essential hypertension. She is being treated with a thiazide diuretic and dietary and lifestyle modifications. The nurse knows that she understands the treatment if she makes which of the following statements?

1. "I will use soy sauce or mustard instead of salt on my food."

2. "I need to cut back to two, 4-ounce glasses of wine a day."
3. "I will stop riding my bike because vigorous exercise will raise my blood pressure."
4. "Smoking helped cause my hypertension, but quitting won't reverse the damage."

41. Hydrochlorothiazide is prescribed to treat high blood pressure. The nurse knows that the client understands the dietary modifications she needs to make if she states that she will increase her intake of

1. fresh oranges.
2. cold cereals.
3. cola drinks.
4. cranberry juice.

42. A client reports an aching pain and cramping sensation that occurs while walking. The pain disappears after cessation of walking. The pain is in both legs. Based on these clinical findings, the nurse suspects the client has (a)

1. deep venous thrombosis (DVT).
2. Raynaud's disease.
3. arteriosclerosis obliterans.
4. thrombophlebitis.

43. An adult has severe arteriosclerosis obliterans and complains of intermittent claudication after walking 20 feet. How should the nurse plan to position the client when she is in bed?

1. Supine with legs elevated.
2. In semi-Fowler's position with knees extended.
3. In reverse Trendelenburg position.
4. In Trendelenburg position.

44. An adult female experiences painful arterial spasms in her hands due to Raynaud's phenomenon. Which of the following should the nurse include in the teaching plan for her?

1. Drink a hot beverage, such as tea or coffee, to relieve spasms.
2. Reduce intake of high fat or high cholesterol foods.
3. Raise the hands above the head to relieve spasms.
4. Wear gloves when handling refrigerated foods.

45. Which assessment finding by the nurse would indicate an abdominal aortic aneurysm?

1. Knifelike pain in the back.
2. Pulsatile mass in the abdomen.

3. Unequal femoral pulses.
4. Boardlike rigid abdomen.

46. A nurse is assessing a post-op femoral popliteal bypass client. Which of the following assessment findings indicates a complication?

1. BP 110/80, HR 86, RR 20.
2. Small amount of dark-red blood on dressing.
3. A decrease in pulse quality in the operated leg.
4. Swelling of the operative leg.

47. An adult has just returned to the surgical unit after a femoral-popliteal bypass on the right leg. The nurse should place the client in what position?

1. Fowler's position with the right leg extended.
2. Supine with the right knee flexed 45°.
3. Supine with the right leg extended and flat on the bed.
4. Semi-Fowler's position with the right leg elevated on two pillows.

48. The client has a large, venous stasis ulcer on her left ankle. Wound care is performed three times a week by a home health nurse. The nurse should teach her to

1. dangle the legs for 5–10 minutes several times a day.
2. wear heavy cotton or wool socks when going outdoors.
3. soak the feet in tepid water three or four times daily.
4. take frequent rest periods with her legs elevated.

49. An adult is hospitalized with deep vein thrombophlebitis. During the first few days of therapy, the nurse should

1. keep the client in Trendelenburg position.
2. apply ice packs three or four times daily to relieve pain.
3. massage the affected leg once a shift.
4. encourage the client to perform active range of motion exercises with both legs each shift.

50. A client is being discharged after treatment of deep venous thrombosis. Coumadin (warfarin) 2.5 mg daily is prescribed. The nurse recognizes that which of the following statements indicates that the client understands the effects of Coumadin?

1. "I'll use an electric razor to shave my legs."
2. "I'll have a podiatrist cut my toenails."
3. "I need to eat more salads and fresh fruits."
4. "I will take aspirin instead of Tylenol for headaches."

51. An adult female, who was admitted 4 hours ago with thrombophlebitis in the left leg, suddenly becomes confused and dyspneic. She begins coughing up blood-streaked sputum and complains of chest pain that worsens on inspiration. The nurse should first

1. apply soft restraints to prevent excessive movement.

2. perform a Heimlich maneuver.

3. place her in bed in semi-Fowler's position.

4. place her in Trendelenburg position on her left side.

52. A client is admitted to rule out pulmonary embolism (PE) from a deep venous thrombosis. A Dextran 70 infusion is ordered for the client. The nurse understands the Dextran is administered to

1. increase blood viscosity.

2. decrease platelet adhesion.

3. decrease plasma volume.

4. increase the hemoglobin.

53. A client reports aching, heaviness, itching, and moderate swelling of the legs. On assessment, the nurse notes dilated tortuous skin veins. Based on this assessment, the nurse suspects the client has

1. thrombophlebitis.

2. venous thrombosis.

3. varicose veins.

4. chronic venous insufficiency.

54. An adult had an above-the-knee amputation of the left leg 2 days ago. The nurse should include which of the following in the care plan?

1. Resting in a prone or supine position with the stump extended several times a day.

2. Using a rolled towel or small pillow to elevate the stump at all times.

3. Applying warm soaks to the stump to reduce phantom limb pain.

4. Avoiding turning to the left side until the stump has healed completely.

55. An adult male had a below-the-knee amputation of the right foot 2 days ago. He is complaining of pain in his right foot. The best response by the nurse is to

1. explain to him that this is a common sensation after amputation.

2. remind him that that foot was amputated and therefore cannot have pain.

3. tell him that such pain is a common psychological response to loss of a limb.

4. show him the stump so he will realize his right foot is gone.

ANSWERS AND RATIONALES

1. 1. Anginal pain is of short duration and is usually relieved by rest.

2. 3. The nurse should assess both spouses' understanding of the disease and rehabilitation processes. They both exhibit the need for information in order to be able to make rational decisions.

3. 1. The Swan-Ganz catheter measures pulmonary artery and capillary wedge pressures, which are good indicators of increase in pulmonary pressure caused by increase in left ventricular pressure.

4. *An increase in cardiac output should be checked. This is an appropriate goal.*
   An elevation in renal blood flow should be checked. This is an appropriate goal. Renal blood flow will increase as cardiac output increases.
   A reduction in the heart's workload should be checked. Reducing the venous return or the cardiac workload is an appropriate goal.

5. 3. With acute myocardial infarction there is ineffective myocardial perfusion, resulting in a decrease in the amount of oxygen available for tissue perfusion. Oxygen is administered to improve tissue perfusion in these clients.

6. 3. A regular heart rate is calculated by multiplying the number of QRS complexes in 6 seconds (8 QRS complexes) by 10 (because there are 60 seconds in 1 minute). The heart rate is 80. This method is not accurate if the client's heart rate is irregular.

7. 1. A common side effect of propranolol is slowed pulse rate because the drug is a beta blocker.

8. 3. Pain on dorsiflexion is a common manifestation of deep vein thrombosis.

9. 4. Venous insufficiency is stasis of venous blood flow or poor blood return to the heart. The leg muscles that normally compress the veins to force blood upward are not effective.

10. 3. Swelling is minimized by promoting gravity drainage. This could be accomplished by elevating the extremities.

11. 1. Some of the most common clinical manifestations of cardiovascular disease are shortness of breath, chest pain or discomfort, dyspnea, palpitations, fainting, and peripheral skin changes such as edema.

12. 3. S_4 is an abnormal heart sound. It is indicative of decreased ventricular compliance.

13. 1. Avoid any stimulants such as coffee, tea, or a depressant such as alcohol.

14. 2. Shellfish contains iodine, which is also in the contrast media used during a catheterization. It is *imperative* to obtain information regarding iodine allergies.

15. 1. Assessment of pedal pulses is imperative after a cardiac catheterization. Evaluation of presence and quality of pulses indicates blood flow to the catheterized extremity.

16. 1. The above rhythm is ventricular tachycardia.

17. 2. The above rhythm is ventricular fibrillation.

18. 2. Lidocaine, a class I antidysrhythmic drug, is indicated when the client has six or more PVCs per minute, multifocal PVCs, couplets or triplets, or PVCs occurring on the downslope of the T wave. Any of these situations is likely to progress to the more dangerous ventricular tachycardia or ventricular fibrillation if not treated immediately.

19. 2. A pulmonary artery catheter will show all right and left heart hemodynamic pressures and provide for cardiac output measurements.

20. 4. Smoking has been determined to increase the risk of coronary heart disease.

21. 3. Nitroglycerin dilates peripheral veins, reducing venous return to the heart. This immediately decreases cardiac workload, relieving ischemia and chest pain. It also dilates coronary arteries, improving oxygen supply to the heart.

22. 3. Nitroglycerin reduces cardiac workload and improves myocardial oxygenation. This prevents episodes of anginal pain.

23. 4. Most fruits and vegetables are low in fat and cholesterol-free. Jello also has no fat or cholesterol.

24. 2. 30 ml is 2 mg/h.
1000 mg = 1 g. 2 g is 200 mg.
2000 mg:500 ml::2 mg: x ml
$2000x = 1000$
x = 0.5 ml/hr
60drops = 1 ml. 60drops × 0.5 ml. = 30 ml/hr.

25. 2. To improve activity tolerance, supervised walks for gradually increasing distances are encouraged when the client is transferred out of the coronary care unit.

26. 1. Assessment is important to identify the probable cause of the pain so that definitive intervention can be planned. Dysrhythmias are a common complication of MI. Crackles in the lungs and an S_3 gallop may indicate heart failure.

27. 3. Nitroglycerin is used prophylactically before activities that are known to cause chest pain, including sexual intercourse.

28. 4. PTCA is also called balloon angioplasty because a balloon-tipped catheter is used. When the balloon is inflated, the plaque is compressed, leaving the artery unobstructed.

29. 2. Aerobic exercise, such as walking, helps to slow formation of atherosclerotic plaques in coronary artery disease. The client needs to make the necessary lifestyle changes to prevent further progression of his disease. Riding instead of walking would not provide aerobic exercise. Therefore, this statement shows that the client needs further teaching.

30. 3. Jugular venous distention is seen in right ventricular failure as volume overload occurs. This overload is reflected upward into the jugulars.

31. 2. With left ventricular heart failure, carbon dioxide and oxygen exchange is impaired due to fluid overload and leads to hypoxia.

32. 4. Crackles in the lungs are a sign of pulmonary edema due to HF. Improved cardiac output due to digoxin and reduced extracellular fluid volume due to furosemide should result in reduction of pulmonary edema.

33. 1. This is the beneficial effect of morphine in pulmonary edema.

34. 4. Metal detectors generate strong magnetic fields that can alter pacemaker settings or produce interference that causes malfunction.

35. 2. The ventricular pacemaker stimulates the ventricle if no atrial impulse is transmitted through the AV node. The appearance of the QRS complex shows that the ventricle has responded to the stimulus.

36. 1. The nurse must make sure both verbally and visually that all health care providers are clear.

37. 3. This hand position would depress the lower half of the sternum, which would compress the heart effectively.

38. 3. The pain of pericarditis is exacerbated with respirations. Rotating the trunk and sitting up frequently relieves the pain.

39. 2. First dose syncope occurs with prazocin. To reduce the risk of fainting, the client should take the first dose at bedtime.

40. 2. Moderation in alcohol intake is an important lifestyle change for controlling high blood pressure. Alcohol adds empty calories to the diet and elevates arterial blood pressure.

41. 1. Oranges are high in potassium. Thiazide diuretics, such as hydrochlorothiazide, deplete body potassium by increasing urinary excretion, so potassium intake should be increased.

42. 3. Intermittent claudication is the main symptom of narrowing of the arteries.

43. 3. Gravity facilitates improved arterial blood flow. The reverse Trendelenburg position, in which the feet are below heart level, is used to improve circulation to the lower extremities.

44. 4. Cold induces arterial spasms. When the hands will be exposed to cold, warm gloves or mittens should be worn.

45. 2. A pulsating abdominal mass is a common finding of an abdominal aortic aneurysm.

46. 3. A decrease in pulse quality signifies a decrease in the patency of the artery.

47. 3. The best position for the affected leg is extended and flat in the bed. Elevating the leg would allow gravity to impede circulation. Having the leg dependent would promote development of edema, which could also impair circulation.

48. 4. Elevating the legs improves venous drainage and reduces edema, which will promote wound healing.

49. 1. Elevation of the legs by raising the foot of the bed 6 inches (Trendelenburg position) reduces venous stasis, decreasing the risk of further thrombus formation.

50. 1. Warfarin is an anticoagulant, which increases the risk of bleeding from any injury. Use of an electric razor reduces the risk of a cut, which might bleed excessively.

51. 3. Her symptoms suggest that the client has pulmonary emboli. Her activity should be limited to prevent further embolization, and her head should be elevated to promote lung expansion and ease dyspnea.

52. 2. Dextran coats the platelet surface to decrease adhesion. In doing so, the plasma volume expands, and viscosity is decreased.

53. 3. This describes varicose veins.

54. 1. It is essential to prevent contractures of the hip joint so that the client will be able to walk with a prosthesis. Lying supine or prone with the stump extended helps to prevent hip contractures.

55. 1. Phantom limb pain is common after amputation. It is a real sensation and needs to be acknowledged by the nurse.

7

The Hematologic System

OVERVIEW OF ANATOMY AND PHYSIOLOGY

CHAPTER OUTLINE

The structures of the hematologic or hematopoietic system include the blood, blood vessels, and blood-forming organs (bone marrow, spleen, liver, lymph nodes, and thymus gland). The major function of blood is to carry necessary materials (oxygen, nutrients) to cells and to remove carbon dioxide and metabolic waste products. The hematologic system also plays an important role in hormone transport, the inflammatory and immune responses, temperature regulation, fluid-electrolyte balance, and acid-base balance.

Bone Marrow

A. Contained inside all bones, occupies interior of spongy bones and center of long bones; collectively one of the largest organs of the body (4–5% of total body weight)
B. Primary function is hematopoiesis (the formation of blood cells)
C. Two kinds of bone marrow, red and yellow
  1. Red (functioning) marrow
    a. Carries out hematopoiesis; production site of erythroid, myeloid, and thrombocytic components of blood; one source of lymphocytes and macrophages
    b. Found in ribs, vertebral column, other flat bones
  2. Yellow marrow: red marrow that has changed to fat; found in long bones; does not contribute to hematopoiesis
D. All blood cells start as stem cells in the bone marrow; these mature into the different, specific types of cells, collectively referred to as formed elements of blood or blood components: erythrocytes, leukocytes, and thrombocytes.

Blood

A. Composed of plasma (55%) and cellular components (45%)
B. *Hematocrit*
  1. Reflects portion of blood composed of red blood cells

2. Centrifugation of blood results in separation into top layer of plasma, middle layer of leukocytes and platelets, and bottom layer of erythrocytes.
3. Majority of formed elements is erythrocytes; volume of leukocytes and platelets is negligible.

C. Distribution
1. 1300 ml in pulmonary circulation
 a. 400 ml arterial
 b. 60 ml capillary
 c. 840 ml venous
2. 3000 ml in systemic circulation
 a. 550 ml arterial
 b. 300 ml capillary
 c. 2150 ml venous

Plasma

A. Liquid part of blood; yellow in color because of pigments
B. Consists of serum (liquid portion of plasma) and fibrinogen
C. Contains plasma proteins such as albumin, serum globulins, fibrinogen, prothrombin, plasminogen
1. Albumin: largest of plasma proteins, involved in regulation of intravascular plasma volume and maintenance of osmotic pressure
2. Serum globulins: alpha, beta, gamma
 a. Alpha: role in transport of steroids, lipids, bilirubin
 b. Beta: role in transport of iron and copper
 c. Gamma: role in immune response, function of antibodies
3. Fibrinogen, prothrombin, plasminogen

Cellular Components

Cellular components or formed elements of blood are erythrocytes (red blood cells [RBCs]), which are responsible for oxygen transport; leukocytes (white blood cells [WBCs]), which play a major role in defense against microorganisms; and thrombocytes (platelets), which function in hemostasis.

A. *Erythrocytes*
1. Bioconcave disc shape, no nucleus, chiefly sacs of hemoglobin
2. Cell membrane is highly diffusible to $O_2$and CO_2
3. RBCs are responsible for oxygen transport via *hemoglobin* (*Hgb*)
 a. Two portions: iron carried on heme portion; second portion is protein
 b. Normal blood contains 12–18 g Hgb/100 ml blood; higher (14–18 g) in men than in women (12–14 g)
4. Production
 a. Start in bone marrow as stem cells, released as reticulocytes (immature cells), mature into erythrocytes

- **b.** Erythropoietin stimulates differentiation; produced by kidneys and stimulated by hypoxia
- **c.** Iron, vitamin B_{12}, folic acid, pyridoxine (vitamin B_6), and other factors required for erythropoiesis

5. Hemolysis (destruction)
- **a.** Average life span 120 days
- **b.** Immature RBCs destroyed in either bone marrow or other reticuloendothelial organs (blood, connective tissue, spleen, liver, lungs, and lymph nodes)
- **c.** Mature cells removed chiefly by liver and spleen
- **d.** *Bilirubin:* by-product of Hgb released when RBCs destroyed, excreted in bile
- **e.** Iron: freed from Hgb during bilirubin formation; transported to bone marrow via transferrin and reclaimed for new Hgb production
- **f.** Premature destruction: may be caused by RBC membrane abnormalities, Hgb abnormalities, extrinsic physical factors (such as the enzyme defects found in G6PD)
- **g.** Normal age RBCs may be destroyed by gross damage as in trauma or extravascular hemolysis (in spleen, liver, bone marrow)

B. *Leukocytes:* granulocytes and mononuclear cells: involved in protection from bacteria and other foreign substances

1. Granulocytes: eosinophils, basophils, and neutrophils
- **a.** *Eosinophils:* involved in phagocytosis and allergic reactions
- **b.** *Basophils:* involved in prevention of clotting in microcirculation and allergic reactions
- **c.** Eosinophils and basophils are reservoirs of histamine, serotonin, and heparin
- **d.** *Neutrophils:* involved in short-term phagocytosis
  - **1)** mature neutrophils: polymorphonuclear leukocytes
  - **2)** immature neutrophils: band cells (bacterial infection usually produces increased numbers of band cells)

2. Mononuclear cells: monocytes and lymphocytes: large nucleated cells
- **a.** *Monocytes:* involved in long-term phagocytosis; play a role in immune response
  - **1)** largest leukocyte
  - **2)** produced by bone marrow: give rise to histiocytes (Kupffer cells of liver), macrophages, and other components of reticuloendothelial system
- **b.** *Lymphocytes:* immune cells; produce substances against foreign cells; produced primarily in lymph tissue (B cells) and thymus (T cells)

C. *Thrombocytes (platelets)*

1. Fragments of megakaryocytes formed in bone marrow

2. Production regulated by thrombopoietin

3. Essential factor in coagulation via adhesion, aggregation, and plug formation
4. Release substances involved in coagulation

Blood Groups

A. Erythrocytes carry antigens, which determine the different blood groups.
B. Blood-typing systems are based on the many possible antigens, but the most important are the antigens of the ABO and Rh blood groups because they are most likely to be involved in transfusion reactions.
   1. ABO typing
      a. Antigens of system are labelled A and B.
      b. Absence of both antigens results in type O blood.
      c. Presence of both antigens is type AB.
      d. Presence of either A or B results in type A and type B, respectively.
      e. Nearly half the population is type O, the *universal donor*.
      f. Antibodies are automatically formed against the ABO antigens not on person's own RBCs; transfusion with mismatched or incompatible blood results in a transfusion reaction (Table 7-1).
   2. Rh typing
      a. Identifies presence or absence of Rh antigen (Rh positive or Rh negative).
      b. Anti-Rh antibodies not automatically formed in Rh-negative person, but if Rh-positive blood is given, antibody formation starts and a second exposure to Rh antigen will trigger a transfusion reaction.
      c. Important for Rh-negative woman carrying Rh-positive baby; first pregnancy not affected, but in a subsequent pregnancy with an Rh-positive baby, mother's antibodies attack baby's RBCs.

Blood Coagulation

Conversion of fluid blood into a solid clot to reduce blood loss when blood vessels are ruptured.

A. Systems that initiate clotting
   1. *Intrinsic system:* initiated by contact activation following endothelial injury ("intrinsic" to vessel itself)
      a. Factor XII initiates as contact made between damaged vessel and plasma protein
      b. Factors VIII, IX, and XI activated
   2. *Extrinsic system*
      a. Initiated by tissue thromboplastins, released from injured vessels ("extrinsic" to vessel)
      b. Factor VII activated

TABLE 7-1 Complications of Blood Transfusion

Type	Causes	Mechanism	Occurrence	Signs and Symptoms	Intervention
Hemolytic	ABO incompatibility; Rh incompatibility;use of dextrose solutions; wide temperature fluctuations	Antibodies in recipient plasma react with antigen in donor cells. Agglutinated cells block capillary blood flow to organs. Hemolysis (Hgb into plasma and urine).	*Acute:* first 5 min after completion of transfusion *Delayed:* days to 2 weeks after	Headache, lumbar or sternal pain, nausea, vomiting, diarrhea, fever, chills, flushing, heat along vein, restlessness, anemia, jaundice, dyspnea, signs of shock, renal shutdown, DIC	Stop transfusion. Continue saline IV. Send blood unit and client blood sampleto lab. Watch for hemoglobinuria. Treat or prevent shock, DIC, and renal shutdown.
Allergic	Transfer of an antigen or antibody from donor to recipient; allergic donors	Immune sensitivity to foreign serum protein	Within 30 min of start of transfusion	Urticaria, laryngeal edema, wheezing, dyspnea, bronchospasm, headache, anaphylaxis	Stop transfusion. Administer antihistamine and/or epinephrine. Treat life-threatening reactions.

Continued

Table 7-1 **Continued**

Type	Causes	Mechanism	Occurrence	Signs and Symptoms	Intervention
Pyrogenic	Recipient possesses antibodies directed against WBCs; bacterial contamination; multitransfused clients; multiparous clients	Leukocyte agglutination Bacterial organisms	Within 15–90 min after initiation of transfusion	Fever, chills, flushing, palpitations, tachycardia, occasional lumbar pain	Stop transfusion. Treat temperature. Transfuse with leukocyte-poor blood or washed RBCs. Administer antibiotics prn.
Circulatory overload	Too rapid infusion in susceptible clients	Fluid volume overload	During and after transfusion	Dyspnea, tachycardia, orthopnea, increased blood pressure, cyanosis, anxiety	Slow infusion rate. Use packed cells instead of whole blood. Monitor CVP through a separate line.
Air embolism	Blood given under air pressure following severe blood loss	Bolus of air blocks pulmonary artery outflow	Anytime	Dyspnea, increased pulse, wheezing, chest pain, decreased blood pressure, apprehension	Clamp tubing. Turn client on left side.

Thrombocytopenia	Use of large amounts of banked blood	Platelets deteriorate rapidly in stored blood	When large amounts of blood given over 24 hr	Abnormal bleeding	Assess for signs of bleeding. Initiate bleeding precautions. Use fresh blood.
Citrate intoxication	Large amounts of citrated blood in clients with decreased liver function	Citrate binds ionic calcium	After large amounts of banked blood	Neuromuscular irritability Bleeding due to decreased calcium	Monitor/treat hypocalcemia. Avoid large amounts of citrated blood. Monitor liver function.
Hyperkalemia	Potassium levels increase in stored blood	Release of potassium into plasma with red cell lysis	In clients with renal insufficiency	Nausea, colic, diarrhea, muscle spasms, ECG changes (tall peaked T-wave, short Q-T segment)	Administer blood less than 5–7 days old in clients with impaired potassium excretion.

B. Common pathway: activated by either intrinsic or extrinsic pathways
   1. Platelet factor 3 (PF3) and calcium react with factors X and V.
   2. Prothrombin converted to thrombin via thromboplastin.
   3. Thrombin acts on fibrinogen, forming soluble fibrin.
   4. Soluble fibrin polymerized by factor XIII to produce a stable, insoluble fibrin clot.

C. Clot resolution: takes place via fibrinolytic system by plasmin and proteolytic enzymes; clot dissolves as tissue repairs.

Spleen

A. Largest lymphatic organ: functions as blood filtration system and reservoir

B. Vascular, bean shaped; lies beneath the diaphragm, behind and to the left of the stomach; composed of a fibrous tissue capsule surrounding a network of fiber

C. Contains two types of pulp
   1. Red pulp: located between the fibrous strands, composed of RBCs, WBCs, and macrophages
   2. White pulp: scattered throughout the red pulp, produces lymphocytes and sequesters lymphocytes, macrophages, and antigens

D. 1%–2% of red cell mass or 200 ml blood/minute stored in spleen; blood comes via the splenic artery to the pulp for cleansing, then passes into splenic venules that are lined with phagocytic cells, and finally to the splenic vein to the liver.

E. Important hematopoietic site in fetus; postnatally produces lymphocytes and monocytes

F. Important in phagocytosis; removes misshapen erythrocytes, unwanted parts of erythrocytes

G. Also involved in antibody production by plasma cells and iron metabolism (iron released from Hgb portion of destroyed erythrocytes returned to bone marrow)

H. In the adult, functions of the spleen can be taken over by the reticuloendothelial system.

Liver

A. Involved in bile production (via erythrocyte destruction and bilirubin production) and erythropoiesis (during fetal life and when bone marrow production is insufficient).

B. Kupffer cells of liver have reticuloendothelial function as histiocytes; phagocytic activity and iron storage.

C. Liver also involved in synthesis of clotting factors, synthesis of antithrombins.

ASSESSMENT

Health History

A. Presenting problem
   1. Nonspecific symptoms may include chills, fatigue, fever, weakness, weight loss, night sweats, delayed wound healing, malaise, lethargy, depression, cold/heat intolerance
   2. Note specific signs and symptoms
      a. Skin: prolonged bleeding, petechiae, jaundice, ecchymosis, pruritus, pallor
      b. Eyes: visual disturbance, yellowed sclera
      c. Ears: vertigo, tinnitus
      d. Mouth and nose: epistaxis; gingival bleeding, ulceration, pain; dysphagia, hoarseness
      e. Neck: nuchal rigidity, lymphadenopathy
      f. Respiratory: dyspnea, orthopnea, palpitations, chest discomfort or pain, cough (productive or dry), hemoptysis
      g. GI: melena, abdominal pain, change in bowel habits
      h. GU: hematuria, recurrent infection, amenorrhea, menorrhagia
      i. CNS: confusion, headache, paresthesias, syncope
      j. Musculoskeletal: joint, back, or bone pain

B. Lifestyle: exposure to chemicals, occupational exposure to radiation

C. Use of medications
   1. Iron, vitamins (B_6, B_{12}, folic acid)
   2. Corticosteroids
   3. Anticoagulants
   4. Antibiotics
   5. Aspirin or aspirin-containing compounds
   6. Cold or allergy preparations
   7. Antiarrhythmics
   8. Blood transfusions (cryoprecipitates)
   9. Cancer chemotherapy drugs
   10. Immunosuppressant drugs

D. Medical history
   1. Surgery: splenectomy, tumor resection, cardiac valve replacement, GI tract resection
   2. Allergies: multiple transfusions with whole blood or blood products, other known allergies
   3. Mononucleosis; radiation therapy; recurrent infections; malabsorption syndrome; anemia; delayed wound healing; thrombophlebitis, pulmonary embolism, deep venous thrombosis (DVT); liver disease, ETOH abuse, vitamin K deficiency; angina pectoris, atrial fibrillation

E. Family history; jaundice, anemia, bleeding disorders (hemophilia, polycythemia), malignancies, congenital blood dyscrasias

Physical Examination

A. Auscultate for heart murmurs; bruits (cerebral, cardiac, carotid); pericardial or pleural friction rubs; bowel sounds.

B. Inspect for

1. Flush or pallor of mucous membranes, nail beds, palms, soles of feet
2. Infection or pallor of sclera, conjunctiva
3. Cyanosis
4. Jaundice of skin, mucous membranes, conjunctiva
5. Signs of bleeding, petechiae, ecchymoses, oral mucosal bleeding (especially gums), epistaxis, hemorrhage from any orifice
6. Ulcerations or lesions
7. Swelling or erythema
8. Neurologic changes: pain and touch, position and vibratory sense, superficial and deep tendon reflexes

C. Palpate lymph nodes; note location, size, texture, sensation, fixation; palpate the ribs for sternal, bone tenderness.

D. Evaluate joint range of motion and tenderness.

E. Percuss for lung excursion, splenomegaly, hepatomegaly.

Laboratory/Diagnostic Tests

A. Blood

1. Complete blood count (CBC) with differential and peripheral smear
   - **a.** White blood cell count (WBC) with differential
   - **b.** Hgb and hct
   - **c.** Platelet and reticulocyte count
   - **d.** Red blood cell count (RBC) with peripheral smear
2. Coagulation studies
   - **a.** Prothrombin time (PT)
   - **b.** Partial thromboplastin time (PTT)
   - **c.** Fibrin split products (FSP)
   - **d.** Lee-White clotting time (whole blood clotting time)
3. Blood chemistry
   - **a.** Blood urea nitrogen (BUN)
   - **b.** Creatinine
   - **c.** Bilirubin: direct and indirect
   - **d.** Uric acid
4. Miscellaneous
   - **a.** Erythrocyte sedimentation rate (ESR)
   - **b.** Serum protein electrophoresis
   - **c.** Serum iron and total iron-binding capacity
   - **d.** Plasma protein assays
   - **e.** Direct and indirect Coombs' tests

B. Urine and stool
   1. Urinalysis
   2. Hematest
   3. Bence-Jones protein assay (urine)
C. Radiologic
   1. Chest or other X-ray as indicated by history and physical exam
   2. Radionuclide scans (e.g., bone scan)
   3. Lymphangiography
D. *Bone marrow aspiration and biopsy*
   1. Puncture of iliac crest (preferred site), vertebrae body, sternum, or tibia (in infants) to collect tissue from bone marrow
   2. Purpose: study cells involved in blood production
   3. Nursing care
      a. Confirm that consent form has been signed.
      b. Allay client anxiety; prepare client for a sharp, brief pain when bone marrow is aspirated into syringe.
      c. Position client and assist physician to maintain sterile field.
      d. Immediately after the aspiration, apply pressure to the site for at least 5 minutes and longer, if necessary.
      e. Check the site frequently for signs of bleeding or infection.
      f. Send specimen to laboratory.

ANALYSIS

Nursing diagnoses for clients with disorders of the hematologic system may include

A. Imbalanced nutrition
B. Risk for infection
C. Ineffective tissue perfusion: cerebral, peripheral
D. Impaired gas exchange
E. Ineffective protection
F. Risk for impaired skin integrity
G. Impaired oral mucous membrane
H. Risk for activity intolerance
I. Acute pain
J. Anxiety

PLANNING AND IMPLEMENTATION

Goals

A. Optimal nutrition will be maintained.
B. Client will be free from infection.
C. Adequate cerebral and peripheral tissue perfusion will be maintained.
D. Client will maintain optimal respiratory function.
E. Client will maintain adequate protective mechanisms.
F. Optimal skin integrity will be maintained.

G. Client maintains optimal health of oral mucous membranes.
H. Client will have increased strength and endurance.
I. Client's pain will be relieved/controlled.
J. Client's anxiety will be relieved/reduced.

Interventions

Blood Transfusion and Component Therapy

A. Purpose: improve oxygen transport (RBCs); volume expansion (whole blood, plasma, albumin); provision of proteins (fresh frozen plasma, albumin, plasma protein fraction); provision of coagulation factors (cryoprecipitate, fresh frozen plasma, fresh whole blood); provision of platelets (platelet concentrate, fresh whole blood)
B. Blood and blood products
   1. Whole blood; provides all components
      a. Large volume can cause difficulty: 12–24 hours for Hgb and hct to rise
      b. Complications: volume overload, transmission of hepatitis or AIDS, transfusion reaction, infusion of excess potassium and sodium, infusion of anticoagulant (citrate) used to keep stored blood from clotting, calcium binding and depletion (citrate) in massive transfusion therapy
   2. Red blood cells
      a. Provide twice the amount of Hgb as an equivalent amount of whole blood
      b. Indicated in cases of blood loss, pre- and post-op clients, and those with incipient congestive failure
      c. Complications: transfusion reaction (less common than with whole blood due to removal of plasma proteins)
   3. Fresh frozen plasma
      a. Contains all coagulation factors including V and VIII
      b. Can be stored frozen for 12 months; takes 20 minutes to thaw
      c. Hang immediately upon arrival to unit (loses its coagulation factors rapidly)
   4. Platelets
      a. Will raise recipient's platelet count by 10,000/mm^3
      b. Pooled from 4–8 units of whole blood
      c. Single-donor platelet transfusions may be necessary for clients who have developed antibodies; compatibility testing may be necessary
   5. Factor VIII fractions (cryoprecipitate): contains Factors VIII, fibrinogen, and XIII
   6. Granulocytes
      a. Do not increase WBC; increase marginal pool (at tissue level) rather than circulating pool

   b. Premedication with steroids, antihistamines, and acetaminophen
   c. Respiratory distress with shortness of breath, cyanosis, and chest pain may occur; requires cessation of transfusion and immediate attention
   d. Shaking chills or rigors common, require brief cessation of therapy, administration of meperidine IV until rigors are diminished, and resumption of transfusion when symptoms relieved
7. Volume expanders: albumin; percentage concentration varies (50–100 ml/unit); hyperosmolar solutions should not be used in dehydrated clients.

C. Nursing care
1. Assess client for history of previous blood transfusions and any adverse reactions.
2. Ensure that the adult client has an 18- or 19-gauge IV catheter in place.
3. Use 0.9% sodium chloride.
4. At least two nurses should verify the ABO group, Rh type, client and blood numbers, and expiration date.
5. Take baseline vital signs before initiating transfusion.
6. Start transfusion slowly (2 ml/minute).
7. Stay with the client during the first 15 minutes of the transfusion and take vital signs frequently.
8. Maintain the prescribed transfusion rate.
   a. Whole blood: approximately 3–4 hours
   b. RBCs: approximately 2–4 hours
   c. Fresh frozen plasma: as quickly as possible
   d. Platelets: as quickly as possible
   e. Cryoprecipitate: rapid infusion
   f. Granulocytes: usually over 2 hours
   g. Volume expanders: volume-dependent rate
9. Monitor for adverse reactions (see Table 7-1).
10. Document the following
   a. Blood component unit number (apply sticker if available)
   b. Date infusion starts and ends
   c. Type of component and amount transfused
   d. Client reaction and vital signs
   e. Signature of transfusionist

EVALUATION

A. Client maintains normal weight; no evidence of malnutrition.
B. Client's temperature is within normal range; no signs of infection.
C. Client neuro status is within normal limits.
D. Client demonstrates adequate peripheral capillary refill, sensation, and movement; palpable peripheral pulses; skin warm, dry, and usual color.

E. Client's respirations are of normal rate, rhythm, and depth; lungs clear to auscultation.
F. Client verbalizes signs and symptoms of infection and preventive measures; reports signs and symptoms of infection immediately.
G. Client's skin remains clear and intact.
H. Client's oral mucous membranes are healthy and intact.
I. Client experiences increased strength and endurance.
J. Client reports relief/control of pain.
K. Client expresses relief/reduction in anxiety.

DISORDERS OF THE HEMATOLOGIC SYSTEM

Anemias

Iron-Deficiency Anemia

A. General information
   1. Chronic microcytic, hypochromic anemia caused by either inadequate absorption or excessive loss of iron
   2. Acute or chronic bleeding principal cause in adults (chiefly from trauma, dysfunctional uterine bleeding, and GI bleeding)
   3. May also be caused by inadequate intake of iron-rich foods or by inadequate absorption of iron (from chronic diarrhea, malabsorption syndromes, high cereal-product intake with low animal protein ingestion, partial or complete gastrectomy, pica)
   4. Incidence related to geographic location, economic class, age group, and sex
      a. More common in developing countries and tropical zones (blood-sucking parasites)
      b. Women between ages 15 and 45 and children affected more frequently, as are the poor
   5. In iron-deficiency states, iron stores are depleted first, followed by a reduction in Hgb formation.

B. Assessment findings
   1. Mild cases usually asymptomatic
   2. Palpitations, dizziness, and cold sensitivity
   3. Brittleness of hair and nails; pallor
   4. Dysphagia, stomatitis, and atrophic glossitis
   5. Dyspnea, weakness
   6. Laboratory findings
      a. RBCs small (microcytic) and pale (hypochromic)
      b. Hgb markedly decreased
      c. Hct moderately decreased
      d. Serum iron markedly decreased
      e. Hemosiderin absent from bone marrow
      f. Serum ferritin decreased
      g. Reticulocyte count decreased

C. Nursing interventions
   1. Monitor for signs and symptoms of bleeding through hematest of all elimination including stool, urine, and gastric contents.
   2. Provide for adequate rest: plan activities so as not to overtire.
   3. Provide a thorough explanation of all diagnostic tests used to determine sources of possible bleeding (helps allay anxiety and ensure cooperation).
   4. Administer iron preparations as ordered.
      a. Oral iron preparations: route of choice
         1) give following meals or a snack.
         2) dilute liquid preparations well and administer using a straw to prevent staining teeth.
         3) when possible administer with orange juice as vitamin C (ascorbic acid) enhances iron absorption.
         4) warn clients that iron preparations will change stool color and consistency (dark and tarry) and may cause constipation.
         5) Antacid ingestion will decrease oral iron effectiveness.
      b. Parenteral: used in clients intolerant to oral preparations, who are noncompliant with therapy, or who have continuing blood losses.
         1) use one needle to withdraw and another to administer iron preparations as tissue staining and irritation are a problem.
         2) use the Z-track injection technique to prevent leakage into tissues
         3) do not massage injection site but encourage ambulation as this will enhance absorption; advise against vigorous exercise and constricting garments.
         4) observe for local signs of complications: pain at the injection site, development of sterile abscesses, lymphadenitis as well as fever, headache, urticaria, hypotension, or anaphylactic shock.
   5. Provide dietary teaching regarding foods high in iron.
   6. Encourage ingestion of roughage and increase fluid intake to prevent constipation if oral iron preparations are being taken.

Pernicious Anemia

A. General information
   1. Chronic progressive, macrocytic anemia caused by a deficiency of intrinsic factor; the result is abnormally large erythrocytes and hypochlorhydria (a deficiency of hydrochloric acid in gastric secretions)
   2. Characterized by neurologic and GI symptoms; death usually results if untreated
   3. Lack of intrinsic factor is caused by gastric mucosal atrophy (possibly due to heredity, prolonged iron deficiency, or an autoimmune

disorder); can also result in clients who have had a total gastrectomy if vitamin B_{12} not administered

4. Usually occurs in men and women over age 50, with an increase in blue-eyed persons of Scandinavian descent
5. Pathophysiology
   - a. Intrinsic factor is necessary for the absorption of vitamin B_{12} into the small intestine.
   - b. B_{12} deficiency diminishes DNA synthesis, which results in defective maturation of cells (particularly rapidly dividing cells such as blood cells and GI tract cells).
   - c. B_{12} deficiency can alter structure and function of peripheral nerves, spinal cord, and the brain.

B. Medical management

1. Drug therapy
   - a. Vitamin B_{12} injections: monthly maintenance
   - b. Iron preparations (if Hgb level inadequate to meet increased numbers of erythrocytes)
   - c. Folic acid
     - 1) Controversial
     - 2) reverses anemia and GI symptoms but may intensify neurologic symptoms
     - 3) may be safe if given in small amounts in addition to vitamin B_{12}
2. Transfusion therapy

C. Assessment findings

1. Anemia, weakness, pallor, dyspnea, palpitations, fatigue
2. GI symptoms: sore mouth; smooth, beefy, red tongue; weight loss; dyspepsia; constipation or diarrhea; jaundice
3. CNS symptoms; tingling, paresthesias of hands and feet, paralysis, depression, psychosis
4. Laboratory tests
   - a. Erythrocyte count decreased
   - b. Blood smear: oval, macrocytic erythrocytes with a proportionate amount of Hgb
   - c. Bone marrow
     - 1) increased megaloblasts (abnormal erythrocytes)
     - 2) few normoblasts or maturing erythrocytes
     - 3) defective leukocyte maturation
   - d. Bilirubin (indirect): elevated unconjugated fraction
   - e. Serum LDH elevated
   - f. Positive *Schilling test*
     - 1) measures absorption of radioactive vitamin B_{12} both before and after parenteral administration of intrinsic factor
     - 2) definitive test for pernicious anemia
     - 3) used to detect lack of intrinsic factor

4) fasting client is given radioactive vitamin B_{12} by mouth and nonradioactive vitamin B_{12} IM to saturate tissue binding sites and to permit some excretion of radioactive vitamin B_{12} in the urine if it is absorbed
5) 24–48 hour urine collection is obtained; client is encouraged to drink fluids
6) if indicated, second stage Schilling test performed 1 week after first stage. Fasting client is given radioactive vitamin B_{12} combined with human intrinsic factor and test is repeated.

g. Gastric analysis: decreased free hydrochloric acid

h. Large numbers of reticulocytes in the blood following parenteral vitamin B_{12} administration

D. Nursing interventions

1. Provide a nutritious diet high in iron, protein, and vitamins (fish, meat, milk/milk products, and eggs).
2. Avoid highly seasoned, coarse, or very hot foods if client has mouth sores.
3. Provide mouth care before and after meals using a soft toothbrush and nonirritating rinses.
4. Bed rest may be necessary if anemia is severe.
5. Provide safety when ambulating (especially if carrying hot items, etc.).
6. Provide client teaching and discharge planning concerning
   - **a.** Dietary instruction
   - **b.** Importance of lifelong vitamin B_{12} therapy
   - **c.** Rehabilitation and physical therapy for neurologic deficits, as well as instruction regarding safety

Aplastic Anemia

A. General information

1. Pancytopenia or depression of granulocyte, platelet, and erythrocyte production due to fatty replacement of the bone marrow
2. Bone marrow destruction may be idiopathic or secondary
3. Secondary aplastic anemia may be caused by
   - **a.** Chemical toxins (e.g., benzene)
   - **b.** Drugs (e.g., chloramphenicol, cytotoxic drugs)
   - **c.** Radiation
   - **d.** Immunologic injury

B. Medical management

1. Blood transfusions: key to therapy until client's own marrow begins to produce blood cells
2. Aggressive treatment of infections
3. Bone marrow transplantation
4. Drug therapy

NURSING ALERT

Life-threatening hemorrhage from mucous membranes is the most common complication of aplastic anemia.

a. Corticosteroids and/or androgens to stimulate bone marrow function and to increase capillary resistance (effective in children but usually not in adults)
b. Estrogen and/or progesterone to prevent amenorrhea in female clients

5. Identification and withdrawal of offending agent or drug

C. Assessment findings
1. Fatigue, dyspnea, pallor
2. Increased susceptibility to infection
3. Bleeding tendencies and hemorrhage
4. Laboratory findings: normocytic anemia, granulocytopenia, thrombocytopenia
5. Bone marrow biopsy: marrow is fatty and contains very few developing cells

D. Nursing interventions
1. Administer blood transfusions as ordered.
2. Provide nursing care for client with bone marrow transplantation.
3. Administer medications as ordered.
4. Monitor for signs of infection and provide care to minimize risk.
   a. Maintain neutropenic precautions.
   b. Encourage high-protein, high-vitamin diet to help reduce incidence of infection.
   c. Provide mouth care before and after meals.
5. Monitor for signs of bleeding and provide measures to minimize risk.
   a. Use a soft toothbrush and electric razor.
   b. Avoid intramuscular injections.
   c. Hematest urine and stool.
   d. Observe for oozing from gums, petechiae, or ecchymoses.
6. Provide client teaching and discharge planning concerning
   a. Self-care regimen
   b. Identification of offending agent and importance of avoiding it (if possible) in future

Hemolytic Anemia

A. General information
   1. A category of diseases in which there is an increased rate of RBC destruction.
   2. May be congenital or acquired.
      a. Congenital: includes hereditary spherocytosis, G6PD deficiency, sickle cell anemia, thalassemia
      b. Acquired: includes transfusion incompatibilities, thrombotic thrombocytopenic purpura, disseminated intravascular clotting, spur cell anemia
   3. Cause often unknown, but erythrocyte life span is shortened and hemolysis occurs at a rate that the bone marrow cannot compensate for.
   4. The degree of anemia is determined by the lag between erythrocyte hemolysis and the rate of bone marrow erythropoiesis.
   5. Diagnosis is based on laboratory evidence of an increased rate of erythrocyte destruction and a corresponding compensatory effort by bone marrow to increase production.

B. Medical management
   1. Identify and eliminate (if possible) causative factors
   2. Drug therapy
      a. Corticosteroids in autoimmune types of anemia
      b. Folic acid supplements
   3. Blood transfusion therapy
   4. Splenectomy (see below)

C. Assessment findings
   1. Clinical manifestations vary depending on severity of anemia and the rate of onset (acute vs. chronic)
   2. Pallor, scleral icterus, and slight jaundice (chronic)
   3. Chills, fever, irritability, precordial spasm, and pain (acute)
   4. Abdominal pain and nausea, vomiting, diarrhea, melena
   5. Hematuria, marked jaundice, and dyspnea
   6. Splenomegaly and symptoms of cholelithiasis, hepatomegaly
   7. Laboratory tests
      a. Hgb and hct decreased
      b. Reticulocyte count elevated (compensatory)
      c. Coombs' test (direct): positive if autoimmune features present
      d. Bilirubin (indirect): elevated unconjugated fraction

D. Nursing interventions
   1. Monitor for signs and symptoms of hypoxia including confusion, cyanosis, shortness of breath, tachycardia, and palpitations.
   2. Note that the presence of jaundice may make assessment of skin color in hypoxia unreliable.
   3. If jaundice and associated pruritus are present, avoid soap during bathing and use cool or tepid water.

4. Frequent turning and meticulous skin care are important as skin friability is increased.
5. Teach clients about the nature of the disease and identification of factors that predispose to episodes of hemolytic crisis.

Splenectomy

A. General information
   1. Indications
      a. Rupture of the spleen caused by trauma, accidental tearing during surgery, diseases causing softening or damage (e.g., infectious mononucleosis)
      b. Hypersplenism: excessive splenic damage of cellular blood components
      c. As the spleen is a major source of antibody formation in children, splenectomy is not recommended during the early years of life; if absolutely necessary, client should receive prophylactic antibiotics post-op
   2. Primary hypersplenism can be alleviated with splenectomy; procedure is palliative only in secondary hypersplenism

B. Nursing interventions: pre-op
   1. Provide routine pre-op care and explain what to expect postoperatively.
   2. Administer pneumococcal vaccine as ordered since client will be at increased risk for pneumococcal infections for several years after splenectomy.

C. Nursing interventions: post-op
   1. Be aware that it is crucial to monitor carefully for hemorrhage and shock as clients with pre-op bleeding tendencies will remain at risk post-op.
   2. Monitor post-op temperature elevation: fever may not be the best indicator of post-op complications such as pneumonia or urinary tract infection, as fever without concomitant infection is common following splenectomy.
   3. Observe for abdominal distension and discomfort secondary to expansion of the intestines and stomach; an abdominal binder may reduce distension.
   4. Know that post-op infection in a child is considered life threatening; administer prophylactic antibiotics as ordered.
   5. Ambulate early and provide chest physical therapy as location of the incision makes post-op atelectasis or pneumonia a risk.
   6. Emphasize to client the need to report even minor signs or symptoms of infection immediately to the physician.

NURSING ALERT

Administer pain medication to allow for effective coughing and deep breathing to prevent pulmonary complications.

Disorders of Platelets and Clotting Mechanism

Disseminated Intravascular Coagulation (DIC)

A. General information
   1. Diffuse fibrin deposition within arterioles and capillaries with widespread coagulation all over the body and subsequent depletion of clotting factors.
   2. Hemorrhage from kidneys, brain, adrenals, heart, and other organs.
   3. Cause unknown.
   4. Clients are usually critically ill with an obstetric, surgical, hemolytic, or neoplastic disease.
   5. May be linked with entry of thromboplastic substances into the blood.
   6. Pathophysiology
      a. Underlying disease (e.g., toxemia of pregnancy, cancer) causes release of thromboplastic substances that promote the deposition of fibrin throughout the microcirculation.
      b. Microthrombi form in many organs, causing microinfarcts and tissue necrosis.
      c. RBCs are trapped in fibrin strands and are hemolysed.
      d. Platelets, prothrombin, and other clotting factors are destroyed, leading to bleeding.
      e. Excessive clotting activates the fibrinolytic system, which inhibits platelet function, causing further bleeding.
   7. Mortality rate is high, usually because underlying disease cannot be corrected.

B. Medical management
   1. Identification and control of underlying disease is key
   2. Blood transfusions: include whole blood, packed RBCs, platelets, plasma, cryoprecipitates, and volume expanders
   3. Heparin administration
      a. Somewhat controversial
      b. Inhibits thrombin thus preventing further clot formation, allowing coagulation factors to accumulate

DELEGATION TIP

Initial vital signs assessment and identification of the client must be performed by the RN. Ancillary personnel should be instructed to obtain vital signs on another extremity.

C. Assessment findings
  1. Petechiae and ecchymoses on the skin, mucous membranes, heart, lungs, and other organs
  2. Prolonged bleeding from breaks in the skin (e.g., IV or venipuncture sites)
  3. Severe and uncontrollable hemorrhage during childbirth or surgical procedures
  4. Oliguria and acute renal failure
  5. Convulsions, coma, death
  6. Laboratory findings
     a. PT prolonged
     b. PTT usually prolonged
     c. Thrombin time usually prolonged
     d. Fibrinogen level usually depressed
     e. Platelet count usually depressed
     f. Fibrin split products elevated
     g. Protamine sulfate test strongly positive
     h. Factor assays (II, V, VII) depressed

D. Nursing interventions
  1. Monitor blood loss and attempt to quantify.
  2. Observe for signs of additional bleeding or thrombus formation.
  3. Monitor appropriate laboratory data.
  4. Prevent further injury.
     a. Avoid IM injections.
     b. Apply pressure to bleeding sites.
     c. Turn and position client frequently and gently.
     d. Provide frequent nontraumatic mouth care (e.g., soft toothbrush or gauze sponge).
  5. Provide emotional support to client and significant others.
  6. Administer blood transfusions and medications as ordered.
  7. Teach client the importance of avoiding aspirin or aspirin-containing compounds.

CLIENT TEACHING CHECKLIST

Teach the client about HIV antibody tests.

- Two blood tests commonly used to detect HIV antibodies are ELISA and Western blot
- ELISA: Client's blood sample is incubated with live HIV. If HIV antibodies are present, they react with the test solution.
- Western blot: If findings are positive, a Western blot assay is performed on the same sample to confirm results and identify specific HIV antibodies.

Immunologic Disorders

Acquired Immune Deficiency Syndrome (AIDS)

A. General information
   1. Characterized by severe deficits in cellular immune function; manifested clinically by opportunistic infections and/or unusual neoplasms
   2. Etiologic factors
      a. Results from infection with human immunodeficiency virus (HIV), a retrovirus that preferentially infects helper T-lymphocytes (T_4 cells)
      b. Transmissible through sexual contact, contaminated blood or blood products, and from infected woman to child in utero or possibly through breast-feeding
      c. HIV is present in an infected person's blood, semen, and other body fluids
   3. Epidemiology is similar to that of hepatitis B; increased incidence in populations in which sexual promiscuity is common and in IV drug abusers
   4. Proposed strategies for prevention
      a. Early detection; include HIV testing as routine part of medical care
      b. Expand opportunities for testing outside of the medical settings
      c. Behavior modification with persons diagnosed with HIV and partners
      d. Reduce viral load in pregnant woman with HIV; reduce perinatal transmission of HIV disease to newborn

B. Medical management

1. No effective cure for AIDS at present; several categories of antiretroviral drugs are available

a. Nucleoside Analogues: Didanosine (Videx) (ddl), Lamivudine (3TC) (Epivir), Stavudine (d4T) (Zerit), Zidovudine (AZT) (Retrovir)

b. Nucleoside Analogues: Didanosine (Videx) (ddl), Lamivudine (3TC) (Epivir), Stavudine (d4T) (Zerit), Zidovudine (AZT) (Retrovir)

c. Non Nucleoside Analogues: Delavirdine (DLV) (Rescriptor), Nevirapine (NVP) (Viramune)

d. Protease Inhibitors: Indinavir (Crixivan), Nelfinavir (Viracept), Ritonavir (Norvir), Saquinavir (Invirase)

2. Primary goal of treatment is to treat opportunistic infections and cancers that develop and provide supportive care for the effects of the disease, e.g., diarrhea, malnutrition, mental changes, etc.

3. Drugs used to treat *pneumocystis carinii* pneumonia (PCP) include

a. PO or IV trimethoprim-sulfamethoxazole (Bactrim, Septra); side effects include rash, leukopenia, fever

b. IM or IV pentamidine (Pentam 300); side effects include hepatotoxicity, nephrotoxicity, blood sugar imbalances, abscess or necroses at IM injection site, hypotension

C. Assessment findings (see Table 7-2)

1. Fatigue, weakness, anorexia, weight loss, diarrhea, pallor, fever, night sweats

2. Shortness of breath, dyspnea, cough, chest pain, and progressive hypoxemia secondary to infection (pneumonia)

3. Progressive weight loss secondary to anorexia, nausea, vomiting, diarrhea, and a general wasting syndrome; fatigue, malaise

4. Temperature elevations (persistent or intermittent); night sweats

5. Neurologic dysfunction secondary to acute meningitis, progressive dementia, encephalopathy, encephalitis

6. Presence of opportunistic infection, for example

a. *Pneumocystis carinii* pneumonia

b. Herpes simplex, cytomegalovirus, and Epstein-Barr viruses

c. Candidiasis: oral or esophageal

d. Mycobacterium-avium complex

7. Neoplasms

a. Kaposi's sarcoma

b. CNS lymphoma

c. Burkitt's lymphoma

d. Diffuse undifferentiated non-Hodgkin's lymphoma

8. Laboratory findings: diagnosis based on clinical criteria and positive HIV antibody test—ELISA (enzyme-linked immunosorbent assay) confirmed by Western blot assay. Other lab findings may include

TABLE 7-2 Classification System for HIV Infection

CD4 + T-cell categories	A Asymptomatic, acute HIV or PGL	B Symptomatic, not (A) or (C) conditions	C AIDS-indicator conditions
(1) 500/uL	A1	B1	C1
(2) 200-499/uL	A2	B2	C2
(3) <200/uL	A3	B3	C3

Clinical Category A	Clinical Category B	Clinical Category C
1 or more of the following, confirmed HIV infection, and without conditions in B and C • Asymptomatic HIV infection • Persistent Generalized Lymphadenopathy (PGL) • Acute (primary) HIV infection with accompanying illness or history of acute HIV infection	• Candidiasis (oral or vaginal), frequent or poorly resistant to therapy • Cervical dysplasia/ cervical carcinoma in situ • Fever or diarrhea exceeding 1 month • Hairy leukoplakia, oral • Herpes zoster, involving 2 episodes or more than one dermatome • ITP • PID • Peripheral neuropathy	• Candidiasis of bronchi, trachea, or lungs • Cervical cancer, invasive • Coccidiomycosis • Cryptosporidiosis • Cytomegalovirus • Encephalopathy • Herpes simplex: chronic ulcer-exceeding 1 month duration • Histoplasmosis • Kaposi's sarcoma • Lymphoma • Mycobacterium - avium complex • Mycobacterium tuberculosis • *Pneumocystis carinii* pneumonia • Salmonella • Toxoplasmosis of brain • Wasting syndrome due to HIV

Note: Adapted from 1993 *Revised Classification System for HIV Infections and Expanded Surveillance Case Definition for AIDS Among Adolescents and Adults*, by Centers for Disease Control and Prevention, U.S. Department of Health and Human Services, 1993, Author, Atlanta, GA.

a. Leukopenia with profound lymphopenia
b. Anemia
c. Thrombocytopenia
d. Decreased circulatory T_4 lymphocyte cells
e. Low T_4:T_8 lymphocyte ratio

D. Nursing interventions
1. Administer medications as ordered for concomitant disease; monitor for signs of medication toxicity.
2. Monitor respiratory status; provide care as appropriate for respiratory problems, e.g., pneumonia.
3. Assess neurological status; reorient client as needed; provide safety measures for the confused/disoriented client.
4. Assess for signs and symptoms of fluid and electrolyte imbalances; monitor lab studies; ensure adequate hydration.
5. Monitor client's nutritional intake; provide supplements, total parenteral nutrition, etc., as ordered.
6. Assess skin daily (especially perianal area) for signs of breakdown; keep skin clean and dry; turn q4 hours while in bed.
7. Inspect oral cavity daily for ulcerations, signs of infection; instruct client to rinse mouth with normal saline and hydrogen peroxide or normal saline and sodium bicarbonate rinses.
8. Observe for signs and symptoms of infection; report immediately if any occur.
9. If severe leukopenia develops, institute neutropenic precautions
   a. Prevent trauma to skin and mucous membranes, e.g., avoid enemas, rectal temperatures; minimize all parenteral infections
   b. Do not place client in a room with clients having infections
   c. Screen visitors for colds, infections, etc.
   d. Do not allow fresh fruits, vegetables, or plants in client's room.
   e. Mask client when leaving room for walks, X-rays, etc.
10. Institute blood and body fluid precautions (see page 158)
11. Provide emotional support for client/significant others; help to decrease sense of isolation
12. Provide client teaching and discharge planning concerning
   a. Importance of observing for signs of infections and notifying physician immediately if any occur
   b. Ways to reduce chance of infection
      1) clean kitchen and bathroom surfaces regularly with disinfectants.
      2) avoid direct contact with pet's litter boxes or stool, bird cage droppings, and water in fish tanks.
      3) avoid contact with people with infections, e.g., cold, flu.
      4) Importance of balancing activity with rest.
      5) Need to eat a well-balanced diet with plenty of fluids.

   c. Prevention of disease transmission
      1) Use safer sex practices, e.g., condoms for sexual intercourse.
      2) Do not donate blood, semen, organs.
      3) Do not share razors, toothbrushes, or other items that may draw blood.
      4) Inform all physicians, dentists, sexual partners of diagnosis.
   d. Resources include Public Health Service, National Gay Task Force, American Red Cross, local support groups

Malignancies

Multiple Myeloma

A. General information
   1. A neoplastic condition characterized by the abnormal proliferation of plasma cells in the bone marrow, causing the development of single or multiple tumors composed of abnormal plasma cells. Disease disseminates into lymph nodes, liver, spleen, and kidneys and causes bone destruction throughout the body.
   2. Cause unknown, but environmental factors thought to be involved
   3. Disease occurs after age 40; affects men twice as often as women
   4. Pathophysiology
      a. Bone demineralization and destruction with osteoporosis and a negative calcium balance
      b. Disruption of erythrocyte, leukocyte, and thrombocyte production
B. Medical management
   1. Drug therapy
      a. Analgesics for bone pain
      b. Chemotherapy (melphalan [Alkeran] and cyclophosphamide [Cytoxan]) to reduce tumor mass; may intensify the pancytopenia to which these clients are prone; requires careful monitoring of laboratory studies
      c. Antibiotics to treat infections
      d. Gammaglobulin for infection prophylaxis
      e. Corticosteroids and mithramycin for severe hypercalcemia
   2. Radiation therapy to reduce tumor mass and for palliation of bone pain
   3. Transfusion therapy
C. Assessment findings
   1. Headache and bone pain increasing with activity
   2. Pathologic fractures
   3. Skeletal deformities of sternum and ribs
   4. Loss of height (spinal column shortening)
   5. Osteoporosis
   6. Renal calculi
   7. Anemia, hemorrhagic tendencies, and increased susceptibility to infection

8. Hypercalcemia
9. Renal dysfunction secondary to obstruction of convoluted tubules by coagulated protein particles
10. Neurologic dysfunction: spinal cord compression and paraplegia
11. Laboratory tests
    a. Radiologic: diffuse bone lesions, widespread demineralization, osteoporosis, osteolytic lesions of skull
    b. Bone marrow; many immature plasma cells; depletion of other cell types
    c. CBC: reduced Hgb, WBC, and platelet counts
    d. Serum globulins elevated
    e. Bence-Jones protein: positive (abnormal globulin that appears in the urine of clients with multiple myeloma and other bone tumors)

D. Nursing interventions
1. Provide comfort measures to help alleviate bone pain.
2. Encourage ambulation to slow demineralization process.
3. Promote safety as clients are prone to pathologic and other fractures.
4. Encourage fluids: 3000–4000 ml/day to counteract calcium overload and to prevent protein from precipitating in the renal tubules.
5. Provide nursing care for clients with bleeding tendencies and susceptibility to infection.
6. Provide a supportive atmosphere to enhance communication and reduce anxiety.
7. Provide client teaching and discharge planning concerning
    a. Crucial importance of long-term hydration to prevent urolithiasis and renal obstruction
    b. Safety measures vital to decrease the risk of injury
    c. Avoidance of crowds or sources of infection if leukopenic

Polycythemia Vera

A. General information
1. An increase in both the number of circulating erythrocytes and the concentration of Hgb within the blood
2. Three forms: polycythemia vera, secondary polycythemia, and relative polycythemia
3. Classified as a myeloproliferative disorder (bone marrow overgrowth)
4. Cause unknown, but thought to be a form of malignancy similar to leukemia
5. Usually develops in middle age, common in Jewish men
6. Pathophysiology
    a. A pronounced increase in the production of erythrocytes accompanied by an increase in the production of myelocytes (leukocytes within bone marrow) and thrombocytes.

b. The consequences of this overproduction are an increase in blood viscosity, an increase in total blood volume (2–3 times greater than normal), and severe congestion of all tissues and organs with blood.

B. Assessment findings
1. Ruddy complexion and duskiness of mucosa secondary to capillary congestion in the skin and mucous membranes
2. Hypertension associated with vertigo, headache, and "fullness" in the head secondary to increased blood volume
3. Symptoms of HF secondary to overwork of the heart
4. Thrombus formation: CVA, MI, gangrene of the extremities, DVT, and pulmonary embolism can occur
5. Bleeding and hemorrhage secondary to congestion and overdistension of capillaries and venules
6. Hepatomegaly and splenomegaly
7. Peptic ulcer secondary to increased gastric secretions
8. Gout secondary to increased uric acid released by nucleoprotein breakdown
9. Laboratory tests
a. CBC: increase in all mature cell forms (erythrocytes, leukocytes, and platelets)
b. Hct: increased
c. Bone marrow: increase in immature cell forms
d. Bilirubin (indirect): increase in unconjugated fraction
e. Liver enzymes may be increased
f. Uric acid increased
g. Hematuria and melena possible

C. Nursing interventions
1. Monitor for signs and symptoms of bleeding complications.
2. Force fluids and record I&O.
3. Prevent development of DVT.
4. Monitor for signs and symptoms of CHF.
5. Provide care for the client having a phlebotomy.
6. Prevent/provide care for bleeding or infection complications.
7. Administer medications as ordered.
a. Radioactive phosphorus (^{32}P): reduction of erythrocyte production, produces a remission of 6 months to 2 years
b. Nitrogen mustard, busulfan (Myleran), chlorambucil, cyclophosphamide to effect myelosuppression
c. Antigout and peptic ulcer drugs as needed.
8. Provide client teaching and discharge planning concerning
a. Decrease in activity tolerance, need to space activity with periods of rest
b. Phlebotomy regimens: outclient frequency is determined by hct; importance of long-term therapy

c. High fluid intake
d. Avoidance of iron-rich foods to avoid counteracting the therapeutic effects of phlebotomy
e. Recognition and reporting of bleeding
f. Need to avoid persons with infections, especially in leukopenic clients.

REVIEW QUESTIONS

1. An adult female is admitted to the hospital with a bleeding ulcer. She is to receive 4 units of packed cells. Which nursing intervention is of PRIMARY importance in the administration of blood?

1. Checking the flow rate.

2. Identifying the client.

3. Monitoring the vital signs.

4. Maintaining blood temperature.

2. Within 20 minutes of the start of transfusion, the client develops a sudden fever. The most appropriate INITIAL response by the nurse is to

1. force fluids.

2. continue to monitor the vital signs.

3. increase the flow rate of IV fluids.

4. stop the transfusion.

3. A 37-year-old male is admitted to the hospital with fever, coughs, chills, and shortness of breath. The nursing assessment reveals that he has a history of experimenting with IV drugs and has had several intimate relationships with men. A diagnostic work-up reveals that he is HIV positive and that he has *pneumocystis carinii* pneumonia. When the nurse assessing the client with AIDS has a negative attitude about the client's lifestyle, which action is most appropriate?

1. Share these feelings with the client.

2. Develop a written interview form.

3. Cancel the assessment.

4. Tell other health care professionals the information may be biased.

4. The client at risk for developing AIDS should be advised to

1. abstain from anal intercourse.

2. have an ELISA test for antibodies.

3. have a semen analysis done.
4. inform all sexual contacts.

5. A young man is admitted to the hospital with *pneumocystic carinii* pneumonia. He is HIV positive. Part of the nursing assessment for this client is an examination of his mouth for which oral problem commonly associated with AIDS?
   1. Halitosis.
   2. Carious teeth.
   3. Creamy white patches.
   4. Swollen lips.

6. The nurse is caring for a client who is HIV positive. To prevent the spread of the HIV virus while caring for her, the nurse will implement the Centers for Disease Control and Prevention (CDC) recommendations for
   1. universal blood and body fluid precautions.
   2. laminar flow rooms during active infection.
   3. body systems isolation.
   4. needle and syringe precautions.

7. An adult has been diagnosed with some type of anemia. The results of his blood tests showed: decreased WBC, normal RBC, decreased Hct, decreased Hgb. Based on these data, which of the following nursing diagnoses should the nurse prioritize as being the most important?
   1. Potential for infection.
   2. Alteration in nutrition.
   3. Self-care deficit.
   4. Fluid volume excess.

8. A client has the following blood lab values:platelets 50,000/ul RBCs 3.5 (3×10^6) Hemoglobin 10 g/dl Hematocrit 30% WBCs 10,000/ul Which nursing instruction should be included in the teaching plan?
   1. Bleeding precautions.
   2. Seizure precautions.
   3. Isolation to prevent infection.
   4. Control of pain with analgesics.

9. A hospitalized client has the following blood lab values: WBC 3,000/ul RBC 5.0 ($\times 10^6$) platelets 300,000 Nursing interventions should be aimed at
   1. preventing infection.
   2. controlling blood loss.

3. alleviating pain.
4. monitoring blood transfusion reactions.

10. A man's blood type is AB and he requires a blood transfusion. To prevent complications of blood incompatibilities, the nurse knows that this client may receive
    1. type A or B blood only.
    2. type AB blood only.
    3. type O blood only.
    4. either type A, B, AB, or O blood.
11. Which nursing intervention is appropriate for the nurse to take when setting up supplies for a client who requires a blood transfusion?
    1. Add any needed IV medication in the blood bag within one-half hour of planned infusion.
    2. Obtain blood bag from laboratory and leave at room temperature for at least one hour prior to infusion.
    3. Prime tubing of blood administration set with 0.9% NS solution, completely filling filter.
    4. Use a small-bore catheter to prevent rapid infusion of blood products that may lead to a reaction.
12. A client who is receiving a blood transfusion begins to experience chills, shortness of breath, nausea, excessive perspiration, and a vague sense of uneasiness. The best action for the nurse to initially take is to
    1. report the signs and symptoms to the physician.
    2. stop the transfusion.
    3. monitor the client's vital signs.
    4. assess respiratory status.
13. A client with iron deficiency anemia is ordered parenteral iron to be given intramuscularly. Which of the following actions should the nurse take in the preparation/administration of this medication?
    1. Use the same large (19–20) gauge needle for drawing up the medication and injecting it.
    2. Massage the site after the injection is given to promote absorption.
    3. Use a 1-inch needle to administer the medication.
    4. Use the Z-track technique to administer the medication.
14. The nurse has been teaching an adult who has iron deficiency anemia about those foods that she needs to include in her meal plans. Which of

the following, if selected, would indicate to the nurse that the client understands the dietary instructions?

1. Citrus fruits and green leafy vegetables.
2. Bananas and nuts.
3. Coffee and tea.
4. Dairy products.

15. In assessing clients for pernicious anemia, the nurse should be alert for which of the following risk factors?

1. Positive family history.
2. Acute or chronic blood loss.
3. Infectious agents or toxins.
4. Inadequate dietary intake.

16. A client has been scheduled for a Schilling's test. The nurse should instruct the client to

1. take nothing by mouth for 12 hours prior to the test.
2. collect his urine for 12 hours.
3. administer a fleets enema the evening before the test.
4. empty his bladder immediately before the test.

17. A 40-year-old woman with aplastic anemia is prescribed estrogen with progesterone. The nurse can expect that these medications are given for which of the following reasons?

1. To stimulate bone growth.
2. To regulate fluid balance.
3. To enhance sodium and potassium absorption.
4. To promote utilization and storage of fluids.

18. Which of the following lab value profiles should the nurse know to be consistent with hemolytic anemia?

1. Increased RBC, decreased bilirubin, decreased hemoglobin and hematocrit, increased reticulocytes.
2. Decreased RBC, increased bilirubin, decreased hemoglobin and hematocrit, increased reticulocytes.
3. Decreased RBC, decreased bilirubin, increased hemoglobin and hematocrit, decreased reticulocytes.
4. Increased RBC, increased bilirubin, increased hemoglobin and hematocrit, decreased reticulocytes.

19. In planning care for a client who has had a splenectomy, the nurse should be aware that this client is most prone to developing
    1. infection.
    2. congestive heart failure.
    3. urinary retention.
    4. viral hepatitis.
20. An adult is diagnosed with disseminated intramuscular coagulation (DIC). The nurse should identify that the client is at risk for which of the following nursing diagnoses?
    1. Risk for increased cardiac output related to fluid volume excess.
    2. Disturbed sensory perception related to bleeding into tissues.
    3. Alteration in tissue perfusion related to bleeding and diminished blood flow.
    4. Risk for aspiration related to constriction of the respiratory musculature.
21. The nurse should understand that a heparin order for a client with DIC is given to
    1. prevent clot formation.
    2. increase blood flow to target organs.
    3. increase clot formation.
    4. decrease blood flow to target organs.
22. A 34-year-old client is diagnosed with AIDS. His pharmacologic management includes zidovudine (AZT). During a home visit, the client states, "I don't understand how this medication works. Will it stop the infection?" The nurse's best response is
    1. "The medication helps to slow the disease process, but it won't cure or stop it totally."
    2. "The medication blocks reverse transcriptase, the enzyme required for HIV replication."
    3. "Don't you know? There aren't any medications to stop or cure HIV."
    4. "No, it won't stop the infection. In fact, sometimes the HIV can become immune to the drug itself."
23. Which statement, from a participant attending a class on AIDS prevention, indicates an understanding of how to reduce transmission of HIV?
    1. "Mothers who are HIV-positive should still be encouraged to breastfeed their babies because breast milk is superior to cow's milk."
    2. "I think a needle exchange program, where clean needles are exchanged for dirty needles, should be offered in every city."

3. "Orgasms are necessary for the heterosexual transmission of the virus."
4. "It's okay to use natural skin condoms since they offer the same protection as the latex condoms."

24. What should be included in the teaching plan to young adults about the spread of AIDS?

1. Heterosexual transmission of HIV is on the rise.
2. The increase of HIV in children is primarily attributed to the rise in sexual abuse.
3. The greatest increase of HIV infection is by homosexual transmission.
4. Transmission of HIV by IV drug users is prominent even when sterile equipment is used.

25. In planning care for a client with multiple myeloma, the nurse should be aware that the client may have orders for

1. bed rest.
2. corticosteroid therapy.
3. fluid restrictions.
4. calcium replacement therapy.

26. Which client statement would indicate to the nurse that the client with polycythemia vera is in need of further instruction?

1. "I'll be flying overseas to see my son and grandchildren for the holidays."
2. "I plan to do my leg exercises at least three times a week."
3. "I'm going to be walking in the mall every day to build up my strength."
4. "At night when I sleep, I like to use two pillows to raise my head up."

ANSWERS AND RATIONALES

1. 2. The most important consideration in transfusion therapy is to give the correct blood product to the correct client.

2. 4. Sudden development of fever during a blood transfusion may be indicative of a pyrogenic reaction. The most appropriate nursing action is to discontinue the blood flow to prevent a more severe reaction.

3. 4. When obtaining a sexual history it is important to communicate an attitude of trust and acceptance. If the nurse performing the assessment recognizes that personal feelings are biasing the accuracy of the assessment, then it is necessary to share this with other health care professionals. This provides the opportunity to communicate with another nurse, who will obtain a more accurate assessment. This strategy also provides the nurse with the opportunity to seek the counsel of others.

4. 2. The ELISA test detects the presence of antibodies to the AIDS virus and is a useful screening tool. It is not a definitive diagnostic test but provides additional information for the high-risk individual.

5. 3. Creamy white patches indicating an opportunistic infection (candidiasis) are often seen in the client with AIDS.

6. 1. Universal blood and body fluid precautions, general infection control outlines, and disease-specific measures are recommended by the CDC for AIDS and AIDS-related infections.

7. 1. These blood values are consistent with a diagnosis of aplastic anemia in which the nurse's primary goals are to prevent complications from infection and hemorrhage. Whenever WBC blood levels are low, this should cue the nurse to recognize that the client's immune system is weakened and the potential for infection is great.

8. 1. The RBCs are decreased (normal 4.5–5.0), which is associated with either the decreased production of RBCs, increased destruction of RBCs, or blood loss. Both hemoglobin (normal 12–18) and hematocrit (normal 38–54) values are subsequently decreased. Low platelets (normal 150,000–400,000) are most frequently associated with a tendency to bleed. These factors support the need for the nurse to monitor the client closely for bleeding problems.

9. 1. The WBC is very low (normal 4,000–11,000). This indicates that the client's immune system is deficient and the client is subject to infection.

10. 4. Persons with type AB blood, because they are universal blood recipients, are able to receive either type A, B, AB, or O blood. People with any blood type other than AB, are restricted as to the type of blood they can receive.

11. 3. The tubing is primed with 0.9% NS solution. If the filter is not completely primed, debris will coagulate in the filter and the transfusion will be slowed. In addition, saline is prepared to infuse in case a transfusion reaction occurs.

12. 2. The signs and symptoms the client is experiencing are indicative of a transfusion reaction and the transfusion must first be discontinued.

13. 4. A Z-track injection technique should be used to prevent leakage of the iron to subcutaneous tissues.

14. 1. Dark, leafy green vegetables (as well as meats, eggs, legumes, and whole-grain or enriched breads and cereals) are rich in iron. In addition,

both citrus foods and green leafy vegetables are high in vitamin C, which aids in iron absorption.

15. 1. There is a familial predisposition for pernicious anemia, and although the disease cannot be prevented, it can be controlled if detected and treated early. Pernicious anemia occurs as a result of the lack of the protein intrinsic factor that is secreted by the gastric mucosa.

16. 1. The client is to fast for 12 hours prior to the test. No food or drink is permitted. Following administration of the vitamin B_{12} dose, food is delayed for 3 hours.

17. 1. In aplastic anemia, the bone marrow elements (erythrocytes, leukocytes, and platelets) are suppressed. Treatments include, but are not limited to, bone marrow transplantation, transfusions to reduce symptomatology, and drugs to stimulate bone marrow function. Drugs like estrogen and progesterone work to stimulate bone growth. Estrogen and progesterone also stop menstruation so there is less blood loss.

18. 2. Decreased RBCs are a result of the excessive destruction of the red blood cells. With this destruction, there is a subsequent decrease in both hemoglobin and hematocrit. In addition, this increased destruction causes an elevation in bilirubin levels. The reticulocyte count is high because the numbers of immature RBCs are increased when RBCs are being destroyed. This count reflects the bone marrow activity, which is active in producing RBCs to compensate for the destruction.

19. 1. Following a splenectomy, immunologic deficiencies may develop, and vulnerability to infection is greatly increased. The postsplenectomy client is highly susceptible to infection from organisms such as *Pneumococcus. A preventive measure is immunization with Pneumovax.*

20. 3. Cerebral, cardiopulmonary, and peripheral tissue perfusion is affected by DIC. The many clots can cause obstruction to blood flow and tissue damage can subsequently occur.

21. 1. In DIC, the paradoxical events of hemorrhage and clotting occur. Although it may seem counterproductive to administer heparin while a client is bleeding, it is necessary to prevent the clotting that is simultaneously occurring in the microcirculation. It is critical that the client be monitored closely.

22. 1. This statement answers the client's question in a simple, matter of fact manner that is truthful and to the point.

23. 2. Although needle exchange programs are very controversial, it is evident the transmission of HIV can be significantly reduced when needle exchange programs are introduced.

24. 1. Heterosexual transmission of HIV is a concern, especially in this age group. It is on the rise and this is often overlooked because the more known transmissions take place among homosexuals and IV drug abusers.

25. 2. Corticosteroids may be added to the chemotherapy regime because of their antitumor effect. In addition, they assist in the excretion of calcium, which helps to treat the hypercalcemia that occurs in clients who have multiple myeloma.

26. 1. With polycythemia vera, maintaining oxygenation is critical. High altitudes can precipitate hypoxia. This client needs further instruction.

8

The Respiratory System

OVERVIEW OF ANATOMY AND PHYSIOLOGY

Upper Respiratory Tract

Structures of the respiratory system, primarily an air conduction system, include the nose, pharynx, and larynx. Air is filtered, warmed, and humidified in the upper airway before passing to lower airway (see Figure 8-1).

CHAPTER OUTLINE

Nose

A. External nose is a framework of bone and cartilage, internally divided into two passages or *nares* (*nasal cavities*) by the septum; air enters the system through the nares.
B. The septum is covered with a mucous membrane, where the olfactory receptors are located. Turbinates, located internally, assist in warming and moistening the air.
C. The major functions of the nose are warming, moistening, and filtering the air.

Pharynx

A. Muscular passageway commonly called the throat.
B. Air passes through the nose to the pharynx, composed of three sections
   1. *Nasopharynx:* located above the soft palate of the mouth, contains the adenoids and openings to the eustachian tubes.
   2. *Oropharynx:* located directly behind the mouth and tongue, contains the palatine tonsils; air and food enter body through oropharynx.
   3. *Laryngopharynx:* extends from the epiglottis to the sixth cervical level.

Larynx

A. Sometimes called "voice box," connects upper and lower airways; framework is formed by the hyoid bone, epiglottis, and thyroid, cricoid, and arytenoid cartilages. The opening of the larynx is called the glottis.
B. Larynx opens to allow respiration and closes to prevent aspiration when food passes through the pharynx.
C. Vocal cords of larynx permit speech and are involved in the cough reflex.

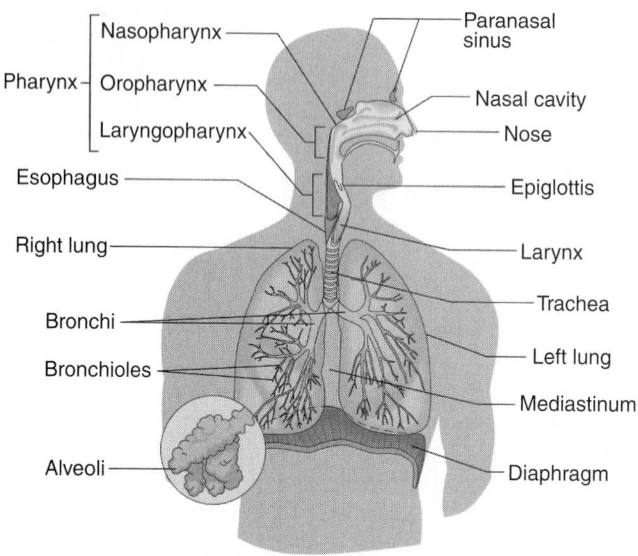

FIGURE 8-1 The respiratory system

Lower Respiratory Tract

Consists of the trachea, bronchi and branches, and the lungs and associated structures (see Figure 8-1).

Trachea

A. Air moves from the pharynx to larynx to trachea (length 11–13 cm, diameter 1.5–2.5 cm in adult).
B. Extends from the larynx to the second costal cartilage, where it bifurcates and is supported by 16–20 C-shaped cartilage rings.
C. The area where the trachea divides into two branches is called the *carina*.

Bronchi

A. Formed by the division of the trachea into two branches (bronchi)
   1. *Right mainstem bronchus:* larger and straighter than the left; further divides into three lobar branches (upper, middle, and lower lobar bronchi) to supply the three lobes of right lung. If passed too far, endotracheal tube might enter right mainstem bronchus; only right lung is then intubated.
   2. *Left mainstem bronchus:* divides into the upper and lower lobar bronchi, to supply two lobes of left lung.

B. At the point a bronchus reaches about 1 mm in diameter it no longer has a connective tissue sheath and is called a *bronchiole*.

Bronchioles

A. In the bronchioles, airway patency is primarily dependent upon elastic recoil formed by network of smooth muscles.

B. The tracheobronchial tree ends at the terminal bronchioles. Distal to the terminal bronchioles the major function is no longer air conduction, but gas exchange between blood and alveolar air. The *respiratory bronchioles* serve as the transition to the alveolar epithelium.

Lungs (Right and Left)

A. Main organs of respiration, lie within the thoracic cavity on either side of the heart.

B. Broad area of lung resting on diaphragm is called the base; the narrow, superior portion is the apex.

C. Each lung is divided into lobes: three in the right lung, two in the left.

D. *Pleura:* serous membrane covering the lungs; continuous with the parietal pleura that lines the chest wall.

E. Lungs and associated structures are protected by the chest wall.

Chest Wall

A. Includes the rib cage, intercostal muscles, and diaphragm.

B. Parietal pleura lines the chest wall and secretes small amounts of lubricating fluid into the intrapleural space (space between the visceral and parietal pleura). This fluid holds the lung and chest wall together as a single unit while allowing them to move separately.

C. The chest is shaped and supported by 12 pairs of ribs and costal cartilages; the ribs have several attached muscles.

1. Contraction of the external intercostal muscles raises the rib cage during inspiration and helps increase the size of the thoracic cavity.
2. The internal intercostal muscles tend to pull ribs down and in and play a role in forced expiration.

D. The *diaphragm* is the major muscle of ventilation (the exchange of air between the atmosphere and the alveoli). Contraction of muscle fibers causes the dome of the diaphragm to descend, thereby increasing the volume of the thoracic cavity. As exertion increases, additional chest muscles or even abdominal muscles may be employed in moving the thoracic cage.

Pulmonary Circulation

A. Provides for reoxygenation of blood and release of CO_2; gas transfer occurs in the pulmonary capillary bed.

B. Pulmonary arteries arise from the right ventricle of the heart and continue to the bronchi and alveoli, gradually decreasing in size to capillaries.

C. The capillaries, after contact with the gas-exchange surface of the alveoli, reform to form the pulmonary veins.

D. The two pulmonary veins, superior and inferior, empty into the left atrium.

Gas Exchange

Alveolar Ducts and Alveoli

A. Alveolar ducts arise from the respiratory bronchioles and lead to the alveoli.

B. *Alveoli* are the functional cellular units of the lungs; about half arise directly from the alveolar ducts and are responsible for about 35% of alveolar gas exchange.

C. Alveoli produce *surfactant*, a phospholipid substance found in the fluid lining the alveolar epithelium. Surfactant reduces surface tension and increases the stability of the alveoli and prevents their collapse.

D. *Alveolar sacs* form the last part of the airway; functionally the same as the alveolar ducts, they are surrounded by alveoli and are responsible for 65% of the alveolar gas exchange.

ASSESSMENT

Health History

A. Presenting problem
   1. Nose/nasal sinuses: symptoms may include colds, discharge, epistaxis, sinus problems (swelling, pain)
   2. Throat: symptoms may include sore throat, hoarseness, difficulty swallowing, strep throat
   3. Lungs: symptoms may include
      a. Cough: note duration; frequency; type (dry, hacking, bubbly, barky, hoarse, congested); sputum (productive vs nonproductive); circumstances related to cough (time of day, positions, talking, anxiety); treatment.
      b. Dyspnea: note onset, severity, duration, efforts to treat, whether associated with radiation, if accompanied by cough or diaphoresis, time of day when it most likely occurs, interference with ADL, whether precipitated by any specific activities, whether accompanied by cyanosis.
      c. Wheezing
      d. Chest pain
      e. Hemoptysis

B. Lifestyle: smoking (note type of tobacco, duration, number per day, number of years of smoking, inhalation, related cough, desire to quit); occupation (work conditions that could irritate respiratory system [asbestos, chemical irritants, dry-cleaning fumes] and monitoring or protection of exposure conditions), geographical location (environmental conditions that could irritate respiratory system [chemical plants/industrial pollutants]); type and frequency of exercise/recreation.

C. Nutrition/diet: fluid intake per 24-hour period; intake of vitamins

D. Past medical history: immunizations (yearly immunizations for colds/flu; frequency and results of tuberculin skin testing); allergies (foods, drugs, contact or inhalant allergens, precipitating factors, specific treatment, desensitization)

Physical Examination

A. Inspect for configuration of the chest (kyphosis, scoliosis, barrel chest) and cyanosis.

B. Determine rate and pattern of breathing (normal rate 12–18/minute); note tachypnea, hyperventilation, or labored breathing pattern.

C. Palpate skin, subcutaneous structures, and muscles for texture, temperature, and degree of development.

D. Palpate for tracheal position, respiratory excursion (symmetric or asymmetric movement of the chest), and for fremitus.

1. Fremitus is normally increased in intensity at second intercostal spaces at sternal border and interscapular spaces only.
2. Increased intensity elsewhere may indicate pneumonia, pulmonary fibrosis, or tumor.
3. Decreased intensity may indicate pneumothorax, pleural effusion, COPD.

E. Percuss lung fields (should find resonance over normal lung tissue, note hyperresonance or dullness) and for diaphragmatic excursion (normal distance between levels of dullness on full expiration and full inspiration is 6–12 cm).

F. Auscultate for normal (vesicular, bronchial, bronchovesicular) and adventitious (rales or crackles, rhonchi, pleural friction rub) breath sounds (see Figure 8-2).

Laboratory/Diagnostic Tests

A. *Arterial blood gases (ABGs)*

1. Measure base excess/deficit, blood pH, CO_2, total CO_2, O_2 content, O_2 saturation (SaO_2), pCO_2 (partial pressure of carbon dioxide), pO_2 (partial pressure of oxygen)
2. Nursing care
   - **a.** If drawn by arterial stick, place a 4×4 bandage over puncture site after withdrawal of needle and maintain pressure with two fingers for at least 2 minutes.
   - **b.** Gently rotate sample in test tube to mix heparin with the blood.
   - **c.** Place sample in ice-water container until it can be analyzed.

B. *Pulmonary function studies*

1. Evaluation of lung volume and capacities by spirometry: tidal volume (TV), vital capacity (VC), inspiratory and expiratory reserve volume (IRV and ERV), residual volume (RV), inspiratory capacity (IC), functional residual capacity (FRC)
2. Involves use of a spirometer to diagram movement of air as client performs various respiratory maneuvers; shows restriction or obstruction to airflow, or both

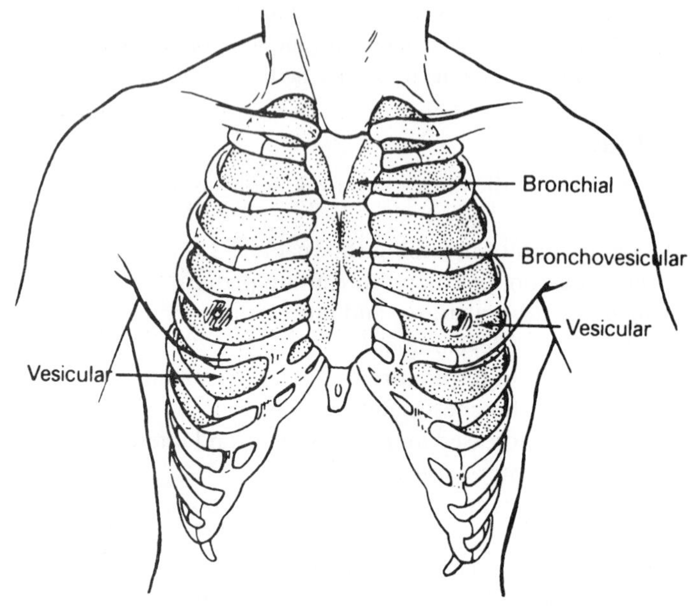

FIGURE 8-2 Locations for hearing normal breath sounds

3. Nursing care
   a. Carefully explaining procedure will help allay anxiety and ensure cooperation.
   b. Perform tests before meals.
   c. Withhold medication that may alter respiratory function unless otherwise ordered.
   d. After procedure assess pulse and provide for rest period.

C. Hematologic studies (ESR, Hgb and hct, WBC)

D. *Sputum culture and sensitivity*
   1. Culture: isolation and identification of specific microorganism from a specimen
   2. Sensitivity: determination of antibiotic agent effective against organism (sensitive or resistant)
   3. Nursing care
      a. Explain necessity of effective coughing.
      b. If client unable to cough, heated aerosol will assist with obtaining a specimen.
      c. Collect specimen in a sterile container that can be capped afterwards.
      d. Volume need not exceed 1–3 ml.
      e. Deliver specimen to lab rapidly.

E. *Tuberculin skin test*

1. Intradermal test done to detect tuberculosis infection; does not differentiate active from dormant infections
2. Purified protein derivative (PPD) tuberculin administered to determine any previous sensitization to tubercle bacillus
3. Several methods of administration
   a. *Mantoux test:* 0.1 ml solution containing 0.5 tuberculin units of PPD-tuberculin is injected into the forearm.
   b. *Tine test:* a stainless steel disc with 4 tines impregnated with PPD-tuberculin is pressed into the skin.
4. Results: read within 48–72 hours; inspect skin and circle zone of induration with a pencil; measure diameter in mm
   a. Negative: zone diameter less than 5 mm
   b. Doubtful or probable: zone diameter 5–10 mm
   c. Positive: zone diameter 10 mm or more

F. *Thoracentesis*

1. Insertion of a needle through the chest wall into the pleural space to obtain a specimen for diagnostic evaluation, removal of pleural fluid accumulation, or to instill medication into the pleural space
2. Nursing care: prior to procedure
   a. Confirm that a signed permit has been obtained.
   b. Explain procedure; instruct client not to cough or talk during procedure.
   c. Position client at side of bed, with upper torso supported on overbed table, feet and legs well supported.
   d. Assess vital signs.
3. Nursing care: following procedure
   a. Observe for signs and symptoms of pneumothorax, shock, leakage at puncture site.
   b. Auscultate chest to ascertain breath sounds.

G. *Bronchoscopy*

1. Insertion of a fiber-optic scope into the bronchi for diagnosis, biopsy, specimen collection, examination of structures/tissues, removal of foreign bodies
2. Nursing care: prior to procedure
   a. Confirm that a signed permit has been obtained.
   b. Explain procedure, remove dentures, and provide good oral hygiene.
   c. Keep client NPO 6–12 hours pretest.
3. Nursing care: following procedure
   a. Position client on side or in semi-Fowler's.
   b. Keep NPO until return of gag reflex.
   c. Assess for and report frank bleeding.
   d. Apply ice bags to throat for comfort; discourage talking, coughing, smoking for a few hours to decrease irritation.

ANALYSIS

Nursing diagnoses for the client with a respiratory dysfunction may include

A. Impaired gas exchange
B. Ineffective airway clearance
C. Ineffective breathing pattern
D. Impaired verbal communication
E. Activity intolerance
F. Anxiety
G. Imbalanced nutrition: less than body requirements
H. Risk for infection

PLANNING AND IMPLEMENTATION

Goals

A. Adequate ventilation will be maintained.
B. Maintenance of patent airway.
C. Effective breathing patterns will be maintained.
D. Client will communicate in an effective manner.
E. Client will demonstrate increased tolerance for activity.
F. Anxiety will be reduced.
G. Adequate nutritional status will be maintained.
H. Client remains free from infection.

Interventions

Chest Drainage Systems

A. Insertion of a catheter into the intrapleural space to maintain constant negative pressure when air/fluid have accumulated.
B. Chest tube is attached to underwater drainage to allow for the escape of air/fluid and to prevent reflux of air into the chest.
C. For evacuation of air, chest tube is placed in the second or third intercostal space, anterior or midaxillary line (air rises to the upper chest).
D. For drainage of fluid, chest tube is placed in the eighth or ninth intercostal space, midaxillary line.
E. Chest tube is connected to tubing for the collection system; the distal end of the collection tubing must be placed below the water level in order to prevent atmospheric air from entering the pleural space.
F. Traditional water-seal drainage; also known as wet suction; can be set up using one, two, or three bottles. No longer used in the United States because it has been replaced by the newer technology of dry-suction water-seal drainage. For explanatory purposes it is included here. Also may be used in other countries.

   1. *One-bottle system* (Figure 8-3A)

      a. Operates by gravity, not suction; the bottle serves as both collection chamber and water seal.

   b. Two hollow tubes (glass rods) are inserted into the stopper of the bottle; the drainage tube is connected to the glass rod that is submerged approximately 2 cm below the water level; the second glass tube allows for the escape of air.
   c. If considerable drainage accumulates it is difficult for the client to expel air and fluid from the pleural space. If this occurs, the glass rod may be pulled up or a new drainage bottle may be set up (according to physician's orders).
2. *Two-bottle system* (Figure 8-3B,C)
   a. One bottle serves as a drainage collection chamber, the other as a water seal.

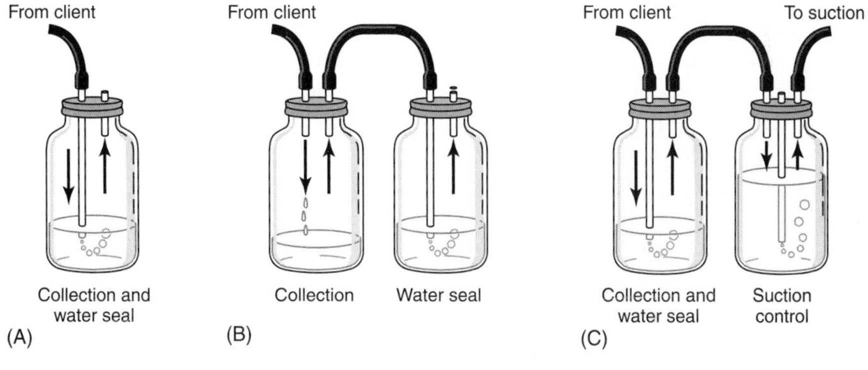

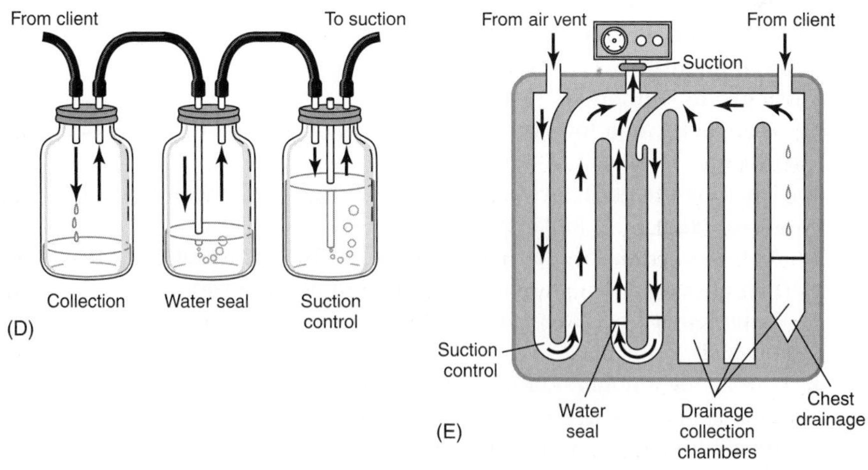

FIGURE 8-3 Water-seal drainage systems. (A) One-bottle system; (B) two-bottle system; (C) two-bottle system with suction; (D) three-bottle system; (E) underwater seal chest drainage device.

  b. The first bottle is the drainage collection chamber and has two short tubes in the rubber stopper. One of these tubes is attached to the drainage tubing coming from the client; the other is attached to the underwater tube of the second bottle (the water-seal bottle). The air vent of the water-seal bottle must be left open to atmospheric air. If suction is used, the first bottle serves as drainage collection and water-seal chamber, and the second bottle serves as the suction chamber.
3. *Three-bottle system* (Figure 8-3D)
   a. This system has a drainage collection, a water-seal, and a suction-control bottle.
   b. The third bottle controls the amount of pressure in the system. The suction-control bottle has three tubes inserted in the stopper, two short and one long. One short tube is joined with the tubing to the former air vent of the water-seal bottle; the second short tube is connected to suction. The third (long) tube (or suction-control tube) is located between the short tubes and has one end open to the atmosphere and the other below the water level.
   c. The depth to which the suction-control tube is immersed controls the amount of pressure within the system. The pressure is determined by the physician.

G. Dry-suction water-seal drainage; also referred to as dry suction; has three chambers (collection chamber, water seal chamber, and wet suction control chamber) (see Figure 8-3E).

H. Dry-suction one-way valve system (also known as Heimlich Flutter Valve); allows unidirectional flow of air and fluid from pleural space, prevents reflux, sets up quickly in emergency, works when knocked over, works well for ambulatory clients.

I. Nursing care: without suction
1. Prepare the unit for use and connect the chest catheter to the drainage tubing.
2. Examine the entire system to ensure airtightness and absence of obstruction from kinks or dependent loops of tubing.
3. Note oscillation of the fluid level within the water-seal tube. It will rise on inspiration and fall on expiration due to changes in the intrapleural pressure. If oscillation stops and system is intact, notify physician.
4. Check the amount, color, and characteristics of the drainage. If drainage ceases and system is not blocked, assess for signs of respiratory distress from fluid/air accumulation.
5. Always keep drainage system lower than the level of the client's chest.
6. Keep Vaseline gauze at bedside at all times in case chest tube falls out.
7. Keep clamps at bedside in case of accidental disconnection. Clamp, troubleshoot, and immediately reconnect.

DELEGATION TIP

Managing chest tube systems is your responsibility. Instruct ancillary personnel to report all concerns and client complaints immediately to you.

8. Encourage coughing and deep breathing to facilitate removal of air and drainage from pleural cavity.
9. Provide ROM exercises.

J. Nursing care: with suction
   1. Attach suction tubing to suction apparatus, and chest catheter to drainage tubing.
   2. Open suction slowly until a stream of bubbles is seen in the suction chamber. There should be continuous bubbling in this chamber and intermittent bubbling in the water seal. Check for an air leak in the system if bubbling in water seal is constant; notify physician if air leak.
   3. Check drainage, keep drainage system below level of client's chest, keep Vaseline gauze at bedside, encourage coughing and deep breathing, and provide ROM exercises as noted above.

K. General principles of chest tube management:
   1. Never clamp chest tubes over an extended period of time unless a specific order is written by the physician. Clamping the chest tubes of a client with air in the pleural space will cause increased pressure buildup and possible tension pneumothorax.
   2. Removal of the chest tube: instruct the client to perform Valsalva maneuver; apply a Vaseline or gauze dressing to the site (per hospital protocol).
   3. If the water-seal bottle should break, immediately obtain some type of fluid-filled container to create an emergency water seal until a new unit can be obtained.

Heimlich Flutter Valve

A. This disposable valve allows a unidirectional flow of air and fluid from the pleural space into a drainage bag and prevents any reflux of air or fluid. A water-seal drainage system is not necessary.

B. Controlled suction can be attached if ordered.

C. The valve is encased in clear plastic, which eliminates the possibility of kinks. Its small size, approximately 7 inches, permits greater mobility.

Chest Physiotherapy

A. General information
   1. Used for individuals with increased production of secretions or thick, sticky secretions, and for clients with impaired removal of secretions or with ineffective cough. May also be used as a preventive measure for clients with weakness of the muscles of respiration or a predisposition to increased production or thickness of secretions.
   2. Includes the techniques of postural drainage, percussion, and vibration.
      a. *Postural drainage:* uses gravity and various positions to stimulate the movement of secretions.
         1) postural drainage positions are determined by the areas of involved lung, assessed by chest X-ray and physical assessment findings.
         2) careful positioning is required to help secretions flow from smaller airways into the segmental bronchus and larger airways where secretions can be coughed up.
      b. *Percussion:* involves clapping with cupped hands on the chest wall over the segment to be drained.
         1) the hand is cupped by holding the fingers together so that the shape of the hand conforms with chest wall.
         2) clapping should be vigorous but not painful.
      c. *Vibration:* in this technique the hand is pressed firmly over the appropriate segment of chest wall, and muscles of upper arm and shoulder are tensed (isometric contraction); done with flattened, not cupped hand.

B. Nursing care
   1. Perform procedure before or 3 hours after meals.
   2. Administer bronchodilators about 20 minutes before procedure.
   3. Remove all tight/constricting clothing.
   4. Have all equipment available (tissues, emesis basin, towel, paper bag).
   5. Assist client to correct prescribed position for postural drainage (client to assume each postural drainage position for approximately 3–5 minutes).
   6. Place towel over area to be percussed.
   7. Instruct client to take several deep breaths.
   8. Percuss designated area for approximately 3 minutes during inspiration and expiration.
   9. Vibrate same designated area during exhalations of 4–5 deep breaths.
   10. Assist client with coughing when in postural drainage position; some clients may need to sit upright to produce a cough.
   11. Repeat the same procedure in all designated positions.
   12. After procedure, assist client to comfortable position and provide good oral hygiene.

Mechanical Ventilation

A. General information
   1. Ventilation is performed by mechanical means in individuals who are unable to maintain normal levels of oxygen and carbon dioxide in the blood.
   2. Indicated in clients with COPD, obesity, neuromuscular disease, severe neurologic depression, thoracic trauma, ARDS; clients who have undergone thoracic or open-heart surgery are likely to be maintained on mechanical ventilation post-op.
B. Types (positive pressure ventilators)
   1. Positive pressure-cycled ventilator: pushes air into the lungs until a predetermined pressure is reached within the tracheobronchial tree; expiration occurs by passive relaxation of the diaphragm.
   2. Volume-cycled ventilator: most popular type for intubated adults and older children; delivers air into the lungs until a certain predetermined tidal volume is reached before terminating inspiration.
   3. Time-cycled ventilator: terminates inspiration after a preset time; tidal volume is regulated by adjusting length of inspiration and flow rate of pressurized gas.
C. Modes of mechanical ventilation
   1. *Assist/control mode*: client's inspiratory effort triggers ventilator, which then delivers breath; may be set to deliver breath automatically if client does not trigger it. The same tidal volume is delivered with each breath.
   2. *Intermittent mandatory ventilation (IMV)*: client may breathe at own rate. IMV breaths are delivered under positive pressure; however, all other respirations taken by the client are delivered at ambient pressure and tidal volume is of client's own determination.
   3. *Positive end expiratory pressure (PEEP)*: ventilator delivers additional positive pressure at the end of expiration, which maintains the alveoli in an expanded state.
   4. *Controlled mandatory ventilation (CMV)*: all breaths initiated by ventilator as there is no pressure sensed by the machine. Same tidal volume is delivered with each breath.
   5. *Continuous positive airway pressure (CPAP)*: achieves the same results as PEEP, except CPAP is used on adult clients who are on a T-piece.
   6. *Pressure support (PS)*: client's inspiratory efforts trigger each breath; every breath ventilator assisted without dyssynchrony, which can occur with SIMV. Often used prior to extubation.
D. Nursing care
   1. Assess for decreased cardiac output and administer appropriate nursing care.
   2. Monitor for positive water balance. Pressure breathing may cause increase in antidiuretic hormone (ADH) and retention of water.
      a. Maintain accurate I&O.
      b. Assess daily weights.
      c. Take PCWP readings as ordered.

d. Palpate for peripheral edema.
e. Auscultate chest for altered breath sounds.

3. Monitor for barotrauma.
   a. Assess ventilator settings every 4 hours.
   b. Auscultate breath sounds every 2 hours.
   c. Monitor ABGs.
   d. Perform complete pulmonary physical assessment every shift.
4. Monitor for GI problems (stress ulcer).
5. Administer muscle relaxants, tranquilizers, analgesics or paralyzing agents as ordered to increase client-machine synchrony by relaxing the client.

Oxygen Therapy

A. Most common therapy for clients with respiratory disease
B. Indications include arterial hypoxemia; COPD; ARDS; tissue, cellular, and circulatory hypoxia
C. Delivery systems
   1. *Low-flow system:* delivers oxygen at variable liter flows designed to add to client's inspired air.
      a. *Nasal cannula*
         1) most common mode of oxygen delivery; consists of delivering 100% oxygen through two prongs inserted 1 cm into each nostril; general flow rates of 1–4 liters/minute are used with desired FiO_2 range of 24%–40%.
         2) nursing care
            a) instruct client to breathe through the nose.
            b) remove cannula and clean nares every 8 hours.
            c) provide mouth care every 2–3 hours.
            d) use gauze pads behind ears to decrease irritation.
            e) assess arterial pO_2 frequently.
      b. *Standard mask*
         1) simple face mask that covers the nose and mouth and provides an additional area for oxygen collection; ranges: 6–12 liters/minute; FiO_2: 40%–65%.
         2) nursing care
            a) instruct client to breathe through the nose.
            b) remove and clean mask every 2–3 hours.
            c) monitor carefully in clients who are prone to develop obstructed airways.
            d) replace mask with nasal cannula during meals and reposition mask immediately after eating.
      c. Nonrebreathing mask
         1) standard mask with a reservoir bag designed to deliver 90%–100% oxygen; a one-way valve between reservoir bag and mask allows the client to inhale only from the reservoir

bag and exhale through separate valves on the side of the mask; ranges: 6–15 liters/minute; FiO_2: 60%–90%.

2) Nursing care
   a) instruct client to breathe through the nose.
   b) ensure that bag does not collapse completely with each inspiration.
   c) remove and clean mask every 2–3 hours.

2. *High-flow system:* client receives entire inspired gas from the apparatus, flow rates must exceed the volume of air required for a person's minute ventilation; *Venturi mask* commonly used.
   a. Provides precise delivery of oxygen concentrations of 24–50%.
   b. Nursing care
      1) provide supplemental oxygen by cannula during meals and other activities where mask interferes.
      2) remove and clean mask every 2–3 hours.

Tracheobronchial Suctioning

A. Suction removal of secretions from the tracheobronchial tree using a sterile catheter inserted into the airway.

B. Catheters may be inserted through various routes: nasopharyngeal, oropharyngeal, or via an artificial airway.

C. Purposes
   1. Maintain a patent airway through removal of secretions
   2. Promote adequate exchange of oxygen/carbon dioxide
   3. Substitute for effective coughing
   4. Obtain a specimen for analysis

D. Procedure
   1. Gather suctioning equipment (receptacle for secretions, sterile catheter, sterile gloves, and container of sterile normal saline), or use inline device for endotracheal tube suctioning.
   2. Turn vacuum on and test suction system.
   3. Place client in semi- to high-Fowler's position.
   4. Apply sterile glove, fill sterile cup with solution, and attach sterile catheter to connecting tube.
   5. Increase inspired oxygen concentration to highest point and hyperinflate the lungs before and after each catheter insertion by using self-inflating bag; have client deep breathe if able.
   6. Use gloved hand to insert catheter.
      a. Oral route
         1) if oral airway in place, slide the catheter alongside it and back to the pharynx; if no oral airway in place, have client protrude the tongue and guide the catheter into the oropharynx.
         2) insert during inspiration until cough is stimulated or secretion obtained.

   b. Nasal route: advance catheter along the floor of the nares or pass it through an artificial nasal airway until cough is stimulated or secretions obtained.
   c. Artificial airway: insert the catheter into the artificial airway until cough is stimulated or secretions obtained.
7. Do not cover the thumb control and do not apply suction during insertion of the catheter.
8. During withdrawal, rotate the catheter while applying intermittent suction.
9. Whole suctioning procedure including insertion and removal of the catheter should not exceed 10 seconds.
10. If it is necessary to continue the suctioning process, hyperinflate the lungs, allow the client to rest briefly, and repeat the process.
11. Discard catheter, glove, and cup; record amount, color, characteristics of the secretions obtained; note client's tolerance of procedure.
12. Auscultate for changes in breath sounds.

Tracheostomy Care

A. Performed to avoid bacterial contamination and obstruction of tracheostomy tube; frequency varies depending on amount of secretions
B. Procedure
   1. Explain procedure and provide reassurance to the client.
   2. If not contraindicated, place client in semi-Fowler's position to promote lung reexpansion.
   3. Disconnect ventilator or humidification device.
   4. Suction trachea to clear secretions.
   5. Reconnect ventilator or humidifier.
   6. Remove all tracheostomy dressing.
   7. Assemble equipment ("trach care kit").
   8. Set up sterile field and put on sterile glove.
      a. For a single-cannula tube
         1) with sterile gloved hand, wipe client's neck under trach tube flanges with presoaked sterile sponge.
         2) wipe skin around tracheostomy with a second sponge until cleansed thoroughly (may use wet cotton-tipped applicators to cleanse around stoma).
         3) use each sponge or applicator only once.
         4) allow area to dry and apply a new sterile dressing (free of lint and fibers).
         5) change tracheostomy ties as needed.
      b. For a double-cannula tube (nondisposable inner cannula)
         1) disconnect ventilator or humidification device and unlock the inner cannula of trach tube using ungloved hand.
         2) place inner cannula in basin containing H2O2 to remove encrustations.

3) if client on a ventilator, insert another inner cannula while old one is being cleaned and reconnect client to ventilator.
4) cleanse stomal area and trach tube flanges with presoaked gauze sponges.
5) clean inner cannula.
6) remove excess liquid by gentle shaking.
7) if client not on a ventilator, gently reinsert inner cannula into tracheostomy tube and lock in place.
8) allow area to dry, apply dressing and new tracheostomy ties as described above.

C. For a double-cannula tube (disposable inner cannula)
1. disconnect ventilator tube.
2. remove inner cannula.
3. insert replacement cannula.
4. cleanse stomal area and trach tube flanges with presoaked gauze sponges.
5. allow area to dry, apply dressing and new tracheostomy ties as described above.

EVALUATION

A. Client demonstrates ABGs or O_2 saturation within normal limits; absence of dyspnea and cyanosis; usual or improved breath sounds and usual mentation.

B. Client demonstrates effective coughing with expectoration of secretions; absence of dyspnea; rate and depth of ventilation within normal range; improved breath sounds.

C. ABGs or O_2 saturation within normal range; lungs clear to auscultation; rate and depth of respirations within client's normal range; effective use of muscles of respiration.

D. Client identifies plans for appropriate alternate speech methods.

E. Client demonstrates increased activity tolerance with absence of dyspnea and excessive fatigue and vital signs within normal limits.

F. Improved rest/sleep patterns; respiratory rate and rhythm within client's normal range; demonstrates effective problem-solving abilities.

G. Client demonstrates behaviors/lifestyle changes to regain and maintain appropriate body weight. Verbalizes importance of nutrition to general well-being. Stable weight; improved anthropometric measurements.

H. Vital signs within client's normal range; client verbalizes understanding of causative/risk factors and utilizes techniques to promote a safe environment.

DISORDERS OF THE RESPIRATORY SYSTEM

Chronic Obstructive Pulmonary Disease (COPD)

Refers to respiratory conditions that produce obstruction of airflow; includes emphysema, bronchitis, bronchiectasis, and asthma.

NURSING ALERT

Between 20 and 25% of the patients with COPD develop peptic ulcer.

Emphysema

A. General information
   1. Enlargement and destruction of the alveolar, bronchial, and bronchiolar tissue with resultant loss of recoil, air trapping, thoracic overdistension, sputum accumulation, and loss of diaphragmatic muscle tone
   2. These changes cause a state of carbon dioxide retention, hypoxia, and respiratory acidosis.
   3. Caused by cigarette smoking, infection, inhaled irritants, heredity, allergic factors, aging
B. Assessment findings
   1. Anorexia, fatigue, weight loss
   2. Feeling of breathlessness, cough, sputum production, flaring of the nostrils, use of accessory muscles of respiration, increased rate and depth of breathing, dyspnea
   3. Decreased respiratory excursion, resonance to hyperresonance, decreased breath sounds with prolonged expiration, normal or decreased fremitus
   4. Diagnostic tests: pCO_2 elevated or normal; pO_2 normal or slightly decreased
C. Nursing interventions
   1. Administer medications as ordered.
      a. Bronchiodilators: aminophylline, isoproterenol (Isuprel), terbutaline (Brethine), metaproterenol (Alupent), theophylline, isoetharine (Bronkosol); used in treatment of bronchospasm
      b. Antimicrobials: tetracycline, ampicillin to treat bacterial infections
      c. Corticosteroids: prednisone
   2. Facilitate removal of secretions.
      a. Ensure fluid intake of at least 3 liters/day.
      b. Provide (and teach client) chest physical therapy, coughing and deep breathing, and use of hand nebulizers.
      c. Suction as needed.
      d. Provide oral hygiene after expectoration of sputum.
   3. Improve ventilation.
      a. Position client in semi- or high-Fowler's.
      b. Instruct client to use diaphragmatic muscle to breathe.

c. Encourage productive coughing after all treatments (splint abdomen to help produce more expulsive cough).
d. Employ pursed-lip breathing techniques (prolonged, slow relaxed expiration against pursed lips).

4. Provide client teaching and discharge planning concerning
   a. Prevention of recurrent infections
      1) avoid crowds and individuals with known infection.
      2) adhere to high-protein, high-carbohydrate, increased vitamin C diet.
      3) receive immunizations for influenza and pneumonia.
      4) report changes in characteristics and color of sputum immediately.
      5) report worsening of symptoms (increased tightness of chest, fatigue, increased dyspnea).
   b. Control of environment
      1) use home humidifier at 30–50% humidity.
      2) wear scarf over nose and mouth in cold weather to prevent bronchospasm.
      3) avoid smoking and contact with environmental smoke.
      4) avoid abrupt changes in temperature.
   c. Avoidance of inhaled irritants
      1) stay indoors if pollution levels are high.
      2) use air conditioner with high-efficiency particulate air filter to remove particles from air.
   d. Increasing activity tolerance
      1) start with mild exercises, such as walking, and gradually increase amount and duration.
      2) use breathing techniques (pursed lip, diaphragmatic) during activities/exercises to control breathing.
      3) have oxygen available as needed to assist with activities.
      4) plan activities that require low amounts of energy.
      5) plan rest periods before and after activities.

Bronchitis

A. General information
   1. Excessive production of mucus in the bronchi with accompanying persistent cough.
   2. Characteristic changes include hypertrophy/hyperplasia of the mucus-secreting glands in the bronchi, decreased ciliary activity, chronic inflammation, and narrowing of the small airways.
   3. Caused by the same factors that cause emphysema.

B. Medical management: drug therapy includes bronchodilators, antimicrobials, expectorants (e.g., Robitussin)

C. Assessment findings

1. Productive (copious) cough, dyspnea on exertion, use of accessory muscles of respiration, scattered rales and rhonchi
2. Feeling of epigastric fullness, slight cyanosis, distended neck veins, ankle edema
3. Diagnostic tests: increased pCO_2, decreased pO_2

D. Nursing interventions: same as for emphysema

Bronchiectasis

A. General information
   1. Permanent abnormal dilation of the bronchi with destruction of muscular and elastic structure of the bronchial wall
   2. Caused by bacterial infection; recurrent lower respiratory tract infections; congenital defects (altered bronchial structures); lung tumors; thick, tenacious secretions

B. Medical management: same as for emphysema

C. Assessment findings
   1. Chronic cough with production of mucopurulent sputum, hemoptysis, exertional dyspnea, wheezing
   2. Anorexia, fatigue, weight loss
   3. Diagnostic tests
      a. Bronchoscopy reveals sources and sites of secretions
      b. Possible elevation of WBC

D. Nursing interventions: same as for emphysema

Pulmonary Tuberculosis

A. General information
   1. Bacterial infectious disease caused by *M. tuberculosis* and spread via airborne droplets when infected persons cough, sneeze, or laugh.
   2. Once inhaled, the organisms implant themselves in the lung and begin dividing slowly, causing inflammation, development of the primary tubercle, and eventual caseation and fibrosis.
   3. Infection spreads via the lymph and circulatory systems.
   4. Half of the cases occur in inner-city neighborhoods, and incidence is highest in areas with a large population of native Americans. Nonwhites affected four times more often than whites. Men affected more often than women. The greatest number of cases occur in persons age 65 and over. Socially and economically disadvantaged, alcoholic, and malnourished individuals affected more often.
   5. The causative agent, *M. tuberculosis*, is an acid-fast bacillus spread via droplet nuclei from infected persons.

NURSING ALERT

Anti-tuberculosis therapy with daily oral doses for at least 6 months usually cures tuberculosis. Finishing the course of treatment prevents the occurrence of multidrug-resistant TB.

B. Assessment findings
   1. Cough (yellow mucoid sputum), dyspnea, hemoptysis, rales or crackles
   2. Anorexia, malaise, weight loss, afternoon low-grade fever, pallor, pain, fatigue, night sweats
   3. Diagnostic tests
      a. Chest X-ray indicates presence and extent of disease process but cannot differentiate active from inactive form
      b. Skin test (PPD) positive; area of induration 10 mm or more in diameter after 48 hours
      c. Sputum positive for acid-fast bacillus (three samples is diagnostic for disease)
      d. Culture positive
      e. WBC and ESR increased

C. Nursing interventions
   1. Administer medications as ordered.
   2. Prevent transmission.
      a. Strict isolation not required if client/significant others adhere to special respiratory precautions for tuberculosis.
      b. Client should be in a well-ventilated private room, with the door kept closed at all times.
      c. All visitors and staff should wear masks when in contact with the client and should discard the used masks before leaving the room; client should wear a mask when leaving the room for tests.
      d. All specimens should be labeled "AFB precautions."
      e. Handwashing is required after direct contact with the client or contaminated articles.
   3. Promote adequate nutrition.
      a. Make ongoing assessments of client's appetite and do kcal counts for 3 days; consult dietitian for diet guidelines.
      b. Offer small, frequent feedings and nutritional supplements; assist client with menu selection stressing balanced nutrition.
      c. Weigh client at least twice a week.
      d. Encourage activity as tolerated to increase appetite.
   4. Prevent social isolation.
      a. Impart a comfortable, confident attitude when caring for the client.

b. Explain the nature of the disease to the client, significant others, and visitors in simple terms.
c. Stress that visits are important, but isolation precautions must be followed.

5. Vary the client's routine to prevent boredom.
6. Discuss the client's feelings and assess for boredom, depression, anxiety, fatigue, or apathy; provide support and encourage expression of concerns.
7. Provide client teaching and discharge planning concerning
   a. Medication regimen: prepare a sheet with each drug name, dosage, time due, and major side effects; stress importance of following medication schedule for prescribed period of time (usually 9 months); include significant others
   b. Transmission prevention: client should cover mouth when coughing, expectorate into a tissue and place it in a paper bag; client should also wash hands after coughing or sneezing; stress importance of plenty of fresh air; include significant others
   c. Importance of notifying physician at the first sign of persistent cough, fever, or hemoptysis (may indicate recurrence)
   d. Need for follow-up care including physical exam, sputum cultures, and chest X-rays
   e. Availability of community health services
   f. Importance of high-protein, high-carbohydrate diet with inclusion of supplemental vitamins

Histoplasmosis

A. General information: a systemic fungal disease caused by inhalation of dust contaminated by Histoplasma capsulatum which is transmitted through bird manure.

B. Medical management: antifungal agent Amphotericin B
   1. Very toxic: toxicity includes anorexia, chills, fever, headache, and renal failure
   2. Acetaminophen, Benadryl, and steroids given with Amphotericin B to prevent reactions

C. Assessment findings
   1. Symptoms similar to tuberculosis or pneumonia
      a. Cough
      b. Fever
      c. Joint pain
      d. Malaise
   2. Sometimes asymptomatic
   3. Diagnostic tests
      a. Chest X-ray (often appears similar to tuberculosis)
      b. Histoplasmin skin test (read the same as PPD)

D. Nursing interventions
   1. Monitor respiratory status
   2. Administer medications as ordered; observe for severe side effects of Amphotericin B: fever (acetaminophen given prophylactically), anaphylactic reaction (Benadryl and steroids given prophylactically), abnormal renal function with hypokalemia and azotemia.

Chest Trauma

Fractured Ribs

A. General information
   1. Common chest injury resulting from blunt trauma.
   2. Ribs 4–8 are most commonly fractured because they are least protected by chest muscles. Splintered or displaced fractured ribs may penetrate the pleura and lungs.
B. Medical management: drug therapy consists of narcotics, intercostal nerve block (injection of intercostal nerves above and below the injury with an anesthetic agent) for pain relief.
C. Assessment findings
   1. Pain, especially on inspiration
   2. Point tenderness and bruising at injury site, splinting with shallow respirations, apprehensiveness
   3. Diagnostic tests
      a. Chest X-ray reveals area and degree of fracture
      b. pCO_2 elevated; pO_2 decreased (later)
D. Nursing interventions
   1. Provide pain relief/control.
      a. Administer ordered narcotics and analgesics cautiously and monitor effects.
      b. Place client in semi- or high-Fowler's position to ease pain associated with breathing.
   2. Monitor client closely for complications.
      a. Assess for bloody sputum (indicative of lung penetration).
      b. Observe for signs and symptoms of pneumothorax or hemothorax.

Flail Chest

A. General information
   1. Fracture of several ribs and resultant instability of the affected chest wall.
   2. Chest wall is no longer able to provide the bony structure necessary to maintain adequate ventilation; consequently, the flail portion and underlying tissue move paradoxically (in opposition) to the rest of the chest cage and lungs.
   3. The flail portion is sucked in on inspiration and bulges out on expiration.
   4. Result is hypoxia, hypercarbia, and increased retained secretions.

5. Caused by trauma (sternal rib fracture with possible costochondral separations).

B. Medical management
   1. Internal stabilization with a volume-cycled ventilator
   2. Drug therapy (narcotics, sedatives)

C. Assessment findings
   1. Severe dyspnea; rapid, shallow, grunty breathing; paradoxical chest motion
   2. Cyanosis, possible neck vein distension, tachycardia, hypotension
   3. Diagnostic tests
      a. pO_2 decreased
      b. pCO_2 elevated
      c. pH decreased

D. Nursing interventions
   1. Maintain an open airway: suction secretions/blood from nose, throat, mouth, and via endotracheal tube; note changes in amount, color, characteristics.
   2. Monitor mechanical ventilation.
   3. Encourage turning, coughing, and deep breathing.
   4. Monitor for signs of shock.

Pneumothorax/Hemothorax

A. General information
   1. Partial or complete collapse of the lung due to an accumulation of air or fluid in the pleural space
   2. Types
      a. *Spontaneous pneumothorax:* the most common type of closed pneumothorax; air accumulates within the pleural space without an obvious cause. Rupture of a small bleb on the visceral pleura most frequently produces this type of pneumothorax.
      b. *Open pneumothorax:* air enters the pleural space through an opening in the chest wall; usually caused by stabbing or gunshot wound.
      c. *Tension pneumothorax:* air enters the pleural space with each inspiration but cannot escape; causes increased intrathoracic pressure and shifting of the mediastinal contents to the unaffected side (mediastinal shift).
      d. *Hemothorax:* accumulation of blood in the pleural space; frequently found with an open pneumothorax resulting in a hemopneumothorax.

B. Assessment findings
   1. Sudden sharp pain in the chest, dyspnea, diminished or absent breath sounds on affected side, decreased respiratory excursion on affected

side, hyperresonance on percussion, decreased vocal fremitus, tracheal shift to the opposite side (tension pneumothorax accompanied by mediastinal shift)

2. Weak, rapid pulse; anxiety; diaphoresis
3. Diagnostic tests
    a. Chest X-ray reveals area and degree of pneumothorax
    b. pCO_2 elevated
    c. pO_2, pH decreased

C. Nursing interventions
1. Provide nursing care for the client with an endotracheal tube: suction secretions, vomitus, blood from nose, mouth, throat, or via endotracheal tube; monitor mechanical ventilation.
2. Restore/promote adequate respiratory function.
    a. Assist with thoracentesis and provide appropriate nursing care.
    b. Assist with insertion of a chest tube to water-seal drainage and provide appropriate nursing care.
    c. Continuously evaluate respiratory patterns and report any changes.
3. Provide relief/control of pain.
    a. Administer narcotics/analgesics/sedatives as ordered and monitor effects.
    b. Position client in high-Fowler's position.

Atelectasis

A. General information
1. Collapse of part or all of a lung due to bronchial obstruction
2. May be caused by intrabronchial obstruction (secretions, tumors, bronchospasm, foreign bodies); extrabronchial compression (tumors, enlarged lymph nodes); or endobronchial disease (bronchogenic carcinoma, inflammatory structures)

B. Assessment findings
1. Signs and symptoms may be absent depending upon degree of collapse and rapidity with which bronchial obstruction occurs
2. Dyspnea, decreased breath sounds on affected side, decreased respiratory excursion, dullness to flatness upon percussion over affected area
3. Cyanosis, tachycardia, tachypnea, elevated temperature, weakness, pain over affected area
4. Diagnostic tests
    a. Bronchoscopy: may or may not reveal an obstruction
    b. Chest X-ray shows diminished size of affected lung and lack of radiance over atelectic area
    c. pO_2 decreased

C. Nursing interventions (prevention of atelectasis in hospitalized clients is an important nursing responsibility)
   1. Turn and reposition every 1–2 hours while client is bedridden or obtunded.
   2. Encourage mobility (if permitted).
   3. Promote liquification and removal of secretions.
   4. Avoid administration of large doses of sedatives and opiates that depress respiration and cough reflex.
   5. Prevent abdominal distension.
   6. Administer prophylactic antibiotics as ordered to prevent respiratory infection.

Pleural Effusion

A. General information
   1. Collection of fluid in the pleural space
   2. A symptom, not a disease; may be produced by numerous conditions
   3. Classification
      a. Transudative: accumulation of protein-poor, cell-poor fluid
      b. Suppurative (empyema): accumulation of pus
   4. May be found in clients with liver/kidney disease, pneumonia, tuberculosis, lung abscess, bronchial carcinoma, leukemia, trauma, pulmonary edema, systemic infection, disseminated lupus erythematosus, polyarteritis nodosa
B. Medical management
   1. Identification and treatment of the underlying cause
   2. Thoracentesis
   3. Drug therapy
      a. Antibiotics: either systemic or inserted directly into pleural space
      b. Fibrinolytic enzymes: trypsin, streptokinase-streptodornase to decrease thickness of pus and dissolve fibrin clots
   4. Closed chest drainage
   5. Surgery: open drainage
C. Assessment findings
   1. Dyspnea, dullness over affected area upon percussion, absent or decreased breath sounds over affected area, pleural pain, dry cough, pleural friction rub
   2. Pallor, fatigue, fever, and night sweats (with empyema)
   3. Diagnostic tests
      a. Chest X-ray positive if greater than 250 ml pleural fluid
      b. Pleural biopsy may reveal bronchogenic carcinoma
      c. Thoracentesis may contain blood if cause is cancer, pulmonary infarction, or tuberculosis; positive for specific organism in empyema

D. Nursing interventions: vary depending on etiology
   1. Assist with repeated thoracentesis.
   2. Administer narcotics/sedatives as ordered to decrease pain.
   3. Assist with instillation of medication into pleural space (reposition client every 15 minutes to distribute the drug within the pleurae).
   4. Place client in high-Fowler's position to promote ventilation.

Pneumonia

A. General information
   1. An inflammation of the alveolar spaces of the lung, resulting in consolidation of lung tissue as the alveoli fill with exudate.
   2. The various types of pneumonias are classified according to the offending organism.
   3. Bacterial pneumonia accounts for 10% of all hospital admissions; affects infants and elderly most often, and most often occurs in winter and early spring.
   4. Caused by various organisms: *D. pneumoniae, S. aureus, E. coli, H. influenzae*.

B. Assessment findings
   1. Cough with greenish to rust-colored sputum production; rapid, shallow respirations with an expiratory grunt; nasal flaring; intercostal rib retraction; use of accessory muscles of respiration; dullness to flatness upon percussion; possible pleural friction rub; high-pitched bronchial breath sounds; rales or crackles (early) progressing to coarse (later)
   2. Fever, chills, chest pain, weakness, generalized malaise
   3. Tachycardia, cyanosis, profuse perspiration, abdominal distension
   4. Diagnostic tests
      a. Chest X-ray shows consolidation over affected areas
      b. WBC increased
      c. pO_2 decreased
      d. Sputum specimens reveal particular causative organism

C. Nursing interventions
   1. Facilitate adequate ventilation.
      a. Administer oxygen as needed and assess its effectiveness.
      b. Place client in semi-Fowler's position.
      c. Turn and reposition frequently clients who are immobilized/obtunded.
      d. Administer analgesics as ordered to relieve pain associated with breathing (codeine is drug of choice).
      e. Auscultate breath sounds every 2–4 hours.
      f. Monitor ABGs.
   2. Facilitate removal of secretions (general hydration, deep breathing and coughing, tracheobronchial suctioning as needed, expectorants as

ordered, aerosol treatments via nebulizer, humidification of inhaled air, chest physical therapy).

3. Observe color, characteristics of sputum and report any changes; encourage client to perform good oral hygiene after expectoration.
4. Provide adequate rest and relief/control of pain.
   a. Provide bed rest with limited physical activity.
   b. Limit visits and minimize conversations.
   c. Plan for uninterrupted rest periods.
   d. Institute nursing care in blocks to ensure periods of rest.
   e. Maintain pleasant and restful environment.
5. Administer antibiotics as ordered, monitor effects and possible toxicity.
6. Prevent transmission (respiratory isolation may be required for clients with staphylococcal pneumonia).
7. Control fever and chills: monitor temperature and administer antipyretics as ordered, maintain increased fluid intake, provide frequent clothing and linen changes.
8. Provide client teaching and discharge planning concerning prevention of recurrence.
   a. Medication regimen/antibiotic therapy
   b. Need for adequate rest, limited activity, good nutrition with adequate fluid intake, and good ventilation
   c. Need to continue deep breathing and coughing for at least 6–8 weeks after discharge
   d. Availability of vaccines (pneumonococcal pneumonia, influenza)
   e. Techniques that prevent transmission (use of tissues when coughing, adequate disposal of secretions)
   f. Avoidance of persons with known respiratory infections
   g. Need to report signs and symptoms of respiratory infection (persistent or recurrent fever; changes in characteristics, color of sputum; chills; increased pain; difficulty breathing; weight loss; persistent fatigue)
   h. Need for follow-up medical care and evaluate

Bronchogenic Carcinoma

A. General information
   1. The majority of primary pulmonary tumors arise from the bronchial epithelium and are therefore referred to as bronchogenic carcinomas.
   2. Characteristic pathologic changes include nonspecific inflammation with hypersecretion of mucus, desquamation of cells, hyperplasia, and obstruction.
   3. Metastasis occurs primarily by direct extension and via the circulatory or lymphatic system.
   4. Men over age 40 affected most often; 1 out of every 10 heavy smokers; affects right lung more often than left.

CLIENT TEACHING CHECKLIST

For the client having a bronchoscopy:

- Test takes 45–60 minutes.
- No food for 6 hours prior to test.
- May be placed in a supine or upright position
- Nothing by mouth post-procedure until gag reflex returns; usually in about 2 hours.
- Client should report any bloody mucous, dyspnea, wheezing, or chest pain immediately.

5. Caused by inhaled carcinogens (primarily cigarette smoke but also asbestos, nickel, iron oxides, air silicone pollution; preexisting pulmonary disorders [TB, COPD]).

B. Medical management: depends on cell type, stage of disease, and condition of client; may include

1. Radiation therapy
2. Chemotherapy: usually includes cyclophosphamide, methotrexate, vincristine, doxorubicin, and procarbazine; concurrently in some combination
3. Surgery: when entire tumor can be removed

C. Assessment findings

1. Persistent cough (may be productive or blood tinged), chest pain, dyspnea, unilateral wheezing, friction rub, possible unilateral paralysis of the diaphragm
2. Fatigue, anorexia, nausea, vomiting, pallor
3. Diagnostic tests
   a. Chest X-ray may show presence of tumor or evidence of metastasis to surrounding structures
   b. Sputum for cytology reveals malignant cells
   c. Bronchoscopy: biopsy reveals malignancy
   d. Thoracentesis: pleural fluid contains malignant cells
   e. Biopsy of scalene lymph nodes may reveal metastasis

D. Nursing interventions

1. Provide support and guidance to client as needed.
2. Provide relief/control of pain.
3. Administer medications as ordered and monitor effects/side effects.
4. Control nausea: administer medications as ordered, provide good oral hygiene, provide small and more frequent feedings.
5. Provide nursing care for a client with a thoracotomy.

6. Provide client teaching and discharge planning concerning
   a. Disease process, diagnostic and therapeutic interventions
   b. Side effects of radiation and chemotherapy
   c. Realistic information about prognosis

Thoracic Surgery

A. General information
   1. Types
      a. *Exploratory thoracotomy:* anterior or posterolateral incision through the fourth, fifth, sixth, or seventh intercostal spaces to expose and examine the pleura and lung
      b. *Lobectomy:* removal of one lobe of a lung; treatment for bronchiectasis, bronchogenic carcinoma, emphysematous blebs, lung abscesses
      c. *Pneumonectomy:* removal of an entire lung; most commonly done as treatment for bronchogenic carcinoma
      d. *Segmental resection:* removal of one or more segments of lung; most often done as treatment for bronchiectasis
      e. *Wedge resection:* removal of lesions that occupy only part of a segment of lung tissue; for excision of small nodules or to obtain a biopsy
   2. Nature and extent of disease and condition of client determine type of pulmonary resection.
B. Nursing interventions: preoperative
   1. Provide routine pre-op care.
   2. Perform a complete physical assessment of the lungs to obtain baseline data.
   3. Explain expected post-op measures: care of incision site, oxygen, suctioning, chest tubes (except if pneumonectomy performed).
   4. Teach client adequate splinting of incision with hands or pillow for turning, coughing, and deep breathing.
   5. Demonstrate ROM exercises for affected side.
   6. Provide chest physical therapy to help remove secretions.
C. Nursing interventions: postoperative
   1. Provide routine post-op care.
   2. Promote adequate ventilation.
      a. Perform complete physical assessment of lungs and compare with pre-op findings.
      b. Auscultate lung fields every 1–2 hours.
      c. Encourage turning, coughing, and deep breathing every 1–2 hours after pain relief obtained.
      d. Perform tracheobronchial suctioning if needed.
      e. Assess for proper maintenance of chest drainage system (except after pneumonectomy).

   f. Monitor ABGs and report significant changes.
   g. Place client in semi-Fowler's position (if pneumonectomy performed, follow surgeon's orders about positioning, often on back or operative side, but not turned to unoperative side).
3. Provide pain relief.
   a. Administer narcotics/analgesics prior to turning, coughing, and deep breathing.
   b. Assist with splinting while turning, coughing, deep breathing.
4. Prevent impaired mobility of the upper extremities by doing ROM exercises; passive day of surgery, then active.
5. Provide client teaching and discharge planning concerning
   a. Need to continue with coughing/deep breathing for 6–8 weeks post-op and to continue ROM exercises
   b. Importance of adequate rest with gradual increases in activity levels
   c. High-protein diet with inclusion of adequate fluids (at least 2 liters/day)
   d. Chest physical therapy
   e. Good oral hygiene
   f. Need to avoid persons with known upper respiratory infections
   g. Adverse signs and symptoms (recurrent fever; anorexia; weight loss; dyspnea; increased pain; difficulty swallowing; shortness of breath; changes in color, characteristics of sputum) and importance of reporting to physician
   h. Avoidance of crowds and poorly ventilated areas

Acute Respiratory Distress Syndrome (ARDS)

A. General information
   1. A form of pulmonary insufficiency more commonly encountered in adults with no previous lung disorders than in those with existing lung disease.
   2. Initial damage to the alveolar-capillary membrane with subsequent leakage of fluid into the interstitial spaces and alveoli, resulting in pulmonary edema and impaired gas exchange.
   3. There is cell damage, decreased surfactant production, and atelectasis, which in turn produce hypoxemia, decreased compliance, and increased work of breathing.
   4. Predisposing conditions include shock, trauma, infection, fluid overload, aspiration, oxygen toxicity, smoke inhalation, pneumonia, DIC, drug allergies, drug overdoses, neurologic injuries, fat emboli.
   5. Has also been called shock lung.
B. Assessment findings
   1. Dyspnea, cough, tachypnea with intercostal/suprasternal retraction, scattered to diffuse rales/rhonchi

2. Changes in orientation, tachycardia, cyanosis (rare)
3. Diagnostic tests
   a. pCO_2 increased and pO_2 decreased
   b. Hypoxemia
   c. Hgb and hct possibly decreased
   d. pO_2 and O_2 saturation not reflective of high O_2 administration

C. Nursing interventions
1. Promote optimal ventilatory status.
   a. Perform ongoing assessment of lungs with auscultation every 1–2 hours.
   b. Elevate head and chest.
   c. Administer/monitor mechanical ventilation with PEEP.
   d. Assist with chest physical therapy as ordered.
   e. Encourage coughing and deep breathing every hour.
   f. Monitor ABGs, O_2 saturation, and report significant changes.
2. Promote rest by spacing activities and treatments.
3. Maintain fluid and electrolyte balance.
4. Treat cause.

Cancer of the Larynx

A. General information
1. Most common upper respiratory malignancy.
2. The majority of laryngeal malignancies are squamous cell carcinomas.
3. Types
   a. Supraglottic (also called extrinsic laryngeal cancer): involves the epiglottis and false cords and is likely to produce no symptoms until advanced stages.
   b. Glottic (also referred to as intrinsic laryngeal cancer): affects the true vocal cords; the most frequently occurring laryngeal cancer; produces early symptoms.
4. Occurs most often in white men in middle or later life
5. Caused by cigarette smoking, excessive alcohol consumption, chronic laryngitis, vocal abuse, family predisposition to cancer of larynx

B. Medical management
1. Radiation therapy: may be effective in cases of localized disease, affecting only one vocal cord
2. Chemotherapy: used as adjuvant therapy to help shrink tumor and eradicate metastases (experimental)
3. Surgery
   a. Partial laryngectomy: a lesion on the true cord on one side is removed along with adjoining tissue. Useful in early, intrinsic lesions. Client is able to talk and has a normal airway post-op.

b. Total laryngectomy (see below)

c. Radical neck dissection

1) performed when metastasis from cancer of the larynx is suspected

2) includes removal of entire larynx, lymph nodes, sternocleidomastoid muscle, internal jugular vein, and spinal accessory nerve

3) may also involve removal of the mandible, submaxillary gland, part of the thyroid and parathyroid gland

4) nursing care: same as for total laryngectomy, below

C. Assessment findings

1. Supraglottic: localized throat pain; burning when drinking hot liquids or orange juice; lump in the neck; eventual dysphagia; dyspnea; weight loss; debility; cough; hemoptysis; muffled voice

2. Glottic: progressive hoarseness (more than 2-week duration), eventual dyspnea

3. Enlarged cervical lymph nodes

D. Nursing interventions: provide care for the client with a laryngectomy.

Total Laryngectomy

A. General information: consists of removal of the entire larynx, hyoid bone, pre-epiglottic space, cricoid cartilage, and 3–4 rings of trachea. The pharyngeal opening to the trachea is closed and remaining trachea brought out to the neck to form a permanent tracheostomy. The result is loss of normal speech and breathing and loss of olfaction.

B. Nursing care: preoperative

1. Provide routine pre-op care.

2. Explain expected procedures after surgery including suctioning, humidification, coughing and deep breathing, IV fluids, nasogastric tube feedings, tracheostomy or laryngectomy tube.

3. Reinforce physician's teaching regarding loss of normal speech, breathing patterns, and sense of smell.

4. Encourage client/significant others to talk about fears and hopes following surgery.

5. Introduce client to changes in modes of communication (esophageal speech, artificial larynx).

6. Establish method of communication to be used immediately post-op (Magic Slate, gestures).

C. Nursing interventions: postoperative

1. Promote optimum ventilatory status.

2. Suction nose frequently because of rhinitis.

3. Assess function of tracheostomy/laryngectomy tube and suction as needed.

4. Promote pain relief.

a. Elevate head of bed to decrease pressure on suture line.

   b. Administer analgesics as needed and monitor effects.
   c. Assist with moving head and turning by supporting back of neck with hands.
5. Promote wound drainage.
   a. Elevate head of bed to promote lymphatic drainage from head.
   b. Monitor amount, characteristics of drainage.
6. Promote nutrition.
   a. Institute and monitor tube feedings as ordered.
   b. Increase fluid intake as tolerated to improve hydration.
   c. Encourage self-feeding.
   d. Advance to normal diet as soon as client able to tolerate.
7. Prevent infection.
   a. Assess WBC and report significant increases.
   b. Take temperature every 4 hours.
   c. Maintain sterile technique when suctioning and performing tracheostomy care.
   d. Observe stoma/suture lines for signs of infection.
   e. Provide frequent oral hygiene.
   f. Monitor sputum and drainage for changes in color, odor, characteristics.
8. Enhance communication.
   a. Carry out modes of communication determined pre-op.
   b. Assess nonverbal behavior.
   c. Allow client time to ask questions and do not anticipate answers.
   d. Arrange for volunteer laryngectomy client to visit client and assist with esophageal speech, artificial larynx, and living with a laryngectomy.
   e. Consult with speech therapist if needed.
   f. Progress to normal diet as soon as possible to regain muscle tone of throat and abdomen.
9. Support client during adaptation to altered physical status.
   a. Encourage client to discuss feelings about changes in appearance, body functioning, and lifestyle; be aware of nonverbal responses to the changes.
   b. Assist to identify and use coping techniques that have been helpful in past.
   c. Suggest flattering clothing styles that don't emphasize chest or neck configuration.
   d. Monitor for and support behaviors indicative of positive adaptation to changes (e.g., interest in appearance).
10. Assess for respiratory complications (dyspnea, cyanosis, tachycardia, tachypnea, restlessness).
11. Provide client teaching and discharge planning concerning
   a. Tracheostomy/laryngectomy and stomal care
   b. Proper administration of nasogastric tube feedings and maintenance of nasogastric tube

c. Control of dryness/crusting of tongue by brushing tongue regularly with soft toothbrush and toothpaste and using mouthwashes
d. Need for humidified air at home
e. Importance of protecting the stoma with a shield or towel while showering, directing shower nozzle away from stoma
f. Need to use electric razors only for 6 months after surgery as facial area will be numb
g. Need to lean forward when expectorating secretions and to cover stoma when coughing or sneezing
h. Snorkle devices to enable swimming (caution is advised since drowning can occur rapidly in these clients)
i. Need to wear an identification bracelet indicating that client is a neck breather
j. Types of stoma guards available
k. Necessity of installing smoke detectors since sense of smell is lost
l. Information about prosthetic devices, speech therapy, and reconstructive surgery

REVIEW QUESTIONS

1. A 17-year-old male is admitted following an automobile accident. He is very anxious, dyspneic, and in severe pain. The left chest wall moves in during inspiration and balloons out when he exhales. The nurse understands these symptoms are most suggestive of
   1. hemothorax.
   2. flail chest.
   3. atelectasis.
   4. pleural effusion.
2. A young man is admitted with a flail chest following a car accident. He is intubated with an endotracheal tube and is placed on a mechanical ventilator (control mode, positive pressure).Which physical finding alerts the nurse to an additional problem in respiratory function?
   1. Dullness to percussion in the third to fifth intercostal space, midclavicular line.
   2. Decreased paradoxical motion.
   3. Louder breath sounds on the right chest.
   4. pH of 7.36 in arterial blood gases.

3. The nurse is caring for a client who has had a chest tube inserted and connected to a portable water-seal drainage. The nurse determines the drainage system is functioning correctly when which of the following is observed?
   1. Continuous bubbling in the water-seal chamber.
   2. Fluctuation in the water-seal (U-tube) chamber.
   3. Suction tubing attached to a wall unit.
   4. Vesicular breath sounds throughout the lung fields.
4. The nurse is caring for a client who has just had a chest tube attached to a portable water-seal drainage system. To ensure that the system functions effectively the nurse should
   1. observe for intermittent bubbling in the water-seal chamber.
   2. flush the chest tubes with 30 to 60 ml of NSS q4 to 6 hours.
   3. maintain the client in an extreme lateral position.
   4. strip the chest tubes in the direction of the client.
5. The nurse enters the room of a client who has a chest tube attached to a water-seal drainage system and notices the chest tube is dislodged from the chest. The most appropriate nursing intervention is to
   1. notify the physician.
   2. insert a new chest tube.
   3. cover the insertion site with petroleum gauze.
   4. instruct the client to breathe deeply until help arrives.
6. An adult is ordered oxygen via nasal prongs. The nurse administering oxygen via this low-flow system recognizes that this method of delivery
   1. mixes room air with oxygen.
   2. delivers a precise concentration of oxygen.
   3. requires humidity during delivery.
   4. is less traumatic to the respiratory tract.
7. An adult is receiving oxygen by nasal prongs. Which statement by the client indicates that client teaching regarding oxygen therapy has been effective?
   1. "I was feeling fine so I removed my nasal prongs."
   2. "I've increased my fluids to six glasses of water daily."
   3. "Don't forget to come back quickly when you get me out of bed; I don't like to be without my oxygen for too long."
   4. "My family was angry when I told them they could not smoke in my room."
8. An adult is diagnosed with tuberculosis. Client teaching for this client will include prevention of disease transmission. The most common

means of transmitting the tubercle bacillus from one individual to another is by

1. hands.
2. droplet nuclei.
3. milk products.
4. eating utensils.

9. The treatment plan for a client newly diagnosed with tuberculosis is likely to include which of the following medications as initial treatment?
   1. Ethambutol (Myambutol) and isoniazid (INH).
   2. Streptomycin and penicillin G (Crysticillin).
   3. Tetracycline and thioridazine (Mellaril).
   4. Pyridoxine (Beesix) and tetracycline.

10. A 64-year-old has been smoking since he was 11 years old. He has a long history of emphysema and is admitted to the hospital because of a respiratory infection that has not improved with outpatient therapy. Which finding would the nurse expect to observe during the client's nursing assessment?
    1. Electrocardiogram changes.
    2. Increased anterior-posterior chest diameter.
    3. Slow, labored respiratory pattern.
    4. Weight-height relationship indicating obesity.

11. Supplemental low-flow oxygen therapy is prescribed for a man with emphysema. Which is the most essential action for the nurse to initiate?
    1. Anticipate the need for humidification.
    2. Notify the physician that this order is contraindicated.
    3. Place the client in an upright position.
    4. Schedule nursing care to allow frequent observations of the client.

12. The nurse is assessing the breath sounds of a client. The nurse hears a sound described as a rustling, like the sound of the wind in the trees over the peripheral lung fields. The breath sounds are
    1. crackles.
    2. rhonchi.
    3. wheezes.
    4. vesicular.

13. The nurse's assessment of a client with lung cancer reveals the following: copious secretions, dyspnea, and cough. Based on these findings the most appropriate nursing diagnosis is
    1. impaired gas exchange.
    2. ineffective airway clearance.
    3. pain.
    4. altered tissue perfusion.
14. A client has just had arterial blood gases drawn. When handling the specimen, the nurse's best action is to
    1. gently shake the syringe.
    2. place the sample in a syringe of warm water.
    3. aspirate 0.5 ml of heparin into the syringe.
    4. have the specimen analyzed immediately.
15. The nurse is to obtain a sputum specimen from a client. Select the correct set of statements instructing the client in the proper technique for obtaining a sputum specimen.
    1. "Collect the specimen right before bed. Spit carefully into the container."
    2. "Brush your teeth, then cough into the container. Do this first thing in the morning."
    3. "Right after lunch, cough and spit into the container."
    4. "Spit into the container, then add two tablespoons of water."
16. The nurse is checking tuberculin skin test results at a health clinic. One client has an area of induration measuring 12 mm in diameter. The nurse is aware that this indicates that
    1. this finding is a normal reading.
    2. this finding indicates active TB.
    3. this is a positive reaction and can indicate exposure to TB.
    4. this client needs to come back in two more days and let the nurse look at the area of induration again.
17. An adult has undergone a bronchoscopy. Which assessment findings indicate to the nurse that he is ready for discharge?
    1. Use of accessory muscles for breathing, decreased lung sounds.
    2. Stable vital signs, return of gag and cough reflex.
    3. Hemoptysis, rhonchi.
    4. Development of tachycardia with occasional PVCs, able to eat and drink.

18. An adult has a chest tube to a Pleur-evac® drainage system attached to a wall suction. An order to ambulate the client has been received. To ambulate the client safely, the nurse should:

1. clamp the chest tube and carefully ambulate the client a short distance.

2. question the order to ambulate the client.

3. carefully ambulate the client, keeping the Pleur-evac lower than Mr. E.'s chest.

4. disconnect the Pleur-evac from the client's chest tube, leave it attached to the bed, ambulate the client, and then reconnect the chest tube when he is returned to bed.

19. The nurse is assessing a client who has a chest tube to water seal drainage with a one-bottle drainage system. Which statement best indicates proper functioning of the chest drainage system?

1. The nurse observes bubbling from the straw in the bottle when the client coughs.

2. The nurse observes no fluctuations in the straw in the bottle with respiration.

3. The nurse observes rising and falling of fluid in the bottle's straw with respiration.

4. The nurse observes the air vent is clamped off.

20. The nurse will perform chest physiotherapy (CPT) on a client every 4 hours. It is important for the nurse to

1. gently slap the chest wall.

2. use vibration techniques to move secretions from affected lung areas during the inspiration phase.

3. perform CPT at least 2 hours after meals.

4. plan apical drainage at the beginning of the CPT session.

21. A client is on a ventilator. The ventilator alarm goes off. The nurse assesses the client and observes increased respiratory rate, use of accessory muscles, and agitation. The nurse's best initial action is to

1. remove the client from the ventilator and ambu bag the client, while continuing to assess to determine the cause of the client's distress.

2. call respiratory therapy to check the ventilator.

3. notify the physician.

4. turn off the alarm.

22. A client with respiratory failure is on a ventilator. The alarm goes off. The nurse's initial reaction should be to

1. notify the physician.
2. assess the client to determine the cause of the alarm.
3. turn off the alarm.
4. disconnect the client and use the ambu bag to ventilate the client.

23. A nurse is setting up oxygen for an adult male. He is to receive oxygen at 2 L per nasal cannula. It is important for the nurse to

1. adjust the flow rate to keep the reservoir bag inflated ⅔ full during inspiration.
2. monitor the client carefully for risk of aspiration.
3. make sure the valves and rubber flaps are patent, functional, and not stuck.
4. remind the client and his wife of the smoking policy.

24. A long-term COPD client is receiving oxygen at 1 L/minute. Her visiting cousin decides she "doesn't look too good" and increases her oxygen to 7 L/minute. What should the nurse's initial action be?

1. Thank the client's cousin and continue to observe the client.
2. Immediately decrease the oxygen.
3. Notify the physician.
4. Elevate the client's head and take vital signs.

25. An adult is receiving oxygen per face mask at 40%. The nurse should include which of the following in her plan of care?

1. Provide good skin care, making sure the mask fits well.
2. Provide water-soluble jelly to the nares.
3. Instruct the client's husband to smoke away from the bed.
4. Assess for signs and symptoms of oxygen toxicity.

26. An adult has a new tracheostomy in place. He has a small amount of thin, white secretions. The stoma is pink with no drainage noted. The nurse should expect to provide trach care every:

1. 4 hours.
2. 8 hours.
3. 24 hours.
4. hour.

27. A 64-year-old female is admitted to the hospital. She has smoked two packs per day for 30 years. While providing her history, she becomes breathless, pauses frequently between words, and appears very anxious. She has a cough with thick white sputum production. Her chest is barrel shaped. Based on these data, the nurse will need to develop a plan of care for a client with

1. pneumonia.
2. chronic obstructive pulmonary disease.
3. tuberculosis.
4. asthma.

28. A 68-year-old male is being admitted to the hospital for an exacerbation of his COPD. The nurse is developing his plan of care. The nurse can expect that this client will

1. be placed on 10 L of oxygen per nasal cannula.
2. be placed in respiratory isolation.
3. require frequent rest periods throughout the day.
4. be placed on fluid restriction.

29. A client with suspected tuberculosis will most likely relate which clinical manifestations?

1. Fatigue, weight loss, low grade fevers, night sweats.
2. Dyspnea, chest pain, cough.
3. Rapid shallow breathing, prolonged labored expiration, stridor.
4. Dyspnea, hypoxemia, decreased pulmonary compliance.

30. An adult is being admitted to the nursing unit with a diagnosis of pneumonia. She has a history of arrested TB. When planning care for this client, the nurse's initial action should be to

1. place the client in respiratory isolation.
2. encourage cough and deep breathing.
3. force fluids.
4. administer O_2.

31. An adult is being followed in the outpatient clinic for a diagnosis of active TB. She is receiving isoniazid 200 mg po qd, rifampin 500 mg po qd, and streptomycin 1500 mg IM twice weekly. Which statement by the client best indicates she understands her therapeutic regime?

1. "I'm glad I only have to take these drugs for a couple of weeks."
2. "I need to take these two drugs every day and come back to the clinic once a week for the shot."
3. "It may work best to take these pills in the evening right before bed."
4. "I'm glad my birth control pills aren't affected by these drugs—the doctor told me not to get pregnant!"

32. The nurse is counseling the family of an 18-year-old with active TB, about measures to prevent transmission of the disease. Which statement by the family best indicates understanding of these instructions?
   1. "I won't let her and her sister share clothes."
   2. "We will have to keep her in her room."
   3. "We all need to wash our hands carefully, but especially our daughter."
   4. "We cannot get TB from exposure to her sputum."
33. An 86-year-old has fallen and broken her eighth rib on her left side. The nurse should include which of the following when developing the plan of care?
   1. Bind the client's chest with a 6-inch Ace bandage.
   2. Keep the client on bed rest for 3 days.
   3. Encourage the client to use her incentive spirometer and cough and deep breathe.
   4. Administer large doses of narcotic analgesic so that the client will be able to more fully participate in pulmonary care.
34. A man is injured in an industrial accident. The industrial nurse assesses him and observes use of accessory muscles, severe chest pain, agitation, shortness of breath. The nurse also notices one side of his chest moving differently than the other. The nurse suspects flail chest. Based on these observations, the nurse's best initial action is to
   1. apply a sandbag to the flail side of his chest.
   2. prepare for intubation and mechanical ventilation.
   3. prepare for chest tube placement.
   4. administer pain medication.
35. A client with a pleural effusion most often presents to the hospital with
   1. pain.
   2. swelling.
   3. dyspnea.
   4. increased sputum production.
36. An 86-year-old female was admitted to the hospital two days ago with pneumonia. She now has an order to be up in the chair as much as possible. The nurse plans to get her up and help her with her morning care. The best plan to accomplish this would be to
   1. get her up before breakfast. Have her eat in the chair, then bathe while still up.

2. allow her to eat breakfast in bed, rest for 30 minutes, get up in the chair, and rest for a few minutes. Allow her to wash her hands and face—nurse to complete bath.
3. Allow her to eat in bed, get her up, and provide her with a pan of water for her to bathe.
4. get her up before breakfast, have her bathe before breakfast, eat in the chair, then a rest in the chair.

37. A client has been admitted to the hospital. Lung assessment reveals the following: bronchial breath sounds over (L) lower lobe, diminished breath sounds (L) lower lobe, tactile fremitus present, percussion dulled in this area. Based on the assessment findings the nurse can expect to plan care for a client with
    1. pneumonia.
    2. asthma.
    3. emphysema.
    4. early left-sided heart failure.

38. A nurse is teaching a class in a community center about lung cancer. Which statement best demonstrates the client's understanding of the risk factors for lung cancer?
    1. "My husband smokes, but I don't! So, I really don't need to worry about getting lung cancer."
    2. "I guess I will need to eat more green and yellow vegetables."
    3. "Just because I have COPD doesn't mean that I have a higher risk."
    4. "I've worked with asbestos all my life and have never had any problems."

39. An adult male was diagnosed with lung cancer 18 months ago. He is now in the terminal stages and is experiencing severe generalized pain. He has ordered morphine sulfate 10 mg IM q 4–6 h prn. When planning his care, the nurse's best action is to
    1. teach him that the pain medicine prescribed will take away all his pain and he will have no discomfort.
    2. counsel him about the addictive qualities of his prescribed narcotic.
    3. inform him that he may only ask for the pain medicine every 4 hours and there is nothing else you can offer in between medication times.
    4. encourage him to ask for the pain medicine before the pain becomes too severe.

40. A 52-year-old client is admitted to the nursing unit from the recovery room following a left pneumonectomy. When planning his care, the nurse can expect this client to

1. have a chest tube to water seal.
2. have a chest tube to suction.
3. be monitored closely for respiratory and cardiac complications.
4. have his left arm maintained in a sling to prevent pain and discomfort.

41. An adult who has had a right thoracotomy for a wedge resection of his lung repeatedly refuses to do breathing or arm exercises because of the pain. What should the nurse include on the client's plan of care?

1. Offer the client pain medication immediately after arm exercises are completed.
2. Offer the client sips of ice water prior to a deep breathing and coughing session.
3. Schedule the client's activity 30–45 minutes after his IM injection of pain medication.
4. Have the client hold a pillow against his abdomen for support.

42. The nurse may expect a client with suspected early ARDS to exhibit which of the following?

1. PaO_2 of 90, PCO_2 of 45, X-ray showing enlarged heart, bradycardia.
2. Thick green sputum production, PaO_2 of 75, pH 7.45.
3. Restlessness, suprasternal retractions, PaO_2 of 65.
4. Wheezes, slow deep respirations, PCO_2 of 55, pH of 7.25.

43. The nurse caring for a client who has had a removal of the larynx and a permanent opening made into the trachea will plan care for a client who has undergone a

1. total laryngectomy.
2. tracheostomy.
3. radical neck dissection.
4. partial laryngectomy.

44. An adult will undergo a total laryngectomy tomorrow. She is concerned about communicating post-op. The nurse should plan for her to communicate by which method the first 24–48 hours after surgery?

1. Using the artificial larynx.
2. Writing or pointing on a communication board.
3. Using esophageal speech.
4. Using a voice button.

45. An adult has had a total laryngectomy. The nurse is discussing options for verbal communication with the client. Which statement indicates the client understands the available options for verbal communication?

1. "Because of the arthritis in my hands, I think the voice button method would be easiest to use."
2. "By the time I leave the hospital, I will be able to talk."
3. "If I use the esophageal speech, my voice will be high pitched and soft."
4. "Using an artificial larynx will make me sound sort of monotone."

46. An adult is ready for discharge after undergoing a total laryngectomy. The nurse is discussing safety aspects of his home care. Which statement by the client best indicates that he understands the safety aspects of his care at home?

1. "It is okay to swim as long as I'm careful."
2. "I should use paper tissues to cover my stoma when I'm coughing."
3. "I should not wear anything to cover my stoma."
4. "I will need to use a humidifier in my home."

ANSWERS AND RATIONALES

1. 2. Paradoxical breathing movements (opposite the normal) are characteristic of flail chest. The flail portion is sucked in on inspiration and bulges out on expiration. Flail chest occurs when there are multiple rib fractures due to trauma.

2. 3. Louder breath sounds on the right side of the chest indicate that the endotracheal tube may be misplaced and is aerating only one lung.

3. 2. Fluctuation in the water-seal chamber demonstrates that the tubing system is patent.

4. 1. Intermittent bubbling in the water-seal chamber indicates that air is leaving the thoracic cavity. If there is no bubbling in the water-seal chamber, it indicates either obstruction of the tubing or reexpansion of the lung. Reexpansion of the lung is unlikely, as the tube has just been inserted.

5. 3. Covering the insertion site with petroleum gauze is a priority nursing measure that prevents air from entering the chest cavity.

6. 1. Low-flow oxygen systems provide an oxygen concentration that is determined by the amount of air drawn into the system and the dilution of oxygen with room air.

7. 4. Oxygen is a flammable gas and smoking is not permitted in the area.
8. 2. The most frequent means of transmission of the tubercle bacillus is by droplet nuclei. The bacillus is present in the air as a result of coughing, sneezing, and expectorating by infected persons.
9. 1. Ethambutol, isoniazid, streptomycin, and rifampin are first-line drugs used in the treatment of tuberculosis.
10. 2. An increased anterior-posterior chest diameter, commonly referred to as "barrel chest," is seen in clients with emphysema as a result of chronic hyperinflation of the lungs.
11. 4. The stimulus to breathe in a client with emphysema becomes low oxygen levels rather than rising CO_2 levels. Frequent nursing observations are necessary to see how the client handles low-flow oxygen administration.
12. 4. This is a description of the normal vesicular breath sounds. They are low pitched, soft sounds heard over the peripheral lung fields where air flows through smaller bronchioles.
13. 2. A client with lung cancer demonstrating the assessment findings provided would indicate a nursing diagnosis of ineffective airway clearance. The goal is this client will breathe without dyspnea or discomfort and maintain a patent airway.
14. 4. The sample must be analyzed within 20 minutes, or if the client has leukocytosis immediately, to ensure accurate results.
15. 2. Teeth are brushed to reduce contamination, then the client coughs into the container. Sputum is best collected in the morning when it is more plentiful.
16. 3. A positive reaction is present when the induration is greater than 10 mm in diameter. The positive reaction indicates exposure to TB or the presence of inactive disease, not active disease.
17. 2. Vital signs are taken frequently. Nothing is given by mouth until the cough and swallow reflexes have returned. Both are important criteria for discharge.
18. 3. The Pleur-evac must not be raised above chest level because it can cause backflow of the fluid into the pleural space precipitating collapse of the lung or mediastinal shift. The Pleur-evac must remain upright and the chest tube should not have traction on it.
19. 3. Fluctuations of 5–10 cm during normal breathing are common. These fluctuations provide continuous manometer of pressure changes in the pleural space and are a reliable indicator of overall respiratory effort.

20. 3. Chest physiotherapy should be performed at least 2 hours after meals to reduce the risk of vomiting and aspiration.

21. 1. The nurse's best initial action should be to remove the client from the ventilator, ventilating the client with an ambu bag. Obviously, the client is experiencing respiratory distress and is not receiving adequate ventilation. The nurse should continue to closely assess to determine the cause and determine if the respiratory distress is related to ventilator malfunction or change in client status.

22. 2. It is important for the nurse to quickly assess the client and determine the cause of the alarm. Once the cause has been determined, the nurse must intervene promptly to prevent complications. See below for examples of causes of ventilator alarms.

23. 4. Oxygen supports combustion. Smoking is not permitted in the room while O_2 is set up or being administered. A sign should be posted to that effect.

24. 2. The COPD client's drive to breathe is hypoxia. In COPD the CO_2 level gradually rises over time and central chemoreceptors are no longer sensitive to high CO_2 levels. Instead, the peripheral chemoreceptors found in the carotid and aortic arch bodies become the major stimuli for breathing. When the client with COPD receives high levels of O_2, the hypoxic drive to breathe is eliminated. The client experiences respiratory depression that may lead to apnea.

25. 1. The mask must fit properly, as a poor fitting mask reduces the amount of oxygen delivered. The mask may also cause skin breakdown, so it is very important to provide skin care. Loosen the strap holding the mask frequently and assess the skin.

26. 2. Trach care should be provided once every 8 hours.

27. 2. These are signs and symptoms of COPD. The nurse would also need to evaluate breathing rate/pattern, use of accessory muscles for breathing, cyanosis, capillary refill, and clubbing of fingernails.

28. 3. A major goal for the COPD client is that the client will use a breathing pattern that does not lead to tiring and to plan activities so that the client does not become overtired. Care should be spaced, allowing frequent rest periods, and preventing fatigue.

29. 1. Typically, the client with TB will present with fatigue, lethargy, nausea, anorexia, weight loss, low grade fever, and night sweats.

30. 1. The client should be placed in respiratory isolation until active TB is ruled out. TB is spread by droplet infection, thus her sputum should be handled according to respiratory isolation protocol.

31. 3. These medications frequently cause nausea. The nausea may be decreased if the medications are taken at bedtime.

32. 3. Handwashing is the best tool for prevention of infection. The client should wash her hands very carefully after any contact with body substances, masks, or soiled tissues. The family should also use good handwashing techniques.

33. 3. Pulmonary care is a vital part of the management of this type of client. Measures are taken to prevent stasis of secretions and promote chest expansion, preventing complications such as atelectasis and pneumonia.

34. 2. Based on the client's symptoms the nurse suspects impending respiratory failure and should prepare for intubation and mechanical ventilation.

35. 3. With pleural effusions, lung expansion may be restricted and the client will experience dyspnea, primarily on exertion.

36. 2. This plan allows frequent rest periods for the client. The client should not rush through morning care activities as rushing will increase hypoxemia, dyspnea, and fatigue.

37. 1. In a client with pneumonia, bronchial breath sounds are heard over areas of density or consolidation. Breath sounds are diminished when the airflow is decreased as is typical with pneumonia. Tactile fremitus is increased over the affected area. Percussion is dulled. In pneumonia, the alveoli fill with fluid, red cells, and white cells creating consolidation.

38. 2. Research has shown that there may be a correlation between vitamin A deficiency in the diet and the development of lung cancer. Daily consumption of green and yellow vegetables is encouraged.

39. 4. A preventive approach to pain control provides a more consistent level of relief and reduces client anxiety, which in turn can reduce discomfort and pain.

40. 3. Post-op respiratory insufficiency may result from an altered level of consciousness related to anesthesia, pain medications, decreased respiratory effort secondary to pain, or inadequate airway clearance. So the client must be monitored very closely with frequent vital sign checks and respiratory assessments.

41. 3. Thirty or 45 minutes after the administration of IM pain medication is the time when the pain medication is most effective. Thus, this is the best time to schedule coughing and deep breathing and arm exercises.

42. It is common for the client to have suprasternal and intercostal retractions as the client loses lung capacity. The nurse should anticipate restlessness, apprehension, agitation, sluggishness, disorientation, and tachycardia.

43. A total laryngectomy is the removal of the larynx and formation of the tracheostomy. The esophagus remains attached to the pharynx. No air will enter through the nose. The client will breathe through the tracheostomy. The procedure is indicated for large glottic tumors with fixation of vocal cords.

44. For the first few days after surgery, the client should communicate by writing. If the client is very tired, a communication board may be used allowing the client to point to statements.

45. An artificial larynx is an electronic device held along the neck and vibration produces mechanical speech. The speech quality is monotone and artificial.

46. To substitute for the nose and pharynx, where air is usually warmed and humidified, a humidifier, pans of water, or houseplants should be used to increase the humidity in the home.

9

The Gastrointestinal System

■ OVERVIEW OF ANATOMY AND PHYSIOLOGY

The organs of the digestive system are grouped into the alimentary canal (GI tract), consisting of the mouth, esophagus, stomach, and small and large intestine; and the accessory digestive organs, including the liver, pancreas, gallbladder, and ductal system (Figure 9-1). The primary functions of this system are movement of food, digestion, absorption, elimination, and provision of a continuous supply of nutrients, electrolytes, and water.

CHAPTER OUTLINE

Mouth

A. Consists of the lips and oral cavity: provides entrance and initial processing for nutrients and sensory data, such as taste, texture, and temperature.
B. Oral cavity contains the teeth, used for mastication, and the tongue, which assists in deglutition, taste sensation, and mastication.
C. The salivary glands, located in the mouth, produce secretions containing ptyalin for starch digestion and mucus for lubrication.
D. The pharynx aids in swallowing and functions in ingestion by providing a route for food to pass from the mouth to the esophagus.

Esophagus

Muscular tube that receives food from the pharynx and propels it into the stomach by peristalsis.

Stomach

A. Located on the left side of the abdominal cavity, occupying the hypochondriac, epigastric, and umbilical regions.
B. Stores and mixes food with gastric juices and mucus, producing chemical and mechanical changes in the bolus of food.

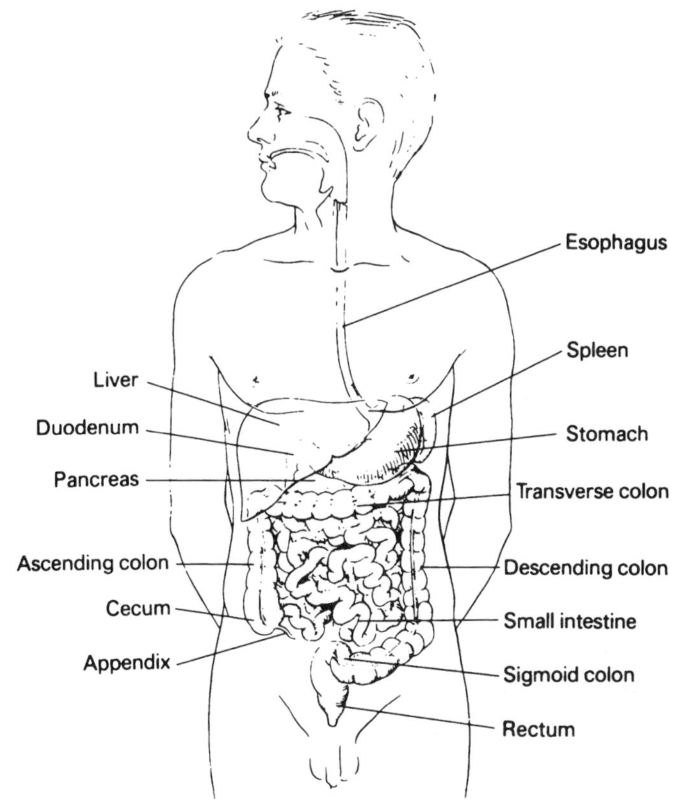

FIGURE 9-1 Anterior view of the structures of the GI tract

1. The secretion of digestive juices is stimulated by smelling, tasting, and chewing food, which is known as the cephalic phase of digestion.
2. The gastric phase is stimulated by the presence of food in the stomach; regulated by neural stimulation via the PNS and hormonal stimulation through secretions of gastrin by the gastric mucosa.
3. After processing in the stomach, the food bolus, called *chyme*, is released into the small intestine through the duodenum.

C. Two sphincters control the rate of food passage.
   1. *Cardiac sphincter:* located at the opening between the esophagus and stomach
   2. *Pyloric sphincter:* located between the stomach and duodenum

D. Three anatomic divisions: fundus, body, and antrum.

E. Gastric secretions
   1. *Pepsinogen:* secreted by chief cells, located in fundus, aids in protein digestion
   2. *Hydrochloric acid:* secreted by parietal cells, functions in protein digestion, released in response to gastrin
   3. *Intrinsic factor:* secreted by parietal cells,promotes absorption of vitamin B_{12}
   4. Mucoid secretions: coat stomach wall and prevent autodigestion

Small Intestine

A. Composed of the duodenum, jejunum, and ileum
B. Extends from the pylorus to the *ileocecal valve*, which regulates flow into the large intestine and prevents reflux into the small intestine.
C. Major functions of the small intestine are digestion and absorption of the end products of digestion.
D. Structural features
   1. *Villi* (functional units of the small intestine): fingerlike projections located in the mucous membrane; contain goblet cells that secrete mucus and absorptive cells that absorb digested foodstuffs.
   2. *Crypts of Lieberkuhn:* produce secretions containing digestive enzymes.
   3. *Brunner's glands:* found in the submucosa of the duodenum, secrete mucus.

Large Intestine

A. Divided into four parts: cecum (with appendix), colon (ascending, transverse, descending, sigmoid), rectum, and anus.
B. Serves as a reservoir for fecal material until defecation occurs; functions to absorb water and electrolytes.
C. Microorganisms present in the large intestine are responsible for a small amount of further breakdown and also make some vitamins.
   1. Amino acids are deaminated by bacteria, resulting in ammonia, which is converted to urea in the liver.
   2. Bacteria in the large intestine aid in the synthesis of vitamin K and some of the vitamin B groups.
D. Feces (solid waste) leave the body via the rectum and anus.
   1. Anus contains internal sphincter (under involuntary control) and external sphincter (voluntary control)
   2. Fecal matter usually 75% water and 25% solid wastes (roughage, dead bacteria, fat, protein, inorganic matter)

Liver

A. Largest internal organ; located in the right hypochondriac and epigastric regions of the abdomen.

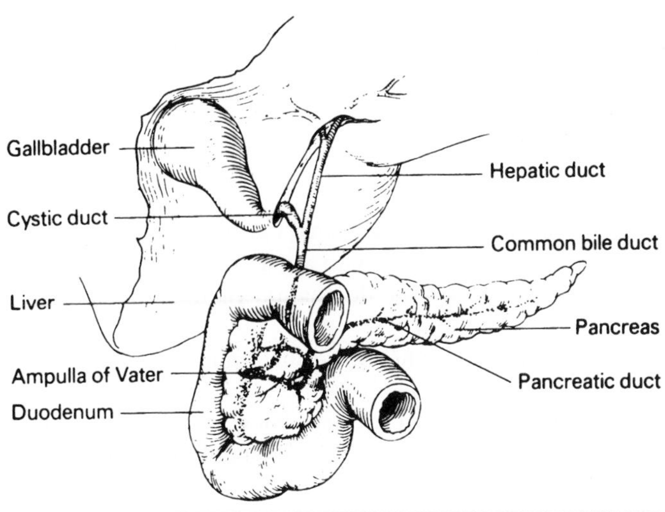

FIGURE 9-2 Gallbladder and ductal system

B. *Liver lobules:* functional units of the liver, composed of hepatic cells.

C. Hepatic sinusoids (capillaries) are lined with Kupffer cells, which carry out the process of phagocytosis.

D. Portal circulation brings blood to the liver from the stomach, spleen, pancreas, and intestines.

E. Functions

1. Metabolism of fats, carbohydrates, and proteins; oxidizes these nutrients for energy and produces compounds that can be stored
2. Production of bile
3. Conjugation and excretion (in the form of glycogen, fatty acids, minerals, fat-soluble and water-soluble vitamins) of bilirubin
4. Storage of vitamins A, D, B_{12}, and iron
5. Synthesis of coagulation factors
6. Detoxification of many drugs and conjugation of sex hormones

Biliary System

Consists of the gallbladder and associated ductal system (bile ducts), see Figure 9-2.

A. *Gallbladder:* lies on the undersurface of the liver, functions to concentrate and store bile.

B. *Ductal system:* provides a route for bile to reach the intestines.

1. Bile is formed in the liver and excreted into the hepatic duct.

2. Hepatic duct joins with the cystic duct (which drains the gallbladder) to form the *common bile duct*.
3. If sphincter of Oddi is relaxed, bile enters the duodenum. If contracted, bile is stored in gallbladder.

Pancreas

A. Positioned transversely in the upper abdominal cavity.
B. Consists of a head, body, and tail along with a pancreatic duct, which extends along the gland and enters the duodenum via the common bile duct.
C. Has both exocrine and endocrine functions; function in GI system is exocrine.
   1. Exocrine cells in the pancreas secrete trypsinogen and chymotrypsin for protein digestion, amylase to break down starch to disaccharides, and lipase for fat digestion.
   2. Endocrine function is related to islets of Langerhans.

Physiology of Digestion and Absorption

A. Digestion: physical and chemical breakdown of food into absorptive substances
   1. Initiated in the mouth where food mixes with saliva and starch is broken down.
   2. Food then passes into the esophagus where it is propelled into the stomach.
   3. In the stomach, food is processed by gastric secretions into a substance called *chyme*.
   4. In the small intestine, carbohydrates are hydrolyzed to monosaccharides, fats to glycerol, and fatty acids and proteins to amino acids to complete the digestive process.
      a. When chyme enters the duodenum, mucus is secreted to neutralize hydrochloric acid; in response to release of *secretin*, pancreas releases bicarbonate to neutralize acid chyme.
      b. *Cholecystokinin and pancreozymin* (*CCK-PZ*) are also produced by the duodenal mucosa; stimulate contraction of the gallbladder along with relaxation of the sphincter of Oddi (to allow bile to flow from the common bile duct into the duodenum), and stimulate release of pancreatic enzymes.

■ ASSESSMENT

Health History

A. Presenting problem
   1. Mouth: symptoms may include dental caries, bleeding gums, dryness or increased salivation, odors, difficulty chewing (note use of dentures)

2. Ingestion: symptoms may include
   a. Changes in appetite: anorexia or hyperorexia; note food preferences/dislikes.
   b. Food intolerances: allergies, fluid, fatty foods.
   c. Weight gain/loss: note symptoms/situations that might interfere with appetite (stress, deliberate weight reduction, dental problems); note average weight and percent gain/loss within past 2–9 months.
   d. Dysphagia: note level of sensation where problem occurs, whether it occurs with foods/fluids.
   e. Nausea: note onset and duration, existence of associated symptoms (weakness, headache, vomiting), occurrence before or after meals.
   f. Vomiting: note onset and duration; foods/fluids that can be maintained; associated symptoms (fever, diarrhea).
   g. Regurgitation (reflux): note whether occurs with ingestion of certain foods, any associated symptoms (vomiting), occurrence with certain positions (supine, recumbent).
3. Digestion/absorption: symptoms may include
   a. Dyspepsia (indigestion): note location of discomfort, whether associated with certain foods, time of day/night of occurrence, associated symptoms (vomiting).
   b. Heartburn (pyrosis): note location, whether pain radiates, whether it occurs before or after meals, time of day when discomfort is most noticeable, foods that aggravate or eliminate symptoms.
   c. Pain: character, frequency, location, duration, distribution, aggravating or alleviating factors.
4. Bowel habits: symptoms may include
   a. Constipation: note number of stools/day or week, changes in size or color of stool, alterations in food/fluid intake, presence of tenesmus, painful defecation, associated symptoms (abdominal pain, cramps)
   b. Diarrhea: note number of stools/day, consistency, quantity, odor, interference with ADL, associated symptoms (nausea, vomiting, flatus, abdominal distension)
5. Hepatic/biliary problems: symptoms may include
   a. Jaundice: note location, duration, notable increase/decrease in degree.
   b. Pruritus: note location, distribution, onset.
   c. Urine changes: note color, onset, notable increase or decrease in color change, associated symptoms (pain).
   d. Clay-colored stools: note onset, number/day, associated symptoms (pain, problems with ingestion/digestion).
   e. Increased bleeding: note ecchymoses, purpura, bleeding gums, hematuria.

B. Lifestyle: eating behaviors (rapid ingestion, skipping meals, snacking), cultural/religious values (vegetarian, kosher foods), ingestion of alcohol, smoking

C. Use of medications: note use of antacids, antiemetics, antiflatulents, vitamin supplements; aspirin and anti-inflammatory agents

D. Past medical history: childhood, adult, psychiatric illness; surgery; bleeding disorders; menstrual history; exposure to infectious agents; allergies

Physical Examination

A. Mouth: inspect/palpate

1. Outer/inner lips: color, texture, moisture
2. Buccal mucosa: color, texture, lesions, ulcerations
3. Teeth/gums: missing teeth, cavities, tenderness, swelling
4. Tongue: protrusion without deviation, texture, color, moisture
5. Palates (hard and soft): color

B. Abdomen: divided into regions and quadrants (Figure 9-3); note specific location of any abnormality.

1. Inspect skin: color, scars, striae, pigmentation, lesions, vascularity.
2. Inspect architecture: contour, symmetry, distension, umbilicus.
3. Inspect movement: peristalsis, pulsations.
4. Auscultate peristaltic sounds.
    - **a.** Normal: bubbling, gurgling, 5–30 times/minute
    - **b.** Increased: may indicate diarrhea, gastroenteritis, early intestinal obstruction
    - **c.** Decreased: may indicate constipation, late intestinal obstruction, use of anticholinergics, post-op anesthesia
5. Auscultate arterial sounds: note presence or absence of bruits in aorta/renal arteries.
6. Percuss for tenderness/masses; determine distribution of tympany and dullness
    - **a.** Liver span: normal 6–12 cm dullness at the midclavicular line; determine shifting dullness (ascites)
    - **b.** Stomach: normal tympany
    - **c.** Spleen: normal tympany, dullness only if enlarged
    - **d.** Small/large intestine: normal tympany
    - **e.** Bladder: normal tympany, dullness if full
7. Palpate to depth of 1 cm (light palpation) to determine areas of tenderness, muscle guarding, and masses
8. Palpate to a depth of 4–8 cm (deep palpation) to identify rigidity, masses, ascites, tenderness, liver margins, spleen

Laboratory/Diagnostic Tests

A. Blood chemistry and electrolyte analysis: albumin, alkaline phosphatase, ammonia, amylase, bilirubin, chloride, LDH, lipase, potassium, SGOT or AST, serum glutamic pyruvic transaminase (SGPT or ALT), sodium

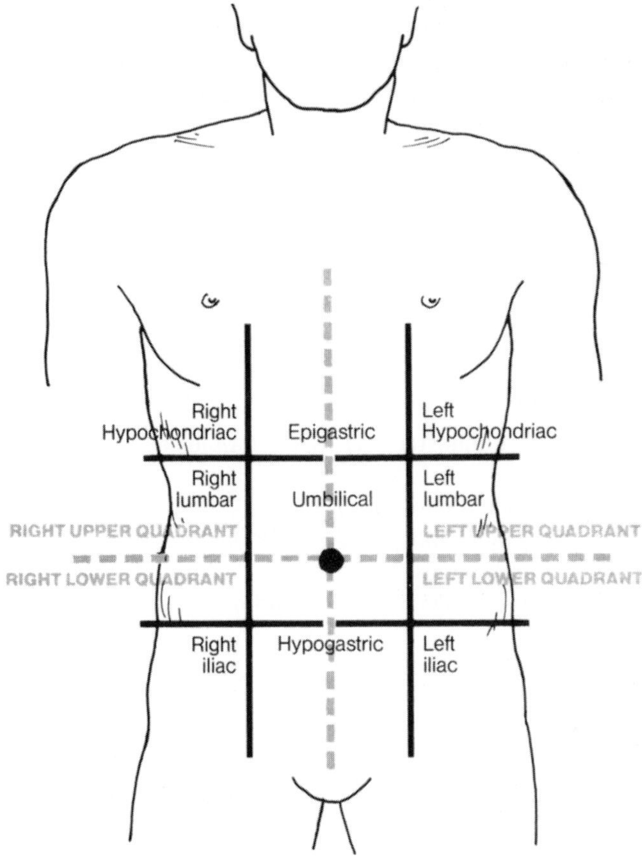

FIGURE 9-3 Abdominal quadrants (broken lines) and regions (solid lines)

B. Hematologic studies: Hgb and hct, PT, WBC

C. Serologic studies: carcinoembryonic antigen (CEA), hepatitis-associated antigens, helicobacter pylori

D. Urine studies: amylase, bilirubin

E. Fecal studies: for blood, fat, infectious organisms

 1. A freshly passed, warm stool is the best specimen.

 2. For fat or infectious organisms collect three separate specimens and label day #1, day #2, day #3.

F. Upper GI series (barium swallow)

 1. Fluoroscopic examination of upper GI tract to determine structural problems and gastric emptying time; client must swallow barium sulfate or other contrast medium; sequential films taken as it moves through the system.

2. Nursing care: pretest
   a. Keep NPO after midnight or 6–8 hours pretest.
   b. Explain that the barium will taste chalky.
3. Nursing care: posttest: administer laxatives to enhance elimination of barium and prevent obstruction or impaction.

G. Lower GI series (barium enema)
1. Barium is instilled into the colon by enema; client retains the contrast medium while X-rays are taken to identify structural abnormalities of the large intestine or colon.
2. Nursing care: pretest
   a. Keep NPO for 8 hours pretest.
   b. Give enemas until clear the morning of test.
   c. Administer laxative or suppository.
   d. Explain that cramping may be experienced during the procedure.
3. Nursing care: posttest: administer laxatives and fluids to assist in expelling barium.

H. Endoscopy (esophagogastroduodenoscopy)
1. Direct visualization of the esophagus, stomach, and duodenum by insertion of a lighted fiberscope
2. Used to observe structures, ulcerations, inflammation, tumors; may include a biopsy
3. Nursing care: pretest
   a. Keep NPO for 6–8 hours.
   b. Ensure consent form has been signed.
   c. Explain that a local anesthetic will be used to ease discomfort and that speaking during the procedure will not be possible; the client should expect hoarseness and a sore throat for several days.
4. Nursing care: posttest
   a. Keep NPO until return of gag reflex.
   b. Assess vital signs and for pain, dysphagia, bleeding.
   c. Administer warm normal saline gargles for relief of sore throat.

I. Colonoscopy
1. Endoscopic visualization of the large intestine: may include biopsy and removal of foreign substances.
2. Nursing care: pretest
   a. Keep NPO for 8 hours pretest.
   b. Administer laxatives for 1–3 days before the exam, and sometimes enemas until clear the night before the test.
   c. Ensure a consent form has been signed.
   d. Explain to client that when the instrument is inserted into the rectum a feeling of pressure might be experienced.
3. Nursing care: posttest
   a. Observe for rectal bleeding and signs of perforation.
   b. Schedule planned rest periods for the client.

J. Sigmoidoscopy
  1. Endoscopic visualization of the sigmoid colon
  2. Used to identify inflammation or lesions, or remove foreign bodies.
  3. Nursing care: pretest
    a. Offer a light supper and light breakfast.
    b. Do bowel prep.
    c. Explain to client that the sensation of an urge to defecate or abdominal cramping might be experienced.
  4. Nursing care: posttest: assess for signs of bowel perforation.

K. Gastric analysis
  1. Insertion of a nasogastric tube to examine fasting gastric contents for acidity and volume
  2. Nursing care: pretest
    a. Keep NPO 6–8 hours pretest.
    b. Advise client about no smoking, anticholinergic medications, antacids for 24 hours prior to test.
    c. Inform client that tube will be inserted into the stomach via the nose, and instruct to expectorate saliva to prevent buffering of secretions.
  3. Nursing care: posttest: provide frequent mouth care.

L. Oral cholecystogram
  1. Injection of a radiopaque dye and X-ray examination to visualize the gallbladder
  2. Used to determine the gallbladder's ability to concentrate and store the dye and to assess patency of the biliary duct system
  3. Nursing care: pretest
    a. Offer a low-fat meal the evening before the test and black coffee, tea, or water the morning of the exam.
    b. Check for iodine sensitivity and administer dye tablets (Telepaque) as ordered.
  4. Nursing care: posttest: observe for side effects of the dye (nausea, vomiting, diarrhea).

M. Liver biopsy (closed needle)
  1. Invasive procedure where a specially designed needle is inserted into the liver to remove a small piece of tissue for study
  2. Nursing care: pretest
    a. Ensure client has signed consent form.
    b. Keep NPO 6–8 hours pretest.
    c. Instruct client to hold breath during the biopsy.
  3. Nursing care: posttest
    a. Assess vital signs every hour for 8–12 hours.
    b. Place client on right side for a few hours with a pillow against the abdomen to provide pressure on the liver.
    c. Observe puncture site for hemorrhage.
    d. Assess for complications of shock and pneumothorax.

ANALYSIS

Nursing diagnoses for the client with a disorder of the digestive system may include

- **A.** Risk for deficient fluid volume
- **B.** Disturbed body image
- **C.** Imbalanced nutrition: less than body requirements
- **D.** Diarrhea
- **E.** Constipation
- **F.** Pain
- **G.** Ineffective breathing pattern
- **H.** Impaired verbal communication
- **I.** Impaired skin integrity

PLANNING AND IMPLEMENTATION

Goals

- **A.** Restoration of fluid and electrolyte balance.
- **B.** Client will express feelings of self-worth.
- **C.** Adequate nutritional status will be maintained.
- **D.** Client will experience decreased frequency of regular bowel habits.
- **E.** Client will establish regular bowel habits of appropriate amount and consistency.
- **F.** Client will be free from pain.
- **G.** Effective breathing patterns will be maintained.
- **H.** Effective communication methods will be established.
- **I.** Skin integrity will be restored/maintained.

Interventions

Enemas

- **A.** General information
  1. Instillation of fluid into the rectum, usually for the purpose of stimulating defecation. The various types include
     - **a.** *Cleansing enema* (tap water, normal saline, or soap): used to treat constipation or feces impaction, as bowel cleansing prior to diagnostic procedures or surgery, to help establish regular bowel functions.
     - **b.** *Retention enema* (mineral oil, olive oil, cottonseed oil): usually administered to lubricate or soften a hard fecal mass to facilitate defecation.
- **B.** Nursing care for a cleansing enema
  1. Explain procedure and that breathing through the mouth relaxes abdominal musculature and helps to avoid cramps; explain the need to take adequate time to defecate.

2. Assemble equipment: prepare solution at 105°–110°F and have bedpan, commode, or nearby bathroom ready for use.
3. Position client and drape adequately.
4. Place waterproof pad under buttocks.
5. Lubricate tube and allow solution to fill the tubing, displacing air.
6. Insert rectal tube 4–5 inches without using force; request that client take several deep breaths.
7. Administer 500–100 ml of solution over 5–10 minutes; if cramping occurs slow the speed of instillation.
8. After administration, have the client retain solution until the urge to defecate becomes strong.
9. Document amount, color, characteristics of stool, and client's reaction during procedure.
10. Assess for dizziness, light-headedness, abdominal cramps, nausea.
11. Monitor electrolyte levels if client is to receive repeated enemas.

C. Nursing care for a retention enema: same as for a cleansing enema except
   1. Oil is used instead of water (comes prepared in commercial kits and is given at body temperature).
   2. Administer 150–200 ml of prepared solution.
   3. Instruct client to retain oil for at least 30 minutes in order for it to take effect.

Gastrostomy

A. General information
   1. Insertion of a catheter through an abdominal incision into the stomach where it is secured with sutures.
   2. Used as an alternative method of feeding, either temporary or permanent, for clients who have problems with swallowing, ingestion, and digestion.

B. Nursing care
   1. Maintain skin integrity: inspect and cleanse skin around stoma frequently; keep deep area dry to avoid excoriation.
   2. Maintain patency of the gastrostomy tube.
      a. Assess for residual before each feeding (check orders concerning withholding feeding).
      b. Irrigate tube before and after meals.
      c. Measure/record any drainage.
   3. Promote adequate nutrition.
      a. Administer feeding with client in high-Fowler's and keep head of bed elevated for 30 minutes after meals to prevent regurgitation.
      b. Maintain feeding at room temperature.
      c. Ensure that prescribed amount of feeding be given within prescribed amount of time.
      d. Weigh client daily.

CLIENT TEACHING CHECKLIST

Teach clients and their families who receive enteral feedings at home how to:

1. Place formula in feeding bag.
2. Set up enteral feeding pump or bag.
3. Obtain formula and related supplies.

   e. Monitor I&O until feedings are well tolerated.
   f. Monitor for signs of dehydration.

Nasogastric (NG) Tubes

A. General information
   1. Soft rubber or plastic tube inserted through a nostril and into the stomach for gastric decompression, feeding, or obtaining specimens for analysis of stomach contents
   2. Types
      a. Levin: single-lumen, nonvented
      b. Salem: a tube within a tube; vented to provide constant inflow of atmospheric air
B. Nursing care
   1. Insertion of the tube
      a. Explain the purpose of the tube and the procedure for insertion.
      b. Measure the tube: distance on the tube from the tip of the nose to the ear lobe plus the distance from the ear lobe to the tip of the xiphoid.
      c. Instruct client to bend head forward if possible during insertion.
   2. Monitor functioning of system and ensure patency of the NG tube: abdominal discomfort/distension, nausea and vomiting, and little or no drainage in collection bottle are all signs that system is not functioning properly.
      a. Assess the position: aspirate gastric contents to confirm that tube is in stomach; inject 10 ml air through tube and auscultate for rapid influx.
      b. Check that tubing is free of kinks; irrigate as per physician order.
      c. Record amount, color, and odor of drainage.
   3. Provide measures to ensure maximal comfort.
      a. Apply water-soluble lubricant to lips to prevent dryness.
      b. Keep nares free from secretions.
      c. Provide periodic warm saline gargles to prevent dryness.
      d. Provide frequent mouth care with toothbrush/toothpaste or flavored mouthwashes.

DELEGATION TIP

You may delegate skin care of the client's nose and oral hygiene to assistive personnel.

   e. If allowed, give client hard candy or gum to stimulate the flow of saliva and prevent dryness.
   f. Elevate head and chest during and for 1–2 hours after feedings to prevent reflux (most comfortable position when suction is used).
4. Monitor/maintain fluid and electrolyte balance.
   a. Assess for signs of metabolic alkalosis (suctioning causes excessive loss of hydrochloric acid and potassium).
   b. Administer IV fluids as ordered.
   c. If suction used, irrigate NG tube with normal saline to decrease sodium loss.
   d. Keep accurate I&O.
   e. If suction used provide ice chips sparingly (if allowed) to avoid dilution of electrolytes.
   f. Monitor lab values and electrolytes frequently.

Intestinal Tubes

A. General information
   1. Tube is inserted via a nostril through the stomach and into the intestine for decompression proximal to an obstruction, relief of an obstruction, decompression of post-op edema at the surgical site.
   2. Types
      a. Cantor tube: single lumen
      b. Harris tube: single lumen
      c. Miller-Abbott: double lumen
B. Nursing care
   1. Facilitate placement of the tube.
      a. Position client in high-Fowler's while tube is being passed from the nose to the stomach; then place client on right side to aid in advancing the tube from the stomach to duodenum.
      b. Continuously monitor tube markings.
      c. Tape tube in place only after placement in duodenum is confirmed.
   2. Provide measures for maximal comfort, as for NG tube.

EVALUATION

A. Adequate urine output; stable vital signs; moist mucous membranes; adequate skin turgor and mobility; electrolyte levels within normal range.

B. Client expresses interest in personal well-being; actively participates in ADL, treatments, and care.

C. Stable weight; improved anthropometric measurements; laboratory values within normal limits; client verbalizes types of foods that should be included or eliminated from prescribed diet.

D. Client reports reduction in frequency of stools and return to more normal stool consistency; laboratory values within normal range.

E. Client reports increased frequency with improved consistency of stool.

F. Relaxed facial expression; decreased abdominal distension; healed mouth ulcers.

G. Improved respiratory rate, depth, and rhythm; lungs clear to auscultation; effective use of muscles of respiration.

H. Client effectively uses artificial means of communication (artificial larynx, sign language, or esophageal speech).

I. No redness, irritation, or breakdown; client demonstrates techniques to prevent skin breakdown.

DISORDERS OF THE GASTROINTESTINAL SYSTEM

Nausea and Vomiting

A. General information
   1. *Nausea:* a feeling of discomfort in the epigastrium with a conscious desire to vomit; occurs in association with and prior to vomiting.
   2. *Vomiting:* forceful ejection of stomach contents from the upper GI tract. Emetic center in medulla is stimulated (e.g., by local irritation of intestine or stomach or disturbance of equilibrium), causing the vomiting reflex.
   3. Nausea and vomiting are the two most common manifestations of GI disease.
   4. Contributing factors
      a. GI disease
      b. CNS disorders (meningitis, CNS lesions)
      c. Circulatory problems (HF)
      d. Metabolic disorders (uremia)
      e. Side effects of certain drugs (chemotherapy, antibiotics)
      f. Pain
      g. Psychic trauma
      h. Response to motion

B. Assessment findings
   1. Weakness, fatigue, pallor, possible lethargy
   2. Dry mucous membrane and poor skin turgor/mobility (if prolonged with dehydration)

3. Serum sodium, calcium, potassium decreased
4. BUN elevated (if severe vomiting and dehydration)

C. Nursing interventions
1. Maintain NPO until client able to tolerate oral intake.
2. Administer medications as ordered and monitor effects/side effects.
   a. Phenothiazines: chlorpromazine (Thorazine), perphenazine (Trilafon), prochlorperazine (Compazine), trifluoperazine (Stelazine)
   b. Antihistamines: benzquinamide (Emete-con), dimenhydrinate (Dramimine), diphenhydramine (Benadryl), hydroxyzine (Atarax, Vistaril), cyclizine (Marezine), meclizine (Antivert), promethazine (Phenergan)
   c. Other drugs to help control nausea and vomiting: thiethylperazine (Torecan), trimethobenzamide (Tigan), metoclopramide (Reglan)
3. Notify physician if vomiting pattern changes.
4. Maintain fluid and electrolyte balance.
   a. Administer IV fluids as ordered, keep accurate record of I&O.
   b. Record amount/frequency of vomitus.
   c. Assess skin tone/turgor for degree of hydration.
   d. Monitor laboratory/electrolyte values.
   e. Test NG tube drainage or vomitus for blood, bile; monitor pH.
5. Provide measures for maximum comfort.
   a. Institute frequent mouth care with tepid water/saline mouthwashes.
   b. Remove encrustations around nares.
   c. Keep head of bed elevated and avoid sudden changes in position.
   d. Eliminate noxious stimuli from environment.
   e. Keep emesis basin clean.
   f. Maintain quiet environment and avoid unnecessary procedures.
6. When vomiting subsides provide clear fluids (ginger ale, warm tea) in small amounts, gradually introduce solid foods (toast, crackers), and progress to bland foods (baked potato), in small amounts.
7. Provide client teaching and discharge planning concerning
   a. Avoidance of situations, foods, or liquids that precipitate nausea and vomiting
   b. Need for planned, uninterrupted rest periods
   c. Medication regimen, including side effects
   d. Signs of dehydration
   e. Need for daily weights with frequent anthropometric measurements

Diarrhea

A. General information

1. Increase in peristaltic motility, producing watery or loosely formed stools. Diarrhea is a symptom of other pathologic processes.
2. Causes
   a. Chronic bowel disorders
   b. Malabsorption problems
   c. Intestinal infections
   d. Biliary tract disorders
   e. Hyperthyroidism
   f. Saline laxatives
   g. Magnesium-based antacids
   h. Stress
   i. Antibiotics
   j. Neoplasms
   k. Highly seasoned foods

B. Assessment findings
1. Abdominal cramps/distension, foul-smelling watery stools, increased peristalsis
2. Anorexia, thirst, tenesmus, anxiety
3. Decreased potassium and sodium if severe

C. Nursing interventions
1. Administer antidiarrheals: diphenoxylate with atropine (Lomotil), paregoric, loperamide (Imodium), Kaopectate as ordered; monitor effects.
2. Control fluid/food intake.
   a. Avoid milk and milk products.
   b. Provide liquids with gradual introduction of bland, high-protein, high-calorie, low-fat, low-bulk foods.
3. Monitor and maintain fluid and electrolyte status; record number, characteristics, and amount of each stool.
4. Prevent anal excoriation.
   a. Cleanse rectal area after each bowel movement with mild soap and water and pat dry.
   b. Apply A and D ointment or Desitin to promote healing.
   c. Use a local anesthetic as needed.
5. Provide client teaching and discharge planning concerning
   a. Medication regimen
   b. Adherence to prescribed diet and avoidance of foods that are known to produce diarrhea
   c. Importance of perineal hygiene and care and daily assessment of skin changes
   d. Importance of good handwashing techniques after each stool
   e. Need to report worsening of symptoms (increased abdominal cramps, increased frequency or amount of stool)
   f. Need to assess daily weights with frequent anthropometric measurements

Constipation

A. General information

1. Lengthening of normal (for individual) time period between bowel movements; small volume of dry, hard stool; results from decreased motility of the colon or from retention of feces in the colon or rectum
2. Causes
   a. Inadequate bulk/liquids in the diet
   b. Lack of physical activity
   c. Retention of barium after radiographic exam
   d. Prolonged use of constipation medications (aluminum-based antacids, anticholinergics, antihistamines, antidepressants, phenothiazines, calcium, iron)

B. Assessment findings

1. Feeling of abdominal fullness, pressure in the rectum; abdominal distension, dyschezia; increased flatus
2. Hardened stool upon digital examination

C. Nursing interventions

1. Promote adequate intake of fluids/foods and dietary modification: increase fluid intake to at least 3000 ml/day; include high-fiber foods in diet.
2. Administer medications as ordered
   a. Cathartics: milk of magnesia, castor oil, cascara sagrada, senna (Senokot), bisacodyl (Dulcolax), psyllium (Metamucil)
   b. Stool softeners: docusate calcium (Surfak), docusate sodium (Colace)
3. Prevent accumulation of stool in the colon/rectum.
   a. Instruct client not to suppress urge to defecate.
   b. Gently massage abdomen to promote stimulation and movement of feces.
4. Provide client teaching and discharge planning concerning
   a. Need to establish and maintain a regular time to defecate
   b. Diet modification
   c. Medication regimen
   d. Need to assume position of comfort when sitting on toilet

Cancer of the Mouth

A. General information

1. Cancer of the mouth may occur on the lips or within the mouth (tongue, floor of mouth, buccal mucosa, hard/soft palate, pharynx, tonsils).
2. Most common type of oral tumor is squamous cell carcinoma; most malignancies occur on the lower lip.

3. More common in men.
4. Caused by
   a. Excessive sun exposure
   b. Tobacco (cigar, pipe, cigarette, snuff)
   c. Excessive alcohol intake
   d. Constant irritation (dental caries)
5. Early detection is very important; most discovered by dentists in routine checkups.

B. Medical management
   1. Radiation therapy: both primary lesion and affected lymph nodes; radioactive implants
   2. Chemotherapy: sometimes indicated, not used as often as radiation therapy and surgery
   3. Surgery: type depends on location and extent of the tumor
      a. Mandibulectomy: removal of the mandible
      b. Hemiglossectomy: removal of half the tongue
      c. Glossectomy: removal of the entire tongue
      d. Radical neck dissection

C. Assessment findings
   1. Ulcerations (often painless) on the lip, tongue, or buccal mucosa
   2. Pain or soreness of the tongue upon eating hot or highly seasoned foods
   3. Erythroplakia, leukoplakia
   4. Difficulty chewing/speaking, dysphagia
   5. Positive oral exfoliative cytology
   6. Positive toluidine blue test

D. Nursing interventions
   1. Provide nursing care for the client receiving radiation therapy
   2. Prepare client for surgery: in addition to routine pre-op care
      a. Inform client of expected changes post-op.
      b. Provide explanation of anticipated post-op suctioning, NG tube, drains.
   3. In addition to routine post-op care
      a. Promote drainage.
         1) place in side-lying position initially, then Fowler's.
         2) suction mouth (except for lip surgery).
         3) maintain patency of drainage tubes.
      b. Promote oral hygiene/comfort.
         1) provide mouth irrigations with sterile water, diluted peroxide, normal saline, or sodium bicarbonate.
         2) avoid use of commercial mouthwashes, lemon and glycerine swabs.
      c. Monitor/promote optimum nutritional status.
         1) provide tube feedings following a hemiglossectomy.

2) place oral fluids in back of the throat with an asepto syringe.
3) provide foods/fluids that are nonirritating and facilitate swallowing (yogurt, puddings).

d. Monitor for signs and symptoms of facial nerve damage (drooping, uneven smile, circumoral numbness or tingling).

Cancer of the Esophagus

A. General information
   1. Malignant tumors of the esophagus usually appear as ulcerated lesions, most often in middle and lower portions of the esophagus.
   2. Penetration of the muscular layers with extension to the outer wall of the esophagus is commonly found. Metastases may cause eventual esophageal obstruction.
   3. More common in men than in women (4:1); usually between ages 50-70.
   4. Cause unknown; contributing factors include cigarette smoking, excessive alcohol intake, trauma, poor oral hygiene, achalasia, diverticula, and lye burns.

B. Medical management
   1. Radiation therapy: used for inoperable tumors, has been found to alleviate symptoms
   2. Chemotherapy: not found effective
   3. Surgery
      a. Esophagectomy: removal of part or all of the esophagus using a Dacron graft to replace the resected portion
      b. Esophagogastrostomy: resection of a portion of the esophagus (usually middle third) and anastomosis of the remaining portion of the stomach
      c. Esophagoenterostomy: resection of portion of the esophagus and anastomosis of a segment of colon to the remaining portion
      d. Palliative gastrostomy: done for the purpose of feeding the client

C. Assessment findings
   1. Substernal burning after drinking hot fluids
   2. Pain located in the substernal and epigastric areas; usually intensified with swallowing
   3. Weight loss
   4. Barium swallow reveals narrowing of the esophagus at the area of the tumor
   5. Diagnostic test: esophagoscopy with a biopsy reveals malignant cells

D. Nursing interventions
   1. Provide nursing care for the client receiving radiation therapy.
   2. Prepare client for surgery: in addition to routine pre-op care
      a. Provide meticulous oral hygiene including teeth, gums, tongue, and mouth.

NURSING ALERT

Encourage clients to eat slowly and ingest small meals as a method to reduce reflux of food.

   b. Explain that client may have a chest tube if thoracic approach is used.
   c. Prepare client for feedings through a gastrostomy.
3. In addition to routine post-op care
   a. Monitor NG tube: expect bloody drainage for approximately 12 hours with gradual change to green, then to yellow.
   b. Prevent gastric reflux: place client in semi-Fowler's position; maintain upright position for 2 hours after meals when client is able to take fluids/food orally.
4. Provide emotional support to client/significant others; prognosis is grave.
5. Provide client teaching and discharge planning concerning
   a. Gastrostomy and proper dietary measures
   b. Importance of cessation of smoking and elimination of alcohol consumption
   c. Maintain good oral hygiene.
   d. Maintain a high-calorie, high-protein diet

Hiatal Hernia

A. General information
   1. Sliding hiatal hernia occurs when a portion of the stomach and vagus nerve slide upward into the thorax through an enlarged hiatus in the diaphragm.
   2. Result is reflux of gastric juices and inflammation of the lower portion of the esophagus.
   3. Occurs more often in women ages 40–70.
   4. May be caused by congenital weakening of the muscles in the diaphragm around the esophagogastric opening; increased intra-abdominal pressure (obesity, pregnancy, ascites); trauma.
B. Medical management
   1. Drug therapy: antacids to reduce acidity and relieve discomfort, cholinergics
   2. Modification of diet: elimination of spicy foods and caffeine
   3. Surgery: reduction of the hiatal hernia via an abdominal or thoracic approach

C. Assessment findings
  1. Heartburn, especially after meals, at night, or with position changes (particularly recumbent), dysphagia, regurgitation several hours after meals without vomiting
  2. Barium swallow displays protrusion of the gastric mucosa through a hiatus
  3. Esophagoscopy reveals an incompetent cardiac sphincter

D. Nursing interventions
  1. Provide a bland diet with six small feedings/day, as ordered.
  2. Administer medications as ordered.
  3. Prepare client for surgery: in addition to routine pre-op care
    a. Inform client about chest tubes (if thoracic approach to be used).
    b. Provide information regarding NG intubation.
  4. In addition to routine post-op care
    a. Decrease/avoid gastric distension.
    b. Promote pulmonary expansion: chest tubes if a thoracic approach; semi-Fowler's position.
  5. Provide client teaching and discharge planning concerning
    a. Modification of diet
    b. Sitting up for meals and for 2 hours after meals will help reduce gastric acid reflux
    c. Use of antacids
    d. Eating small, frequent meals slowly to help prevent gastric distension
    e. Need to avoid carbonated beverages and anticholinergic drugs (and OTC medications that contain them)
    f. Avoidance of heavy lifting (to prevent intra-abdominal pressure); bend, kneel, or stoop instead
    g. Importance of treating persistent cough
    h. Adherence to weight-reduction plan if obese

Gastritis

A. General information
  1. An acute inflammatory condition that causes a breakdown of the normal gastric protective barriers with subsequent diffusion of hydrochloric acid into the gastric lumen
  2. Results in hemorrhage, ulceration, and adhesions of the gastric mucosa
  3. Present in some form (mild to severe) in 50% of all adults
  4. Caused by excessive ingestion of certain drugs (salicylates, steroids, Butazolidin), alcohol; food poisoning; large quantities of spicy, irritating foods in diet

B. Assessment findings
  1. Anorexia, nausea and vomiting, hematemesis, epigastric fullness/ discomfort, epigastric tenderness

2. Decreased Hgb and hct (if anemic)
3. Endoscopy: inflammation and ulceration of gastric mucosa
4. Gastric analysis: hydrochloric acid usually increased, except in atrophic gastritis

C. Nursing interventions
1. Monitor and maintain fluid and electrolyte balances.
2. Control nausea and vomiting (NPO until able to tolerate foods, then bland diet).
3. Administer medications as ordered: antiemetics, antacids, sedatives.
4. Maintain patency of NG tube.
5. Provide client teaching and discharge planning concerning avoidance of foods/medications such as coffee, spicy foods, alcohol, salicylates, ibuprofen, steroids.

Peptic Ulcer Disease

Gastric Ulcers

A. General information
1. Ulceration of the mucosal lining of the stomach; most commonly found in the antrum
2. Gastric secretions and stomach emptying rate usually normal
3. Rapid diffusion of gastric acid from the gastric lumen into gastric mucosa, however, causes an inflammatory reaction with tissue breakdown
4. Also characterized by reflux into the stomach of bile containing duodenal contents
5. Occurs more often in men, in unskilled laborers, and in lower socioeconomic groups; peak age 40–55 years
6. Predisposing factors include smoking, alcohol abuse, emotional tension, and drugs (salicylates, steroids, Butazolidin)
7. Caused by bacterial infection (*Helicobacter pylori*)

B. Medical management
1. Supportive: rest, bland diet, stress management
2. Drug therapy: antacids, histamine (H_2) receptor antagonists, anticholinergics, omeprazole (Prilosec), sucralfate (Carafate); also metronidazole and amoxacillin for ulcers caused by *Helicobacter pylori*
3. Surgery: various combinations of gastric resections and anastomosis

C. Assessment findings
1. Pain located in left epigastrium, with possible radiation to the back; usually occurs 1–2 hours after meals
2. Weight loss
3. Hgb and hct decreased (if anemic)
4. Endoscopy reveals ulceration; differentiates ulcers from gastric cancer

TABLE 9-1 Drug Therapy for Peptic Ulcer

Drug Type	Action	Side Effects	Nursing Implications
TRANQUILIZERS			
• Combination drug (Librax); chlordiazepoxide (Librium) and clidinium bromide (Quarzan)	Decrease vagal activity and reduce anxiety	Sedation, headache, mental depression, blurred vision, nausea, vomiting, diarrhea, physical/psychological dependence	Contraindicated with other CNS depressants, antidepressants; avoid alcohol use, narcotic analgesics.
ANTICHOLINERGICS			
• Belladonna tincture	Decreases acetylcholine, block cholinergic receptors	Dry mouth, constipation	Contraindicated in narrow-angle glaucoma, myasthenia gravis, paralytic ileus, urinary retention.
• Pirenzepine (Gastrozepine)	Blocks muscarinic receptors that regulate gastric acid secretion	No severe anticholinergic side effects	
• Propantheline bromine (Pro-Banthine)	Decreases gastric secretions; used in irritable bowel syndrome, pancreatitis, urinary bladder spasm	Standard anticholinergic effects: dry mouth, decreased secretions, tachycardia, urinary retention	
• Tridihexethyl chloride (Pathilon)	Decreases gastric secretions		
ANTACIDS			
• Aluminum hydroxide, aluminum carbonate (Amphogel, Alternagel)	Neutralize gastric acid and reduce pepsin activity	Prolonged use may cause hypophosphatemia	

Continued

Table 9-1 Continued

Drug Type	Action	Side Effects	Nursing Implications
• Magnesium hydroxide, magnesium trisilicate, magnesium phosphate (Maalox, Gaviscon)		Hypermagnesemia	Contraindicated in impaired renal function.
HISTAMINE (H_2) BLOCKERS			
• Cimetadine (Tagamet) • Rantadine (Zantac) • Famotidine (Pepcid) • Nizatidine (Axid)	Block H_2 receptor sites of parietal cells of stomach	Headaches, dizziness, constipation, pruritus, skin rash, gynecomastia, decreased libido, impotence	Do not give within 1 hour of antacids. Cimetidine may enhance effects of oral anticoagulants, theophylline, caffeine, phenytoin, diazepam, propranolol, phenobarbital, calcium channel blockers; rantadine and famotidine have fewer side effects.
PROTON PUMP INHIBITORS (PPIs)			
• Esomeprazole magnesium (Nexium) • Iansoprazole (Prevacid)	Inhibit gastric secretion regardless of acetylcholine or histamine release; used in treatment of erosive		

• Omeprazole (Prilosec) • Pantoprazole (Protonix) • Rabeprazole (Aciphex)	esophagitis/GERD, gastric and duodenal ulcers, *H. pylori*		
PEPSIN INHIBITOR			
• Sucralfate (Carafate)	Reacts with acid to form a paste that binds to ulcerated tissue to prevent further destruction by digestive enzyme pepsin	Dizziness, nausea, constipation, dry mouth, rash, pruritus, back pain, sleepiness	Mucosal protective drug; must be given 30 minutes before meals and at bedtime.
PROSTAGLANDIN E_1 ANALOGUE			
• Misoprostol (Cytotec)	Synthetic prostaglandin replacement product that blocks secretion of excess acid and protects stomach mucosa; used adjunctively with long-term NSAIDS or ASA	Diarrhea, abdominal pain, flatulence, nausea, vomiting, constipation, menstrual spotting	
ANTI-INFECTIVES			
• Metronidazole hydrochloride (Flagyl, Protostat) • Amoxicillin (Amoxil) • Clarithromycin (Biaxin) • Tetracycline	Used in dual, triple, quadruple combination therapy for treatment of *H. pylori*		

5. Gastric analysis: normal gastric acidity in gastric ulcer, increased in duodenal ulcer
6. Upper GI series: presence of ulcer confirmed

D. Nursing interventions
1. Administer medications as ordered.
2. Provide nursing care for the client with ulcer surgery.
3. Provide client teaching and discharge planning concerning
a. Medical regimen
1) take medications at prescribed times.
2) have antacids available at all times.
3) recognize situations that would increase the need for antacids.
4) avoid ulcerogenic drugs (salicylates, steroids).
5) know proper dosage, action, and side effects.
b. Proper diet
1) bland diet consisting of six small meals/day.
2) eat meals slowly.
3) avoid acid-producing substances (caffeine, alcohol, highly seasoned foods).
4) avoid stressful situations at mealtime.
5) plan for rest periods after meals.
6) avoid late bedtime snacks.
c. Avoidance of stress-producing situations and development of stress-reduction methods (relaxation techniques, exercises, biofeedback).

Duodenal Ulcers

A. General information
1. Most commonly found in the first 2 cm of the duodenum
2. Occur more frequently than gastric ulcers
3. Characterized by gastric hyperacidity and a significant increased rate of gastric emptying
4. Occur more often in younger men; more women affected after menopause; peak age 35–45 years
5. Predisposing factors include smoking, alcohol abuse, psychological stress, bacterial infection (*Helicobacter pylori*)

B. Medical management: same as for gastric ulcers

C. Assessment findings
1. Pain located in midepigastrium and described as burning, cramping; usually occurs 2–4 hours after meals and is relieved by food.
2. Diagnostic tests: same as for gastric ulcer.

D. Nursing interventions: same as for gastric ulcer

Gastric Surgery

A. General information
   1. Surgery is performed when peptic ulcer disease does not respond to medical management or for gastric cancer
   2. Types
      a. *Vagotomy:* severing of part of the vagus nerve innervating the stomach to decrease gastric acid secretion
      b. *Antrectomy:* removal of the antrum of the stomach to eliminate the gastric phase of digestion
      c. *Pyloroplasty:* enlargement of the pyloric sphincter with acceleration of gastric emptying
      d. *Gastroduodenostomy (Billroth I)*: removal of the lower portion of the stomach with anastomosis of the remaining portion of the duodenum
      e. *Gastrojejunostomy (Billroth II)*: removal of the antrum and distal portion of the stomach and duodenum with anastomosis of the remaining portion of the stomach to the jejunum
      f. *Gastrectomy:* removal of 60–80% of the stomach
      g. *Esophagojejunostomy (total gastrectomy)*: removal of the entire stomach with a loop of jejunum anastomosed to the esophagus
   3. Dumping syndrome
      a. Abrupt emptying of stomach contents into the intestine
      b. Common complications of gastric surgery
      c. Associated with the presence of hyperosmolar chyme in the jejunum, which draws fluid by osmosis from the extracellular fluid into the bowel. Decreased plasma volume and distension of the bowel stimulates increased intestinal motility.
      d. Signs and symptoms include weakness, faintness, palpitations, diaphoresis, feeling of fullness, or discomfort, nausea, and occasionally diarrhea; appear 15–30 minutes after meals and last for 20–60 minutes.

B. Nursing interventions: routine preoperative care

C. Nursing interventions: postoperative
   1. Provide routine post-op care.
   2. Ensure adequate function of NG tube.
      a. Measure drainage accurately to determine necessity for fluid and electrolyte replacement; notify physician if there is no drainage.
      b. Anticipate frank, red bleeding for 12–24 hours.
   3. Promote adequate pulmonary ventilation.
      a. Place client in mid- or high-Fowler's position to promote chest expansion.
      b. Teach client to splint high upper abdominal incision before turning, coughing, and deep breathing.
   4. Promote adequate nutrition.
      a. After removal of NG tube, provide clear liquids with gradual introduction of small amounts of bland food at frequent intervals.

   b. Monitor weight daily.
   c. Assess for regurgitation; if present, instruct client to eat smaller amounts of food at a slower pace.
5. Provide client teaching and discharge planning concerning
   a. Gradually increasing food intake until able to tolerate three meals/day
   b. Daily monitoring of weight
   c. Stress-reduction measures
   d. Need to report signs of complications to physician immediately (hematemesis, vomiting, diarrhea, pain, melena, weakness, feeling of abdominal fullness/distension)
   e. Methods of controlling symptoms associated with dumping syndrome
      1) avoidance of concentrated sweets
      2) adherence to six, small, dry meals/day
      3) maintenance of modified diet
      4) refraining from taking fluids during meals but rather 2 hours after meals
      5) Assuming a recumbent position for ½ hour after meals

Cancer of the Stomach

A. General information
   1. Most often develops in the distal third and may spread through the walls of the stomach into adjacent tissues, lymphatics, regional lymph nodes, and other abdominal organs, or through the bloodstream to the lungs and bones.
   2. Affects men twice as often as women; more frequent in African Americans and Orientals; most commonly occurs between ages 50 and 70
   3. Causes
      a. Excessive intake of highly salted or smoked foods
      b. Diet low in quantity of vegetables and fruits
      c. Atrophic gastritis
      d. Achlorhydria
      e. Helicobacterpylori infection
B. Medical management
   1. Chemotherapy
   2. Radiation therapy
   3. Treatment for anemia, gastric decompression, nutritional support, fluid and electrolyte maintenance
   4. Surgery: type depends on location and extent of lesion.
      a. Subtotal gastrectomy (Billroth I or II)
      b. Total gastrectomy
C. Assessment findings
   1. Fatigue, weakness, dizziness, shortness of breath, nausea and vomiting, hematemesis, weight loss, indigestion, epigastric fullness, feeling of early satiety when eating, epigastric pain (later)

2. Pallor, lethargy, poor skin turgor and mobility, palpable epigastric mass
3. Diagnostic tests
   a. Stool for occult blood positive
   b. CEA positive
   c. Hgb and hct decreased
   d. SGOT (AST), SGPT (ALT), LDH, serum amylase elevated (if liver and pancreatic involvement)
   e. Gastric analysis reveals histologic changes

D. Nursing interventions
1. Give consistent nutritional assessment and support.
2. Provide care for the client receiving chemotherapy.
3. Provide care for the client with gastric surgery (see Gastric Surgery, page 323).

Hernias

A. General information
1. Protrusion of a viscus from its normal cavity through an abnormal opening/weakened area
2. Occurs anywhere but most often in the abdominal cavity
3. Types
   a. *Reducible:* can be manually placed back into the abdominal cavity.
   b. *Irreducible:* cannot be placed back into the abdominal cavity.
   c. *Inguinal:* occurs when there is weakness in the abdominal wall where the spermatic cord in men and round ligament in women emerge.
   d. *Femoral:* protrusion through the femoral ring; more common in females.
   e. *Incisional:* occurs at the site of a previous surgical incision as a result of inadequate healing postoperatively.
   f. *Umbilical:* most commonly found in children.
   g. *Strangulated:* irreducible, with obstruction to intestinal flow and blood supply.

B. Medical management
1. Manual reduction, use of a truss (firm support)
2. Bowel surgery if strangulated
3. Herniorrhaphy: surgical repair of the hernia by suturing the defect

C. Assessment findings
1. Vomiting, protrusion of involved area (more obvious after coughing), and discomfort at site of protrusion
2. Crampy abdominal pain and abdominal distention (if strangulated with a bowel obstruction)

D. Nursing interventions
1. Observe client for complications such as strangulation.
2. Prepare client for herniorrhaphy, provide routine pre-op care.

3. In addition to routine post-op care
   a. Assess for possible distended bladder, particularly with inguinal hernia repair.
   b. Discourage coughing, but deep breathing and turning should be done.
   c. Assist to splint incision when coughing or sneezing.
   d. Apply ice bags to scrotal area (if inguinal repair) to decrease edema.
   e. Scrotal (athletic) support may be ordered in some cases.
4. Provide client teaching and discharge planning concerning
   a. Need to avoid strenuous physical activities (e.g., heavy lifting, pulling, pushing) for at least 6 weeks.
   b. Need to report any difficulty with urination.

Intestinal Obstructions

A. General information
   1. Mechanical intestinal obstruction: physical blockage of the passage of intestinal contents with subsequent distension by fluid and gas; caused by adhesions, hernias, volvulus, intussusception, inflammatory bowel disease, foreign bodies, strictures, neoplasms, fecal impaction
   2. *Paralytic ileus* (*neurogenic or adynamic ileus*): interference with the nerve supply to the intestine resulting in decreased or absent peristalsis; caused by abdominal surgery, peritonitis, pancreatic toxic conditions, shock, spinal cord injuries, electrolyte imbalances (especially hypokalemia)
   3. Vascular obstructions: interference with the blood supply to a portion of the intestine, resulting in ischemia and gangrene of the bowel; caused by an embolus, atherosclerosis
B. Assessment findings
   1. Small intestine: nonfecal vomiting; colicky intermittent abdominal pain
   2. Large intestine: cramplike abdominal pain, occasional fecal-type vomitus; client will be unable to pass stools or flatus
   3. Abdominal distension, rigidity, high-pitched bowel sounds above the level of the obstruction, decreased or absent bowel sounds distal to obstruction
   4. Diagnostic tests
      a. Flat-plate (X-ray) of the abdomen reveals the presence of gas/fluid
      b. Hct increased
      c. Serum sodium, potassium, chloride decreased
      d. BUN increased
C. Nursing interventions
   1. Monitor fluid and electrolyte balance, prevent further imbalance; keep client NPO and administer IV fluids as ordered.
   2. Accurately measure drainage from NG/intestinal tube.

3. Place client in Fowler's position to alleviate pressure on the diaphragm and encourage nasal breathing to minimize swallowing of air and further abdominal distension.
4. Institute comfort measures associated with NG intubation and intestinal decompression.
5. Prevent complications.
   a. Measure abdominal girth daily to assess for increasing abdominal distension.
   b. Assess for signs and symptoms of peritonitis.
   c. Monitor urinary output.

Chronic Inflammatory Bowel Disorders

Regional Enteritis (Crohn's Disease)

A. General information
   1. Chronic inflammatory bowel disease that can affect both the large and small intestine; terminal ileum, cecum, and ascending colon most often affected
   2. Characterized by granulomas that may affect all the bowel wall layers with resultant thickening, narrowing, and scarring of the intestinal wall
   3. Both sexes affected equally; more common in the Jewish population; two age peaks: 20–30 years and 40–60 years
   4. Cause unknown; contributing factors include food allergies, autoimmune reaction, psychologic disorders
B. Medical management
   1. Diet: high calorie, high vitamin, high protein, low residue, milk free; supplementary iron preparations
   2. Drug therapy: antimicrobials (especially sulfasalazine) to prevent or control infection, corticosteroids, antidiarrheals, anticholinergics
   3. Supplemental parenteral nutrition
   4. Surgery: resection of diseased portion of bowel and temporary or permanent ileostomy
C. Assessment findings
   1. Right, lower quadrant tenderness and pain; abdominal distension
   2. Nausea and vomiting, 3–4 semisoft stools/day with mucus and pus
   3. Decreased skin turgor, dry mucus membranes
   4. Increased peristalsis
   5. Pallor
   6. Diagnostic tests
      a. Hgb and hct (if anemic) decreased
      b. Sigmoidoscopy negative or reveals scattered ulcers
      c. Barium enema shows narrowing with areas of strictures separated by segments of normal bowel

D. Nursing interventions

1. Provide appropriate nutrition while reducing bowel motility.
   a. Administer/monitor TPN.
   b. Provide high-protein, high-calorie, low-residue diet with no milk products (if able to tolerate oral foods/fluids).
   c. Weigh daily, monitor kcal counts, and take periodic anthropometric measurements.
   d. Record number and characteristics of stools daily.
   e. Administer antidiarrheals, antispasmodics, and anticholinergics as ordered.
   f. Provide tepid fluids to avoid stimulation of the bowel.
   g. Omit gas-producing foods/fluids from diet.
   h. Administer/monitor enteral tube feedings as ordered.
2. Promote comfort/rest: provide good perineal care with frequent washing and adequate drying after each bowel movement; apply analgesic or protective ointment as needed; provide sitz baths as needed.
3. Provide care for the client with bowel surgery.

Ulcerative Colitis

A. General information

1. Inflammatory disorder of the bowel characterized by inflammation and ulceration that starts in the rectosigmoid area and spreads upward. The mucosa of the bowel becomes edematous, thickened with eventual scar formation. The colon consequently loses its elasticity and absorptive capabilities.
2. Occurs more often in women and the Jewish population, usually between ages 15 and 40.
3. Cause unknown; contributing factors include autoimmune factors, viral infection, allergies, emotional stress, insecurity.

B. Medical management

1. Mild to moderate form
   a. Low-roughage diet with no milk products
   b. Drug therapy (antimicrobials, corticosteroids, anticholinergics, antidiarrheals, immunosuppressives, hematinic agents)
2. Severe form: client kept NPO with IVs and electrolyte replacements, NG tube with suction, blood transfusions, surgery

C. Assessment findings

1. Severe diarrhea (15–20 liquid stools/day containing blood, mucus, and pus); severe tenesmus, weight loss, anorexia, weakness, crampy discomfort
2. Decreased skin turgor, dry mucous membranes
3. Low-grade fever, abdominal tenderness over the colon

4. Diagnostic tests
   a. Sigmoidoscopy reveals mucosa that bleeds easily with ulcer development
   b. Hgb and hct decreased

D. Nursing interventions: same as for Crohn's disease

Diverticulosis/Diverticulitis

A. General information
   1. A diverticulum is an outpouching of the intestinal mucosa, most commonly found in the sigmoid colon.
   2. *Diverticulosis:* multiple diverticula of the colon
   3. *Diverticulitis:* inflammation of the diverticula
   4. Men affected more often than women, more common in obese individuals; usually occurs between ages 40 and 45
   5. Caused by stress, congenital weakening of muscular fibers of intestine, and dietary deficiency of roughage and fiber

B. Medical management
   1. High-residue diet with no seeds for diverticulosis; low residue diet for diverticulitis
   2. Drug therapy: bulk laxatives, stool softeners, anticholinergics, antibiotics
   3. Surgery (rare): resection of diseased portion of colon with temporary colostomy may be indicated

C. Assessment findings
   1. Intermittent lower left quadrant pain and tenderness over rectosigmoid area
   2. Alternating constipation and diarrhea with blood and mucus
   3. Diagnostic tests
      a. Barium enema indicates an inflammatory process
      b. Hgb and hct decreased (if anemic)

D. Nursing interventions
   1. Administer medications as ordered.
   2. Provide nursing care for the client with bowel surgery.
   3. Provide client teaching and discharge planning concerning
      a. Importance of adhering to dietary regimen.
      b. Prevention of increased intraabdominal pressure.
      c. Signs and symptoms of peritonitis and need to notify physician immediately if they occur.

Cancer of the Colon/Rectum

A. General information
   1. Adenocarcinoma is the most common type of colon cancer and may spread by direct extension through the walls of the intestine or

NURSING ALERT

CEA is used to monitor the effectiveness of colorectal cancer therapy. It is useful for assessing the adequacy of a surgical resection; it is also called a tumor marker.

through the lymphatic or circulatory system. Metastasis is most often to the liver.

2. Second most common site for cancer in men and women; usually occurs between ages 50 and 60
3. May be caused by diverticulosis, chronic ulcerative colitis, familial polyposis

B. Medical management: chemotherapy, radiation therapy, bowel surgery

C. Assessment findings
   1. Alternating diarrhea/constipation, lower abdominal cramps, abdominal distension
   2. Weakness, anorexia, weight loss, pallor, dyspnea
   3. Diagnostic tests
      a. Stool for occult blood positive
      b. Hgb and hct decreased
      c. CEA positive
      d. Sigmoidoscopy reveals a mass
      e. Barium enema shows a colon mass
      f. Digital rectal exam indicates a palpable mass

D. Nursing interventions
   1. Administer chemotherapy agents as ordered, provide care for the client receiving chemotherapy.
   2. Provide care for the client receiving radiation therapy.
   3. Provide care for the client with bowel surgery.

Bowel Surgery

A. General information: type of surgery varies depending on location and extent of lesion; may be indicated in Crohn's disease, ulcerative colitis, intestinal obstructions, colon/rectal cancer.

B. Types: Table 9-2.

C. Nursing interventions common to all bowel surgery
   1. In addition to routine pre-op care
      a. Ensure adherence to dietary restrictions.
         1) offer clear liquids only on day before surgery.
         2) provide high-calorie, low-residue diet 3–5 days before surgery.
      b. Assist with bowel preparation.

TABLE 9-2 Bowel Surgeries

Type	Procedures
Abdominoperineal	Distal sigmoid colon, rectum, and anus resection are removed through a perineal incision and a permanent colostomy is created. Surgery of choice for cancer of the colon/rectum.
Ileostomy	Opening of the ileum onto the abdominal surface; most frequently done for treatment of ulcerative colitis, but may also be done for Crohn's disease.
Continent ileostomy (Kock's pouch)	An intra-abdominal reservoir with a nipple valve is formed from the distal ileum. The pouch acts as a reservoir for fecal material and is cleaned at regular intervals by insertion of a catheter.
Cecostomy	An opening between the cecum and the abdominal base temporarily diverts the fecal flow to rest the distal portion of the colon after some types of surgery.
Temporary colostomy	Usually located in the ascending or transverse colon; most often done to rest the bowel.
Double-barreled colostomy	The colon is resected and both ends are brought through the abdominal wall creating two stomas, a proximal and a distal; done most often for an obstruction or tumor in the descending or transverse colon.
Loop colostomy	Often a temporary procedure whereby a loop of bowel is brought out above the skin surface and held in place by a glass rod. There is one stoma but two openings, a proximal and a distal.
Permanent colostomy	Consists of a single stoma made when the distal portion of the bowel is removed; most often located in the sigmoid or descending colon.
Resection with anastomosis	Diseased part of the bowel is removed and remaining portions anastomosed, allowing elimination through the rectum.

1) administer antibiotics 3–5 days pre-op to decrease bacteria in intestine.
2) administer enemas (possibly with added antibiotics) to further cleanse the bowel.

c. Administer vitamins C and K (decreased by bowel cleansing) to prevent post-op complications.

2. In addition to routine post-op care
   a. Promote elimination.
      1) assess for signs of returning peristalsis.
      2) monitor characteristics of initial stools.
   b. Monitor and maintain fluid and electrolyte balance.

D. Additional nursing interventions specific to abdominoperineal resection
   1. Reinforce and change perineal dressings as needed.
   2. Record type, amount, color of drainage.
   3. Irrigate with normal saline or hydrogen peroxide.
   4. Provide warm sitz baths 4 times/day.
   5. Cover wound with dry dressing.

E. Additional nursing interventions specific to colostomy
   1. Prevent skin breakdown.
      a. Cleanse skin around stoma with mild soap and water and pat dry.
      b. Use a skin barrier to protect skin around the stoma.
      c. Assess skin regularly for irritation.
      d. Avoid the use of adhesives on irritated skin.
   2. Control odor, maintain pleasant environment.
      a. Change pouch/seal whenever necessary.
      b. Empty or clean bag frequently, and provide ventilation afterwards; use deodorizer in bag/room if needed.
      c. Avoid gas-producing foods.
   3. Promote adequate stomal drainage.
      a. Assess stoma for color and intactness.
      b. Expect mucoid/serosanguinous drainage during the first 24 hours, then liquid type.
      c. Assess for flatus indicating return of intestinal function.
      d. Monitor for changing consistency of fecal drainage.
   4. Irrigate colostomy as needed.
      a. Position client on toilet or in high-Fowler's if client on bed rest.
      b. Fill irrigation bag with desired amount of water (500–1000 ml) and hang bag so the bottom is at shoulder height.
      c. Remove air from tubing and lubricate the tip of the catheter or cone.
      d. Remove old pouch and clean skin and stoma with water.
      e. Gently dilate stoma and insert the irrigation catheter or cone snugly.

f. Open tubing and allow fluid to enter the bowel.
g. Remove catheter or cone and allow fecal contents to drain.
h. Observe and record amount and character of fecal return.

5. Promote adequate nutrition.
   a. Assess return of peristalsis.
   b. Advance diet as tolerated, add new foods gradually.
   c. Avoid constipating foods.
6. Provide at least 2500 ml liquid/day.
7. Encourage client to discuss concerns and feelings about surgery.
8. Provide client teaching and discharge planning concerning
   a. Recognition of complications and need to report immediately
      1) changes in odor, consistency, and color of stools
      2) bleeding from the stoma
      3) persistent constipation or diarrhea
      4) changes in the contour of the stoma
      5) persistent leakage around the stoma
      6) skin irritation despite treatment
   b. Proper procedure for colostomy irrigation.

Peritonitis

A. General information
   1. Local or generalized inflammation of part or all of the parietal and visceral surfaces of the abdominal cavity
   2. Initial response: edema, vascular congestion, hypermotility of the bowel and outpouring of plasmalike fluid from the extracellular, vascular, and interstitial compartments into the peritoneal space
   3. Later response: abdominal distension leading to respiratory compromise, hypovolemia results in decreased urinary output
   4. Intestinal motility gradually decreases and progresses to paralytic ileus
   5. Caused by trauma (blunt or penetrating), inflammation (ulcerative colitis, diverticulitis), volvulus, intestinal ischemia, or intestinal obstruction

B. Medical management
   1. NPO with fluid replacement
   2. Drug therapy: antibiotics to combat infection, analgesics for pain
   3. Surgery
      a. *Laparotomy:* opening made through the abdominal wall into the peritoneal cavity to determine the cause of peritonitis
      b. Depending on cause, bowel resection may be necessary

C. Assessment findings
   1. Severe abdominal pain, rebound tenderness, muscle rigidity, absent bowel sounds, abdominal distension (particularly if large bowel obstruction)
   2. Anorexia, nausea, and vomiting

3. Shallow respirations; decreased urinary output; weak, rapid pulse; elevated temperature
4. Diagnostic tests
   a. WBC elevated
   b. Hct elevated (if hemoconcentration)

D. Nursing interventions
1. Assess respiratory status for possible distress.
2. Assess characteristics of abdominal pain and changes over time.
3. Administer medications as ordered.
4. Perform frequent abdominal assessment.
5. Monitor and maintain fluid and electrolyte balance; monitor for signs of septic shock.
6. Maintain patency of NG or intestinal tubes.
7. Place client in Fowler's position to localize peritoneal contents.
8. Provide routine pre- and post-op care if surgery ordered.

Hemorrhoids

A. General information
1. Congestion and dilation of the veins of the rectum and anus; usually result from impairment of flow of blood through the venous plexus
2. May be internal (above the anal sphincter) or external (outside anal sphincter)
3. Most commonly occur between ages 20 and 50
4. Predisposing conditions include occupations requiring long periods of standing; increased intra-abdominal pressure caused by prolonged constipation, pregnancy, heavy lifting, obesity, straining at defecation; portal hypertension

B. Medical management
1. Stool softeners, local anesthetics, or anti-inflammatory creams
2. Diet modification: high fiber, adequate liquids
3. Hemorrhoidectomy: surgical excision of hemorrhoids indicated when there is prolapse, severe pain, and excessive bleeding

C. Assessment findings
1. Bleeding with defecation, hard stools with streaks of blood
2. Pain with defecation, sitting, or walking
3. Protrusion of external hemorrhoids upon inspection
4. Diagnostic tests
   a. Proctoscopy reveals presence of internal hemorrhoids
   b. Hgb and hct decreased if bleeding excessive, prolonged

D. Nursing interventions: preoperative
1. Prepare client for hemorrhoidectomy.
2. In addition to routine pre-op care, provide laxatives/enemas to promote cleansing of the bowel.

E. Nursing interventions: postoperative
   1. Provide routine post-op care.
   2. Assess for rectal bleeding: inspect rectal area/dressings every 2–3 hours and report significant increases in bloody drainage.
   3. Promote comfort.
      a. Assist client to side-lying or prone position, provide flotation pad when sitting.
      b. Administer analgesics as ordered and monitor effects.
   4. Promote elimination: administer stool softeners as ordered and, if possible, administer analgesic before first post-op bowel movement.
   5. Provide client teaching and discharge planning concerning
      a. Dietary modifications (high fiber and ingestion of at least 2000 ml/day)
      b. Need to defecate when urge is felt
      c. Use of stool softeners as needed until healing occurs
      d. Sitz baths after each bowel movement for at least 2 weeks after surgery
      e. Perineal care
      f. Recognition and reporting immediately to physician of the following signs and symptoms
         1) rectal bleeding
         2) continued pain on defecation
         3) puslike drainage from rectal area

DISORDERS OF THE LIVER

Hepatitis

A. General information
   1. Widespread inflammation of the liver tissue with liver cell damage due to hepatic cell degeneration and necrosis; proliferation and enlargement of the Kupffer cells; inflammation of the periportal areas (may cause interruption of bile flow)
   2. *Hepatitis A*
      a. Incubation period: 15–45 days
      b. Transmitted by fecal/oral route: often occurs in crowded living conditions; with poor personal hygiene; or from contaminated food, milk, water, or shellfish
   3. *Hepatitis B*
      a. Incubation period: 50–180 days
      b. Transmitted by blood and body fluids (saliva, semen, vaginal secretions): often from contaminated needles among IV drug abusers; intimate/sexual contact
   4. *Hepatitis C*
      a. Incubation period: 7–50 days
      b. Transmitted by parenteral route: through blood and blood products, needles, syringes

5. *Hepatitis D*
   a. Incubation period: 14–56 days
   b. Transmitted by blood and body fluids; seen in persons who have hepatitis B
6. *Hepatitis E*
   a. Incubation period: 15–64 days
   b. Transmitted by fecal/oral route; usually water-borne; seen in travelers returning from underdeveloped countries

B. Assessment findings
1. Preicteric stage
   a. Anorexia, nausea and vomiting, fatigue, constipation or diarrhea, weight loss
   b. Right upper quadrant discomfort, hepatomegaly, splenomegaly, lymphadenopathy
2. Icteric stage
   a. Fatigue, weight loss, light-colored stools, dark urine
   b. Continued hepatomegaly with tenderness, lymphadenopathy, splenomegaly
   c. Jaundice, pruritus
3. Posticteric stage
   a. Fatigue, but an increased sense of well-being
   b. Hepatomegaly gradually decreasing
4. Diagnostic tests
   a. Hepatitis A, B, C
      1) SGPT (ALT), SGOT (AST), alkaline phosphatase, bilirubin, ESR: all increased (preicteric)
      2) leukocytes, lymphocytes, neutrophils: all decreased (pericteric)
      3) prolonged PT
   b. Hepatitis A
      1) hepatitis A virus (HAV) in stool before onset of disease
      2) anti-HAV (IgG) appears soon after onset of jaundice; peaks in 1–2 months and persists indefinitely
      3) anti-HAV (IgM): positive in acute infection; lasts 4–6 weeks
   c. Hepatitis B
      1) HBsAg (surface antigen): positive, develops 4–12 weeks after infection
      2) anti-HBsAG: negative in 80% of cases
      3) anti-HBc: associated with infectivity, develops 2–16 weeks after infection
      4) HBeAg: associated with infectivity and disappears before jaundice
      5) anti-HBe: present in carriers, represents low infectivity
   d. Hepatitis C
      1) initial screening test enzyme-linked immunoabsorbent assay (ELISA) test

2) if ELISA test is positive and ALT is normal then recombinant immunoblot assay (RIBA) done
3) reverse transcription polymerase chain reaction (RT-PCR) test can pick up virus 2–3 weeks after exposure

e. Hepatitis D: rise in hepatitis D virus antibodies (anti-HDV) titer
f. Hepatitis E: testing usually done only for symptomatic persons who have traveled to high-risk areas; hepatitis E antibodies (anti-HEV) present

C. Nursing interventions
1. Promote adequate nutrition.
   a. Administer antiemetics as ordered, 30 minutes before meals to decrease occurrence of nausea and vomiting.
   b. Provide small, frequent meals of a high-carbohydrate, moderate- to high-protein, high-vitamin, high-calorie diet.
   c. Avoid very hot or very cold foods.
2. Ensure rest/relaxation: plan schedule for rest and activity periods, organize nursing care to minimize interruption.
3. Monitor/relieve pruritus (see Cirrhosis of the Liver).
4. Administer corticosteroids as ordered.
5. Institute isolation procedures as required; pay special attention to good hand-washing technique and adequate sanitation.
6. In hepatitis A administer immune serum globulin (ISG) early to exposed individuals as ordered.
7. In hepatitis B
   a. Screen blood donors for HBsAg.
   b. Use disposable needles and syringes.
   c. Instruct client/others to avoid sexual intercourse while disease is active.
   d. Administer ISG to exposed individuals as ordered.
   e. Administer hepatitis B immunoglobulin (HBIG) as ordered to provide temporary and passive immunity to exposed individuals.
   f. To produce active immunity, administer hepatitis B vaccine to those individuals at high risk.
8. In non-A, non-B: use disposable needles and syringes; ensure adequate sanitation.
9. Provide client teaching and discharge planning concerning
   a. Importance of avoiding alcohol
   b. Avoidance of persons with known infections
   c. Balance of activity and rest periods
   d. Importance of not donating blood
   e. Dietary modifications
   f. Recognition and reporting of signs of inadequate convalescence: anorexia, jaundice, increasing liver tenderness/discomfort
   g. Techniques/importance of good personal hygiene

Cirrhosis of the Liver

A. General information
   1. Chronic, progressive disease characterized by inflammation, fibrosis, and degeneration of the liver parenchymal cells
   2. Destroyed liver cells are replaced by scar tissue, resulting in architectural changes and malfunction of the liver
   3. Types
      a. *Laënnec's cirrhosis:* associated with alcohol abuse and malnutrition; characterized by an accumulation of fat in the liver cells, progressing to widespread scar formation.
      b. *Postnecrotic cirrhosis:* results in severe inflammation with massive necrosis as a complication of viral hepatitis.
      c. *Cardiac cirrhosis:* occurs as a consequence of right-sided heart failure; manifested by hepatomegaly with some fibrosis.
      d. *Biliary cirrhosis:* associated with biliary obstruction, usually in the common bile duct; results in chronic impairment of bile excretion.
   4. Occurs twice as often in men as in women; ages 40–60

B. Assessment findings
   1. Fatigue, anorexia, nausea and vomiting, indigestion, weight loss, flatulence, irregular bowel habits
   2. Hepatomegaly (early): pain located in the right upper quadrant; atrophy of liver (later); hard, nodular liver upon palpation; increased abdominal girth
   3. Changes in mood, alertness, and mental ability; sensory deficits; gynecomastia, decreased axillary and pubic hair in males; amenorrhea in young females
   4. Jaundice of the skin, sclera, and mucous membranes; pruritus
   5. Easy bruising, spider angiomas, palmar erythema
   6. Muscle atrophy
   7. Diagnostic tests
      a. SGOT (AST), SGPT (ALT), LDH alkaline phosphatase increased
      b. Serum bilirubin increased
      c. PT prolonged
      d. Serum albumin decreased
      e. Hgb and hct decreased

C. Nursing interventions
   1. Provide sufficient rest and comfort.
      a. Provide bed rest with bathroom privileges.
      b. Encourage gradual, progressive, increasing activity with planned rest periods.
      c. Institute measures to relieve pruritus.
         1) do not use soaps and detergents.
         2) bathe in tepid water followed by application of an emollient lotion.

3) provide cool, light, nonrestrictive clothing.
4) keep nails short to avoid skin excoriation from scratching.
5) apply cool, moist compresses to pruritic areas.

2. Promote nutritional intake.
   a. Encourage small frequent feedings.
   b. Promote a high-calorie, low- to moderate-protein, high-carbohydrate, low-fat diet, with supplemental vitamin therapy (vitamins A, B-complex, C, D, K, and folic acid).
3. Prevent infection.
   a. Prevent skin breakdown by frequent turning and skin care.
   b. Provide reverse isolation for clients with severe leukopenia; pay special attention to handwashing technique.
   c. Monitor WBC.
4. Monitor/prevent bleeding.
5. Administer diuretics as ordered.
6. Provide client teaching and discharge planning concerning
   a. Avoidance of agents that may be hepatotoxic (sedatives, opiates, or OTC drugs detoxified by the liver)
   b. How to assess for weight gain and increased abdominal girth
   c. Avoidance of persons with upper respiratory infections
   d. Recognition and reporting of signs of recurring illness (liver tenderness, increased jaundice, increased fatigue, anorexia)
   e. Avoidance of all alcohol
   f. Avoidance of straining at stool, vigorous blowing of nose and coughing, to decrease the incidence of bleeding

Ascites

A. General information
   1. Accumulation of free fluid in the abdominal cavity
   2. Most frequently caused by cirrhotic liver damage, which produces hypoalbuminemia, increased portal venous pressure, and hyperaldosteronism
   3. May also be caused by HF

B. Medical management
   1. Supportive: modify diet, bed rest, salt-poor albumin
   2. Diuretic therapy
   3. Surgery
      a. *Paracentesis:* insertion of a needle into the peritoneal cavity through the abdomen to remove abnormally large amounts of peritoneal fluid.
         1) peritoneal fluid assessed for cell count, specific gravity, protein, and microorganisms.
         2) used in clients with acute respiratory or abdominal distress secondary to ascites.

   b. *LeVeen shunt (peritoneal-venous shunt)*: used in chronic, unmanageable ascites
      1) permits continuous reinfusion of ascitic fluid back into the venous system through a silicone catheter with a one-way pressure-sensitive valve.
      2) one end of the catheter is implanted into the peritoneal cavity and is channeled through the subcutaneous tissue to the superior vena cava, where the other end of the catheter is implanted; the valve opens when pressure in the peritoneal cavity is 3–5 cm of water higher than in superior vena cava, thereby allowing ascitic fluid to flow into the venous system.

C. Assessment findings
   1. Anorexia, nausea and vomiting, fatigue, weakness, changes in mental functioning
   2. Positive fluid wave and shifting dullness on percussion, flat or protruding umbilicus, abdominal distension/tautness with striae and prominent veins, abdominal pain
   3. Peripheral edema, shortness of breath
   4. Diagnostic tests
      a. Potassium and serum albumin decreased
      b. PT prolonged
      c. LDH, SGOT (AST), SGPT (ALT), BUN, sodium increased

D. Nursing interventions
   1. Monitor nutritional status/provide adequate nutrition with modified diet.
      a. Restrict sodium to 200–500 mg/day.
      b. Restrict fluids to 1000–1500 ml/day.
      c. Promote high-calorie foods/snacks.
   2. Monitor/prevent increasing edema.
      a. Administer diuretics as ordered and monitor for effects.
      b. Measure I&O.
      c. Monitor peripheral pulses.
      d. Measure abdominal girth.
      e. Inspect/palpate extremities, sacrum.
      f. Administer salt-poor albumin to replace vascular volume.
   3. Monitor/promote skin integrity.
      a. Reposition frequently.
      b. Apply lotions to stretched areas.
      c. Assess for redness, breakdown.
   4. Promote comfort: place client in mid- to high-Fowler's and reposition frequently.
   5. Provide nursing care for the client undergoing paracentesis.
      a. Confirm that client has signed a consent form.
      b. Instruct client to empty bladder before the procedure to prevent inadvertent puncture of the bladder during insertion of trocar.

c. Inform client that a local anesthetic will be provided to decrease pain.
d. Place in sitting position to facilitate the flow of fluid by gravity.
e. Measure abdominal girth and weight before and after the procedure.
f. Record color, amount, and consistency of fluid withdrawn and client tolerance during procedure.
g. Assess insertion site for leakage.

6. Provide routine pre- and post-op care for the client with LeVeen shunt.

Esophageal Varices

A. General information
1. Dilation of the veins of the esophagus, caused by portal hypertension from resistance to normal venous drainage of the liver into the portal vein
2. Causes blood to be shunted to the esophagogastric veins, resulting in distension, hypertrophy, and increased fragility.
3. Caused by portal hypertension, which may be secondary to cirrhosis of the liver (alcohol abuse), swallowing poorly masticated food, increased intra-abdominal pressure

B. Medical management
1. Iced normal saline lavage
2. Transfusions with fresh whole blood
3. Vitamin K therapy
4. Sengstaken-Blakemore tube: a three-lumen tube used to control bleeding by applying pressure on the cardiac portion of the stomach and against bleeding esophageal varices. One lumen serves as NG suction, a second lumen is used to inflate the gastric balloon, the third to inflate the esophageal balloon.
5. Intra-arterial or IV vasopressin
6. Injection sclerotherapy
7. Surgery for portal hypertension (decompresses esophageal varices and helps to maintain optimal portal perfusion)
   a. Ligation of esophageal and gastric veins to stop acute bleeding
   b. *Portacaval shunt:* end-to-side or side-to-side anastomosis of the portal vein to the inferior vena cava
   c. *Splenorenal shunt:* end-to-side or side-to-side anastomosis of the splenic vein to the left renal vein
   d. *Mesocaval shunt:* end-to-side or use of a graft to anastomose the inferior vena cava to the side of the superior mesenteric vein

C. Assessment findings
1. Anorexia, nausea and vomiting, hematemesis, fatigue, weakness
2. Splenomegaly, increased splenic dullness, ascites, caput medusae, peripheral edema, bruits

3. Diagnostic tests
   a. PT prolonged
   b. Hematest of vomitus positive
   c. Serum albumin, RBC, Hgb, and hct decreased
   d. LDH, SGOT (AST), SGPT (ALT), BUN, increased

D. Nursing interventions
1. Monitor/provide care for client with Sengstaken-Blakemore tube.
   a. Facilitate placement of the tube: check and lubricate tip and elevate head of bed.
   b. Prevent dislodgment of the tube by placing client in semi-Fowler's position; maintain traction by securing the tube to a piece of sponge or foam rubber placed on the nose.
   c. Keep scissors at bedside at all times.
   d. Monitor respiratory status; assess for signs of distress and if respiratory distress occurs cut the tubing to deflate the balloons and remove tubing immediately.
   e. Label each lumen to avoid confusion; maintain prescribed amount of pressure on esophageal balloon and deflate balloon as ordered to avoid necrosis.
   f. Observe nares for skin breakdown and provide mouth and nasal care every 1–2 hours (encourage client to expectorate secretions, suction gently if unable).
2. Promote comfort: place client in semi-Fowler's position (if not in shock); provide mouth care.
3. Monitor for further bleeding and for signs and symptoms of shock; hematest all secretions.
4. Administer vasopressin as ordered and monitor effects.
5. Provide routine pre- and post-op care if the client has portasystemic or portacaval shunt.
6. Provide client teaching and discharge planning concerning
   a. Minimizing esophageal irritation (avoidance of salicylates, alcohol; use of antacids as needed; importance of chewing food thoroughly)
   b. Avoidance of increased abdominal, thoracic, and portal pressure
   c. Recognition and reporting of signs of hemorrhage

Hepatic Encephalopathy

A. General information
1. Frequent terminal complication in liver disease
2. Diseased liver is unable to convert ammonia to urea, so that large quantities remain in the systemic circulation and cross the blood/brain barrier, producing neurologic toxic symptoms.
3. Caused by cirrhosis, GI hemorrhage, hyperbilirubinemia, transfusions (particularly with stored blood), thiazide diuretics, uremia, dehydration

B. Assessment findings
   1. Early in course of disease: changes in mental functioning (irritability); insomnia, slowed affect; slow slurred speech; impaired judgment; slight tremor; Babinski's reflex, hyperactive reflexes
   2. Progressive disease: asterixis, disorientation, apraxia, tremors, fetor hepaticus, facial grimacing
   3. Late in disease: coma, absent reflexes
   4. Diagnostic tests
      a. Serum ammonia levels increased (particularly later)
      b. PT prolonged
      c. Hgb and hct decreased

C. Nursing interventions
   1. Conduct ongoing neurologic assessment and report deteriorations.
   2. Restrict protein in diet; provide high carbohydrate intake and vitamin K supplements.
   3. Administer enemas, cathartics, intestinal antibiotics, and lactulose as ordered to reduce ammonia levels.
   4. Protect client from injury: keep side rails up; provide eye care with use of artificial tears/eye patch.
   5. Avoid administration of drugs detoxified in liver (phenothiazines, gold compounds, methyldopa, acetaminophen).
   6. Maintain client on bed rest to decrease metabolic demands on liver.

Cancer of the Liver

A. General information
   1. Primary cancer of the liver is extremely rare, but it is a common site for metastasis because of liver's large blood supply and portal drainage. Primary cancers of the colon, rectum, stomach, pancreas, esophagus, breast, lung, and melanomas frequently metastasize to the liver.
   2. Enlargement, hemorrhage, and necrosis are common occurrences; primary liver tumors often metastasize to the lung.
   3. Higher incidence in men.
   4. Prognosis poor; disease well advanced before clinical signs evident.

B. Medical management
   1. Chemotherapy and radiotherapy (palliative) to decrease tumor size and pain
   2. Resection of liver segment or lobe if tumor is localized

C. Assessment findings
   1. Weakness, anorexia, nausea and vomiting, weight loss, slight increase in temperature
   2. Right upper quadrant discomfort/tenderness, hepatomegaly, blood-tinged ascites, friction rub over liver, peripheral edema, jaundice
   3. Diagnostic tests: same as cirrhosis of the liver plus

a. Blood sugar decreased
b. Alpha fetoprotein increased
c. Abdominal X-ray, liver scan, liver biopsy all positive

D. Nursing interventions: same as for cirrhosis of the liver plus
1. Provide emotional support for client/significant others regarding poor prognosis.
2. Provide care of the client receiving radiation therapy or chemotherapy.
3. Provide care of client with abdominal surgery plus
a. Preoperative
1) Perform bowel prep to decrease ammonium intoxication.
2) Administer vitamin K to decrease risk of bleeding.
b. Postoperative
1) Administer 10% glucose for first 48 hours to avoid rapid blood sugar drop.
2) Monitor for hyper/hypoglycemia.
3) Assess for bleeding (hemorrhage is most threatening complication).
4) Assess for signs of hepatic encephalopathy.

DISORDERS OF THE GALLBLADDER

Cholecystitis/Cholelithiasis

A. General information
1. Cholecystitis: acute or chronic inflammation of the gallbladder, most commonly associated with gallstones. Inflammation occurs within the walls of the gallbladder and creates a thickening accompanied by edema. Consequently, there is impaired circulation, ischemia, and eventual necrosis.
2. Cholelithiasis: formation of gallstones, cholesterol stones most common variety
3. Most often occurs in women after age 40, in postmenopausal women on estrogen therapy, in women taking oral contraceptives, and in the obese; Caucasians and Native Americans are also more commonly affected.
4. Stone formation may be caused by genetic defect of bile composition, gallbladder/bile stasis, infection.
5. Acute cholecystitis usually follows stone impaction, adhesions; neoplasms may also be implicated.

B. Medical management
1. Supportive treatment: NPO with NG intubation and IV fluids
2. Diet modification with administration of fat-soluble vitamins
3. Drug therapy
a. Narcotic analgesics (Demerol is drug of choice) for pain. Morphine sulfate is contraindicated because it causes spasms of the sphincter of Oddi.

   b. Anticholinergics (atropine) for pain. (Anticholinergics relax smooth muscle and open bile ducts.)
   c. Antiemetics
4. Surgery: cholecystectomy/choledochostomy

C. Assessment findings
1. Epigastric or right upper quadrant pain, precipitated by a heavy meal or occurring at night
2. Intolerance for fatty foods (nausea, vomiting, sensation of fullness)
3. Pruritus, easy bruising, jaundice, dark amber urine, steatorrhea
4. Diagnostic tests
   a. Direct bilirubin transaminase, alkaline phosphatase, WBC, amylase, lipase: all increased
   b. Oral cholecystogram (gallbladder series): positive for gallstone

D. Nursing interventions
1. Administer pain medications as ordered and monitor for effects.
2. Administer IV fluids as ordered.
3. Provide small, frequent meals of modified diet (if oral intake allowed).
4. Provide care to relieve pruritus.
5. Provide care for the client with a cholecystectomy or choledochostomy.

Cholecystectomy/Choledochostomy

A. General information
1. Cholecystectomy: removal of the gallbladder with insertion of a T-tube into the common bile duct if common bile duct exploration is performed
2. Choledochostomy: opening of common duct, removal of stone, and insertion of a T-tube
3. Cholecystectomy performed via laparoscopy for uncomplicated cases when client has not had previous abdominal surgery

B. Nursing interventions: routine preoperative care

C. Nursing interventions: postoperative
1. Provide routine post-op care.
2. Position client in semi-Fowler's or side-lying positions; reposition frequently.
3. Splint incision when turning, coughing, and deep breathing.
4. Maintain/monitor functioning of T-tube.
   a. Ensure that T-tube is connected to closed gravity drainage.
   b. Avoid kinks, clamping, or pulling of the tube.
   c. Measure and record drainage every shift.
   d. Expect 300–500 ml bile-colored drainage first 24 hours, then 200 ml/24 hours for 3–4 days.

   e. Monitor color of urine and stools (stools will be light colored if bile is flowing through T-tube but normal color should reappear as drainage diminishes).
   f. Assess for signs of peritonitis.
   g. Assess skin around T-tube; cleanse frequently and keep dry.
5. Provide client teaching and discharge planning concerning
   a. Adherence to dietary restrictions
   b. Resumption of ADL (avoid heavy lifting for at least 6 weeks; resume sexual activity as desired unless ordered otherwise by physician); clients having laparoscopy cholecystectomy usually resume normal activity within 2 weeks.
   c. Recognition and reporting of signs of complications (fever, jaundice, pain, dark urine, pale stools, pruritus)

Appendicitis

See page 499.

DISORDERS OF THE PANCREAS

Pancreatitis

A. General information
   1. An inflammatory process with varying degrees of pancreatic edema, fat necrosis, or hemorrhage
   2. Proteolytic and lipolytic pancreatic enzymes are activated in the pancreas rather than in the duodenum, resulting in tissue damage and autodigestion of the pancreas
   3. Occurs most often in the middle aged
   4. Caused by alcoholism, biliary tract disease, trauma, viral infection, penetrating duodenal ulcer, abscesses, drugs (steroids, thiazide diuretics, and oral contraceptives), metabolic disorders (hyperparathyroidism, hyperlipidemia)
B. Medical management
   1. Drug therapy
      a. Analgesics to relieve pain. Note: Morphine is contraindicated due to the spasmodic effects of opiates on the sphincter of Oddi, which will cause exacerbation of symptoms.
      b. Smooth-muscle relaxants (papaverine, nitroglycerin) to relieve pain
      c. Anticholinergics (atropine, propantheline bromide [Pro-Banthine]) to decrease pancreatic stimulation
      d. Antacids to decrease pancreatic stimulation
      e. H_2 antagonists, vasodilators, calcium gluconate
   2. Diet modification
   3. NPO (usually)
   4. Peritoneal lavage
   5. Dialysis

C. Assessment findings
  1. Pain located in left upper quadrant with radiation to back, flank, or substernal area; may be accompanied by difficulty breathing and is aggravated by eating
  2. Vomiting, shallow respirations (with pain), tachycardia, decreased or absent bowel sounds, abdominal tenderness with muscle guarding, positive Grey Turner's spots (ecchymoses on flanks) and positive Cullen's sign (ecchymoses of periumbilical area)
  3. Diagnostic tests
    a. Serum amylase and lipase, urinary amylase, blood sugar, lipid levels: all increased
    b. Serum calcium decreased
    c. CT scan shows enlargement of the pancreas

D. Nursing interventions
  1. Administer analgesics, antacids, anticholinergics as ordered, monitor effects.
  2. Withhold food/fluid and eliminate odor and sight of food from environment to decrease pancreatic stimulations.
  3. Maintain NG tube and assess for drainage.
  4. Institute nonpharmacologic measures to decrease pain.
    a. Assist client to positions of comfort (knee-chest; fetal position).
    b. Teach relaxation techniques and provide a quiet, restful environment.
  5. Provide client teaching and discharge planning concerning
    a. Dietary regimen when oral intake permitted
      1) high-carbohydrate, high-protein, low-fat diet
      2) eating small, frequent meals instead of three large ones
      3) avoiding caffeine products
      4) eliminating alcohol consumption
      5) maintaining relaxed atmosphere after meals
    b. Recognition and reporting of signs of complications
      1) continued nausea and vomiting
      2) abdominal distension with increasing fullness
      3) persistent weight loss
      4) severe epigastric or back pain
      5) frothy/foul-smelling bowel movements
      6) irritability, confusion, persistent elevation of temperature (2 days)

Cancer of the Pancreas

A. General information
  1. Most pancreatic tumors are adenocarcinomas and half occur in the head of the pancreas
  2. Tumor growth results in common bile duct obstruction with jaundice

3. Occurs more often in men and in the African American and Jewish populations; ages 45–65
4. Contributing factors: chemical carcinogens, cigarette smoking, high-fat diet, diabetes mellitus
5. Prognosis generally poor

B. Medical management
1. Radiation therapy
2. Whipple's procedure (pancreatoduodenectomy): resection of the proximal pancreas, adjoining duodenum, distal portion of the stomach, and distal segment of the common bile duct
3. Drug therapy
   a. Pancreatic enzymes; oral hypoglycemic agents or insulin, bile salts necessary after surgery
   b. Chemotherapy may also be used

C. Assessment findings
1. Anorexia; rapid, progressive weight loss; dull abdominal pain located in upper abdomen or left hypochondriacal region with radiation to the back, related to eating; jaundice
2. Diagnostic tests
   a. Increased serum lipase (early)
   b. Increased bilirubin (conjugated)
   c. Increased serum amylase

D. Nursing interventions
1. See Pancreatitis.
2. Provide care for the client receiving radiation therapy or chemotherapy.
3. Routine pre- and post-op care (for clients undergoing Whipple's procedure).
4. Provide emotional support to client/significant others.
5. Provide client teaching and discharge planning concerning
   a. Need to eat small frequent meals of a low-fat, high-calorie diet with vitamin supplements.
   b. Importance of adhering to medication regimen after surgery.

REVIEW QUESTIONS

1. An adult client has a nasogastric tube in place to maintain gastric decompression. Which nursing action will relieve discomfort in the nostril with the NG tube?
   1. Remove any tape and loosely pin the tube to his gown.
   2. Lubricate the NG tube with viscous xylocaine.

3. Loop the NG tube to avoid pressure on the nares.
4. Replace the NG tube with a smaller diameter tube.

2. An adult client has just returned to his room following a bowel resection and end-to-end anastomosis. The nurse can expect the drainage from the NG tube in the early post-op period to be
   1. clear.
   2. mucoid.
   3. scant.
   4. discolored.

3. A 23-year-old man with a long history of ulcerative colitis is experiencing an exacerbation of the disease and is admitted with severe diarrhea, electrolyte disturbances, and severe abdominal pain. He questions the nurse about his prognosis. The best response to this inquiry is
   1. Ask your physician.
   2. It is rarely fatal.
   3. It depends on the form of the disease.
   4. You sound concerned.

4. The physician inserts a central venous catheter; the nurse should assist the client to assume which of the following positions?
   1. Supine.
   2. Trendelenburg.
   3. Reverse Trendelenburg.
   4. High-Fowler's.

5. A 35-year-old man has a history of peptic ulcer disease. He has had numerous bleeding episodes in the past and is admitted to the hospital for evaluation. His physician has prescribed cimetidine (Tagamet). The nurse recognizes that the primary reason this client is taking Tagamet is that it
   1. blocks the secretion of gastric hydrochloric acid.
   2. coats the gastric mucosa with a protective membrane.
   3. increases the sensitivity of H_2 receptors.
   4. releases basal gastric acid.

6. An adult has a Billroth II procedure and does well postoperatively. The nurse knows the client understands discharge teaching when the client recognizes that symptoms of dizziness, sweating, and weakness in the weeks following the surgery are usually associated with
   1. afferent loop syndrome.
   2. dumping syndrome.

3. pernicious anemia.
4. marginal ulcers.

7. A 56-year-old man has had a significant problem with alcohol abuse for the past 15 years. His wife brings him to the emergency department because he is increasingly confused and is coughing blood. His medical diagnosis is cirrhosis of the liver. He has ascites and esophageal varices. This client is least likely to have
   1. bulging flanks.
   2. protruding umbilicus.
   3. abdominal distension.
   4. bluish discoloration of the umbilicus.
8. The major dietary treatment for ascites calls for
   1. high protein.
   2. increased potassium.
   3. restricted fluids.
   4. restricted sodium.
9. Which laboratory value would the nurse expect to find in a client as a result of liver failure?
   1. Decreased serum creatinine.
   2. Decreased sodium.
   3. Increased ammonia.
   4. Increased calcium.
10. A man is admitted with bleeding esophageal varices. A Sengstaken-Blakemore tube is inserted in an effort to stop the bleeding. After the Sengstaken-Blakemore tube is inserted, the client has difficulty breathing. Based on this information, the first action the nurse should take is to
    1. deflate the esophageal balloon.
    2. encourage him to take deep breaths.
    3. monitor his vital signs.
    4. notify the physician.
11. A 35-year-old is scheduled for a esophagoduo-denoscopy. In planning for his postprocedural care, the nurse recognizes that the *most effective* nursing action for preventing respiratory complications is to
    1. keep the client positioned on his left side for 8–10 hours.
    2. assess for a gag reflex before offering the client anything to eat or drink.

3. provide throat lozenges for complaints of a sore throat.
4. position the client in high Fowler's until he is fully awake and alert.

12. A 52-year-old is being evaluated for cancer of the colon. In preparing the client for a barium enema, the nurse can expect that the client will be

1. placed on a low-residue diet 1 to 2 days before the study.
2. given an oil retention enema the morning of the study.
3. instructed to swallow six radiopaque tablets the evening before the study.
4. positioned in a high Fowler's position immediately following the procedure.

13. A 45-year-old complains of excessive weight loss and anorexia. Laboratory studies show that he is anemic. Hepatocellular carcinoma is suspected. A liver biopsy is performed at the bedside. The nurse can expect that after the procedure the client will be

1. encouraged to ambulate to prevent the formation of venous thrombosis.
2. asked to turn, cough, and deep breathe every 2 hours for the next 8 hours.
3. placed in a high Fowler's position to maximize thoracic expansion.
4. positioned on his right side with a pillow under the costal margin, and immobile for several hours.

14. A client has a fecal impaction. The physician orders an oil-retention enema followed by a cleansing enema. The nurse would administer the oil-retention enema initially to

1. lubricate the walls of the intestinal tract.
2. soften the fecal mass and lubricate the walls of the rectum and colon.
3. reduce bacterial content of the fecal mass.
4. coat the walls of the intestines to prevent irritation by the hardened fecal mass.

15. A 30-year-old has amyotrophic lateral sclerosis. His neurologic status has continued to deteriorate. He is receiving enteral feedings through a gastrostomy tube. The nurse recognizes that the *priority* assessment before administering a bolus feeding is

1. check the expiration date of the prepared enteral feeding.
2. confirm the presence of a gag reflex.
3. check placement of feeding tube.
4. review laboratory studies for indications of electrolyte imbalances.

16. An adult is 8 hours post-op a Billroth II (gastric resection) for an intractable gastric ulcer. The drainage from his nasogastric decompression tube is thickened and the volume of secretions has dramatically reduced in the last 2 hours. The client complains that he feels like he is going to vomit. The *most* appropriate nursing action is to

    1. reposition the nasogastric tube by advancing it gently.
    2. notify the physician of your findings.
    3. irrigate the nasogastric tube with 50 ml of sterile normal saline.
    4. discontinue the low-intermittent suctioning.

17. A 47-year-old is receiving chemotherapy for cancer of the liver. Her physician has prescribed metoclopramide for the nausea and vomiting associated with the chemotherapy. Metoclopramide has anticholinergic and extrapyramidal side effects. The nurse recognizes that these side effects put the client at high risk for

    1. hyperglycemia related to increased gastric emptying.
    2. injury related to decreased visual acuity and ataxia.
    3. decreased cardiac output related to reduced heart rate.
    4. fluid volume deficit related to frequent episodes of diarrhea.

18. An adult develops diarrhea secondary to hyperosmolar enteral therapy. The care plan now includes giving the client water every 4 to 6 hours and after feedings. Which of the following findings would indicate that fluid therapy was effective?

    1. Dry mucous membranes.
    2. Hyperactive bowel sounds.
    3. Increased urinary output.
    4. Hypokalemia.

19. An elderly client complains of frequent episodes of constipation. An effective strategy for preventing constipation is

    1. reducing fluid intake to encourage bulk formation in the intestinal lumen.
    2. use of laxatives daily to establish a regular elimination pattern.
    3. a regimen of exercises directed at toning the abdominal muscles.
    4. setting a routine for bowel elimination just before bedtime.

20. A 55-year-old is scheduled for a resection of the lower thoracic esophagus to remove a malignant tumor. In planning for postoperative care, the nurse would expect to

1. keep the client in a supine position to encourage thoracic expansion.
2. carefully advance the nasogastric tube past the anastomosis site.
3. frequently assess the client's breath sounds.
4. provide a regular diet high in protein.

21. A 46-year-old client has been experiencing frequent episodes of "heartburn" and regurgitation of acrid, sour-tasting fluid. These episodes tend to occur especially after a heavy meal. The client is diagnosed with a hiatal hernia. The nurse knows that the client had a good understanding of her treatment regimen when she states she will
    1. elevate her legs when she is sleeping.
    2. increase the roughage in her diet.
    3. drink more fluids with her meals.
    4. avoid caffeine, alcohol, and chocolate.
22. A 35-year-old stockbroker has recently been diagnosed with peptic ulcer disease. Diagnostic studies confirm the presence of the gram-negative bacteria *Helicobacter pylori* in his gastrointestinal tract. If the client has a duodenal ulceration, the nurse would expect him to describe the "ulcer pain" as
    1. located in the upper right epigastric area radiating to his right shoulder or back.
    2. relieved by vomiting.
    3. occurring 2 to 3 hours after a meal, often awakening him between 1:00 and 2:00 A.M.
    4. worsening with the ingestion of food.
23. A 42-year-old has been diagnosed with peptic ulcer disease. Her medication regimen includes misoprostol. The nurse understands that misoprostol exerts its therapeutic effect by
    1. neutralizing excess gastric acid.
    2. inhibiting gastric acid production.
    3. increasing mucous production and bicarbonate levels.
    4. increasing gastric emptying time.
24. A 56-year-old has Billroth II (gastrojejunostomy) for intractable peptic ulcer disease. The nurse is instructing the client concerning the potential complication of dumping syndrome. The nurse can expect that the client's dietary and activity instructions would include
    1. a high carbohydrate diet.
    2. exercise after mealtime to promote the digestive process.

3. limit drinking fluids with meals.
4. a protein-restricted diet.

25. A 45-year-old underwent a total gastrectomy for gastric cancer. The nurse has been giving the client post-op instructions about his diet, activities, and medications. Which of the following statements indicates that he understands his post-op care?
    1. "I should take a walk after meals to aid my digestion."
    2. "Drinking more water with my meals will prevent indigestion."
    3. "I need more carbohydrates in my diet for an extra energy source."
    4. "The visiting nurse will come monthly to give an injection of vitamin B_{12}."
26. A 72-year-old has a direct inguinal hernia. The nurse caring for the client should be alert for
    1. hypoactive bowel sounds.
    2. passage of semi-liquid, brown stools.
    3. vomiting of bile-stained gastric contents.
    4. complaints of constant, localized abdominal pain.
27. An adult has developed peritonitis related to a perforated duodenal ulceration. During the nursing assessment, the nurse would expect to find
    1. decreased or absent bowel sounds.
    2. colicky abdominal pain.
    3. high-pitched bowel sounds.
    4. alternating episodes of constipation and diarrhea.
28. A nursing diagnosis appropriate for a client who has ulcerative colitis is
    1. abdominal pain, related to decreased peristalsis.
    2. diarrhea related to hyperosmolar intestinal contents.
    3. excess fluid volume related to increased water absorption by intestinal mucosa.
    4. activity intolerance related to fatigue.
29. The nurse is caring for a 26-year-old recently diagnosed with ulcerative colitis. The nurse has been giving dietary instructions to help prevent exacerbation of his inflammatory bowel disease. Which dietary choice indicates that the client understands the dietary instructions?
    1. apple.
    2. celery.

3. refined cereals.
4. hard cheeses.

30. When a client is diagnosed with ulcerative colitis, the nurse should be alert for the complication of

1. intestinal obstruction.
2. toxic megacolon.
3. malnutrition from malabsorption.
4. fistula formation.

31. A client with diverticulosis is admitted to the hospital. The nurse can expect that this client will be placed on

1. a bland, low residue diet.
2. a low protein, high carbohydrate diet.
3. a soft, but high fiber diet.
4. saline cathartics to increase intestinal peristalsis.

32. An adult has been diagnosed with colon cancer. The nursing assessment would *most* likely reveal

1. epigastric pain that intensifies when the stomach is empty.
2. stools that are fatty and foul-smelling.
3. alternating episodes of diarrhea and constipation.
4. a rigid, board-like abdomen.

33. The nurse has been instructing a client regarding identifying and alleviating the risk factors associated with colon cancer. The nurse recognizes that the client has a good understanding of the means to reduce the chances of colon cancer when he states,

1. "I will exercise daily."
2. "I will include more red meat in my diet."
3. "I will have an annual chest X-ray."
4. "I will include more fresh fruits and vegetables in my diet."

34. An adult has a sigmoid colostomy. The nurse is performing peristomal skin care and changing the stoma pouch. The most appropriate nursing action is to

1. empty the ostomy pouch when it is full.
2. pull flange and pouch off together to prevent spillage of stomach pouch contents.

3. leave ¼ inch of skin exposed around stoma when determining size to cut new skin barrier.
4. apply liquid deodorant to mucous membrane of protruding stoma.

35. An adult has a double-barreled, transverse colostomy. The nurse has formulated the nursing diagnosis: risk for impaired skin integrity related to irritation of the peristomal skin by the effluent. The *most* appropriate nursing action relevant to this nursing diagnosis is
    1. strict measurement and recording of intake and output.
    2. assessing for bowel sounds when changing ostomy appliance.
    3. wash peristomal skin with an astringent solution to reduce bacterial contamination.
    4. apply skin barrier before applying flange and ostomy pouch.

36. An adult is brought to the emergency room with severe, constant, localized abdominal pain. Abdominal muscles are rigid and rebound tenderness is present. Peritonitis is suspected. The client is hypotensive and tachycardiac. The nursing diagnosis *most* appropriate to the signs/symptoms is
    1. deficient fluid volume related to depletion of intravascular volume.
    2. disturbed thought process related to toxic effects of elevated ammonia levels.
    3. abdominal pain related to increased intestinal peristalsis.
    4. imbalanced nutrition, less than body requirements, related to malabsorption.

37. A 28-year-old has had a hemorrhoidectomy. The nurse recognizes that the client understands post-op discharge instructions when she states that she will
    1. reduce her fluid intake for several weeks after her surgery.
    2. include more fresh fruits and vegetables in her diet.
    3. vigorously clean her perianal area with soap and water after every bowel movement.
    4. limit her activities to bed rest for at least 6 hours a day.

38. The client with hepatitis may be anicteric and symptomless. The nurse recognizes that if symptoms are present early in the hepatic inflammatory disorder, the *most likely* symptom/sign is
    1. dark urine.
    2. ascites.

3. occult blood in stools.
4. anorexia.

39. A 22-year-old visits her physician with flu-like symptoms that have persisted for nearly a month. She complains of headaches, malaise, anorexia, and fever. She is a childcare worker at a local daycare center with children ranging in ages from 6 months to 5 years. Based on the associated risk factors and mode of transmission, the nurse recognizes that the client is most likely experiencing

1. hepatitis A.
2. hepatitis B.
3. hepatitis C.
4. hepatitis D.

40. A 25-year-old laboratory technician in a community health clinic has been experiencing fatigue, headaches, diminished appetite, and a yellowish discoloration of sclera for the past 2 months. He is diagnosed with hepatitis B and asks the nurse how he contracted hepatitis. The nurse's *most* appropriate response is

1. airborne droplets carry the infectious hepatitis B virus.
2. the hepatitis B virus is transmitted parenterally and through intimate contact.
3. an individual may contract hepatitis B by using contaminated eating utensils.
4. hepatitis B may be transmitted through eating shellfish from contaminated water sources.

41. A 56-year-old client with hepatic cirrhosis related to 10-year history of alcohol abuse is at risk for injury related to portal hypertension. The *most* appropriate nursing action to decrease his risk of injury is

1. keep his fingernails short.
2. offer small, frequent feedings.
3. observe stools for color and consistency.
4. assess for jaundice of skin and sclera.

42. A 52-year-old is diagnosed with Laennec's cirrhosis. He has massive ascites formation. His respirations are rapid and shallow. The physician decides to perform a paracentesis. The nurse caring for the client during the procedure gives the *highest priority* to

1. gathering the appropriate sterile equipment.
2. labeling samples of abdominal fluid and sending them to the laboratory.

3. positioning the client upright on the edge of the bed.
4. measuring and recording blood pressure and pulse frequently during the procedure.

43. An adult who has a 7-year history of hepatic cirrhosis was brought to the emergency room because he began vomiting large amounts of dark-red blood. A Sengstaken-Blakemore tube was inserted to tamponade the bleeding esophageal varices. While the balloon tamponade is in place, the nurse caring for him gives the highest priority to
    1. assessing his stools for occult blood.
    2. evaluating capillary refill in extremities.
    3. performing frequent mouth care.
    4. auscultating breath sounds.

44. A 52-year-old is experiencing advanced hepatic cirrhosis now complicated by hepatic encephalopathy. He is confused, restless, and demonstrating asterixis. The nurse has formulated the nursing diagnosis: disturbed thought processes related to
    1. massive ascites formation.
    2. increased serum ammonia levels.
    3. fluid volume excess.
    4. altered clotting mechanism.

45. A 45-year-old has choledocholithiasis. During the nursing admission, the nurse notes that the client's sclera and skin are jaundiced. He also complains of abdominal distention and pain, which he is *most likely* to describe as
    1. an intermittent, colicky pain in his left flank.
    2. pain which awakens him during the night, and is relieving by eating.
    3. a vise-like pressure over his sternum.
    4. right upper quadrant pain that often radiates to his right shoulder.

46. A 40-year-old is admitted to the hospital for acute cholecystitis. She is now 6 hours post-op abdominal cholecystectomy with a choledochostomy and has a T-tube in place. The nurse understands that proper management of the T-tube includes
    1. hanging the T-tube drainage below the bed.
    2. notifying the physician if T-tube drainage is 75 ml for the first 24 hours after surgery.
    3. irrigating the T-tube with sterile normal saline q2h to prevent obstruction.
    4. clamping the T-tube if the client develops sudden, severe abdominal pain.

47. A 40-year-old has experienced repeated episodes of acute pancreatitis. He has continued to consume alcohol. The nurse observes that he is doubled-over, rocking back-and-forth in pain. The nurse understands that morphine and morphine derivatives are contraindicated for the pain associated with acute pancreatitis because

1. it causes severe respiratory depression.

2. depression of GI peristalsis may cause constipation.

3. spasms of the sphincter of Oddi may occur.

4. it is rapidly metabolized by the liver.

48. A 56-year-old has a 5-year history of alcohol abuse. He appears acutely ill. He is vomiting bile-stained emesis. The nurse notes signs of severe, hemorrhagic pancreatitis that is accurately documented as

1. the presence of a positive fluid wave in the abdominal area.

2. a yellowish color of the sclera and skin.

3. ecchymosis in the flank and around the umbilical area.

4. bloody, foul-smelling stools.

49. A 66-year-old with a 10-year history of alcohol abuse has recently been diagnosed with chronic pancreatitis. The physician has prescribed pancrelipase, a pancreatic enzyme replacement. The nurse will recognize that the client understands his medication regimen when he states,

1. "I will take this medication with a glass of milk."

2. "If my stools appear yellowish with a foul odor, I will call my doctor."

3. "I will take my medication with some antacid so it will not bother my stomach."

4. "I will be sure to thoroughly chew the capsule contents before swallowing the medication."

50. A 60-year-old has been diagnosed with a malignant tumor of the head of the pancreas. A pancreatoduodenectomy (Whipple's procedure) was done to resect the tumor. The nurse recognizes that hemorrhage is a potentially major complication of a Whipple procedure. Which of the following assessment findings suggest this complication?

1. Jaundice of the skin and sclera.

2. Hyperglycemia.

3. Oliguria.

4. Bradycardia.

ANSWERS AND RATIONALES

1. 3. Looping the NG tube will prevent pressure on the nares that can cause pain and eventual necrosis.
2. 4. The drainage following abdominal surgery is discolored as it is evacuating stomach and intestinal contents, not mucoid material.
3. 4. The nurse should explore the client's motivation for posing the question and establish this current knowledge.
4. 2. The client is placed in Trendelenburg position to aid in the filling of the subclavian veins.
5. 1. Cimetidine (Tagemet) is a histamine antagonist that blocks the secretion of hydrochloric acid.
6. 2. Signs of dumping syndrome include vertigo, pallor, sweating, palpitations, and weakness. Dumping syndrome occurs after a gastric resection because ingested foods rapidly enter the jejunum without proper mixing and without the normal duodenal processing. It subsides in 6–12 months.
7. 4. Bluish discoloration of the umbilicus (Cullen's sign) is present in massive gastrointestinal hemorrhage resulting from free blood present in the abdomen. This is not consistent with cirrhosis of the liver.
8. 4. Sodium restriction is most important for a client with cirrhosis because fluid retention contributes to ascites.
9. 3. Increased ammonia levels could be seen because ammonia is a by-product of protein metabolism, and a diseased liver is unable to convert ammonia into urea to be excreted in the urine.
10. 1. If the client's airway is obstructed by the Sengstaken-Blakemore tube, the esophageal balloon must be deflated so the client can breathe.
11. 2. The client's throat is sprayed with a local anesthetic agent. Until the anesthetic agent wears off, the client is at high risk for aspiration.
12. 1. A low-residue diet 1 to 2 days before the study aids in evacuating the lower intestinal tract of all fecal matter.
13. 4. The client experiencing a liver biopsy is at risk for bleeding or hemorrhage related to penetration of the liver capsule. Positioning on the right side acts as a tamponade against the puncture site discouraging bleeding from the site.
14. 2. Oil retention enemas are given to soften the hardened fecal mass and lubricate the walls of the rectum and colon. Cleansing enemas stimulate intestinal peristalsis, thus eliminating the softened fecal mass.

15. 3. A client with altered central nervous system functioning is at high risk for aspiration. Checking for the placement of the feeding tube using several different methods, i.e., aspiration of gastric contents for residual volume, determining pH of aspirated gastric contents, and auscultating for gurgling sounds with injection of air bolus, is the priority nursing assessment to ensure client safety.

16. 2. The nasogastric tube for gastric decompression after a gastric resection is never irrigated without a specific order from the physician. Irrigating the nasogastric tube may rupture the suture line and hemorrhaging may occur.

17. 2. Metoclopramide blocks dopamine receptors in the chemoreceptor trigger zone (CTZ). This action results in the extrapyramidal and anticholinergic side effects that include sedation, dilated pupils and parkinsonian effects.

18. 3. Increased urinary output is related to the resolved dehydration state. Adding fluid to the enteral feedings reduced the osmolarity of the gastrointestinal contents.

19. 3. Exercises to strengthen the abdominal muscles are appropriate to aiding the defecation process.

20. 3. Surgical resection of the esophagus has a relatively high mortality rate related to pulmonary complications.

21. 4. These substances aggravate the episodes of heartburn (pyrosis) and gastroesophageal reflux.

22. 3. Duodenal ulcer pain characteristically occurs 2 to 3 hours after a meal, often awakening the client in the very early morning hours.

23. 3. Misoprostol, a synthetic prostaglandin, is a cytoprotective agent. By increasing mucous production and bicarbonate levels, the mucosal barrier better resists the erosive action of the gastric acid-pepsin complex.

24. 3. Fluids with meals cause rapid emptying of the gastric contents. Fluids with meals should be limited.

25. 4. A total gastrectomy results in a loss of intrinsic factor, which is necessary for the absorption of vitamin B_{12}.

26. 3. A direct inguinal hernia is most likely to cause a small bowel obstruction. Therefore, the nurse must monitor closely for the signs/symptoms of a small bowel mechanical obstruction, including vomiting of bile-stained gastric contents from reverse peristalsis.

27. 1. A paralytic ileus is related to disturbance of the neural stimulation of the bowel. There is decreased or absence of bowel sounds.

28. 4. Anorexia, weight loss, fever, vomiting, and blood loss are conditions that will cause the client to become easily fatigued. Activities are planned or restricted to conserve energy.

29. 3. Oral fluids and a low-residue, high-protein, and high-calorie diet are prescribed to meet nutritional requirements.

30. 2. Toxic megacolon is a serious complication of ulcerative colitis. Excessive dilation of the colon may lead to intestinal perforation and death.

31. 3. A soft, high-fiber diet is indicated to increase the bulk of the stool, thereby promoting defecation. Fluid intake of 2 L/day is recommended unless otherwise contraindicated. Seeds are not allowed.

32. 3. A change in bowel habits such as alternating episodes of diarrhea and constipation is a common manifestation of colon cancer.

33. 4. A diet low in fiber is a major risk factor for colon cancer. Fresh fruits and vegetables increase the fiber content of the diet, thereby, reducing the risk of colon cancer.

34. 3. Leaving ¼ inch of skin exposed around stoma when determining size to cut skin barrier prevents trauma to stoma.

35. 4. A skin barrier applied helps prevent enzymatic activity, which is a risk for peristomal skin breakdown.

36. 1. Hypovolemia occurs because massive amounts of fluid and electrolytes move from intestinal lumen into peritoneal cavity and deplete intravascular volume. Hypotension and tachycardia are manifestations of this massive fluid shift.

37. 2. Post-hemorrhoidectomy diet is modified to include increased fluid and fiber intake. This promotes regular bowel elimination and reduces the occurrence of constipation.

38. 4. Anorexia is often an early and severe symptom of hepatitis.

39. 1. Hepatitis A is transmitted through the fecal-oral route. Childcare workers are in a high risk group because of potentially poor hygiene/sanitation practices.

40. 2. Hepatitis B is transmitted parenterally or through intimate sexual contact with a carrier.

41. 3. Portal hypertension puts the client at risk for injury related to bleeding/hemorrhaging esophageal varices. Monitoring stools permits early detection of bleeding in the GI tract.

42. 4. A serious complication of a paracentesis is hypovolemic shock or vascular collapse. Early detection of this cardiovascular complication through monitoring blood pressure and pulse is a nursing priority intervention.

43. 4. Airway obstruction and aspiration of gastric contents are potential serious complications of balloon tamponade. Frequent assessment of the client's respiratory status is the priority.

44. 2. Hepatic cirrhosis leads to elevated serum ammonia levels, which have an adverse toxic effect on cerebral metabolism.

45. 4. Pain related to gallstones in the common duct is located in the right upper quadrant and often radiates to the right shoulder or back.

46. 2. The T-tube usually drains 200–500 ml in the first 24 hours. Decreased bile drainage may indicate an obstruction to bile flow or bile may be leaking into the peritoneum.

47. 3. Morphine sulfate causes spasms of the sphincter of Oddi, which will exacerbate the episode of acute pancreatitis.

48. 3. Bruising (ecchymosis) in the flank and umbilical area is known as Cullen's sign, which indicates severe, hemorrhagic pancreatitis.

49. 2. The presence of steatorrhea indicates that the dosage of pancrelipase needs to be adjusted.

50. 3. Oliguria is a primary sign of hypovolemic shock related to hemorrhage.

10

The Genitourinary System

■ OVERVIEW OF ANATOMY AND PHYSIOLOGY

The genitourinary system includes the kidneys, ureters, urinary bladder, urethra, and the male and female genitalia. This section discusses only the male genitalia; the female reproductive system is covered in Unit 6.

CHAPTER OUTLINE

Urinary System

Kidneys

See Figure 10-1.

A. Two bean-shaped organs that lie in the retroperitoneal space on either side of the vertebral column; adrenal glands located on top of each kidney

B. *Renal parenchyma*

1. Cortex: outermost layer; site of glomeruli and proximal and distal tubules of nephron
2. Medulla: middle layer; formed by collecting tubules and ducts

C. *Renal sinus and pelvis*

1. Papillae: projections of renal tissues located at the tips of the renal pyramids
2. Calices
    - **a.** Minor calyx: collects urine flow from collecting duct
    - **b.** Major calyx: directs urine from renal sinus to renal pelvis
3. Urine flows from renal pelvis to ureters

D. *Nephron:* the functional unit of the kidney (Figure 10-2)

1. Renal corpuscle (vascular system of nephron)
    - **a.** Bowman's capsule: a portion of the proximal tubule, surrounds the glomerulus
    - **b.** Glomerulus: a capillary network permeable to water, electrolytes, nutrients, and wastes; impermeable to large protein molecules

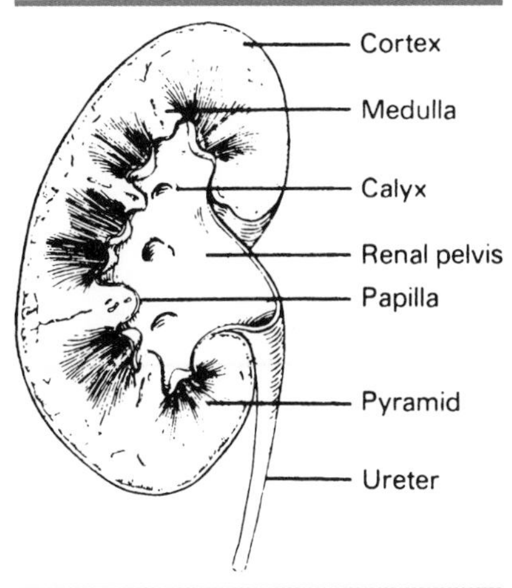

FIGURE 10-1 Anatomy of the kidney

2. Renal tubule: divided into proximal convoluted tubule, descending loop of Henle, ascending loop of Henle, distal convoluted tubule, and collecting duct

Ureters

A. Two tubes approximately 25–35 cm long
B. Extend from the renal pelvis to the pelvic cavity, where they enter the bladder, convey urine from the kidneys to the bladder
C. Ureterovesical valve prevents backflow of urine into ureters

Bladder

A. Located behind the symphysis pubis; composed of muscular, elastic tissue that makes it distensible
B. Serves as a reservoir of urine (capable of holding 1000–1800 ml; moderately full bladder usually holds about 500 ml)
C. Internal and external urethral sphincters control the flow of urine; urge to void stimulated by passage of urine past the internal sphincter (involuntary) to the upper part of the urethra. Relaxation of external sphincter (voluntary) produces emptying of the bladder (voiding, micturition).

Urethra

A. A small tube that extends from the bladder to the exterior of the body
B. In females, located behind the symphysis pubis and anterior to the vagina; approximately 3–5 cm long
C. In males, extends the entire length of the penis; approximately 20 cm long

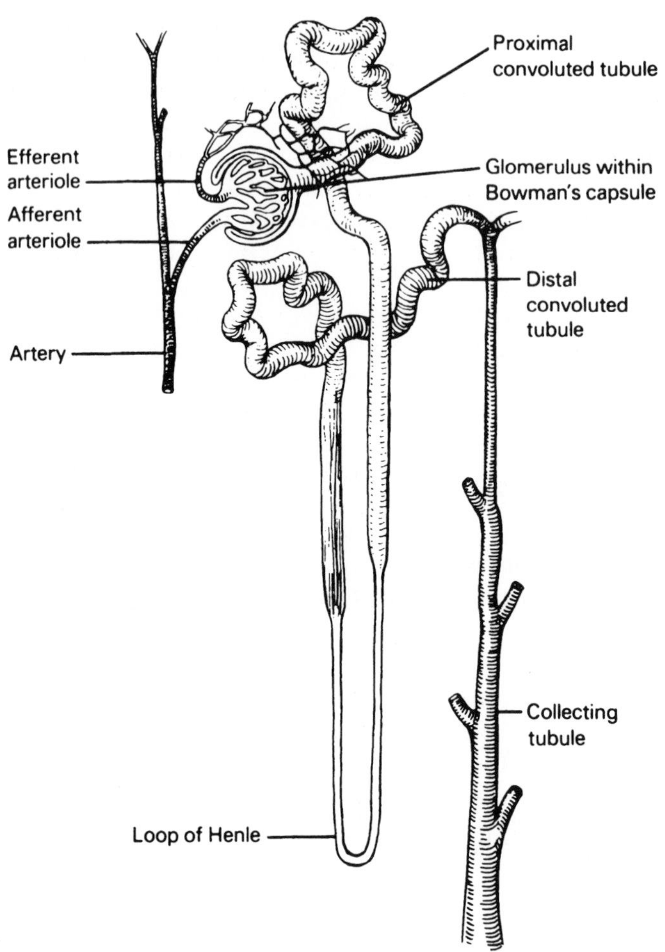

FIGURE 10-2 The nephron

Regulatory Functions of Kidney

Kidneys and urinary system play a major role in maintenance of homeostatic control of the body. Kidneys remove nitrogenous wastes and regulate fluid and electrolyte balance and acid-base balance. Urine is the end product of these mechanisms.

Formation of Urine

A. Glomerular filtration
   1. Ultrafiltration of blood by the glomerulus; beginning of urine formation
      a. Requires hydrostatic pressure (supplied by the heart and assisted by vascular resistance [glomerular hydrostatic pressure]) and sufficient circulating volume.

   b. Pressure in Bowman's capsule opposes hydrostatic pressure and filtration; if glomerular pressure insufficient to force substances out of the blood into the tubules, filtrate formation stops.
2. Glomerular filtration rate (GFR): amount of blood filtrated by the glomeruli in a given time; normal is 125 ml/min
3. Filtrate formed has essentially same composition as blood plasma without the proteins; blood cells and proteins are usually too large to pass the glomerular membrane.

B. Tubular function: the tubules and collecting ducts carry out the functions of reabsorption, secretion, and excretion. Reabsorption of water and electrolytes is controlled by antidiuretic hormone (ADH), released by the pituitary, and aldosterone, secreted by the adrenal glands (see Table 10-1).
   1. Proximal convoluted tubule: reabsorption of certain constituents of the glomerular filtrate: 80% of electrolytes and H_2O, all glucose and amino acids, and bicarbonate; secretes organic substances and wastes.
   2. Loop of Henle: reabsorption of sodium and chloride in the ascending limb; reabsorption of water in the descending limb; concentrates/dilutes urine.
   3. Distal convoluted tubule: secretes potassium, hydrogen ions, and ammonia; reabsorbs H_2O (regulated by ADH) and bicarbonate; regulates calcium and phosphate concentrations.
   4. Collecting ducts: receive urine from distal convoluted tubules and reabsorb water (regulated by ADH).

C. Normal adult produces 1 liter/day of urine.

Blood Pressure Control

A. Kidneys regulate blood pressure partly through maintenance of volume (formation/excretion of urine).

B. The renin-angiotensin system is the other kidney-controlled mechanism that can contribute to rise in blood pressure. When blood pressure drops, the cells of the glomerulus release renin, which then activates angiotensin to cause vasoconstriction.

Penis

A. An external structure that serves as a passageway for urine and semen

B. Capable of distension during sexual excitement

C. Distal portion, glans penis, is covered by a prepuce or foreskin that may or may not be removed (circumcised)

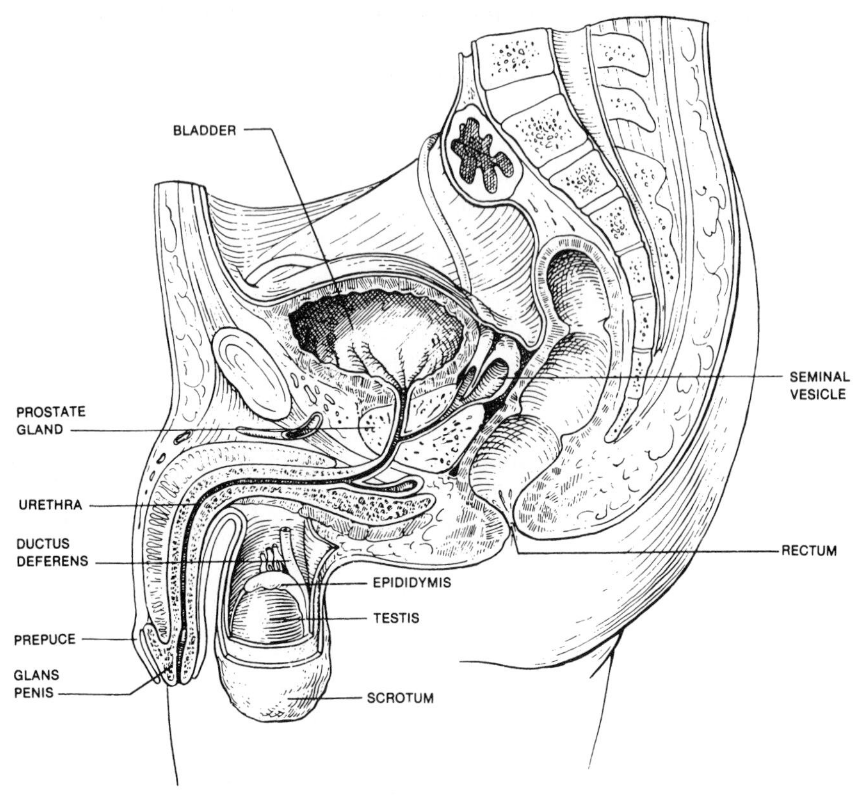

FIGURE 10-3 The male reproductive system

Scrotum

A. Saclike structure that hangs from the root of the penis

B. Contains the testes and epididymis, and helps to regulate temperature conducive to sperm production

Testes

A. Small oval structures suspended in the scrotum

B. Produce sperm (exocrine function) and male hormones (endocrine function, see Table 10-2).

Ductal System

A. Epididymis: first part of ductal system

1. Soft cordlike structure that lies along the posterolateral surface of each testis

   2. Head is attached to the top of the testis, tail is continuous with vas deferens; stores spermatozoa while they mature.
B. Spermatic cord: consists of vas deferens, arteries, veins, nerves, and lymphatic vessels. Vas deferens joins the duct of the seminal vesicles to become the ejaculatory duct.

Accessory Glands

A. Prostate: located below the bladder and in front of the rectum; approximately 4–6 cm long
   1. Enclosed in firm, fibrous capsule; connected to the urethra and ejaculatory ducts
   2. Secretes a milky fluid that aids in the passage of spermatozoa and helps keep them viable
B. Cowper's glands: lie on each side of the urethra and just below the prostate; secrete a small amount of lubricating fluid.
C. Seminal vesicles: paired structures parallel to the bladder; secrete a portion of the ejaculate and may contribute to nutrition and activation of sperm.

ASSESSMENT

Health History

A. Presenting problem: symptoms may include
   1. Pain in flank, groin; dysuria
   2. Changes in urination patterns: frequency, nocturia, hesitancy of stream, urgency, dribbling, incontinence, retention
   3. Changes in urinary output: polyuria, oliguria, anuria
   4. Changes in color/consistency of urine: dilute, concentrated, malodorous; hematuria, pyuria
B. Lifestyle: occupation (type of employment, exposure to chemicals such as carbon tetrachloride, ethylene glycol); level of activity, exercise
C. Nutrition/diet: water, calcium, dairy product intake
D. Past medical history: hypertension; diabetes mellitus; gout; cystitis; kidney infections; connective tissue diseases (systemic lupus erythematosus); infectious diseases; drug use (prescribed/OTC); previous catheterizations, hospitalizations, or surgery for renal problems
E. Family history: hypertension, diabetes mellitus, renal disease, gout, connective tissue disorders, urinary tract infections (UTIs), renal calculi

Physical Examination

A. Inspect skin for color, turgor, and mobility; purpuric lesions; integrity.
B. Inspect mouth for color, moisture, odor, ulcerations.
C. Inspect face for edema, particularly periorbital edema.

D. Inspect abdomen and palpate bladder for distension; percuss bladder for tympany or dullness (if full).
E. Inspect extremities for edema.
F. Determine rate, rhythm, and depth of respirations.
G. Inspect muscles for tremors, atrophy.
H. Palpate right and left kidneys for tenderness, pain, enlargement; percuss costovertebral angles for tenderness/pain; fist percuss kidneys for tenderness/pain.
I. Palpate flank area for pain and prostate for size, shape, consistency.
J. Auscultate aorta and renal arteries for bruits.

Laboratory/Diagnostic Tests

A. Urine studies
  1. Urinalysis: examination to assess the nature of the urine produced
    a. Evaluates color, pH, and specific gravity.
    b. Determines presence of glucose (glycosuria), protein, blood (hematuria), ketones (ketonuria).
    c. Analyzes sediment for cells (presence of WBC called pyuria), casts, bacteria, crystals.
  2. Urine culture and sensitivity: diagnoses bacterial infections of the urinary tract
  3. Residual urine: amount of urine left in bladder after voiding measured via catheter (permanent or temporary) in bladder
  4. Creatinine clearance: determines amount of creatinine (waste product of protein breakdown) in the urine over 24 hours, measures overall renal function
B. Urine collection methods: nursing care
  1. Routine urinalysis: wash perineal area if soiled, obtain first voided morning specimen; send to lab immediately (should be examined within 1 hour of voiding).
  2. Clean catch (midstream) specimen for urine culture.
    a. Cleanse perineal area.
      1) females: spread labia and cleanse meatus front to back using antiseptic sponges.
      2) males: retract foreskin (if uncircumsized) and cleanse glans with antiseptic sponges.
    b. Have client initiate urine stream then stop.
    c. Collect specimen in a sterile container.
    d. Have client complete urination but not in specimen container.
  3. 24-hour specimen (preferred method for creatinine clearance test)
    a. Have client void and discard specimen; note time.
    b. Collect all subsequent urine specimens for 24 hours.
    c. If specimen is accidentally discarded, the test must be restarted.
    d. Record exact start and finish of collection; include date and times.

C. Blood studies
   1. Bicarbonate
   2. BUN: measures renal ability to excrete urea nitrogen
   3. Calcium
   4. Serum creatinine: specific test for renal disorders; reflects ability of kidneys to excrete creatinine
   5. Phosphorus
   6. Potassium
   7. Sodium
   8. Prostate-specific antigen (PSA)
D. KUB/plain film: an abdominal flat-plate X-ray showing the kidneys, ureters, and bladder; may identify the number and size of kidneys with tumors, malformations, and calculi
E. Intravenous pyelogram (IVP)
   1. Fluoroscopic visualization of the urinary tract after injection with a radiopaque dye
   2. Nursing care: pretest
      a. Assess for iodine sensitivity.
      b. Inform client he will lie on a table throughout procedure.
      c. Administer cathartic or enema the night before.
      d. Keep client NPO for 8 hours pretest.
   3. Nursing care: posttest: force fluids
F. Cystoscopy
   1. Use of a lighted scope (cystoscope) to inspect the bladder
      a. Inserted into the bladder via the urethra
      b. May be used to remove tumors, stones, or other foreign material (use of electrical current to remove tumors is called fulguration); or to implant radium, place catheters in ureters
   2. Nursing care: pretest
      a. Explain to client that procedure will be done under general or local anesthesia.
      b. Confirm consent form is signed.
      c. Administer sedatives 1 hour before test, as ordered.
      d. General anesthesia: keep client NPO.
      e. Local anesthesia: offer liquid breakfast.
      f. Give enemas as ordered.
   3. Nursing care: posttest
      a. Provide warm sitz baths, mild analgesics to relieve discomfort after test.
      b. Monitor I&O and vital signs (especially temperature, as elevation may indicate infection).
      c. Expect mild hematuria at first; urine will be pink tinged, subsiding over 24–48 hours; monitor for large clots.
      d. Advise client that burning on urination is normal and will subside.
      e. Force fluids.

ANALYSIS

Nursing diagnoses for the client with a disorder of the genitourinary system may include

A. Deficient fluid volume
B. Fluid volume excess
C. Fatigue
D. Risk for injury
E. Disturbed thought processes
F. Impaired oral mucous membrane
G. Imbalanced nutrition: less than body requirements
H. Risk for infection
I. Impaired skin integrity
J. Urinary retention
K. Sexual dysfunction

PLANNING AND IMPLEMENTATION

Goals

A. Fluid imbalance will be resolved.
B. Client will exhibit improved sense of energy.
C. Client will not exhibit unusual bleeding.
D. Thought processes will improve.
E. Integrity of mucous membranes will be maintained.
F. Adequate nutritional status will be maintained.
G. Client will remain free from infection.
H. Adequate skin integrity will be maintained.
I. Client will demonstrate restored urinary flow.
J. Changes in sexual functioning will be accepted.

Interventions

Urinary Catheterization

A. General information
1. Insertion of a catheter through the external meatus and the urethra into the bladder
2. Purposes include relief from urinary retention, bladder decompression, prevention of bladder obstruction, instillation of medications into the bladder, splinting the bladder, and output monitoring.

B. Nursing care: insertion
1. Explain procedure to client and collect necessary equipment (catheter set).
2. Wash hands and position client.
3. Use sterile technique while inserting catheter.
4. Observe for urine return and obtain specimen.
5. Connect drainage tubing to catheter (indwelling) and tape.

DELEGATION TIP

Insertion of a urinary catheter may be delegated to ancillary personnel. Male catheterization is more commonly delegated to properly trained personnel.

C. Nursing care: indwelling catheter
   1. Maintain catheter patency: place drainage tubing properly to avoid kinking or pinching.
   2. Observe for signs of obstruction (e.g., decreased urine in collection bag, voiding around the catheter, abdominal discomfort, bladder distension).
   3. Irrigate catheter as necessary.
   4. Ensure comfort and safety: relieve bladder spasms by administering belladonna suppositories (if ordered); ensure adequate fluid intake and provide perineal care.
   5. Prevent infection: maintain a closed drainage system and prevent backflow of urine by keeping drainage system below level of bladder.
   6. Empty collection bag at least every 8 hours.
   7. Promote acidification of the urine with acid-ash diet and ascorbic acid.
   8. Change catheter/drainage system only when necessary.

Dialysis

A. General information
   1. Removal by artificial means of metabolic wastes, excess electrolytes, and excess fluid from clients with renal failure
   2. Principles
      a. Diffusion: movement of particles from an area of high concentration to one of low concentration across a semipermeable membrane
      b. Osmosis: movement of water through a semipermeable membrane from an area of lesser concentration of particles to one of greater concentration

B. Purposes
   1. Remove the end products of protein metabolism from blood
   2. Maintain safe levels of electrolytes
   3. Correct acidosis and replenish blood bicarbonate system
   4. Remove excess fluid from the blood

C. Types: hemodialysis and peritoneal dialysis

Hemodialysis

A. General information
   1. Shunting of blood from the client's vascular system through an artificial dialyzing system, and return of dialyzed blood to the client's circulation

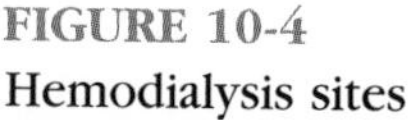

FIGURE 10-4
Hemodialysis sites

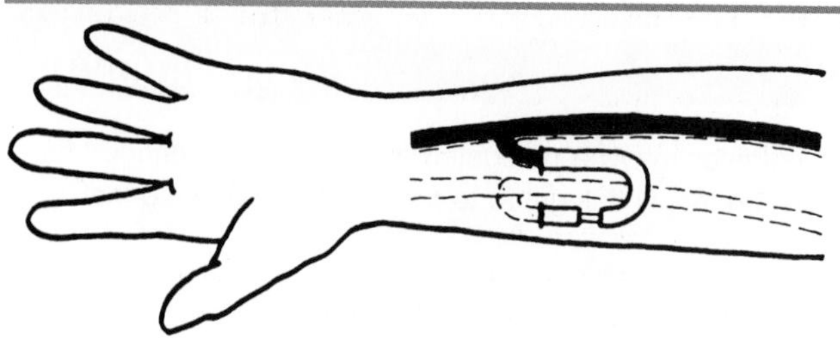

ARTERIOVENOUS SHUNT

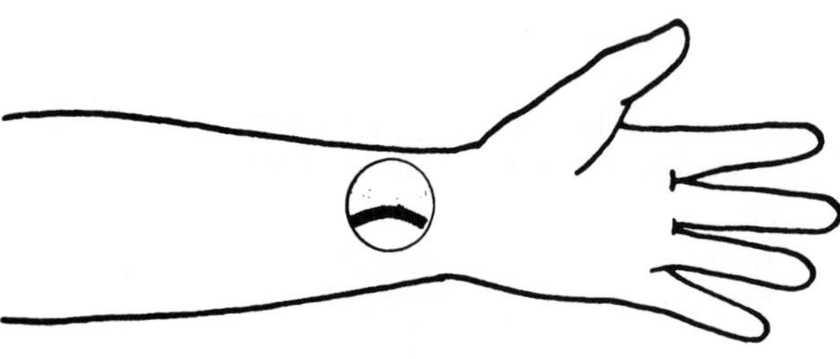

ARTERIOVENOUS FISTULA

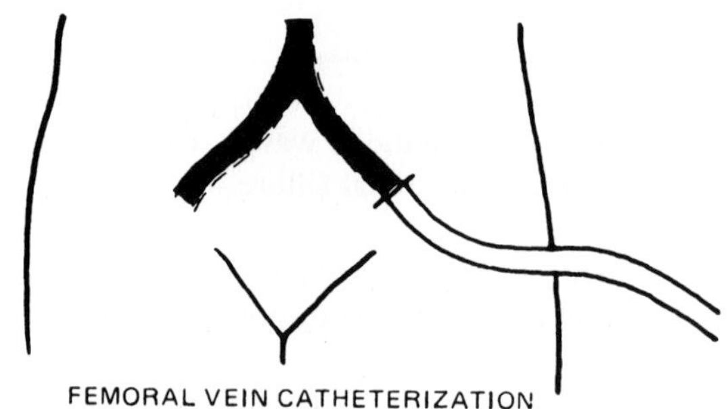

FEMORAL VEIN CATHETERIZATION

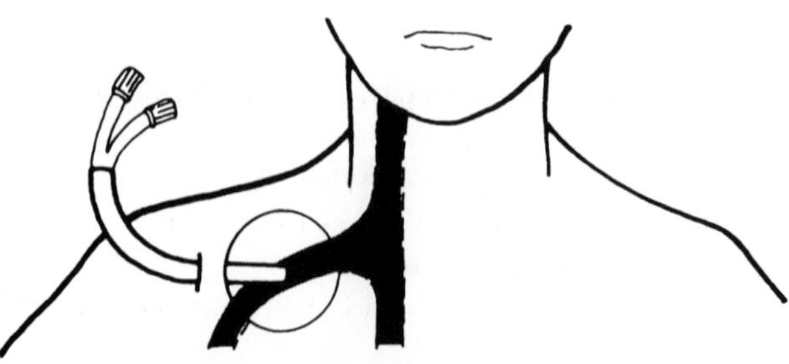

SUBCLAVIAN VEIN CATHETERIZATION

2. Dialysis coil acts as the semipermeable membrane; the dialysate is a specially prepared solution.
3. Access routes (see Figure 10-4)
   a. External AV shunt: one cannula inserted into an artery and the other into a vein; both are brought out to the skin surface and connected by a U-shaped shunt.
   b. AV fistula: internal anastomosis of an artery to an adjacent vein in a sideways position; fistula is accessed for hemodialysis by venipuncture; takes 4–6 weeks to be ready for use.
   c. Femoral/subclavian cannulation: insertion of a catheter into one of these large veins for easy access to circulation; procedure is similar to insertion of a CVP line; temporary.
   d. Graft: piece of bovine artery or vein, Gore-Tex material, or saphenous vein sutured to client's own vessel; used for clients with compromised vascular systems; provides a segment in which to place dialysis needles.

B. Nursing care: external AV shunt
   1. Auscultate for a bruit and palpate for a thrill to ensure patency.
   2. Assess for clotting (color change of blood, absence of pulsations in tubing).
   3. Change sterile dressing over shunt daily.
   4. Avoid performing venipuncture, administering IV infusions, giving injections, or taking a blood pressure with a cuff on the shunt arm.

C. Nursing care: AV fistula.
   1. Auscultate for a bruit and palpate for a thrill to ensure patency.
   2. Report bleeding, skin discoloration, drainage, and pain.
   3. Avoid restrictive clothing/dressings over site.
   4. Avoid administration of IV infusions, giving injections, or taking blood pressure with a cuff on the fistula extremity.

D. Nursing care: femoral/subclavian cannulation
   1. Palpate peripheral pulses in cannulized extremity.
   2. Observe for bleeding/hematoma formation.
   3. Position catheter properly to avoid dislodgment during dialysis.

E. Nursing care: before and during hemodialysis
   1. Have client void.
   2. Chart client's weight.
   3. Assess vital signs before and every 30 minutes during procedure.
   4. Withhold antihypertensives, sedatives, and vasodilators to prevent hypotensive episode (unless ordered otherwise).
   5. Ensure bed rest with frequent position changes for comfort.
   6. Inform client that headache and nausea may occur.
   7. Monitor closely for signs of bleeding since blood has been heparinized for procedure.

F. Nursing care: postdialysis
   1. Chart client's weight.
   2. Assess for complications.

a. Hypovolemic shock: may occur as a result of rapid removal or ultrafiltration of fluid from the intravascular compartment.
b. Dialysis disequilibrium syndrome (urea is removed more rapidly from the blood than from the brain): assess for nausea, vomiting, elevated blood pressure, disorientation, leg cramps, and peripheral paresthesias.

Peritoneal Dialysis

A. General information: introduction of a specially prepared dialysate solution into the abdominal cavity, where the peritoneum acts as a semipermeable membrane between the dialysate and blood in the abdominal vessels
B. Nursing care
   1. Chart client's weight.
   2. Assess vital signs before, every 15 minutes during first exchange, and every hour thereafter.
   3. Assemble specially prepared dialysate solution with added medications.
   4. Have client void.
   5. Warm dialysate solution to body temperature.
   6. Assist physician with trocar insertion.
   7. Inflow: allow dialysate to flow unrestricted into peritoneal cavity (10–20 minutes).
   8. Dwell: allow fluid to remain in peritoneal cavity for prescribed period (30–45 minutes).
   9. Drain: unclamp outflow tube and allow to flow by gravity.
   10. Observe characteristics of dialysate outflow.
       a. Clear pale yellow: normal
       b. Cloudy: infection, peritonitis
       c. Brownish: bowel perforation
       d. Bloody: common during first few exchanges; abnormal if continues
   11. Monitor total I&O and maintain records.
   12. Assess for complications.
       a. Peritonitis resulting from contamination of solution or tubing during exchange
       b. Respiratory difficulty: may occur from upward displacement of diaphragm due to increased pressure in the peritoneal cavity; assess for signs and symptoms of atelectasis, pneumonia, and bronchitis
       c. Protein loss: most serum proteins pass through the peritoneal membrane and are lost in the dialysate fluid; monitor serum protein levels closely

Continuous Ambulatory Peritoneal Dialysis

A. General information
   1. A continuous type of peritoneal dialysis performed at home by the client or significant others.
   2. Dialysate is delivered from flexible plastic containers through a permanent peritoneal catheter.
   3. Following infusion of the dialysate into the peritoneal cavity, the bag is folded and tucked away during the dwell period.

B. Provide client teaching and discharge planning concerning
   1. Need to assess the permanent peritoneal catheter for complications
      a. Dialysate leak
      b. Exit site infection
      c. Bacterial/fungal contamination
      d. Obstruction
   2. Adherence to high-protein (if indicated), well-balanced diet
   3. Importance of periodic blood chemistries
   4. Daily weights

EVALUATION

A. Adequate urinary output with specific gravity/laboratory studies within client's normal range; stable weight; absence of edema; pulmonary congestion.

B. Client verbalizes increased tolerance for activities.

C. Skin and mucous membranes free from ecchymoses/bleeding; improved laboratory values (CBC, platelet count; clotting factors); no signs of bleeding.

D. Client identifies ways to compensate for cognitive impairment; demonstrates improved problem-solving skills.

E. Oral mucosa pink, moist, and intact; no ulcerations; saliva consistency normal; verbalizes interventions to promote/maintain healthy oral mucosa.

F. Stable weight gain; laboratory values within client's normal range; improved anthropometric measurements.

G. Vital signs within normal range; client identifies measures to prevent/reduce the risk of infection.

H. Skin warm and dry; absence of redness and irritation.

I. Voiding in adequate amounts with no palpable bladder distention; postvoid residuals less than 50 ml; absence of dribbling/overflow.

J. Client identifies acceptable sexual practices and explores alternate methods.

K. Client integrates treatment regimens into ADL; shows increased interest in appearance; actively participates in treatments.

DISORDERS OF THE GENITOURINARY SYSTEM

Disorders of the Urinary Tract

Cystitis

A. General information
   1. Inflammation of the bladder due to bacterial invasion
   2. More common in women
   3. Predisposing factors include stagnation of urine, obstruction, sexual intercourse, high estrogen levels
B. Assessment
   1. Abdominal or flank pain/tenderness, frequency and urgency of urination, pain on voiding, nocturia
   2. Fever
   3. Diagnostic tests: urine culture and sensitivity reveals specific organism (80% E. coli)
C. Nursing interventions
   1. Force fluids (3000 ml/day).
   2. Provide warm sitz baths for comfort.
   3. Assess urine for odor, hematuria, sediment.
   4. Administer medications as ordered and monitor effects.
      a. Systemic antibiotics: ampicillin, cephalosporins, aminoglycosides
      b. Sulfonamides: sulfisoxazole (Gantrisin), sulfamethoxazole (Gantanol), trimethoprim-sulfamethoxazole (Bactrim)
      c. Antibacterials: nitrofurantoin (Macrodantin), methenamine mandelate (Mandelamine), nalidixic acid (NegGram)
      d. Urinary tract analgesic: pyridium
   5. Provide client teaching and discharge planning concerning
      a. Importance of adequate hydration
      b. Frequent voiding to avoid stagnation
      c. Proper personal hygiene; women to cleanse from front to back
      d. Voiding after sexual intercourse
      e. Acidification of the urine to decrease bacterial multiplication (acid-ash diet, vitamin C)
      f. Need for follow-up urine cultures

Bladder Cancer

A. General information
   1. Most common site of cancer of the urinary tract
   2. Occurs in men 3 times more often than women; peak age 50–70 years
   3. Predisposing factors include exposure to chemicals (especially aniline dyes), cigarette smoking, chronic bladder infections
B. Medical management: dependent on the staging of cell type; includes
   1. Radiation therapy, usually in combination with surgery

2. Chemotherapy: considerable research on both agents and methods of administration
    a. Methods include direct bladder instillations, intra-arterial infusions, IV infusion, oral ingestion
    b. Agents include 5-fluorouracil, methotrexate, bleomycin, mitomycin-C, hydroxyurea, doxorubicin, cyclophosphamide, cisplatin; results variable
3. Surgery: see Bladder Surgery.

C. Assessment findings
1. Intermittent painless hematuria, dysuria, frequent urination
2. Diagnostic tests
    a. Cytoscopy with biopsy reveals malignancy
    b. Cytologic exam of the urine reveals malignant cells

D. Nursing interventions: provide care for the client receiving radiation therapy or chemotherapy, and for the client with bladder surgery.

Bladder Surgery

A. General information
1. Cystectomy (removal of the urinary bladder) with one of the various types of urinary diversions is the surgical procedure done for bladder cancer
2. Types of urinary diversions
    a. Ureterosigmoidostomy: ureters are excised from the bladder and implanted into sigmoid colon; urine flows through the colon and is excreted via the rectum
    b. Ileal conduit: ureters are implanted into a segment of the ileum that has been resected from the intestinal tract with formation of an abdominal stoma; most common type of urinary diversion
    c. Cutaneous ureterostomy: ureters are excised from the bladder and brought through abdominal wall with creation of a stoma
    d. Nephrostomy: insertion of a catheter into the renal pelvis via an incision into the flank or by percutaneous catheter placement into the kidney

B. Nursing interventions: preoperative
1. Provide routine pre-op care.
2. Assess client's ability to learn prior to starting a teaching program.
3. Discuss social aspects of living with a stoma (sexuality, changes in body image).
4. Assess understanding and emotional response of client/significant others.
5. Perform pre-op bowel preparation for procedures involving the ileum or colon.
6. Inform client of post-op procedures.

C. Nursing interventions: postoperative
 1. Provide routine post-op care.
 2. Maintain integrity of the stoma.
  a. Monitor for and report signs of impaired stomal healing (pale, dark red, or blue-black color; increased stomal height, edema, bleeding).
  b. Maintain stomal circulation by using properly fitted faceplate.
  c. Monitor for signs and symptoms of stomal obstruction (sudden decrease in urine output, increased abdominal tenderness and distension).
 3. Prevent skin irritation and breakdown.
  a. Inspect skin areas for signs of breakdown daily.
  b. Patch test all adhesives, sprays, and skin barriers before use.
  c. Change appliance only when necessary and when production of urine is slowest (early morning).
  d. Place wick (rolled gauze pad) on stomal opening when appliance is off.
  e. Cleanse peristomal skin with mild soap and water.
  f. Remove alkaline encrustations by applying vinegar and water solution to peristomal area.
  g. Implement measures to maintain urine acidity (acid-ash foods, vitamin C therapy, omission of milk/dairy products).
 4. Provide care for the client with an NG tube; will be in place until bowel motility returns.
 5. Assist client to identify strengths and qualities that have a positive effect on self-concept.
 6. Provide client teaching and discharge planning concerning
  a. Maintenance of stomal/peristomal skin integrity
  b. Proper application of appliance
  c. Recommended method of cleaning reusable ostomy equipment (manufacturer's recommendations)
  d. Information regarding prevention of UTIs (adequate fluids; empty pouch when half full; change to bedside collection bag at night)
  e. Control of odor (adequate fluids; avoid foods with strong odor; place small amount of vinegar or deodorizer in pouch)
  f. Reporting signs and symptoms of UTIs.

Nephrolithiasis/Urolithiasis

A. General information
 1. Presence of stones anywhere in the urinary tract; frequent composition of stones: calcium, oxalate, and uric acid
 2. Most often occurs in men age 20–55; more common in the summer
 3. Predisposing factors
  a. Diet: large amounts of calcium, oxalate

NURSING ALERT

Monitor the client for signs of infection, such as rising temperature or chills.

   b. Increased uric acid levels
   c. Sedentary lifestyle, immobility
   d. Family history of gout or calculi; hyperparathyroidism

B. Medical management
   1. Surgery
      a. Percutaneous nephrostomy: tube is inserted through skin and underlying tissues into renal pelvis to remove calculi.
      b. Percutaneous nephrostolithotomy: delivers ultrasound waves through a probe placed on the calculus.
   2. Extracorporeal shock-wave lithotripsy: delivers shock waves from outside the body to the stone, causing pulverization
   3. Pain management and diet modification

C. Assessment findings
   1. Abdominal or flank pain; renal colic; hematuria
   2. Cool, moist skin
   3. Diagnostic tests
      a. KUB: pinpoints location, number, and size of stones
      b. IVP: identifies site of obstruction and presence of nonradiopaque stones
      c. Urinalysis: indicates presence of bacteria, increased protein, increased WBC and RBC

D. Nursing interventions
   1. Strain all urine through gauze to detect stones and crush all clots.
   2. Force fluids (3000–4000 ml/day).
   3. Encourage ambulation to prevent stasis.
   4. Relieve pain by administration of analgesics as ordered and application of moist heat to flank area.
   5. Monitor I&O.
   6. Provide modified diet, depending upon stone consistency.
      a. Calcium stones: limit milk/dairy products; provide acid-ash diet to acidify urine (cranberry or prune juice, meat, eggs, poultry, fish, grapes, whole grains); take vitamin C.
      b. Oxalate stones: avoid excess intake of foods/fluids high in oxalate (tea, chocolate, rhubarb, spinach); maintain alkaline-ash diet to alkalinize urine (milk; vegetables; fruits except prunes, cranberries, and plums).
      c. Uric acid stones: reduce foods high in purine (liver, brains, kidneys, venison, shellfish, meat soups, gravies, legumes); maintain alkaline urine.

7. Administer allopurinol (Zyloprim) as ordered, to decrease uric acid production; push fluids when giving allopurinol.
8. Provide client teaching and discharge planning concerning
   a. Prevention of urinary stasis by maintaining increased fluid intake especially in hot weather and during illness; mobility; voiding whenever the urge is felt and at least twice during the night
   b. Adherence to prescribed diet
   c. Need for routine urinalysis (at least every 3–4 months)
   d. Need to recognize and report signs/symptoms of recurrence (hematuria, flank pain)

Pyelonephritis

A. General information
   1. Inflammation of the renal pelvis; may be unilateral or bilateral, acute or chronic
   2. Acute: infection usually ascends from lower urinary tract
   3. Chronic: thought to be a combination of structural alterations along with infection, major cause is ureterovesical reflux, with infected urine backing up into ureters and renal pelvises; result of recurrent infections is eventual renal parenchymal deterioration and possible renal failure
B. Medical management
   1. Acute: antibiotics, antispasmodics, surgical removal of any obstruction
   2. Chronic: antibiotics and urinary antiseptics (sulfanomides, nitrofurantoin); surgical correction of structural abnormality if possible
C. Assessment findings
   1. Acute: fever, chills, nausea and vomiting; severe flank pain or dull ache
   2. Chronic: client usually unaware of disease; may have bladder irritability, chronic fatigue, or slight dull ache over kidneys; eventually develops hypertension, atrophy of kidneys
D. Nursing interventions: acute pyelonephritis
   1. Provide adequate comfort and rest.
   2. Monitor I&O.
   3. Administer antibiotics as ordered.
   4. Provide client teaching and discharge planning concerning
      a. Medication regimen
      b. Follow-up cultures
      c. Signs and symptoms of recurrence and need to report
E. Nursing interventions: chronic pyelonephritis
   1. Administer medications as ordered.
   2. Provide adequate fluid intake and nutrition.
   3. Support client/significant others and explain possibility of dialysis, transplant options if significant renal deterioration.

Acute Renal Failure

A. General information
   1. Sudden inability of the kidneys to regulate fluid and electrolyte balance and remove toxic products from the body
   2. Causes
      a. Prerenal: factors interfering with perfusion and resulting in decreased blood flow and glomerular filtrate, ischemia, and oliguria; include CHF, cardiogenic shock, acute vasoconstriction, hemorrhage, burns, septicemia, hypotension
      b. Intrarenal: conditions that cause damage to the nephrons; include acute tubular necrosis (ATN), endocarditis, diabetes mellitus, malignant hypertension, acute glomerulonephritis, tumors, blood transfusion reactions, hypercalcemia, nephrotoxins (certain antibiotics, X-ray dyes, pesticides, anesthetics)
      c. Postrenal: mechanical obstruction anywhere from the tubules to the urethra; include calculi, BPH, tumors, strictures, blood clots, trauma, anatomic malformation

B. Assessment findings
   a. Oliguric phase (caused by reduction in glomerular filtration rate)
      1. urine output less than 400 ml/24 hours; duration 1–2 weeks
      2. manifested by hypernatremia, hyperkalemia, hyperphosphatemia, hypocalcemia, hypermagnesemia, and metabolic acidosis
      3. diagnostic tests: BUN and creatinine elevated
   b. Diuretic phase (slow, gradual increase in daily urine output)
      1. diuresis may occur (output 3–5 liters/day) due to partially regenerated tubule's inability to concentrate urine
      2. duration: 2–3 weeks; manifested by hyponatremia, hypokalemia, and hypovolemia
      3. diagnostic tests: BUN and creatinine elevated
   c. Recovery or convalescent phase: renal function stabilizes with gradual improvement over next 3–12 months

C. Nursing interventions
   1. Monitor/maintain fluid and electrolyte balance.
      a. Obtain baseline data on usual appearance and amount of client's urine
      b. Measure I&O every hour; note excessive losses.
      c. Administer IV fluids and electrolyte supplements as ordered.
      d. Weigh daily and report gains.
      e. Monitor lab values; assess/treat fluid and electrolyte and acid-base imbalances as needed (see Tables 10-5 and 10-6).

NURSING ALERT

Monitor the client with renal failure for fluid overload if they are receiving a blood transfusion. Packed red blood cells give the necessary blood constituents without the added volume.

2. Monitor alteration in fluid volume.
   a. Monitor vital signs, PAP, PCWP, CVP as needed.
   b. Weigh client daily.
   c. Maintain strict I&O records.
   d. Assess every hour for hypervolemia; provide nursing care as needed.
      1) maintain adequate ventilation.
      2) decrease fluid intake as ordered.
      3) administer diuretics, cardiac glycosides, and antihypertensives as ordered; monitor effects.
   e. Assess every hour for hypovolemia; replace fluids as ordered.
   f. Monitor ECG and auscultate heart as needed.
   g. Check urine, serum osmolality/osmolarity, and urine specific gravity as ordered.
3. Promote optimal nutritional status.
   a. Weigh daily.
   b. Maintain strict I&O.
   c. Administer TPN as ordered.
   d. With enteral feedings, check for residual and notify physician if residual volume increases.
   e. Restrict protein intake.
4. Prevent complications from impaired mobility (pulmonary embolism, skin breakdown, contractures, atelectasis.
5. Prevent fever/infection.
   a. Take rectal temperature and obtain orders for cooling blanket/ antipyretics as needed.
   b. Assess for signs of infection.
   c. Use strict aseptic technique for wound and catheter care.
6. Support client/significant others and reduce/relieve anxiety.
   a. Explain pathophysiology and relationship to symptoms.
   b. Explain all procedures and answer all questions in easy-to-understand terms.
   c. Refer to counseling services as needed.
7. Provide care for the client receiving dialysis if used.
8. Provide client teaching and discharge planning concerning
   a. Adherence to prescribed dietary regime
   b. Signs and symptoms of recurrent renal disease
   c. Importance of planned rest periods

   d. Use of prescribed drugs only
   e. Signs and symptoms of UTI or respiratory infection, need to report to physician immediately

Chronic Renal Failure

A. General information
   1. Progressive, irreversible destruction of the kidneys that continues until nephrons are replaced by scar tissue; loss of renal function gradual
   2. Predisposing factors: recurrent infections, exacerbations of nephritis, urinary tract obstructions, diabetes mellitus, hypertension
B. Medical management
   1. Diet restrictions
   2. Multivitamins
   3. Hematinics
   4. Aluminum hydroxide gels
   5. Antihypertensives
C. Assessment findings
   1. Nausea, vomiting; diarrhea or constipation; decreased urinary output; dyspnea
   2. Stomatitis, hypotension (early), hypertension (later), lethargy, convulsions, memory impairment, pericardial friction rub, HF
   3. Diagnostic tests: urinalysis
      a. Protein, sodium, and WBC elevated
      b. Specific gravity, platelets, and calcium decreased
D. Nursing interventions
   1. Prevent neurologic complications.
      a. Assess every hour for signs of uremia (fatigue, loss of appetite, decreased urine output, apathy, confusion, elevated blood pressure, edema of face and feet, itchy skin, restlessness, seizures).
      b. Assess for changes in mental functioning.
      c. Orient confused client to time, place, date, and persons; institute safety measures to protect client from falling out of bed.
      d. Monitor serum electrolytes, BUN, and creatinine as ordered.
   2. Promote optimal GI function.
      a. Assess/provide care for stomatitis
      b. Monitor nausea, vomiting, anorexia; administer antiemetics as ordered.
      c. Assess for signs of GI bleeding.
   3. Monitor/prevent alteration in fluid and electrolyte balance.
   4. Assess for hyperphosphatemia (paresthesias, muscle cramps, seizures, abnormal reflexes), and administer aluminum hydroxide gels (Amphojel, AlternaGEL) as ordered.
   5. Promote maintenance of skin integrity.

CLIENT TEACHING CHECKLIST

For clients with chronic renal failure:

- Teach client to take diuretics in the morning rathar than in the evening to avoid sleep disturbances.
- Instruct the client who is anemic to rest frequently.
- Encourage client to report cramps and muscle twitching.
- Encourage client to keep appointment for electrolyte monitoring.

   a. Assess/provide care for pruritus.
   b. Assess for uremic frost (urea crystallization on the skin) and bathe in plain water.
6. Monitor for bleeding complications, prevent injury to client.
   a. Monitor Hgb, hct, platelets, RBC.
   b. Hematest all secretions.
   c. Administer hematinics as ordered.
   d. Avoid IM injections.
7. Promote/maintain maximal cardiovascular function.
   a. Monitor blood pressure and report significant changes.
   b. Auscultate for pericardial friction rub.
   c. Perform circulation checks routinely.
   d. Administer diuretics as ordered and monitor output.
   e. Modify digitalis dose as ordered (digitalis is excreted in kidneys).
8. Provide care for client receiving dialysis.

Kidney Transplantation

A. General information
   1. Transplantation of a kidney from a donor to recipient to prolong the life of person with renal failure
   2. Sources of donor selection
      a. Living relative with compatible serum and tissue studies, free from systemic infection, and emotionally stable
      b. Cadavers with good serum and tissue crossmatching; free from renal disease, neoplasms, and sepsis; absence of ischemia/trauma
B. Nursing interventions: preoperative
   1. Provide routine pre-op care.
   2. Discuss the possibility of post-op dialysis/immunosuppressive drug therapy with client and significant others.

C. Nursing interventions: postoperative
   1. Provide routine post-op care.
   2. Monitor fluid and electrolyte balance carefully.
      a. Monitor I&O hourly and adjust IV fluid administration accordingly.
      b. Anticipate possible massive diuresis.
   3. Encourage frequent and early ambulation.
   4. Monitor vital signs, especially temperature; report significant changes.
   5. Provide mouth care and nystatin (Mycostatin) mouthwashes for candidiasis.
   6. Administer immunosuppressive agents as ordered
      a. Cyclosporine (Sandimmune): does not cause significant bone marrow depression. Assess for hypertension; blood chemistry alterations (hypermagnesemia, hyperkalemia, decreased sodium bicarbonate); neurologic functioning.
      b. Azathioprine (Imuran): assess for manifestations of anemia, leukopenia, thrombocytopenia, oral lesions.
      c. Cyclophosphamide (Cytoxan): assess for alopecia, hypertension, kidney/liver toxicity, leukopenia.
      d. Antilymphocytic globulin (ALG), antithymocytic globulin (ATG): assess for fever, chills, anaphylactic shock, hypertension, rash, headache.
      e. Corticosteroids (prednisone, methylprednisolone sodium succinate [Solu-Medrol]): assess for peptic ulcer and GI bleeding, sodium/water retention, muscle weakness, delayed healing, mood alterations, hyperglycemia, acne.
   7. Assess for signs of rejection. Include decreased urinary output, fever, pain/tenderness over transplant site, edema, sudden weight gain, increasing blood pressure, generalized malaise, rise in serum creatinine, and decrease in creatinine clearance.
   8. Provide client teaching and discharge planning concerning
      a. Medication regimen: names, dosages, frequency, and side effects
      b. Signs and symptoms of rejection and the need to report immediately
      c. Dietary restrictions: restricted sodium and calories, increased protein
      d. Daily weights
      e. Daily measurement of I&O
      f. Resumption of activity and avoidance of contact sports in which the transplanted kidney may be injured

Nephrectomy

A. General information
   1. Surgical removal of an entire kidney
   2. Indications include renal tumor, massive trauma, removal for a donor, polycystic kidneys

B. Nursing interventions: preoperative care
   1. Provide routine pre-op care.
   2. Ensure adequate fluid intake.
   3. Assess electrolyte values and correct any imbalances before surgery.
   4. Avoid nephrotoxic agents in any diagnostic tests.
   5. Advise client to expect flank pain after surgery if retroperitoneal approach (flank incision) is used.
   6. Explain that client will have chest tube if a thoracic approach is used.
C. Nursing interventions: postoperative
   1. Provide routine post-op care.
   2. Assess urine output every hour; should be 30–50 ml/hour.
   3. Observe urinary drainage on dressing and estimate amount.
   4. Weigh daily.
   5. Maintain adequate functioning of chest drainage system; ensure adequate oxygenation and prevent pulmonary complications.
   6. Administer analgesics as ordered.
   7. Encourage early ambulation.
   8. Teach client to splint incision while turning, coughing, deep breathing.
   9. Provide client teaching and discharge planning concerning
      a. Prevention of urinary stasis
      b. Maintenance of acidic urine
      c. Avoidance of activities that might cause trauma to the remaining kidney (contact sports, horseback riding)
      d. No lifting heavy objects for at least 6 months
      e. Need to report unexplained weight gain, decreased urine output, flank pain on unoperative side, hematuria
      f. Need to notify physician if cold or other infection present for more than 3 days
      g. Medication regimen and avoidance of OTC drugs that may be nephrotoxic (except with physician approval)

Disorders of the Male Reproductive System

Epididymitis

A. General information
   1. Inflammation of epididymis, one of the most common intrascrotal infections
   2. May be sexually transmitted, usually caused by N. gonorrhoeae, C. trachomatis; also caused by GU instrumentation, urinary reflux
B. Assessment findings
   1. Sudden scrotal pain, scrotal edema, tenderness over the spermatic cord
   2. Diagnostic test: urine culture reveals specific organism

C. Nursing interventions
   1. Administer antibiotics and analgesics as ordered.
   2. Provide bed rest with elevation of the scrotum.
   3. Apply ice packs to scrotal area to decrease edema.

Prostatitis

A. General information
   1. Inflammatory condition that affects the prostate gland
   2. Several forms: acute bacterial prostatitis, chronic bacterial prostatitis, or abacterial chronic prostatitis
   3. Acute and chronic bacterial prostatitis usually caused by E. coli, N. gonorrhoeae, Enterobacter or Proteus species, and group D streptococci
   4. Most important predisposing factor: lower UTIs
B. Assessment findings
   1. Acute: fever, chills, dysuria, urethral discharge, prostatic tenderness, copious purulent urethral discharge upon palpation
   2. Chronic: backache; perineal pain; mild dysuria; frequency; enlarged, firm, and slightly tender prostate upon palpation
   3. Diagnostic tests
      a. WBC elevated
      b. Bacteria in initial urinalysis specimens
C. Nursing interventions
   1. Administer antibiotics, analgesics, and stool softeners as ordered.
   2. Provide increased fluid intake.
   3. Provide sitz baths/rest to relieve discomfort.
   4. Provide client teaching and discharge planning concerning
      a. Importance of maintaining adequate hydration
      b. Antibiotic therapy regimen (may need to remain on medication for several months)
      c. Activities that drain the prostate (masturbation, sexual intercourse, prostatic massage)

Benign Prostatic Hypertrophy (BPH)

A. General information
   1. Mild to moderate glandular enlargement, hyperplasia, and overgrowth of the smooth muscles and connective tissue
   2. As the gland enlarges, it compresses the urethra, resulting in urinary retention.
   3. Most common problem of the male reproductive system; occurs in 50% of men over age 50; 75% of men over age 75
   4. Cause unknown; may be related to hormonal mechanism
B. Assessment findings
   1. Nocturia, frequency, decreased force and amount of urinary stream, hesitancy (more difficult to start voiding), hematuria

2. Enlargement of prostate gland upon palpation by digital rectal exam
3. Diagnostic tests
   a. Urinalysis: alkalinity increased; specific gravity normal or elevated
   b. BUN and creatinine elevated (if longstanding BPH)
   c. Prostate-specific antigen (PSA) elevated (normal is <4 ng/ml)
   d. Cystoscopy reveals enlargement of gland and obstruction of urine flow

C. Nursing interventions
1. Administer antibiotics as ordered.
2. Provide client teaching concerning medications
   a. Terazosin (Hytrin) relaxes bladder sphincter and makes it easier to urinate. May cause hypotension and dizziness.
   b. Finasteride (Proscar) shrinks enlarged prostate.
3. Force fluids.
4. Provide care for the catheterized client.
5. Provide care for the client with prostatic surgery.

Cancer of the Prostate

A. General information
1. Second most common cause of cancer deaths in American males over age 55
2. Usually an adenocarcinoma; growth related to the presence of androgens
3. Spreads from the prostate to the seminal vesicles, urethral mucosa, bladder wall, external sphincter, and lymphatic system
4. Highest incidence is in African American men age 60 or over
5. Cause is unknown

B. Medical management
1. Drug therapy: estrogens, chemotherapeutic agents
2. Radiation therapy
3. Surgery: radical prostatectomy

C. Assessment findings: same as for BPH above but diagnostic test results are
1. Elevated acid phosphatase (distant metastasis) and alkaline phosphatase (bone metastasis)
2. Bone scan: abnormal in metastatic areas

D. Nursing interventions
1. Administer medications as ordered and provide care for the client receiving chemotherapy.
2. Provide care for the client receiving radiation therapy.
3. Provide care for the client with a prostatectomy.

Prostatic Surgery

A. General information
1. Indicated for benign prostatic hypertrophy and prostatic cancer.

2. Types
   a. Transurethral resection (TUR or TURP): insertion of a resectoscope into the urethra to excise prostatic tissue; good for poor surgical risks, does not require an incision; most common type of surgery for BPH
   b. Suprapubic prostatectomy: the prostate is approached by a low abdominal incision into the bladder to the anterior aspect of the prostate; for large tumors obstructing the urethra
   c. Retropubic prostatectomy: to remove a large mass high in the pelvic area; involves a low midline incision below the bladder and into the prostatic capsule
   d. Perineal prostatectomy: often used for prostatic cancer; the incision is made through the perineum, which facilitates radical surgery if a malignancy is found

B. Nursing interventions: preoperative
   1. Provide routine pre-op care.
   2. Institute and maintain urinary drainage.
   3. Force fluids; administer antibiotics, acid-ash diet to eradicate UTI.
   4. Reinforce what surgeon has told client/significant others regarding effects of surgery on sexual function.

C. Nursing interventions: postoperative
   1. Provide routine post-op care.
   2. Ensure patency of 3-way Foley.
   3. Monitor continuous bladder irrigations with sterile saline solution (removes clotted blood from bladder), and control rate to keep urine light pink changing to clear.
   4. Expect hematuria for 2–3 days.
   5. Irrigate catheter with normal saline as ordered.
   6. Control/treat bladder spasms; encourage short, frequent walks; decrease rate of continuous bladder irrigations (if urine is not red and is without clots); administer anticholinergics (propantheline bromide [Pro-Banthine]) or antispasmodics (B&O suppositories) as ordered.
   7. Prevent hemorrhage: administer stool softeners to discourage straining at stool; avoid rectal temperatures and enemas; monitor Hgb and hct.
   8. Report bright red, thick blood in the catheter; persistent clots, persistent drainage on dressings.
   9. Provide for bladder retraining after Foley removal.
      a. Instruct client to perform perineal exercises (stopping and starting stream during voiding; pressing buttocks together then relaxing muscles) to improve sphincter control.
      b. Limit liquid intake in evening.
      c. Restrict caffeine-containing beverages.
      d. Withhold anticholinergics and antispasmodics (these drugs relax bladder and increase chance of incontinence) if permitted.
   10. Provide client teaching and discharge planning concerning

a. Continued increased fluid intake
b. Signs of UTI and need to report them
c. Continued perineal exercises
d. Avoidance of heavy lifting, straining during defecation, and prolonged travel (at least 8–12 weeks)
e. Measures that promote urinary continence
f. Possible impotence (more common after perineal resection)
    1) discuss ways of expressing sexuality (massage, cuddling)
    2) suggest alternative methods of sexual gratification and use of assistive aids
    3) discuss possibility of penile prosthesis with physician
g. Need for annual and self-exams

REVIEW QUESTIONS

1. A 55-year-old man is hospitalized for bladder cancer. He is scheduled for ileal loop surgery to create a urostomy. Which information is most important for the nurse to include in a teaching plan for this client when learning to change his urostomy appliance?
    1. Change the appliance before going to bed.
    2. Cut the wafer one inch larger than the stoma.
    3. Cleanse the peristomal skin with mild soap and water.
    4. Use firm pressure to attach the wafer to the skin.
2. Which nursing intervention best prevents urinary tract infections in a person who has an ileal conduit?
    1. Allowing the bag to fill completely.
    2. Attaching a larger bag at night.
    3. Restricting fluids to less than 1000 ml daily.
    4. Changing the appliance every 8 hours.
3. An 84-year-old man has just returned to the nursing unit after a transurethral resection. He has a 3-way indwelling urinary catheter for continuous bladder irrigation connected to straight drainage. Immediately after surgery, the nurse would expect his urine to be
    1. clear.
    2. light yellow.
    3. pink or dark red.
    4. bright red.

4. An elderly man has just returned to the nursing care unit following a transurethral resection. He has a three-way indwelling catheter with continuous bladder irrigation. He tells the nurse he has to void. The most appropriate nursing action is to
   1. allow him to void around the catheter.
   2. irrigate the catheter.
   3. notify the physician.
   4. remove the catheter.
5. A 17-year-old is admitted to the hospital with a diagnosis of acute renal failure. She is oliguric and has proteinuria. She asks the nurse, "How long will it be until I start to make urine again?" A correct nursing response would be to tell her that this phase of renal failure will last for approximately
   1. 1–2 days.
   2. 3–7 days.
   3. 1–2 weeks.
   4. 3–4 weeks.
6. A client who is in acute renal failure develops pulmonary edema. Nursing interventions for this person should include which of the following? Check all that apply.
   1. ______ Administering oxygen.
   2. ______ Encouraging coughing and deep breathing.
   3. ______ Placing the client in a semi-sitting position.
   4. ______ Replacing lost fluids.
7. The nurse is caring for a person who is admitted in acute renal failure. The appearance of a U wave on the ECG should alert the nurse to check laboratory values for
   1. hyperkalemia.
   2. hypokalemia.
   3. hypernatremia.
   4. hyponatremia.
8. A young man is admitted in chronic renal failure and placed on hemodialysis three times a week. Which is an attainable short-term goal for this person when he is placed on hemodialysis?
   1. Understanding the treatment and its implications.
   2. Independence in the care of the AV shunt.
   3. Self-monitoring during dialysis.
   4. Recording dialysate composition and temperature.

9. The nurse is caring for a woman who is on hemodialysis. She has an arteriovenous fistula. Which finding is expected when assessing the fistula?
    1. Ecchymotic area.
    2. Enlarged veins.
    3. Pulselessness.
    4. Redness.
10. A female client is to have a urine culture collected. The nurse instructs the client on the procedure for collecting a clean catch urine specimen by telling the client to
    1. separate the labia, clean from front to back with the three wipes impregnated with the cleaning solution, and then start to void in the toilet. Stop, and finally continue to void into the sterile container.
    2. retract the foreskin, cleanse with the three cleansing sponges, and start to void. Stop, and finally continue to void into the sterile container.
    3. separate the labia, clean from back to front with the three wipes impregnated with the cleaning solution, and then start to void in the toilet. Stop, and finally continue to void into the sterile container.
    4. retract the foreskin, clean with soap and water, and then start to void. Stop, and finally continue to void into the sterile container.
11. The nurse is to collect a urine culture specimen from a catheterized client. Which one of the following statements describes the nurse's actions for this procedure?
    1. With a sterile syringe the nurse aspirates 50 ml of urine from the silicone catheter tubing.
    2. With a sterile syringe, the nurse aspirates 1–3 ml from the distal end of the catheter after first cleaning the sampling port with alcohol.
    3. With a sterile syringe, the nurse aspirates 1–3 ml from the distal end of the catheter after first cleaning the sampling port with soap and water.
    4. The nurse disconnects the catheter from the tubing and allows a small volume of urine to drain into a sterile container.
12. The nurse is ordered to perform a urinary catheterization for post-void residual volume (PVR) on a client with urinary incontinence. Several minutes after the client voids, the nurse obtains a residual urine of 30 ml. The nurse interprets this residual volume of urine to be
    1. adequate bladder emptying.
    2. inadequate bladder emptying.

3. decreased urethral pressure.
4. increased urethral pressure.

13. Post cystoscopy, which one of the following assessment findings would the nurse expect to find?
    1. Gross hematuria and pain.
    2. Pink-tinged urine and burning on voiding.
    3. Colicky pain and bladder distention.
    4. Flank pain and bladder distention.

14. A post-op client is unable to void and is ordered to have an indwelling catheter inserted immediately. The nurse performing the catheterization is extremely concerned with
    1. teaching the client deep breathing techniques to decrease post-op pain, preprocedure.
    2. maintaining strict aseptic technique.
    3. medicating the client for pain, before the procedure.
    4. teaching the client the signs and symptoms of urinary tract infection.

15. The nurse is assessing a client with an indwelling catheter and finds the catheter is not draining and the client's bladder is distended. The nurse should immediately plan to
    1. notify the physician.
    2. assess the catheter tubing for kinks and position so downhill flow is initiated.
    3. change the catheter.
    4. aspirate urine for culture.

16. The nurse is teaching a client about the concept of dialysis and how it works for the body. It is the nurse's understanding that dialysis is a technique that
    1. will move blood through a semipermeable membrane into a dialysate that is used to remove waste products as well as correct fluid and electrolyte imbalances.
    2. will add electrolytes and water to the blood when passing through a semipermeable membrane to correct electrolyte imbalances.
    3. will increase potassium to the blood when passing through a semipermeable membrane to correct electrolyte imbalances.
    4. allows the nurse to choose to use either diffusion osmosis or ultrafiltration to correct the client's fluid and electrolyte imbalance.

17. A client with end-stage renal disease (ESRD) receives hemodialysis three times a week. The nurse concludes that dialysis is effective when
    1. the client does not have a large weight gain.
    2. the client has no signs and symptoms of infection.
    3. the client expresses he or she can catch up on rest while on dialysis.
    4. the client is able to return to employment.
18. The nurse is caring for a client going to hemodialysis three times a week. The client receives the following medications every morning: hydrochlorothiazide (Hydrodiuril), nitroglycerin patch (Minitran), vancomycin, and allopurinol (Zyloprim). The nurse expects to withhold which of the above medications until after hemodialysis?
    1. Hydrochlorothiazide (Hydrodiuril) and vancomycin.
    2. Hydrochlorothiazide (Hydrodiuril) and nitroglycerin patch (Minitran).
    3. Nitroglycerin (Minitran) and allopurinol (Zyloprim).
    4. Vancomycin and allopurinol (Zyloprim).
19. The nurse is caring for a client receiving peritoneal dialysis. The nurse is completing the exchange by draining the dialysate and notices the dialysate is cloudy. The nurse best interprets this finding as
    1. the normal appearance of draining dialysate.
    2. a sign of infection.
    3. an indication of an impending lower back problem.
    4. a sign of a vascular access occlusion.
20. The nurse knows the client on continuous ambulatory peritoneal dialysis (CAPD) understands his treatment when the client states,
    1. "I must increase my carbohydrate intake daily."
    2. "I must maintain a positive nitrogen balance by decreasing proteins."
    3. "I must take prophylactic antibiotics to prevent infection."
    4. "I must be aware of the signs and symptoms of peritonitis."
21. A woman presents to the urgent care center with dysuria and hematuria. The woman reveals that she has a history of cystitis. The nurse should also assess for which of the following clinical manifestations suggesting cystitis?
    1. Frequency and urgency of urination, flank pain, nausea, and vomiting.
    2. Abscess formation and flank pain.
    3. Frequency and urgency of urination, suprapubic pain, and foul smelling urine.
    4. Fever, nausea, vomiting, and flank pain.

22. A 3-day post-op client for a ureterosigmoidostomy is complaining of cramping in lower extremities and occasional dizziness. The nurse should give highest priority to

1. assessing for electrolyte imbalance.
2. assessing for cardiac dysrhythmias.
3. observing the client's response to surgery.
4. verifying the temperature of the client's lower extremities.

23. The nurse who is caring for a client with a Kock's pouch should plan to teach the client about

1. decreasing the client's sexual encounters.
2. adhering to catheterization schedules.
3. decreasing fluid intake to avoid embarrassing situations.
4. decreasing fluid intake to manage the urinary diversion.

24. A 35-year-old male presents to the ER with hematuria, flank pain, fever, nausea, and vomiting. He is admitted and passes a "stone." The stone is sent to the laboratory and is found to be composed of uric acid. The client is placed on allopurinol (Zyloprim). The nurse understands that the allopurinol (Zylopri) is prescribed to

1. decrease the client's serum creatinine.
2. reduce the urinary concentration of uric acid.
3. acidify the urine.
4. bind oxalate in the gastrointestinal tract.

25. The nurse is caring for a client who has just been given discharge instruction for kidney stones. Which statement by the client indicates a need for further instruction?

1. "I will decrease my intake of all foods on the list you gave me that are high in purine, calcium, or oxalate."
2. "I will decrease my fluid intake."
3. "I will take my medication daily."
4. "I will return to my doctor in one week for follow-up."

26. Medication will be used in the management of a client with urolithiasis. Based on knowledge of urolithiasis, the nurse should include which of the following in planning nursing care for the client?

1. Place the client in bed with side rails up as a narcotic will be given.
2. Keep the client NPO so there will be no experience of nausea with medication administration.

3. Increase intake of purine-, calcium-, and oxalate-rich food.
4. Add Probenecid to the narcotic to prevent renal tubular excretion of the narcotic.

27. The nurse is performing discharge teaching for a client who was admitted with pyelonephritis. The client asks the nurse, "What is pyelonephritis?" Based on the nurse's knowledge of pyelonephritis the best response would be,
    1. "Pyelonephritis is an inflammation of the bladder."
    2. "Pyelonephritis is a rupture of the bladder."
    3. "Pyelonephritis is an infection of the kidney."
    4. "Pyelonephritis is an infection of the lower urinary tract."
28. On a medical-surgical unit, a client is admitted with acute renal failure. The nurse must continually assess for
    1. hyponatremia and hyperkalemia.
    2. decreased BUN and creatinine.
    3. alkalosis.
    4. hypercalcemia.
29. The client with chronic renal failure complains of irritating white crystals on his skin. The nurse recognizes this finding as uremic frost and takes which of the following nursing actions?
    1. Administers an antihistamine because the doctor would prescribe one to relieve itching.
    2. Increases fluids to prevent crystal formation and decrease itching.
    3. Provides skin care with tepid water and applies lotion on the skin to relieve itching.
    4. Permits the client to soak in a bathtub to remove crystals.
30. The nurse has been working with a client with chronic renal failure. Which of the following behaviors would indicate to the nurse that the client understands his dietary regimen?
    1. He reports eating two bananas for breakfast, rice and beans for lunch, and fruit salad, green beans, and an 8 oz. T-bone steak for dinner.
    2. He reports eating bacon and eggs for breakfast, hot dogs and sauerkraut for lunch, and baked canned ham with green beans for dinner.
    3. He reports eating an apple and oatmeal for breakfast, homemade tomato soup for lunch, and pasta with fish for dinner.

4. He reports eating half a honeydew melon and three eggs for breakfast, a baked potato with processed cheese spread and broccoli for lunch, and chicken, yams, pinto beans, squash, and 8 oz. of pecans for dinner.

31. A client who has been in intensive care, for cardiogenic shock related to a myocardial infarction, is recovering. He is transferred to the renal unit in renal failure. The client's spouse asks the nurse "Is this acute or chronic renal failure?" Based on knowledge of this client's history the nurse's best response is,
    1. "Don't worry; this is an excellent renal unit, so we can treat either acute or chronic failure."
    2. "Acute renal failure always progresses to chronic renal failure."
    3. "Acute renal failure is glomerular degeneration whereas chronic renal failure is the result of cardiovascular collapse."
    4. "Acute renal failure generally results from decreased blood to the kidneys, nephrotoxicity, or muscle injury. The myocardial infarction caused extensive heart muscle damage decreasing blood to the kidneys."

32. A client immediately post kidney transplant should be assessed by the nurse for
    1. fluid and electrolyte imbalances.
    2. infection.
    3. hepatotoxicity.
    4. respiratory complications.

33. An adult had a renal transplant, as a result of glomerulonephritis, and is at the physician's office for a follow-up visit. The client tells the office nurse "I am not worried about rejection. I am not going to come here weekly." The nurse interprets his reaction to constant follow-up care as an example of
    1. projection.
    2. intellectualization.
    3. denial.
    4. regression.

34. The prudent nurse will complete which one of the following initial assessments on the client immediately post-op nephrectomy?
    1. Performing cardiovascular assessment.
    2. Ordering laboratory studies monitoring renal functions and electrolytes.
    3. Inspecting the incision site for bleeding.

4. Obtaining a urine culture.

35. The nurse is completing an admission assessment on a client with benign prostatic hyperplasia (BPH). The nurse should obtain an in-depth assessment about
    1. laboratory studies.
    2. urinary patterns.
    3. electrocardiograms.
    4. internal bleeding.

36. A client with BPH is at the clinic for follow-up. Which of the following statements indicates to the nurse his understanding of management of his condition?
    1. "As soon as I finish this visit I won't ever have to worry about BPH again."
    2. "I don't know how I am going to get used to voiding every 2 to 3 hours."
    3. "I will wear an athletic supporter while I am awake."
    4. "I am going to avoid fluids while at work to prevent dribbling."

37. A client who is 8 hours post-transurethral resection prostatectomy (TURP) asks the nurse "Why is my urine in the bag clotting like blood?" The nurse's best interpretation of this finding is that
    1. after all surgery bleeding is normal.
    2. it is common for blood clots to be irrigated from the bladder for a day or so.
    3. the physician needs to be called as the client is hemorrhaging.
    4. the client is tugging on the catheter causing irritation to the bladder mucosa.

38. A 68-year-old client, 48 hours post-transurethral resection prostatectomy asks "How will my sex life be affected?" The nurse's best response would be,
    1. "I will get the physician to determine if your sex life was affected during surgery."
    2. "Only your doctor can answer that. Why don't you ask him prior to discharge."
    3. "A transurethral prostatectomy does not usually result in erectile dysfunction."
    4. "Don't you remember, before surgery you were told that you would not be able to engage in sexual intercourse but you can express your love for your spouse by alternate acts such as cuddling."

39. Following a prostatectomy, the client has a 3-way, indwelling catheter for continuous bladder irrigation. During evening shift, 2400 ml of irrigant was instilled. At the end of the shift, the drainage bag was drained of 2900 ml of fluid. The nurse calculates the urine output to be

1. 5300 ml.

2. 2900 ml.

3. 240 ml.

4. 500 ml.

ANSWERS AND RATIONALES

1. 3. Cleansing the peristomal skin is critical to maintenance of skin integrity.

2. 2. Attaching a larger bag at night helps to prevent reflux of urine into the stoma during a period when the bag is emptied less frequently.

3. The urine is expected to be pink or dark red for up to 36 hours after a transurethral resection.

4. Blood clots obstructing the catheter can produce the sensation of needing to void. Irrigating the catheter will remove any blood clots, allowing the urine to drain freely.

5. The oliguric period in acute renal failure is usually 1–2 weeks.

6. Administered oxygen should be checked. Oxygenation is seriously compromised in pulmonary edema.
Encouraging coughing and deep breathing should be checked. Coughing and deep breathing may help with oxygenation.Placing the client in a semi-sitting position should be checked. This position facilitates breathing.

7. U waves on an ECG are associated with hypokalemia.

8. Prior to the start of dialysis the client should fully comprehend its meaning and the changes in lifestyle required.

9. Leaking of arterial blood into an AV fistula causes the veins to enlarge so they are easier to access for hemodialysis.

10. Women should separate the labia, clean from front to back, and then proceed to void into the toilet. Stop, and finally continue to void into the sterile container.

11. Several ml's of urine for culture can be aspirated with a 21-gauge needle and 3-ml syringe after the sampling port or the distal catheter has been swabbed with alcohol or iodine swabs. The urinary catheter and drainage system should remain a closed system to prevent infection.

12. Measurement of post-void residual volume (PVR) should be performed for all clients with urinary incontinence. Catheterization is performed several minutes after the client voids. A residual of less than 50 ml signifies adequate bladder emptying.

13. Pink-tinged urine and burning on voiding for a day or two following the procedure are expected.

14. Strict aseptic technique is vital to prevent urinary tract infection. The client is positioned on the back with heels flat on the bed with legs separated. The meatus is cleansed with an iodine solution. The catheter is lubricated with a water-soluble jelly and is inserted through the urethra into the bladder until urine starts to flow. The balloon is inflated and the catheter is taped securely to the leg.

15. Possible signs of indwelling catheter obstruction can be pain, distention, and no urinary output. Possible causes of obstruction include blood clots, mineral sediment, or mucous plugs in the catheter or tubing. The most effective strategies to promote drainage are to place the tubing so downhill flow is unobstructed and to empty the collection system regularly. Irrigation and catheter changes should be performed when all other means fail as they are associated with a high potential for infection.

16. Dialysis allows substances to move from the blood through a semipermeable membrane into a dialysis solution (dialysate) to correct fluid and electrolyte imbalances as well as remove waste products that accumulate when the client is in renal failure. The principles of dialysis include diffusion, osmosis, and ultrafiltration.

17. It is imperative for the client to maintain an adequate fluid status as evidenced by normal weight and also remain infection free. The primary nursing goal is to help the client maintain a positive self-image and continue to be a productive member of society.

18. The morning of dialysis antihypertensives, nitrates, and sedatives are usually withheld as they may precipitate hypotensive episodes.

19. Peritonitis is usually caused by Staphylococcus. The first indication of peritonitis is cloudy dialysate.

20. Peritonitis is a life-threatening complication of CAPD, which is manifested by abdominal pain and distention, diarrhea, vomiting, and fever. Clients are given antibiotics orally or parenterally as necessary, not prophylactically.

21. The signs and symptoms of cystitis are frequency and urgency of urination, suprapubic pain, dysuria, foul-smelling urination, and sometimes pyuria. Some clients with cystitis may be asymptomatic.

22. In this surgical procedure, the client's ureters are anastomosed to the sigmoid colon. This results in the client having drainage from the rectum, which often leads to acidosis and electrolyte imbalance involving potassium, chloride, and magnesium.

23. The client with a Kock's pouch should be taught about living with a stoma, how to self-catheterize and irrigate the appliance, increasing fluid intake to dilute urine to prevent irritation of the stoma, and lastly stoma care. The client will need to self-catheterize at regular intervals.
24. Allopurinol (Zyloprim) reduces the urinary concentration of uric acid to decrease the recurrence of uric acid stones.
25. A high fluid intake of at least 3000 ml/day is needed to remove minerals prior to precipitation.
26. Nursing care priorities for the client with urolithiasis include pain relief and prevention of urinary tract obstruction and recurrence of stones. The nurse can expect to administer narcotics and maintain client safety.
27. Pyelonephritis is an inflammation or infection of the kidney or kidney pelvis.
28. The most common findings in acute renal failure include elevations in BUN and creatinine, metabolic acidosis, hyponatremia, hyperkalemia, hypocalcemia, and hypophosphatemia.
29. Skin care should be provided for the client by bathing with tepid water and oils to reduce dryness and itching.
30. A client with chronic renal failure needs to adhere to a low-protein, low-sodium, and low-potassium diet. This meal plan would fall into these restrictions.
31. A myocardial infarction causes decreased cardiac output, which may cause acute renal failure. The other mechanisms responsible for acute renal failure are nephrotoxicity, trauma, burns, sepsis, and mismatched blood. Chronic renal failure results from irreversible damage to the nephrons and glomeruli. Diseases commonly responsible for chronic renal failure are diabetes, hypertension, and kidney infections.
32. The immediate assessments to be performed for a kidney recipient are fluid and electrolyte status, intake and output, and hypotension.
33. Denial is disowning intolerable thoughts. The client is denying feelings of anxiety and the seriousness of potential rejection of the organ.
34. The renal system is highly vascular; the client is at risk for post-op bleeding.
35. Benign prostatic hyperplasia (BPH) is the growth of new cells in the prostate gland, resulting in urinary obstruction; therefore, assessment of the obstructive symptoms are: decrease in the force of the urinary stream; hesitancy in initiation of urine; dribbling; urinary retention; incomplete bladder emptying; nocturia; dysuria; and urgency.
36. Clients with BPH should void every 2 to 3 hours to flush the urinary tract.

37. Blood clots are normal after a prostatectomy for the first 36 hours. Large quantities of bright red blood may indicate hemorrhage.

38. Prior to surgery, the client should be informed that his sexual functioning will not be hampered other than retrograde ejaculation, which is not physically harmful.

39. Urine output is calculated by subtracting the amount of irrigant instilled from the total fluid removed from the drainage bag (2900 ml drainage - 2400 ml irrigant = 500 ml urine).

11

The Musculoskeletal System

■ OVERVIEW OF ANATOMY AND PHYSIOLOGY

The musculoskeletal system consists of the bones, muscles, joints, cartilage, tendons, ligaments, and bursae. Its major function is to provide a structural framework for the body and to provide a means for movement.

CHAPTER OUTLINE

Bones

A. Functions
   1. Provide support to skeletal framework
   2. Assist in movement by acting as levers for muscles
   3. Protect vital organs and soft tissues
   4. Manufacture RBCs in the red bone marrow (hematopoiesis)
   5. Provide site for storage of calcium and phosphorus

B. Types of bones
   1. Long: central shaft (diaphysis) made of compact bone and two ends (epiphyses) composed of cancellous bone (e.g., femur and humerus)
   2. Short: cancellous bone covered by thin layer of compact bone (e.g., carpals and tarsals)
   3. Flat: two layers of compact bones separated by a layer of cancellous bone (e.g., skull and ribs)
   4. Irregular: sizes and shapes vary (e.g., vertebrae and mandible)

Joints

A. Articulation of bones occurs at joints; movable joints provide stabilization and permit a variety of movements

B. Classification (according to degree of movement)
   1. Synarthroses: immovable joints
   2. Amphiarthroses: partially movable joints
   3. Diarthroses (synovial): freely movable joints
      a. Have a joint cavity (synovial cavity) between the articulating bone surfaces

  b. Articular cartilage covers the ends of the bones
  c. A fibrous capsule encloses the joint
  d. Capsule is lined with synovial membrane that secretes synovial fluid to lubricate the joint and reduce friction

Muscles

A. Functions
  1. Provide shape to the body
  2. Protect the bones
  3. Maintain posture
  4. Cause movement of body parts by contraction
B. Types of muscles
  1. *Cardiac:* involuntary; found only in heart
  2. *Smooth:* involuntary; found in walls of hollow structures (e.g., intestines)
  3. *Striated (skeletal):* voluntary
C. Characteristics of skeletal muscles
  1. Muscles are attached to the skeleton at the point of origin and to bones at the point of insertion.
  2. Have properties of contraction and extension, as well as elasticity, to permit isotonic (shortening and thickening of the muscle) and isometric (increased muscle tension) movement.
  3. Contraction is innervated by nerve stimulation.

Cartilage

A. A form of connective tissue
B. Major functions are to cushion bony prominences and offer protection where resiliency is required

Tendons and Ligaments

A. Composed of dense, fibrous connective tissue
B. Functions
  1. Ligaments attach bone to bone
  2. Tendons attach muscle to bone

■ ASSESSMENT

Health History

A. Presenting problem
  1. Muscles: symptoms may include pain, cramping, weakness
  2. Bones and joints: symptoms may include stiffness, swelling, pain, redness, heat, limitation of movement

B. Lifestyle: usual patterns of activity and exercise (limitations in ADL, use of assistive devices such as canes or walkers), nutrition (obesity) and diet, occupation (sedentary, heavy lifting, or pushing)

C. Use of medications: drugs taken for musculoskeletal problems

D. Past medical history: congenital defects, trauma, inflammations, fractures, back pain

E. Family history: arthritis, gout

Physical Examination

A. Inspect for overall body build, posture, and gait.

B. Inspect and palpate joints for swelling, deformity, masses, movement, tenderness, crepitations.

C. Inspect and palpate muscles for size, symmetry, tone, strength.

Laboratory/Diagnostic Tests

A. Hematologic studies
- **1.** Muscle enzymes: CPK, aldolase, SGOT (AST)
- **2.** Erythrocyte sedimentation rate (ESR)
- **3.** Rheumatoid factor
- **4.** Complement fixation
- **5.** Lupus erythematosus cells (LE prep)
- **6.** Antinuclear antibodies (ANA)
- **7.** Anti-DNA
- **8.** C-reactive protein
- **9.** Uric acid

B. X-rays: detect injury to or tumors of bone or soft tissue

C. Bone scan
- **1.** Measures radioactivity in bones 2 hours after IV injection of a radioisotope; detects bone tumors, osteomyelitis.
- **2.** Nursing care
  - **a.** Have client void immediately before the procedure.
  - **b.** Explain that client must remain still during the scan itself.

D. Arthroscopy
- **1.** Insertion of fiberoptic endoscope (arthroscope) into a joint to visualize it, perform biopsies, or remove loose bodies from the joint
- **2.** Performed in OR using aseptic technique
- **3.** Nursing care
  - **a.** Maintain pressure dressing for 24 hours.
  - **b.** Advise client to limit activity for several days.

E. Arthrocentesis: insertion of a needle into the joint to aspirate synovial fluid for diagnostic purposes or to remove excess fluid

F. Myelography
   1. Lumbar puncture used to withdraw a small amount of CSF, which is replaced with a radiopaque dye; used to detect tumors or herniated intravertebral discs
   2. Nursing care: pretest
      a. Keep NPO after liquid breakfast.
      b. Check for iodine allergy.
      c. Confirm that consent form has been signed and explain procedure to client.
   3. Nursing care: posttest
      a. If oil-based dye (e.g., iophendylate [Pantopaque]) was used, keep client flat for 12 hours.
      b. If water-based dye (e.g., metrizamide [Amipaque]) was used
         1) elevate head of bed 30–45° to prevent upward displacement of dye, which may cause meningeal irritation and possibly seizures.
         2) institute seizure precautions and do not administer any phenothiazine drugs to client, e.g., prochlorperazine (Compazine).

G. Electromyography
   1. Measures and records activity of contracting muscles in response to electrical stimulation; helps differentiate muscle disease from motor neuron dysfunction
   2. Nursing care: explain procedure to the client and advise that some discomfort may occur due to needle insertion

ANALYSIS

Nursing diagnoses for clients with disorders of the musculoskeletal system may include

A. Risk for injury
B. Risk for disuse syndrome
C. Impaired physical mobility
D. Bathing/hygiene self-care deficit
E. Dressing/grooming self-care deficit
F. Toileting self-care deficit
G. Body-image disturbance
H. Pain

PLANNING AND IMPLEMENTATION

Goals

Client will

A. Be free from injury.
B. Be free from complications of immobility.
C. Attain optimal level of mobility.

D. Perform self-care activities at optimal level.
E. Adapt to alterations in body image.
F. Achieve maximum comfort level.

Interventions

Preventing Complications of Immobility

Range-of-Motion (ROM) Exercises

A. Movement of joint through its full ROM to prevent contractures and increase or maintain muscle tone/strength
B. Types
   1. Active: carried out by client; increases and maintains muscle tone; maintains joint mobility
   2. Passive: carried out by nurse without assistance from client; maintains joint mobility only; body part not to be moved beyond its existing ROM
   3. Active assistive: client moves body part as far as possible and nurse completes remainder of movement
   4. Active resistive: contraction of muscles against an opposing force; increases muscle size and strength

Isometric Exercises

A. Active exercise through contraction/relaxation of muscle; no joint movement; length of muscle does not change.
B. Client increases tension in muscle for several seconds and then relaxes.
C. Maintains muscle strength and size.

Assistive Devices for Walking

A. Cane
   1. Types: single, straight-legged cane; tripod cane; quad cane.
   2. Nursing care: teach client to hold cane in hand opposite affected extremity and to advance cane at the same time the affected leg is moved forward.
B. Walker
   1. Mechanical device with four legs for support.
   2. Nursing care: teach client to hold upper bars of walker at each side, then to move the walker forward and step into it.
C. Crutches: teaching the client proper use of crutches is an important nursing responsibility.
   1. Ensure proper length
      a. When client assumes erect position the top of crutch is 2 inches below the axilla, and the tip of each crutch is 6 inches in front and to the side of the feet.
      b. Client's elbows should be slightly flexed when hand is on hand grip.
      c. Weight should not be borne by the axillae.

2. Crutch gaits
   a. Four-point gait: used when weight bearing is allowed on both extremities
      1) advance right crutch.
      2) step forward with left foot.
      3) advance left crutch.
      4) step forward with right foot.
   b. Two-point gait: typical walking pattern, an acceleration of four-point gait
      1) step forward moving both right crutch and left leg simultaneously.
      2) step forward moving both left crutch and right leg simultaneously.
   c. Three-point gait: used when weight bearing is permitted on one extremity only
      1) advance both crutches and affected extremity several inches, maintaining good balance.
      2) advance the unaffected leg to the crutches, supporting the weight of the body on the hands.
   d. Swing-to gait: used for clients with paralysis of both lower extremities who are unable to lift feet from floor
      1) both crutches are placed forward.
      2) client swings forward to the crutches.
   e. Swing-through gait: same indications as for swing-to gait
      1) both crutches are placed forward.
      2) client swings body through the crutches.

Care of the Client with a Cast

A. Types of casts: long arm, short arm, long leg, short leg, walking cast with rubber heel, body cast, shoulder spica, hip spica
B. Casting materials
   1. Plaster of paris—traditional cast
      a. Takes 24–72 hours to dry.
      b. Precautions must be taken until cast is dry to prevent dents, which may cause pressure areas.
      c. Signs of a dry cast: shiny white, hard, resistant.
      d. Must be kept dry since water can ruin a plaster cast.
   2. Synthetic casts, e.g., fiberglass
      a. Strong, lightweight; sets in about 20 minutes.
      b. Can be dried using cast dryer or hair blow-dryer on cool setting; some synthetic casts need special lamp to harden.
      c. Water-resistant; however, if cast becomes wet, must be dried thoroughly to prevent skin problems under cast.
C. Cast drying—plaster cast
   1. Use palms of hands, not fingertips, to support cast when moving or lifting client.

2. Support cast on rubber- or plastic-protected pillows with cloth pillowcase along length of cast until dry.
3. Turn client every 2 hours to reduce pressure and promote drying.
4. Do not cover the cast until it is dry (may use fan to facilitate drying).
5. Do not use heat lamp or hair dryer on plaster cast.

D. Assessment
1. Perform neurovascular checks to area distal to cast.
   a. Report absent or diminished pulse, cyanosis or blanching, coldness, lack of sensation, inability to move fingers or toes, excessive swelling.
   b. Report complaints of burning, tingling, or numbness.
2. Note any odor from the cast that may indicate infection.
3. Note any bleeding on cast in a surgical client.
4. Check for "hot spots" that may indicate inflammation under cast.

E. General care
1. Instruct client to wiggle toes or fingers to improve circulation.
2. Elevate affected extremity above heart level to reduce swelling.
3. Apply ice bags to each side of the cast if ordered.

F. Provide client teaching and discharge planning concerning
1. Isometric exercises when cleared with physician
2. Reinforcement of instructions given on crutch walking
3. Do not get cast wet; wrap cast in plastic bag when bathing or take sponge bath
4. If a cast that has already dried and hardened does become wet, may use blow-dryer on low setting over wet spot; if large area of plaster cast becomes wet, call physician
5. Do not scratch or insert foreign bodies under cast; may direct cool air from blow-dryer under cast for itching
6. Recognize and report signs of impaired circulation or of infection
7. Cast cleaning
   a. Clean surface soil on plaster cast with a slightly damp cloth; mild soap may be used for synthetic cast
   b. To brighten a plaster cast, apply white shoe polish sparingly

Care of the Client in Traction

A. A pulling force exerted on bones to reduce and/or immobilize fractures, reduce muscle spasm, correct or prevent deformities

B. Types
1. Skin traction: weights are attached to a moleskin or adhesive strip secured by elastic bandage or other special device (e.g., foam rubber boot) used to cover the affected limb.
   a. *Buck's extension*
      1) exerts straight pull on affected extremity
      2) generally used to temporarily immobilize the leg in a client with a fractured hip

3) shock blocks at the foot of the bed produce countertraction and prevent the client from sliding down in bed

b. *Russell traction*
   1) knee is suspended in a sling attached to a rope and pulley on a Balkan frame, creating upward pull from the knee; weights are attached to foot of bed (as in Buck's extension) creating a horizontal force exerted on the tibia and fibula
   2) generally used to stabilize fractures of the femoral shaft while client is awaiting surgery
   3) elevating foot of bed slightly provides countertraction
   4) head of bed should remain flat
   5) foot of bed usually elevated by shock blocks to provide countertraction
c. *Cervical traction*
   1) cervical head halter attached to weights that hang over head of bed
   2) used for soft tissue damage or degenerative disc disease of cervical spine to reduce muscle spasm and maintain alignment
   3) usually intermittent traction
   4) elevate head of bed to provide countertraction
d. *Pelvic traction*
   1) pelvic girdle with extension straps attached to ropes and weights
   2) used for low back pain to reduce muscle spasm and maintain alignment
   3) usually intermittent traction
   4) client in semi-Fowler's position with knee bent
   5) secure pelvic girdle around iliac crests

2. Skeletal traction: traction applied directly to the bones using pins, wires, or tongs (e.g., Crutchfield tongs) that are surgically inserted; used for fractured femur, tibia, humerus, cervical spine
3. Balanced suspension traction: produced by a counterforce other than the client's weight; extremity floats or balances in the traction apparatus; client may change position without disturbing the line of traction
4. *Thomas splint and Pearson attachment* (usually used with skeletal traction in fractures of the femur)
   a. Hip should be flexed at 20°
   b. Use footplate to prevent foot drop

C. Nursing care
   1. Check traction apparatus frequently to ensure that
      a. Ropes are aligned and weights are hanging freely.
      b. Bed is in proper position.
      c. Line of traction is within the long axis of the bone.
   2. Maintain client in proper alignment.
      a. Align in center of bed.
      b. Do not rest affected limb against foot of bed.

DELEGATION TIP

Appropriately trained ancillary staff may apply skin traction. The nurse should assure proper body alignment, neurovascular integrity, and proper padding of surfaces.

3. Perform neurovascular checks to affected extremity.
4. Observe for and prevent footdrop.
   a. Provide footplate.
   b. Encourage plantarflexion and dorsiflexion exercises.
5. Observe for and prevent deep venous thrombosis (especially in Russell traction due to pressure on popliteal space).
6. Observe for and prevent skin irritation and breakdown (especially over bony prominences and traction application sites).
   a. Russell traction: check popliteal area frequently and pad the sling with felt covered by stockinette or ABDs.
   b. Thomas splint: pad top of splint with same material as in Russell traction.
   c. Cervical traction: pad chin area and protect ears.
7. Provide pin care for clients in skeletal traction.
   a. Usually consists of cleansing and applying antibiotic ointment, but individual agency policies may vary.
   b. Observe for any redness, drainage, odor.
8. Assist with ADL; provide overhead trapeze to facilitate moving, using bedpan, etc.
9. Prevent complications of immobility.
10. Encourage active ROM exercises to unaffected extremities.
11. Check carefully for orders about turning.
   a. Buck's extension: client may turn to unaffected side (place pillows between legs before turning).
   b. Russell traction and balanced suspension traction: client may turn slightly from side to side without turning body below the waist.
   c. May need to make bed from head to foot.

EVALUATION

A. Client remains free from injury.
B. Client is free from complications of immobility.
   1. Maintains clear, intact skin.
   2. Has regular bowel movements.
   3. Is free from urinary tract infection/retention/calculi.
   4. Has clear breath sounds; normal rate, rhythm, and depth of respiration.

5. Demonstrates adequate peripheral circulation.
6. Maintains joint mobility and muscle tone.
7. Remains oriented to time, place, and person.
8. Is active in decision making regarding own care.

C. Optimum level of mobility is attained.
D. Client attains independence in self-care activities; uses assistive devices as necessary.
E. Client successfully adjusts to alterations in body image; exhibits increased self-esteem.
F. Pain is relieved or is more manageable.

DISORDERS OF THE MUSCULOSKELETAL SYSTEM

Rheumatoid Arthritis (RA)

A. General information
   1. Chronic systemic disease characterized by inflammatory changes in joints and related structures.
   2. Occurs in women more often than men (3:1); peak incidence between ages 35–45.
   3. Cause unknown, but may be an autoimmune process; genetic factors may also play a role.
   4. Predisposing factors include fatigue, cold, emotional stress, infection.
   5. Joint distribution is symmetric (bilateral); most commonly affects smaller peripheral joints of hands and also commonly involves wrists, elbows, shoulders, knees, hips, ankles, and jaw.
   6. If unarrested, affected joints progress through four stages of deterioration: synovitis, pannus formation, fibrous ankylosis, and bony ankylosis.

B. Medical management
   1. Drug therapy
      a. Aspirin: mainstay of treatment, has both analgesic and anti-inflammatory effect.
      b. Nonsteroidal anti-inflammatory drugs (NSAIDs): ibuprofen (Motrin), indomethacin (Indocin), fenoprofen (Nalfon), mefenamic acid (Ponstel), phenylbutazone (Butazolidin), piroxicam (Feldene), naproxen (Naprosyn), sulindac (Clinoril); relieve pain and inflammation by inhibiting the synthesis of prostaglandins
      c. Gold compounds (chrysotherapy)
         1) injectable form: sodium thiomalate (Myochrysine); aurothioglucose (Solganal); given IM once a week; take 3–6 months to become effective; side effects include proteinuria, mouth ulcers, skin rash, aplastic anemia; monitor blood studies and urinalysis frequently.

2) oral form: auranofin (Ridaura); smaller doses are effective; take 3–6 months to become effective; diarrhea also a side effect with oral form; blood and urine studies should also be monitored.

d. Corticosteroids

1) intra-articular injections temporarily suppress inflammation in specific joints.

2) systemic administration used only when client does not respond to less potent anti-inflammatory drugs.

e. Methotrexate, Cytoxan given to suppress immune response; side effects include bone marrow suppression

2. Physical therapy to minimize joint deformities

3. Surgery to remove severely damaged joints (e.g., total hip replacement; knee replacement)

C. Assessment findings

1. Fatigue, anorexia, malaise, weight loss, slight elevation in temperature.

2. Joints are painful, warm, swollen, limited in motion, stiff in morning and after periods of inactivity, and may show crippling deformity in long-standing disease.

3. Muscle weakness secondary to inactivity.

4. History of remissions and exacerbations.

5. Some clients have additional extra-articular manifestations: subcutaneous nodules; eye, vascular, lung, or cardiac problems.

6. Diagnostic tests

a. X-rays show various stages of joint disease

b. CBC: anemia is common

c. ESR elevated

d. Rheumatoid factor positive

e. ANA may be positive

f. C-reactive protein elevated

D. Nursing interventions

1. Assess joints for pain, swelling, tenderness, limitation of motion.

2. Promote maintenance of joint mobility and muscle strength.

a. Perform ROM exercises several times a day; use of heat prior to exercise may decrease discomfort; stop exercise at the point of pain.

b. Use isometric or other exercise to strengthen muscles.

3. Change position frequently; alternate sitting, standing, lying.

4. Promote comfort and relief/control of pain.

a. Ensure balance between activity and rest.

b. Provide 1–2 scheduled rest periods throughout day.

c. Rest and support inflamed joints; if splints used, remove 1–2 times/ day for gentle ROM exercises.

5. Ensure bed rest if ordered for acute exacerbations.

a. Provide firm mattress.

b. Maintain proper body alignment.

   c. Have client lie prone for ½ hour twice a day.
   d. Avoid pillows under knees.
   e. Keep joints mainly in extension, not flexion.
   f. Prevent complications of immobility.
6. Provide heat treatments (warm bath, shower, or whirlpool; warm, moist compresses; paraffin dips) as ordered.
   a. May be more effective in chronic pain.
   b. Reduce stiffness, pain, and muscle spasm.
7. Provide cold treatments as ordered; most effective during acute episodes.
8. Provide psychologic support and encourage client to express feelings.
9. Assist client in setting realistic goals; focus on client strengths.
10. Provide client teaching and discharge planning concerning
    a. Use of prescribed medications and side effects
    b. Self-help devices to assist in ADL and to increase independence
    c. Importance of maintaining a balance between activity and rest
    d. Energy conservation methods
    e. Performance of ROM, isometric, and prescribed exercises
    f. Maintenance of well-balanced diet
    g. Application of resting splints as ordered
    h. Avoidance of undue physical or emotional stress
    i. Importance of follow-up care

Osteoarthritis

A. General information
   1. Chronic, nonsystemic disorder of joints characterized by degeneration of articular cartilage
   2. Women and men affected equally; incidence increases with age
   3. Cause unknown; most important factor in development is aging (wear and tear on joints); others include obesity, joint trauma
   4. Weight-bearing joints (spine, knees, hips) and terminal interphalangeal joints of fingers most commonly affected
B. Assessment findings
   1. Pain (aggravated by use and relieved by rest) and stiffness of joints
   2. Heberden's nodes: bony overgrowths at terminal interphalangeal joints
   3. Decreased ROM, possible crepitation (grating sound when moving joint)
   4. Diagnostic tests
      a. X-rays show joint deformity as disease progresses
      b. ESR may be slightly elevated when disease is inflammatory
C. Nursing interventions
   1. Assess joints for pain and ROM.
   2. Relieve strain and prevent further trauma to joints.
      a. Encourage rest periods throughout day.
      b. Use cane or walker when indicated.

c. Ensure proper posture and body mechanics.
d. Promote weight reduction if obese.
e. Avoid excessive weight-bearing activities and continuous standing.

3. Maintain joint mobility and muscle strength.
   a. Provide ROM and isometric exercises.
   b. Ensure proper body alignment.
   c. Change client's position frequently.
4. Promote comfort/relief of pain.
   a. Administer medications as ordered: aspirin and NSAIDs most commonly used; intra-articular injections of corticosteroids relieve pain and improve mobility.
   b. Apply heat as ordered (e.g., warm baths, compresses, hot packs) or ice to reduce pain.
5. Prepare client for joint replacement surgery if necessary.
6. Provide client teaching and discharge planning concerning
   a. Use of prescribed medications and side effects
   b. Importance of rest periods
   c. Measures to relieve strain on joints
   d. ROM and isometric exercises
   e. Maintenance of a well-balanced diet
   f. Use of heat/ice as ordered

Gout

A. General information
   1. A disorder of purine metabolism; causes high levels of uric acid in the blood and the precipitation of urate crystals in the joints
   2. Inflammation of the joints caused by deposition of urate crystals in articular tissue
   3. Occurs most often in males
   4. Familial tendency

B. Medical management
   1. Drug therapy
      a. Acute attack: Colchicine IV or PO (discontinue if diarrhea occurs); NSAIDs such as indomethacin (Indocin), naproxen (Naprosyn), phenylbutazone (Butazolidin)
      b. Prevention of attacks
         1) uricosuric agents (probenecid [Benemid], sulfinpyrazone [Anturane]) increase renal excretion of uric acid
         2) allopurinal (Zyloprim) inhibits uric acid formation
   2. Low-purine diet may be recommended
   3. Joint rest and protection
   4. Heat or cold therapy

C. Assessment findings
   1. Joint pain, redness, heat, swelling; joints of foot (especially great toe) and ankle most commonly affected (acute gouty arthritis stage)
   2. Headache, malaise, anorexia
   3. Tachycardia; fever; tophi in outer ear, hands, and feet (chronic tophaceous stage)
   4. Diagnostic test: uric acid elevated
D. Nursing interventions
   1. Assess joints for pain, motion, appearance.
   2. Provide bed rest and joint immobilization as ordered.
   3. Administer antigout medications as ordered.
   4. Administer analgesics for pain as ordered.
   5. Increase fluid intake to 2000–3000 ml/day to prevent formation of renal calculi.
   6. Apply local heat or cold as ordered.
   7. Apply bed cradle to keep pressure of sheets off joints.
   8. Provide client teaching and discharge planning concerning
      a. Medications and their side effects
      b. Modifications for low-purine diet: avoidance of shellfish, liver, kidney, brains, sweetbreads, sardines, anchovies
      c. Limitation of alcohol use
      d. Increase in fluid intake
      e. Weight reduction if necessary
      f. Importance of regular exercise

Systemic Lupus Erythematosus (SLE)

A. General information
   1. Chronic connective tissue disease involving multiple organ systems
   2. Occurs most frequently in young women
   3. Cause unknown; immune, genetic, and viral factors have all been suggested
   4. Pathophysiology
      a. A defect in body's immunologic mechanisms produces autoantibodies in the serum directed against components of the client's own cell nuclei.
      b. Affects cells throughout the body resulting in involvement of many organs, including joints, skin, kidney, CNS, and cardiopulmonary system.
B. Medical management
   1. Drug therapy
      a. Aspirin and NSAIDs to relieve mild symptoms such as fever and arthritis
      b. Corticosteroids to suppress the inflammatory response in acute exacerbations or severe disease

   c. Immunosuppressive agents such as azathioprine (Imuran), cyclophosphamide (Cytoxan) to suppress the immune response when client unresponsive to more conservative therapy
2. Plasma exchange to provide temporary reduction in amount of circulating antibodies
3. Supportive therapy as organ systems become involved

C. Assessment findings
1. Fatigue, fever, anorexia, weight loss, malaise, history of remissions and exacerbations
2. Joint pain, morning stiffness
3. Skin lesions
   a. Erythematous rash on face, neck, or extremities may occur
   b. Butterfly rash over bridge of nose and cheeks
   c. Photosensitivity with rash in areas exposed to sun
4. Oral or nasopharyngeal ulcerations
5. Alopecia
6. Renal system involvement (proteinuria, hematuria, renal failure)
7. CNS involvement (peripheral neuritis, seizures, organic brain syndrome, psychosis)
8. Cardiopulmonary system involvement (pericarditis, pleurisy)
9. Increase susceptibility to infection
10. Diagnostic tests
   a. ESR elevated
   b. CBC; anemia; WBC and platelet counts decreased
   c. ANA positive
   d. LE prep positive
   e. Anti-DNA positive
   f. Chronic false-positive test for syphilis

D. Nursing interventions
1. Assess symptoms to determine systems involved.
2. Monitor vital signs, I&O, daily weights.
3. Administer medications as ordered.
4. Institute seizure precautions and safety measures with CNS involvement.
5. Provide psychologic support to client/significant others.
6. Provide client teaching and discharge planning concerning
   a. Disease process and relationship to symptoms
   b. Medication regimen and side effects
   c. Importance of adequate rest
   d. Use of daily heat and exercises as prescribed for arthritis
   e. Need to avoid physical or emotional stress
   f. Maintenance of a well-balanced diet
   g. Need to avoid direct exposure to sunlight (wear hat and other protective clothing)
   h. Need to avoid exposure to persons with infections

   i. Importance of regular medical follow-up
   j. Availability of community agencies

Osteomyelitis

A. General information
   1. Infection of the bone and surrounding soft tissues, most commonly caused by *S. aureus*.
   2. Infection may reach bone through open wound (compound fracture or surgery), through the bloodstream, or by direct extension from infected adjacent structures.
   3. Infections can be acute or chronic; both cause bone destruction.
B. Assessment findings
   1. Malaise, fever
   2. Pain and tenderness of bone, redness and swelling over bone, difficulty with weight bearing; drainage from wound site may be present
   3. Diagnostic tests
      a. CBC: WBC elevated
      b. Blood cultures may be positive
      c. ESR may be elevated
C. Nursing interventions
   1. Administer analgesics and antibiotics as ordered.
   2. Use sterile technique during dressing changes.
   3. Maintain proper body alignment and change position frequently to prevent deformities.
   4. Provide immobilization of affected part as ordered.
   5. Provide psychologic support and diversional activities (depression may result from prolonged hospitalization).
   6. Prepare client for surgery if indicated.
      a. Incision and drainage of bone abscess
      b. Sequestrectomy: removal of dead, infected bone and cartilage
      c. Bone grafting after repeated infections
      d. Leg amputation
   7. Provide client teaching and discharge planning concerning
      a. Use of prescribed oral antibiotic therapy and side effects
      b. Importance of recognizing and reporting signs of complications (deformity, fracture) or recurrence

Fractures

A. General information
   1. A break in the continuity of bone, usually caused by trauma
   2. Pathologic fractures: spontaneous bone break, found in certain diseases or conditions (osteoporosis, osteomyelitis, multiple myeloma, bone tumors)
   3. Types

   a. Complete: separation of bone into two parts
      1) transverse
      2) oblique
      3) spiral
   b. Incomplete (partial): fracture does not go all the way through the bone, only part of the bone is broken.
   c. Comminuted: bone is broken or splintered into pieces.
   d. Closed or simple: bone is broken without break in skin.
   e. Open or compound: break in skin with or without protrusion of bone.

B. Medical management
   1. Traction
   2. Reduction
      a. Closed reduction through manual manipulation followed by application of cast
      b. Open reduction
   3. Application of a cast

C. Assessment findings
   1. Pain, aggravated by motion; tenderness
   2. Loss of motion; edema, crepitus (grating sound), ecchymosis
   3. Diagnostic test: X-ray reveals break in bone

D. Nursing interventions
   1. Provide emergency care of fractures.
   2. Perform neurovascular checks on affected extremity.
   3. Observe for signs of compartment syndrome (swelling causes an increase within muscle compartment which causes edema and more pressure; irreversible neuromuscular damage can occur within 4 to 6 hours); signs include weak pulse, pallor followed by cyanosis, paresthesias and severe pain.
   4. Observe for signs of fat emboli (respiratory distress, mental disturbances, fever, petechiae) especially in the client with multiple long-bone fractures.
   5. Encourage diet high in protein and vitamins to promote healing.
   6. Encourage fluids to prevent constipation, renal calculi, and UTIs.
   7. Provide care for the client in traction, with a cast, or with open reduction.
   8. Provide client teaching and discharge planning concerning
      a. Cast care if indicated
      b. Crutch walking if necessary
      c. Signs of complications and need to report them

Open Reduction and Internal Fixation

A. General information
   1. Open reduction of fractures requires surgery to realign bones; may include internal fixation with pins, screws, wires, plates, rods, or nails

CLIENT TEACHING CHECKLIST

Instruct the client to inspect their environment for possible safety issues such as loose carpeting or rugs, slippery floors, poor lighting, and a slippery tub or shower.

NURSING ALERT

Clients with orthostatic hypotension, impaired vision, lower limb dysfunction, and neurologia are predisposed to falls leading to hip fractures.

2. Indications include
    a. Compound fractures
    b. Fractures accompanied by serious neurovascular injuries
    c. Fractures with widely separated fragments
    d. Comminuted fractures
    e. Fractures of the femur
    f. Fractures of joints

B. Nursing interventions: preoperative
    1. Provide routine pre-op care.
    2. Provide meticulous skin preparation to prevent infection.

C. Nursing interventions: postoperative
    1. Provide routine post-op care.
    2. Maintain affected limb in proper alignment.
    3. Perform neurovascular checks to affected extremity.
    4. Observe for post-op infection.

Fractured Hip

A. General information
    1. Fracture of the head, neck (intracapsular fracture) or trochanteric area (extracapsular fracture) of the femur
    2. Occurs most often in elderly women
    3. Predisposing factors include osteoporosis and degenerative changes of bone

B. Medical management
    1. Buck's or Russell traction as temporary measures to maintain alignment of affected limb and reduce the pain of muscle spasm

2. Surgery
   a. Open reduction and internal fixation with pins, nails, and/or plates
   b. Hemiarthroplasty: insertion of prosthesis (e.g., Austin-Moore) to replace head of femur

C. Assessment findings
   1. Pain in affected limb
   2. Affected limb appears shorter, external rotation
   3. Diagnostic test: X-ray reveals hip fracture

D. Nursing interventions
   1. Provide general care for the client with a fracture.
   2. Provide care for the client with Buck's or Russell traction (page 368).
   3. Monitor for disorientation and confusion in the elderly client; reorient frequently and provide safety measures.
   4. Perform neurovascular checks to affected extremity.
   5. Prevent complications of immobility.
   6. Encourage use of trapeze to facilitate movement.
   7. Administer analgesics as ordered for pain.
   8. In addition to routine post-op care for the client with open reduction and internal fixation
      a. Check dressings for bleeding, drainage, infection: empty Hemovac and note output; keep compressed to facilitate drainage.
      b. Assess client's LOC.
      c. Reorient the confused client frequently.
      d. Avoid oversedating the elderly client.
      e. Turn client every 2 hours.
      f. Turn to unoperative side only.
      g. Place two pillows between legs while turning and when lying on side.
      h. Institute measures to prevent thrombus formation.
         1) apply elastic stockings.
         2) encourage plantarflexion and dorsiflexion foot exercises.
         3) administer anticoagulants such as aspirin if ordered.
      i. Encourage quadriceps setting and gluteal setting exercises when allowed.
      j. Observe for adequate bowel and bladder function.
      k. Assist client in getting out of bed, usually on first or second post-op day.
      l. Pivot or lift into chair as ordered.
      m. Avoid weight bearing until allowed.
   9. Provide care for the client with a hip prosthesis if necessary (similar to care for client with total hip replacement).

Total Hip Replacement

A. General information
   1. Replacement of both acetabulum and head of femur with prostheses

NURSING ALERT

Clients post-hip replacement have venous thromboembolism 57% of the time if anticoagulant therapy is not administered.

2. Indications
   a. Rheumatoid arthritis or osteoarthritis causing severe disability and intolerable pain
   b. Fractured hip with nonunion

B. Nursing interventions
1. Provide routine pre-op care.
2. In addition to routine post-op care for the client with hip surgery
   a. Maintain abduction of affected limb at all times with abductor splint or two pillows between legs.
   b. Prevent external rotation (may vary depending on type of prosthesis and method of insertion) by placing trochanter rolls along leg.
   c. Prevent hip flexion.
      1) keep head of bed flat if ordered.
      2) may raise bed to 45° for meals if allowed.
   d. Turn only to unoperative side if ordered; use abductor splint or two pillows between knees while turning and when lying on side.
   e. Assist client in getting out of bed when ordered.
      1) usually on second post-op day.
      2) avoid weight bearing until allowed.
      3) avoid adduction and hip flexion; do not use low chair.
3. Provide client teaching and discharge planning concerning
   a. Prevention of adduction of affected limb and hip flexion
      1) do not cross legs.
      2) use raised toilet set.
      3) do not bend down to put on shoes or socks.
      4) do not sit in low chairs.
   b. Signs of wound infection
   c. Exercise program as ordered
   d. Partial weight bearing only until full weight bearing allowed

Herniated Nucleus Pulposus (HNP)

A. General information
1. Protrusion of nucleus pulposus (central part of intervertebral disc) into spinal canal causing compression of spinal nerve roots

2. Occurs more often in men
3. Herniation most commonly occurs at the fourth and fifth intervertebral spaces in the lumbar region
4. Predisposing factors include heavy lifting or pulling and trauma

B. Medical management
1. Conservative treatment
   a. Bed rest
   b. Traction
      1) lumbosacral disc: pelvic traction
      2) cervical disc: cervical traction
   c. Drug therapy
      1) anti-inflammatory agents
      2) muscle relaxants
      3) analgesics
   d. Local application of heat and diathermy
   e. Corset for lumbosacral disc
   f. Cervical collar for cervical disc
   g. Epidural injections of corticosteroids
2. Surgery
   a. Discectomy with or without spinal fusion
   b. Chemonucleolysis
      1) injection of chymopapain (derivative of papaya plant) into disc to reduce size and pressure on affected nerve root
      2) used as alternative to laminectomy in selected cases

C. Assessment findings
1. Lumbosacral disc
   a. Back pain radiating across buttock and down leg (along sciatic nerve)
   b. Weakness of leg and foot on affected side
   c. Numbness and tingling in toes and foot
   d. Positive straight-leg raise test: pain on raising leg
   e. Depressed or absent Achilles reflex
   f. Muscle spasm in lumbar region
2. Cervical disc
   a. Shoulder pain radiating down arm to hand
   b. Weakness of affected upper extremity
   c. Paresthesias and sensory disturbances
3. Diagnostic tests: myelogram localizes site of herniation

D. Nursing interventions
1. Ensure bed rest on a firm mattress with bed board.
2. Assist client in applying pelvic or cervical traction as ordered.
3. Maintain proper body alignment.
4. Administer medications as ordered.
5. Prevent complications of immobility.
6. Provide additional comfort measures to relieve pain.

7. Provide pre-op care for client receiving chemonucleolysis.
   a. Administer cimetidine (Tagamet) and diphenhydramine HCl (Benadryl) every 6 hours as ordered to reduce possibility of allergic reaction.
   b. Possibly administer corticosteroids before procedure.
8. Provide post-op care for client receiving chemonucleolysis.
   a. Observe for anaphylaxis.
   b. Observe for less serious allergic reaction (e.g., rash, itching, rhinitis, difficulty in breathing).
   c. Monitor for neurologic deficits (numbness or tingling in extremities or inability to void).
9. Provide client teaching and discharge planning concerning
   a. Back-strengthening exercises as prescribed
   b. Maintenance of good posture
   c. Use of proper body mechanics, how to lift heavy objects correctly
      1) maintain straight spine.
      2) flex knees and hips while stooping.
      3) keep load close to body.
   d. Prescribed medications and side effects
   e. Proper application of corset or cervical collar
   f. Weight reduction if needed

Discectomy/Laminectomy

A. General information
   1. Discectomy: excision of herniated fragments of intervertebral disc.
   2. Laminectomy: excision of lamina to reduce pressure on the spinal cord, spinal nerves, or to provide access for removing the disc.
   3. Indications
      a. Most commonly used for herniated nucleus pulposus not responsive to conservative therapy or with evidence of decreasing sensory or motor status
      b. Also indicated for spinal decompression as with spinal cord injury, to remove fragments of broken bone, or to remove spinal neoplasm or abscess
   4. Spinal fusion may be done at the same time if spine is unstable
B. Nursing interventions: preoperative
   1. Provide routine pre-op care.
   2. Teach client log rolling (turning body as a unit while maintaining alignment of spinal column) and use of bedpan.
C. Nursing interventions: postoperative
   1. Provide routine post-op care.
   2. Position client as ordered.
      a. Lower spinal surgery: generally flat
      b. Cervical spinal surgery: slight elevation of head of bed to prevent edema around airway

3. Maintain proper body alignment; with cervical spinal surgery avoid neck flexion and apply cervical collar as ordered.
4. Turn client every 2 hours.
   a. Use log-rolling technique and turning sheet.
   b. Place pillows between legs while on side.
5. Assess for complications.
   a. Monitor sensory and motor status every 2–4 hours.
   b. With cervical spinal surgery client may have difficulty swallowing and coughing.
      1) monitor for respiratory distress.
      2) keep suction and tracheostomy set available.
6. Check dressings for hemorrhage, CSF leakage, infection.
7. Promote comfort.
   a. Administer analgesics as ordered.
   b. Provide additional comfort measures and positioning.
8. Assess for adequate bladder and bowel function.
   a. Monitor every 2–4 hours for bladder distension.
   b. Assess bowel sounds.
   c. Prevent constipation.
9. Prevent complications of immobility.
10. Assist with ambulation.
    a. Usually out of bed day after surgery.
    b. Apply brace or corset if ordered.
    c. If client allowed to sit, use straight-back chair and keep feet flat on floor.

D. Provide client teaching and discharge planning concerning
   1. Wound care
   2. Maintenance of good posture and proper body mechanics
   3. Activity level as ordered
   4. Recognition and reporting of signs of complications such as wound infection, sensory or motor deficits

Spinal Fusion

A. General information
   1. Fusion of spinous processes with bone graft from iliac crest to provide stabilization of spine
   2. Performed in conjunction with laminectomy or discectomy

B. Nursing interventions
   1. Provide pre-op care as for laminectomy.
   2. In addition to post-op care for laminectomy
      a. Position client correctly.
         1) lumbar spinal fusion: keep bed flat for first 12 hours, then may elevate head of bed 20–30°, keep off back for first 48 hours.
         2) cervical spinal fusion: elevate head of bed slightly.

b. Assist with ambulation.
   1) time varies with surgeon and extent of fusion.
   2) usually out of bed 3–4 days post-op.
   3) apply brace before getting client out of bed.
   4) apply special cervical collar for cervical spinal fusion.
c. Promote comfort: client may experience considerable pain from graft site.

3. In addition to client teaching and discharge planning for laminectomy, advise client that
   a. Brace will be needed for 4 months and lighter corset for 1 year after surgery.
   b. It takes 1 year until graft becomes stable.
   c. No bending, lifting, stooping, or sitting for prolonged periods for 4 months.
   d. Walking without excessive tiring is healthful exercise.
   e. Diet modification will help prevent weight gain resulting from decreased activity.

REVIEW QUESTIONS

1. An adult has been diagnosed with rheumatoid arthritis for the past 8 years. Her condition is deteriorating despite conservative treatment, and intramuscular gold is prescribed by the physician. When teaching her about gold (chrysotherapy), it is important that the nurse emphasize
   1. Cushing's syndrome is common.
   2. improvement may not occur for 3–6 months.
   3. side effects are rare.
   4. the need to take this drug daily.
2. A woman who has had rheumatoid arthritis for several years is admitted to the hospital. Upon physical examination of the client, the nurse should expect to find
   1. asymmetric joint involvement.
   2. Heberden's nodes.
   3. obesity.
   4. small joint involvement.
3. A 92-year-old woman was found at home lying on the floor of her kitchen. She was unable to move without experiencing severe pain in her right hip. She is admitted to the orthopedic unit with a diagnosis of a right intracapsular hip fracture. Buck's extension traction is employed prior to surgery. She complains of numbness in the right foot. The nurse inspects

the foot and notes the traction tapes are lengthwise on opposite sides of the limb. The nurse's response to the client should be

1. "How long has your foot been numb?"
2. "I can adjust it for your comfort."
3. "I'll call your doctor about it."
4. "There is nothing wrong with the traction."

4. An elderly woman had an Austin-Moore prosthesis inserted following an intracapsular hip fracture. During the early postoperative period the nurse teaches the client about maintaining her hip in the proper position. Which of the following statements indicates that the client understands her instructions?
   1. "I shouldn't bend my knees."
   2. "Put a pillow between my legs when you turn me."
   3. "I will be sure to put my shoes on when I go for a walk."
   4. "Put me on the commode chair for my bowel movement."
5. The nurse is caring for an elderly woman who has had a fractured hip repaired. In the first few days following the surgical repair which of the following nursing measures will best facilitate the resumption of activities for this client?
   1. Arranging for a wheelchair.
   2. Asking her family to visit.
   3. Assisting her to sit out of bed in a chair qid.
   4. Encouraging the use of an overhead trapeze.
6. A 90-year-old woman is preparing for transfer to an extended care facility to continue recovery following repair of a fractured hip. She begins to cry and says, "When you're young these things don't happen. Why did I break my hip at this age?" Which response by the nurse indicates the best understanding of risk factors for the elderly?
   1. "As you age you become less aware of your surroundings and careless about safety."
   2. "Nothing works as well when we are older."
   3. "There are no known specific reasons why hip fractures occur more often in your age group."
   4. "Your age and sex are factors in the loss of minerals from your bones, making them more likely to break."
7. An adult is admitted to the hospital. X-rays reveal a fractured tibia and a cast is applied. Of the following, which nursing action would be most important after the cast is in place?
   1. Assessing for capillary refill.
   2. Arranging for physical therapy.

3. Discussing cast care with the client
4. Helping the client to ambulate.

8. A 44-year-old has been complaining of severe low back pain that has been treated conservatively for the past year. She is admitted to the hospital for treatment of a herniated disc. A laminectomy with spinal fusion is scheduled. When she returns to the unit after surgery, she is afraid to turn. Of the following maneuvers the client may use to avoid pain, which is unsafe?
   1. Log rolling.
   2. Asking for pain medication.
   3. Placing pillows between her legs.
   4. Sitting up in bed.
9. A 48-year-old man has suffered low-back pain and sciatica for over 2 years. He is admitted to the hospital for evaluation and treatment of this problem. A thorough assessment of his level of discomfort from low-back pain is important primarily because
   1. this will provide a baseline for later comparison.
   2. this is a method for identifying clients with "low back neurosis."
   3. clients who have pain localized to the back and radiating to one extremity are probably not candidates for surgery.
   4. surgery is contraindicated for clients who have had pain for less than two years.
10. An adult man is scheduled for a lumbar laminectomy. Preoperative teaching regarding postoperative pain management should include which of the following explanations?
    1. Pain and spasm are not expected and therefore there will be minimal need for pain medication.
    2. Pain and spasm are expected and pain medication will be provided as needed.
    3. Pain and spasm are expected but pain medication will interfere with a neurological assessment and will therefore be given sparingly.
    4. Pain and spasm are expected but pain medication will be limited as client tolerance to the medication is feared.
11. A 38-year-old woman is visiting her mother who has been hospitalized for repair of a fractured hip. The physician told her that her mother has severe osteoporosis and that this was a contributing factor to her current problem. The daughter has many questions for the nurse regarding her risk for developing osteoporosis. Which statement by the daughter indicates

that she does not fully understand the relationship between exercise and maintenance of bone mass?

1. I will begin jogging.
2. I will begin jumping rope.
3. I will begin swimming.
4. I will begin walking.

12. In preparing a teaching plan for an adult who has had an arthroscopy, the nurse will include which of the following?
    1. Client should check extremity for color, mobility, and sensation at least every 2 hours after procedure.
    2. Client may return to regular activities immediately after procedure.
    3. Remove compression dressing 6 to 8 hours after procedure.
    4. Keep extremity in flexion for 24 hours after procedure.

13. The nursing care plan for an adult who has had a myelogram using an oil-based contrast medium should include which intervention by the nurse?
    1. Give the client a light meal immediately before the myelogram, to help prevent nausea or lightheadedness.
    2. Restrict fluids for 12 hours after the myelogram.
    3. Keep the client in a recumbent position for 12–24 hours after the myelogram.
    4. Assure the client that stiff neck or photophobia are expected side effects of the contrast medium used during the myelogram.

14. Which statement by the family tells the nurse that they understand how to perform passive range of motion exercises on a bed-bound family member?
    1. "We should put each joint through a full series of exercises until Mother tells us she's fatigued."
    2. "Every day, we should try to move all of her joints a degree or two further than they naturally go."
    3. "If Mother has a muscle spasm, we should stop exercising that limb for a day or two."
    4. "To exercise Mother's elbow, we would hold her upper arm still, and move her forearm."

15. An adult is learning how to use a cane. The nurse knows that the person can use the cane safely when observing which of the following?
    1. The cane is held on the unaffected side; the cane and affected leg are moved forward, then the unaffected leg comes forward.

2. The cane is held on the affected side; the cane is moved forward, then the unaffected leg, then the affected leg.
3. The cane is held on the unaffected side; the cane is moved forward, then the unaffected leg, then the affected leg.
4. The cane is held on the affected side; the cane and unaffected leg are moved forward, then the affected leg comes forward.

16. An adult who has had a total hip replacement is learning how to walk with a standard (not reciprocal) walker. Which description below tells the nurse that he is using the walker correctly?

1. One side of the walker is simultaneously advanced with the opposite foot; the process is repeated on the other side.
2. Each time he steps on his nonaffected side, the client advances the walker; when moving his affected side, he steps into the walker and lifts his nonaffected foot.
3. The client balances on both feet, most weight on his nonaffected side, and lifts the walker forward; he then balances on the walker and swings both feet forward into the walker.
4. The client lifts the walker in front while balancing on both feet, then walks into the walker, supporting his body weight on his hands while advancing his affected side.

17. A man has sprained his knee and the emergency nurse is fitting him with crutches. If the man is measured while he is lying down, how does the nurse ensure the correct crutch length?

1. Measure client from anterior axillary fold to sole of foot and add 2 inches.
2. Add 6 inches to the length of the client's foot and measure the distance from that point to the client's axilla.
3. Measure from the client's axilla to his palm to get the length from the top of the crutch to the hand piece. Measure from palm to sole to determine length of lower part of crutch.
4. Subtract 24 inches from client's height to determine length of crutch from top to tip.

18. The nurse is teaching a client with a broken left ankle how to go up stairs when using crutches. Which statement by the nurse is correct?

1. "Place both crutches on the next step, stand on the right foot and place the left foot on the step next to the crutches."
2. "Place the left crutch and right foot on the next step and push off with both arms then lift the left foot up to the step."
3. "Place the right foot on the next step, then move the crutches and the left foot onto the step."
4. "Place the right crutch and left foot on the next step; move the right crutch up onto the step, then swing the right foot up."

19. A 17-year-old sprained his left ankle playing football. The emergency nurse is teaching the client ambulation with crutches using a four-point gait. Which sequence correctly describes this gait?

1. Weight on both crutches and right foot; crutches and left foot move forward while weight stays on right foot; all weight transferred to crutches, then to right foot; crutches advanced forward for next step.
2. Weight on both crutches and both feet; right crutch advances forward, then left foot is advanced as weight shifts to right foot and both crutches; weight is distributed to both feet and right crutch as left crutch is advanced; right foot is advanced with weight on left foot and both crutches.
3. Weight on both crutches and both feet; left foot and right crutch are advanced simultaneously and weight transferred to them; right foot and left crutch are advanced simultaneously and weight transferred to them; the pattern is continued.
4. Weight on both feet and crutches; both crutches are advanced while weight remains on feet; weight transfers to crutches as feet swing forward and land with heels on line with the crutches; both crutches are advanced and the pattern is continued.

20. Which of the following findings would alert the nurse to notify the physician of a serious complication for the client with a cast on his leg?

1. Itching under the cast.
2. Poor capillary refill of the toes.
3. Ability of client to move toes without difficulty.
4. Pain relieved by application of ice bag to cast.

21. Which intervention below would be appropriate for the nurse to teach the client with a cast on his left arm?

1. "Cover your plaster cast with plastic before taking a long bath or shower."
2. "Repair breaks in the cast with super-glue or epoxy."
3. "Remove surface dirt on your cast with a damp cloth."
4. "If your fiberglass cast gets wet, dry it with the warm setting on your blowdryer."

22. An adult is in Russell traction. It is appropriate for the nurse to make which of the following assessments because of the client's treatment modality?

1. Make sure sling under the affected knee is smooth and doesn't apply pressure in the popliteal space.
2. Ensure that both buttocks clear the mattress.

3. Check that the leg in traction is on the mattress, not elevated.
4. Assess for numbness and tingling of one or more fingers, suggesting radial, ulnar, or median nerve pressure.

23. A client's family asks why the client has been put into pelvic traction for low-back pain. The best response for the nurse to give is,
    1. "He really needs bed rest; the traction will force him to stay in bed."
    2. "By pulling on either side of the pelvis, the lower back muscles are stretched and this gives relief from the crampy back muscles."
    3. "Traction helps to relieve compression of the roots of the nerves."
    4. "By holding the pelvis still, the back muscles can relax and start to heal."
24. An adult's left leg is in Buck's extension traction. She complains of burning under the traction boot and the toes on that foot are cool. The nurse's best first action is to
    1. ask, "What do you mean by 'burning'?"
    2. notify the physician at once.
    3. remove the boot, then reapply and reassess.
    4. apply an ice pack to the boot for 15 minutes.
25. A client whose left leg is in balanced suspension traction for a femur fracture needs to be moved to a new bed. The nurse understands that this can be safely done as long as
    1. all weights are removed from the ends of the traction ropes so the leg moves freely before the move is attempted.
    2. the left leg is kept above the level of the heart.
    3. sufficient time is given to the client to move himself to the new bed at his own rate of tolerance.
    4. the line of pull is maintained on the left leg.
26. Which statement best describes the nurse's assessment of the client with rheumatoid arthritis?
    1. Assessment is done of the musculoskeletal, cardiac, pulmonary, and renal systems.
    2. Pain is best assessed by monitoring the client's facial expression during exam and by observing limitations in the client's own movement.
    3. Vital signs are an adequate assessment of the acuity of the client's level of pain.
    4. The client's health history is not nearly as important as the nurse's findings on physical examination.
27. An adult is admitted to the medical unit with an acute exacerbation of rheumatoid arthritis. Which of the following will the nurse include on his nursing care plan?

1. "Administer analgesics for pain when systolic blood pressure increases 20 mmHg or more or pulse increases 20% or more."
2. "Develop plan with client to meet self-care needs."
3. "Instruct client to stop taking iron supplements that lead to constipation."
4. "Schedule hygiene activities together in one block to provide longer rest periods before and after care."

28. An adult has rheumatoid arthritis and is taking prednisone. In creating a teaching plan, the nurse will be certain to include which of the following?

1. "You should expect to be on corticosteroids for the rest of your life."
2. "It will take 3 to 6 months for you to notice any effect from this medication."
3. "Notify your physician of any stomach upset you may have."
4. "Avoid bananas and spinach while you are taking this drug."

29. Which statement by an adult with osteoarthritis indicates to the nurse that she understands her therapeutic regimen?

1. "I will wait until my pain is very bad before I take my pain medication, or else further on in my disease, the medication won't help at all."
2. "Jogging for short distances is better for my arthritis than walking for longer distances."
3. "It would probably be a good idea for me to lose the 30 pounds my doctor recommended I lose."
4. "I should do all my house cleaning on one day, so I can rest for the remainder of the week."

30. In preparing a teaching plan for the client with osteoarthritis, the nurse would include which of the following?

1. Application of cold packs to affected joints to decrease swelling.
2. Client education regarding self-administration of medications.
3. Progressively increasing activity to point of muscle fatigue to build muscle bulk and improve rate of metabolism.
4. Teaching client that degenerative changes are progressive and that pain is a natural sequela of age.

31. The nurse, assessing a client with systemic lupus erythematosus can expect to find which of the following?

1. Dysphagia.
2. Decreased visual acuity or blindness.
3. Dryness or itching of genitalia.
4. Abnormal lung sounds.

32. A client with systemic lupus erythematosus is taking gold. Which of the following interventions would the nurse include in the teaching plan for this client?

    1. "Stop taking your anti-inflammatory medication as long as you are taking gold preparations."
    2. "You will give yourself intramuscular injections of gold preparations every day for 2 to 4 weeks, then taper down to one injection every 2 months."
    3. "You will be taking a large dose when you start taking gold capsules, and will taper down to a smaller dose as the therapy becomes effective."
    4. "Stay away from crowds during flu season and have your blood tested after every other gold injection."

33. In assessing the client with osteomyelitis, the nurse would expect to find which of the following?

    1. Pale, cool, tender skin at site.
    2. Decreased white blood cell count.
    3. Positive wound cultures.
    4. Decreased erythrocyte sedimentation rate.

34. An adult has a fractured left radius, which has been casted. While performing an assessment of this client, the nurse will correctly identify which of these findings as *emergent*?

    1. Pain at the fracture site.
    2. Swelling of fingers of left hand.
    3. Diminished capillary refill of fingers of left hand.
    4. Warm, dry fingers of left hand.

35. Which intervention by the emergency nurse is critical in caring for the client with a fractured tibia and fibula?

    1. Cutting away clothing on the injured leg.
    2. Palpation of the dorsalis pedis pulses.
    3. Administration of analgesic medications as ordered.
    4. Initiating two, large-bore IV catheters and warmed normal saline at a fast rate.

36. A 20-year-old was brought to the emergency department after an auto accident. There is a strong scent of alcohol about her, and she states she had three beers over 3 hours. Her only injury is an open fracture of the left humerus. Which assessment finding by the emergency nurse is critical?

1. Status of client's tetanus immunization.
2. Current blood alcohol level.
3. Support systems available at home to assist with care.
4. Last time client voided.

37. A firefighter fell off a roof while fighting a house fire and fractured his femur. Approximately 24 hours after the incident, the nurse finds him dyspneic, tachypneic, with scattered crackles in his lung fields; he is coughing up large amounts of thick, white sputum. The nurse correctly interprets this as
    1. respiratory compromise related to inhalation of smoke.
    2. pneumonia related to prolonged bed rest.
    3. fat embolism syndrome related to femur fracture.
    4. hypovolemic shock related to multiple trauma.

38. An adult has had a total right hip replacement. The nurse understands that his operative hip is kept in extension and abduction because this position
    1. reduces the risk for the development of thromboemboli.
    2. promotes circulation to the operative site, reducing the risk of avascular necrosis.
    3. helps to prevent dislocation of the hip prosthesis.
    4. facilitates the drainage of blood and fluid at the operative site.

39. An adult who has had a total right hip replacement asks the nurse about "moving around in this bed." The nurse's best response is based on the knowledge that
    1. the client should remain supine for 48 hours after surgery, with affected leg in a slightly inward-rotation position.
    2. although the client must remain supine, she can cross her legs to change position for comfort.
    3. a side-lying position is undesirable, but the head of the bed can be elevated 60–75° to shift weight off of back and buttocks.
    4. the client will be repositioned using an abductor pillow between the legs.

40. Which statement by a client who has had an open reduction/internal fixation of her fractured left hip indicates to the nurse that the client understands her care?
    1. "My nephew will move my bed down to the first floor so I won't have to go up stairs when I get home."
    2. "I should expect my surgical site to be swollen and red for a week or two after I get home."

3. "The night nurse will take off these thigh-high stockings at bedtime, and the day nurse will put them back on at breakfast time."
4. "I need to limit my fluid intake so I won't be getting on and off the bedpan so often; it's not good for my hip."

41. The nurse teaches an adult woman that because she has osteoporosis, she must take safety precautions to prevent falls, "because you could break a hip." The client asks the nurse what one has to do with the other, and the nurse's best response is based on the knowledge that

1. osteoporosis yields brittle bones which break easily.
2. osteoporosis causes changes in balance, which makes the client more susceptible to falls that could lead to hip fractures.
3. hips are the primary sites of calcium loss in osteoporosis, making them more susceptible to fracture.
4. both osteoporosis and hip fractures are common in elderly women.

42. An adult is diagnosed with a herniated nucleus pulposus at the C5-C6 interspace and a second at the C6-C7 interspace. Which of the following findings would the nurse expect to discover during the assessment?

1. Constant, throbbing headaches.
2. Numbness of the face.
3. Clonus in the lower extremities.
4. Pain in the scapular region.

43. An adult has undergone a cervical laminectomy. Because of the potential complications associated with this procedure, the nurse must perform which of the following assessments?

1. Assess for wheezes and stridor.
2. Check pupils for response to direct and consensual light.
3. Assess gag reflex.
4. Assess shoulder shrug and neck strength.

44. The nurse is caring for a person who just had a cervical laminectomy. The nurse knows that the client will most likely be maintained in what position?

1. Left lateral decubitus with neck flexed to 30°.
2. Supine, with no pillows under the head.
3. Flat, with a neck roll under the neck.
4. Modified Trendelenburg, with a soft cervical collar in place.

45. An adult is being discharged after a lumbar laminectomy. Which statement indicates to the nurse that the client understands her discharge teaching?

1. "I can't wait to sit in my own recliner and rest while I watch my soaps!"
2. "I'll be able to man the refreshment stand at my nephew's baseball game next weekend, won't I?"
3. "My friend is getting me a footstool for in front of my sink."
4. "I have to buy a soft mattress so my spine won't be subjected to any extra pressure."

46. The nurse is planning post-op care for a client undergoing a laminectomy. The nurse needs to know whether or not a spinal fusion is also performed because
    1. the contrast medium used to check the fusion site for grafting could cause an allergic reaction.
    2. the client whose laminectomy is performed with a spinal fusion will be on bed rest longer than the client who does not undergo spinal fusion.
    3. clients undergoing spinal fusion will be in long torso casts for 6 to 8 weeks after surgery.
    4. the client whose laminectomy is performed with a spinal fusion is at greater risk for spontaneous pneumothorax than the client who does not undergo spinal fusion.

ANSWERS AND RATIONALES

1. 2. Chrysotherapy often requires a 3–6 month period before effects are seen.
2. 4. Small joint involvement is common in rheumatoid arthritis. All of the other symptoms are seen in osteoarthritis but not rheumatoid arthritis.
3. 1. Numbness is symptomatic of circulatory or nerve impairment to the extremity. It is important to know the length of time the client has been experiencing this sensation.
4. 2. A pillow placed between the client's legs will keep the affected leg abducted and in good alignment while the client is being turned.
5. 4. Exercise is important to keep the joints and muscles functioning and to prevent secondary complications. Use of the overhead trapeze prevents hazards of immobility by permitting movement in bed and strengthening of the upper extremities in preparation for ambulation.
6. 4. Elderly females are prone to hip fractures because the cessation of estrogen production after menopause contributes to demineralization of bone.
7. 1. Good capillary refill indicates that the cast has not caused a circulatory problem in the extremity. Assessing circulation is a priority of action.

8. 4. The client returning from a lumbar spinal fusion should be kept flat in bed.
9. 1. The importance of an accurate history cannot be overemphasized in assessing the character and location of the pain. A baseline assessment of neurological signs is made so that deviation from the database can be noted. Once a pain assessment is complete a plan for pain management can be developed.
10. 2. Clients should be told that they may experience pain and spasm in the early postoperative period and that pain medication will be provided.
11. 3. Physical compression of weight-bearing joints stimulates osteoblastic deposition of calcium. Swimming does not involve weight bearing and physical compression of joints.
12. 1. Because the joint is distended with saline and the arthroscope is introduced into the joint area, the potential for neurovascular damage exists. Color (indicating adequate vascular perfusion), sensation, and mobility (indicating intact neurologic status) should be assessed, although mobility assessment will likely be limited to "wiggling the digits."
13. 3. If an oil-based contrast medium is used, the client will be kept in a recumbent position for 12–24 hours to reduce cerebrospinal fluid leakage, and thus decrease the likelihood of developing a postprocedure headache. If a water-soluble medium is used, the client will usually remain in bed, with the head elevated 15–30° (to minimize the upward migration of the medium), but some physicians may allow these clients to ambulate.
14. 4. To perform passive range of motion, the joint is supported, the bones above the joint are stabilized, and the body part distal to the joint is exercised through the range of motion. The family's description of how to maneuver the elbow illustrates this well.
15. 1. The cane, held on the unaffected side, will provide a wider base of support for the affected side while the unaffected limb is moving. The client should keep the cane close to the body to prevent leaning.
16. 4. The sequence for using a walker is balance on both feet, lift the walker and place in front of you, walk into the walker (using it for support when standing on affected limb) and then balance on both feet before repeating the sequence.
17. 1. Although measuring the client while he is lying down is not the preferred method of fitting crutches, this formula may be used successfully.
18. 3. The unaffected limb is advanced to the next step, then the crutches and the affected limb move to that step (weight stays on crutches or foot of unaffected side). A handy mnemonic for clients is, "Up with the good leg,

down with the bad,'' meaning the ''good'' leg is used first when going up stairs, and the crutches and ''bad'' leg go to the new step first when going down stairs.

19. 2. A four-point gait is used when partial weight bearing is called for; it provides maximal support.

20. 2. Poor capillary refill (a ''pinking up'' of the toes after the nailbeds are blanched by compression, which takes more than 3 seconds) is indicative of a circulatory compromise. In this scenario, the likely cause is compartment syndrome: an increase of pressure within the cast (''compartment''). Other signs/symptoms include pain unrelieved by usual modalities, disproportional swelling, and inability to move digits.

21. 3. A damp, not wet, cloth can be used to remove superficial dirt. Stained areas can be covered with a thin layer of white shoe polish.

22. 1. Russell traction is a modification of Buck extension, used for a femur fracture that is not appropriate for internal fixation. The modification occurs when a sling is placed under the affected knee, giving more comfort to the client, and preventing some of the rotation tendencies.

23. 3. Although this information may be a bit technical for the lay members of the client's family, it is the only answer that provides correct information. Increased lumbar flexion relieves compression of the lumbar nerve roots, which is why the head of the bed is elevated 30° and the knees are flexed; 15–30 lb of traction increases lumbar flexion and facilitates relief.

24. 2. These are signs of potential neurovascular compromise, an orthopedic emergency. Additionally, the nurse would check the capillary refill of the toes, any peripheral pulses present, and the sensation and mobility of the foot. In addition, the nurse would compare findings on the affected side with those on the nonaffected side.

25. 4. A vertical transfer is permitted, as long as manual traction is applied to maintain the ''line of pull,'' that is, the direction of the traction, or ''pull,'' which the balanced suspension device supplied.

26. 1. Rheumatoid arthritis is a condition with multisystem effects. The cardiopulmonary and renal systems must be assessed as well as the obvious assessment of the musculoskeletal system. Because some of the medications used in treating rheumatoid arthritis can have serious systemic effects (e.g., gold therapy, corticosteroids), this is especially true of the client on aggressive pharmacotherapy.

27. 2. Although this is an exacerbation of an existing problem, it is always appropriate to formulate a plan—with the client's input—as how best to meet his self-care needs. The plan will need to address protection of joints, conservation of energy, and methods to simplify work tasks. Correct use of assistive devices may also be involved in the plan.

28. 3. High dosage or long-term use of corticosteroids is associated with the development of gastric ulcers. Other adverse effects associated with this treatment include hypertension, hyperglycemia, infection susceptibility, and psychiatric disorders.

29. 3. Weight reduction can reduce stress on weight-bearing joints; because the client's physician has recommended it, we can believe that she will benefit from weight loss.

30. 2. Anti-inflammatory medications including salicylates and nonsteroidal anti-inflammatories will be taken by the client indefinitely. The client must understand the regimen; ways to monitor for (and when possible diminish) adverse effects must also be taught.

31. 4. Abnormal lung sounds are indicative of respiratory insufficiency from pleural effusions or infiltrations. Pleural effusions may occur with myocarditis, which might manifest as a pericardial friction rub assessed during the cardiovascular exam.

32. 4. Signs of gold toxicity include bone marrow suppression and hematuria, proteinuria, diarrhea, and stomatitis. The client receiving parenteral gold should expect to have blood and urine monitored after every other injection.

33. 3. Positive wound cultures are used to help determine the causative organisms and indicate which antibiotic therapy is appropriate. Blood cultures may also be positive.

34. 3. Diminished capillary refill suggests vascular compromise, an emergency condition.

35. 2. Neurovascular compromise is possible with fracture; distal pulses should be palpated to ensure circulation is adequate; the dorsalis pedis pulses in both feet should be assessed for comparison purposes. Likewise color, sensation, and mobility should be assessed. These interventions are also to be repeated at frequent intervals during the emergent phase, and especially after any intervention (i.e., splinting, casting).

36. 1. There is a strong risk of infection with an open fracture (a fracture with an open wound through skin surface to bone injury), and the nurse will expect the client to be given antibiotics prophylactically; in addition, tetanus immunization status must be assessed, and tetanus prophylaxis given if needed, or if the status cannot be determined.

37. 3. These are classic observations of the client with fat embolism syndrome, seen within 48 hours of a long-bone fracture. Onset of symptoms is rapid, and often fatal. Any respiratory difficulties, personality changes, or chest pain in clients with recent long-bone fractures must be assessed with fat embolism syndrome in mind.

38. 3. Positioning the client in extension and abduction helps to ensure that the femoral head part of the prosthesis remains in the acetabular cup. The use of wedge pillows or abduction splints helps in maintaining correct position.

39. 4. To maintain the femoral component of the prosthesis in the acetabular cup, an abductor pillow may be used to keep the legs separate; this must be maintained in all repositioning activities. The client is always encouraged to assist with repositioning, as long as the integrity of the hip position is maintained.

40. 1. The client will need to refrain from climbing stairs in the early recovery phase, except as guided during physical therapy sessions. Moving to the first floor is a prudent decision.

41. 1. Osteoporosis is a disorder in which bone formation is slower than bone resorption. The outcome of this disequilibrium is bones that are increasingly porous, brittle, and fragile. Any bone can be broken, but the trauma associated with falls frequently leads to hip fractures in clients with osteoporosis.

42. 4. Sometimes misinterpreted by the client as a heart attack or bursitis, pain with cervical disc herniation at this level may occur between the scapulae, in the neck or the top of the shoulders. Stiffness, paresthesias, or numbness in upper extremities is also possible.

43. 1. The client is assessed for respiratory distress that would be caused by cord edema. The nurse would also look for signs of interstitial edema and/or hematoma.

44. 2. This position will maintain spinal alignment. Occasionally, the physician will approve the use of a pillow under the head, or the head of the bed raised 30° if a soft cervical collar is used, and if the surgical approach was posterior.

45. 3. When standing (for example, while washing dishes at the sink), the client should place one foot on a stool, thus alternating the weight between the feet.

46. 2. Because the bone graft used for fusion is taken from the iliac crest or fibula, the client will have pain and the potential for complications at those sites as well as complications from the laminectomy. Bed rest may be maintained for longer periods of time; lumbar support may be used once the client is ambulating, and pain relief must be directed at the graft site as well as the laminectomy site.

12

The Endocrine System

OVERVIEW OF ANATOMY AND PHYSIOLOGY

The endocrine system is composed of an interrelated complex of glands (pituitary, adrenals, thyroid, parathyroids, islets of Langerhans of the pancreas, ovaries, and testes) that secrete a variety of hormones directly into the bloodstream. Its major function, together with the nervous system, is to regulate body functions.

CHAPTER OUTLINE

Hormone Regulation

A. *Hormones:* chemical substances that act as messengers to specific cells and organs (target organs), stimulating and inhibiting various processes; two major categories
   1. Local: hormones with specific effect in the area of secretion (e.g., secretin, cholecystokinin-pancreozymin [CCK-PZ])
   2. General: hormones transported in the blood to distant sites where they exert their effect (e.g., cortisol)

B. *Negative feedback mechanisms:* major means of regulating hormone levels
   1. Decreased concentration of a circulating hormone triggers production of a stimulating hormone from the pituitary gland; this hormone in turn stimulates its target organ to produce hormones.
   2. Increased concentration of a hormone inhibits production of the stimulating hormone, resulting in decreased secretion of the target organ hormone.

C. Some hormones are controlled by changing blood levels of specific substances (e.g., calcium, glucose).

D. Certain hormones (e.g., cortisol or female reproductive hormones) follow rhythmic patterns of secretion.

E. Autonomic and CNS control (pituitary-hypothalamic axis): hypothalamus controls release of the hormones of the anterior pituitary gland through *releasing and inhibiting factors* that stimulate or inhibit hormone secretion.

Structure and Function of Endocrine Glands

See (Table 12-1) and Figure 12-1.

TABLE 12-1 Hormone Functions

Endocrine Gland	Hormones	Functions
Pituitary		
Anterior lobe	TSH	Stimulates thyroid gland to release thyroid hormones.
	ACTH	Stimulates adrenal cortex to produce and release adrenocorticoids.
	FSH, LH	Stimulate growth, maturation, and function of primary and secondary sex organs.
	GH or somatotropin	Stimulates growth of body tissues and bones.
	Prolactin or LTH	Stimulates development of mammary glands and lactation.
Posterior lobe	ADH	Regulates water metabolism; released during stress or in response to an increase in plasma osmolality to stimulate reabsorption of water and decrease urine output.
	Oxytocin	Stimulates uterine contractions during delivery and the release of milk in lactation.
Intermediate lobe	MSH	Affects skin pigmentation.
Adrenal		
Adrenal cortex	Mineralocorticoids (e.g., aldosterone)	Regulate fluid and electrolyte balance; stimulate reabsorption of sodium, chloride, and water; stimulate potassium excretion.
	Glucocorticoids (e.g., cortisol, corticosterone)	Increase blood glucose levels by increasing rate of glyconeogenesis; increase protein catabolism, increase mobilization of fatty acids; promote sodium and water retention; anti-inflammatory effect; aid body in coping with stress.

Continued

	Sex hormones (androgens, estrogen, progesterone)	Influence development of secondary sex characteristics.
Adrenal medulla	Epinephrine, norepinephrine	Function in acute stress; increase heart rate, blood pressure; dilate bronchioles; convert glycogen to glucose when needed by muscles for energy.
Thyroid	T_3, T_4	Regulate metabolic rate; carbohydrate, fat, and protein metabolism; aid in regulating physical and mental growth and development.
	Thyrocalcitonin	Lowers serum calcium by increasing bone deposition.
Parathyroid	PTH	Regulates serum calcium and phosphate levels.
Pancreas (Islets of Langerhans)		
Beta cells	Insulin	Allows glucose to diffuse across cell membrane; converts glucose to glycogen.
Alpha cells	Glucagon	Increases blood glucose by causing glyconeogenesis and glycogenolysis in the liver; secreted in response to low blood sugar.
Ovaries	Estrogen, progesterone	Development of secondary sex characteristics in the female, maturation of sex organs, sexual functioning, maintenance of pregnancy.
Testes	Testosterone	Development of secondary sex characteristics in the male, maturation of sex organs, sexual functioning.

Pituitary Gland (Hypophysis)

A. Located in sella turcica at the base of the brain

B. "Master gland" of the body, composed of three lobes

  1. Anterior lobe (adenohypophysis)

    a. Secretes tropic hormones (hormones that stimulate target glands to produce their hormone): adrenocorticotropic hormone (ACTH), thyroid-stimulating hormone (TSH), follicle-stimulating hormone (FSH), luteinizing hormone (LH)

    b. Also secretes hormones that have direct effect on tissues: somatotropic or growth hormone, prolactin

    c. Regulated by hypothalamic releasing and inhibiting factors and by negative feedback system

  2. Posterior lobe (neurohypophysis): does not produce hormones; stores and releases antidiuretic hormone (ADH) and oxytocin, produced by the hypothalamus

  3. Intermediate lobe: secretes melanocyte-stimulating hormone (MSH)

Adrenal Glands

A. Two small glands, one above each kidney

B. Consist of two sections

  1. Adrenal cortex (outer portion): produces mineralocorticoids, glucocorticoids, sex hormones

  2. Adrenal medulla (inner portion): produces epinephrine, norepinephrine

Thyroid Gland

A. Located in anterior portion of the neck

B. Consists of two lobes connected by a narrow isthmus

C. Produces thyroxine (T_4), triiodothyronine (T_3), thyrocalcitonin

Parathyroid Glands

A. Four small glands located in pairs behind the thyroid gland

B. Produce parathormone (PTH)

Pancreas

A. Located behind the stomach

B. Has both endocrine and exocrine functions

C. Islets of Langerhans (alpha and beta cells) involved in endocrine function

  1. Beta cells: produce insulin

  2. Alpha cells: produce glucagon

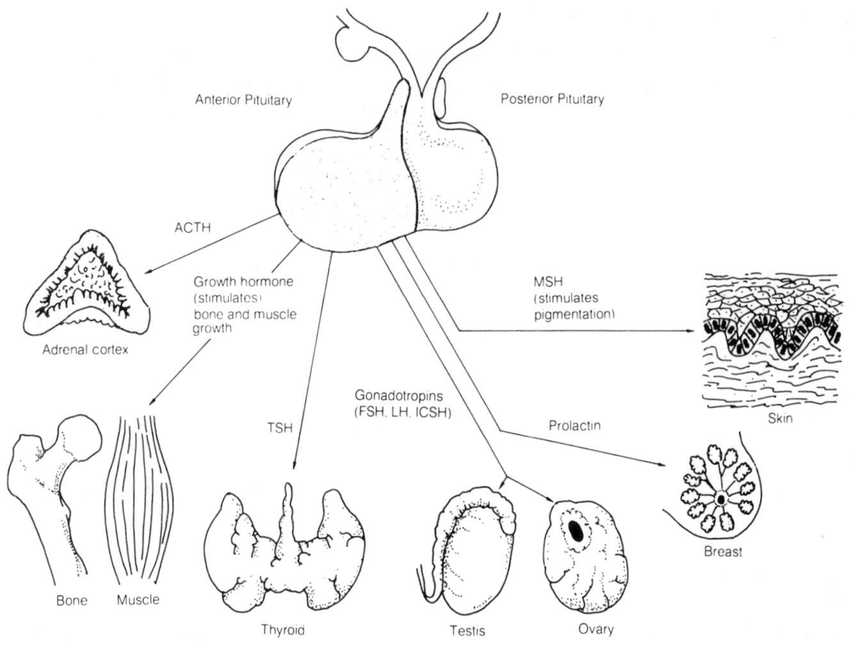

FIGURE 12-1 Hormones secreted by the anterior pituitary gland

Gonads

A. Ovaries: located in pelvic cavity, produce estrogen and progesterone
B. Testes: located in scrotum, produce testosterone

ASSESSMENT

Health History

A. Presenting problem: symptoms may include
1. Change in appearance: hair, nails, skin (change in texture or pigmentation); change in size, shape, or symmetry of head, neck, face, eyes, or tongue
2. Change in energy level
3. Temperature intolerance
4. Development of abnormal secondary sexual characteristics; change in sexual function
5. Change in emotional state, thought pattern, or intellectual functioning
6. Signs of increased activity of sympathetic nervous system (e.g., nervousness, palpitations, tremors, sweating)
7. Change in bowel habits, appetite, or weight; excessive hunger or thirst
8. Change in urinary pattern

B. Lifestyle: any increased stress
C. Past medical history: growth and development (any delayed or excessive growth); diabetes, thyroid disease, hypertension, obesity, infertility
D. Family history: endocrine diseases, growth problems, obesity, mental illness

Physical Examination

A. Check height, weight, body stature, and body proportions.
B. Observe distribution of muscle mass, fat distribution, any muscle wasting.
C. Inspect for hair growth and distribution.
D. Check condition and pigmentation of skin; presence of striae.
E. Inspect eyes for any bulging.
F. Observe for enlargement in neck area and quality of voice.
G. Observe development of secondary sex characteristics.
H. Palpate thyroid gland (normally cannot be palpated): note size, shape, symmetry, any tenderness, presence of any lumps or nodules.

Laboratory/Diagnostic Tests

A variety of tests may be performed to measure the amounts of hormones present in the serum or urine in assessing pituitary, adrenal, and parathyroid functions; these tests will be referred to when appropriate under specific disorders of the endocrine system.

Thyroid Function

A. Serum studies: nonfasting blood studies (no special preparation necessary)
   1. Serum T_4 level: measures total serum level of thyroxine
   2. Serum T_3 level: measures serum triiodothyronine level
   3. TSH: measurement differentiates primary from secondary hypothyroidism

B. Radioactive iodine uptake (RAIU)
   1. Administration of ^{123}I or ^{131}I orally; measurement by a counter of the amount of radioactive iodine taken up by the gland after 24 hours
   2. Performed to determine thyroid function; increased uptake indicates hyperactivity; minimal uptake may indicate hypothyroidism
   3. Nursing care
      a. Take thorough history; thyroid medication must be discontinued 7–10 days prior to test; medications containing iodine, cough preparations, excess intake of iodine-rich foods, and tests using iodine (e.g., IVP) can invalidate this test.
      b. Assure client that no radiation precautions are necessary.

C. Thyroid scan
   1. Administration of radioactive isotope (orally or IV) and visualization by a scanner of the distribution of radioactivity in the gland

2. Performed to determine location, size, shape, and anatomic function of thyroid gland; identifies areas of increased or decreased uptake; valuable in evaluating thyroid nodules
3. Nursing care: same as RAIU

Pancreatic Function

A. Fasting blood sugar: measures serum glucose levels; client fasts from midnight before the test
B. Two-hour postprandial blood sugar: measurement of blood glucose 2 hours after a meal is ingested
   1. Fast from midnight before test
   2. Client eats a meal consisting of at least 75 g carbohydrate or ingests 100 g glucose
   3. Blood drawn 2 hours after the meal
C. Oral glucose tolerance test: most specific and sensitive test for diabetes mellitus
   1. Fast from midnight before test
   2. Fasting blood glucose and urine glucose specimens obtained
   3. Client ingests 100 g glucose; blood sugars are drawn at 30 and 60 minutes and then hourly for 3–5 hours; urine specimens may also be collected
   4. Diet for 3 days prior to test should include 200 g carbohydrate and at least 1500 kcal/day
   5. During test, assess the client for reactions such as dizziness, sweating, and weakness
D. Glycosylated hemoglobin (hemoglobin A_{1c}) reflects the average blood sugar level for the previous 100–120 days. Glucose attaches to a minor hemoglobin (A_{1c}). This attachment is irreversible.
   1. Fasting is not necessary.
   2. Excellent method to evaluate long-term control of blood sugar.

ANALYSIS

Nursing diagnoses for the client with a disorder of the endocrine system may include

A. Imbalanced nutrition: more or less than body requirements
B. Risk for infection
C. Impaired urinary elimination
D. Deficient fluid volume
E. Risk for impaired skin integrity
F. Sexual dysfunction
G. Deficient knowledge
H. Ineffective individual coping
I. Disturbed sleep pattern
J. Disturbed body image

PLANNING AND IMPLEMENTATION

Goals

Client will

A. Regain optimal nutritional status.
B. Be free from infection.
C. Have adequate urinary elimination and fluid volume.
D. Maintain skin integrity.
E. Experience optimum sexual health.
F. Demonstrate and use knowledge of disease process, prescribed medications, treatments, and complications in order to maintain optimal health.
G. Use positive coping behaviors in dealing with the effects of acute and chronic illness.
H. Attain an optimal balance of rest and activity.

Interventions

Care of the Client on Corticosteroid Therapy

A. General information
  1. Types of preparations include cortisone, hydrocortisone, prednisone, dexamethasone (Decadron)
  2. Indications
    a. Replacement therapy in primary and secondary adrenocortical insufficiency
    b. Symptomatic treatment for anti-inflammatory effect of numerous inflammatory, allergic, or immunoreactive disorders (e.g., arthritis, SLE, bronchial asthma, skin diseases, ocular disorders, allergic diseases, inflammatory bowel disorders, cerebral edema and increased ICP, shock, nephrotic syndrome, malignancies, myasthenia gravis, multiple sclerosis)
  3. Common side effects: salt and water retention, sweating, increased appetite
  4. Adverse reactions
    a. Cardiovascular: hypertension, CHF
    b. GI: peptic ulcer, ulcerative esophagitis
    c. Integumentary: petechiae, ecchymoses, purpura, hirsutism, acne, thinning of skin, striae, redistribution of body fat in subcutaneous tissue, abnormal pigmentation, poor wound healing
    d. Endocrine: impaired glucose metabolism, hyperglycemia, menstrual dysfunction, growth retardation
    e. Musculoskeletal: muscle weakness, osteoporosis
    f. Neurologic: personality changes, headache, syncope, vertigo, irritability, insomnia, seizures
    g. Ophthalmologic: cataract formation, glaucoma

   h. Other: hypokalemia, thrombophlebitis, masking of signs of infection, increased susceptibility to infection
   i. Sudden withdrawal may precipitate acute adrenal insufficiency

B. Nursing care
   1. Administer with food or milk; instruct client to report gastric distress (antacids may be necessary).
   2. Give in a single daily dose, preferably before 9 A.M. (corticosteroids suppress adrenal function least when given in early morning, the time of maximal adrenocortical activity).
   3. Instruct client to avoid infections and to report immediately if one is suspected.
   4. Instruct client never to withdraw the drug abruptly, as this may cause acute adrenal insufficiency.
   5. Observe client for any mental changes (e.g., irritability, mood swings, euphoria, depression).
   6. Alert women that menstrual irregularity may develop.
   7. Monitor blood pressure, I&O, weight, blood glucose, and serum potassium.
   8. Advise client to restrict salt intake.
   9. Encourage intake of foods high in potassium.

EVALUATION

A. Client maintains normal weight; no evidence of malnutrition.
B. Client's temperature is within normal limits; no signs of infection.
C. Client has adequate patterns of urinary elimination.
D. Peripheral edema is reduced.
E. Blood pressure and urine output are within normal limits; no signs of dehydration.
F. Skin is intact and free from irritation.
G. Client verbalizes satisfying sexual activity/expression.
H. Client demonstrates and uses knowledge of disease process, prescribed medications, and treatments; reports any complications.
I. Client uses effective coping behaviors to successfully adapt to effects of illness, changes in body image, and loss of function.
J. Client maintains balance between activity and rest.
K. Client demonstrates increased self-esteem.

DISORDERS OF THE ENDOCRINE SYSTEM

Specific Disorders of the Pituitary Gland

Hypopituitarism

A. General information
   1. Hypofunction of the anterior pituitary gland resulting in deficiencies of both the hormones secreted by the anterior pituitary gland and those secreted by the target glands

2. May be caused by tumor, trauma, surgical removal, or irradiation of the gland; or may be congenital

B. Medical management: specific treatment depends on cause
   1. Tumor: surgical removal or irradiation of the gland
   2. Regardless of cause, treatment will include replacement of deficient hormones: e.g., corticosteroids, thyroid hormone, sex hormones, gonadotropins (may be used to restore fertility).

C. Assessment findings
   1. Tumor: bitemporal hemianopia, headache
   2. Varying signs of hormonal disturbances depending on which hormones are being undersecreted (e.g., menstrual dysfunction, hypothyroidism, adrenal insufficiency)
   3. Retardation of growth if condition occurs before epiphyseal closure
   4. Diagnostic tests
      a. Skull X-ray, CT scan may reveal pituitary tumor
      b. Plasma hormone levels may be decreased depending on specific hormones undersecreted

D. Nursing interventions
   1. Provide care for the client undergoing hypophysectomy or radiation therapy if indicated.
   2. Provide client teaching and discharge planning concerning
      a. Hormone replacement therapy
      b. Importance of follow-up care

Hyperpituitarism

A. General information
   1. Hyperfunction of the anterior pituitary gland resulting in oversecretion of one or more of the anterior pituitary hormones
   2. Overproduction of the growth hormone produces acromegaly in adults and gigantism in children (if hypersecretion occurs before epiphyseal closure).
   3. Usually caused by a benign pituitary adenoma

B. Medical management: surgical removal or irradiation of the gland

C. Assessment findings
   1. Tumor: bitemporal hemianopia; headache
   2. Hormonal disturbances depending on which hormones are being excreted in excess
   3. Acromegaly caused by oversecretion of growth hormones: transverse enlargement of bones, especially noticeable in skull and in bones of hands and feet; features become coarse and heavy; lips become heavier; tongue enlarged

4. Diagnostic tests
   a. Skull X-ray, CT scan reveal pituitary tumor
   b. Plasma hormone levels reveal increased growth hormone, oversecretion of other hormones

D. Nursing interventions
   1. Monitor for hyperglycemia and cardiovascular problems (hypertension, angina, HF) and modify care accordingly.
   2. Provide psychologic support and acceptance for alterations in body image.
   3. Provide care for the client undergoing hypophysectomy or radiation therapy if indicated

Hypophysectomy

A. General information
   1. Partial or complete removal of the pituitary gland
   2. Indications: pituitary tumors, diabetic retinopathy, metastatic cancer of the breast or prostate, which may be endocrine dependent
   3. Surgical approaches
      a. Craniotomy: usually transfrontal
      b. Transphenoidal: incision made in inner aspect of upper lip and gingiva; sella turcica is entered through the floor of the nose and sphenoid sinuses

B. Nursing care
   1. In addition to pre-op care of the craniotomy client, explain post-op expectations.
   2. In addition to post-op care of the craniotomy client, observe for signs of target gland deficiencies (diabetes insipidus, adrenal insufficiency, hypothyroidism) due to total removal of the gland or to post-op edema.
      a. Perform hourly urine outputs and specific gravities; alert physician if urine output is greater than 800–900 ml/2 hours or if specific gravity is less than 1.004.
      b. Administer cortisone replacement as ordered.
   3. If transphenoidal approach used
      a. Elevate the head of the bed to 30° to decrease headache and pressure on the sella turcica.
      b. Administer mild analgesics for headache as ordered.
      c. Perform frequent oral hygiene with soft swabs to cleanse the teeth and mouth rinses; no toothbrushing
      d. Observe for and prevent CSF leak from surgical site
         1) warn the client not to cough, sneeze, or blow nose.
         2) observe for clear drainage from nose or postnasal drip (constant swallowing); check drainage for glucose; positive results indicate that drainage is CSF.
         3) if leakage does occur

            a) elevate head of bed and call the physician.
            b) most leaks will resolve in 72 hours with bed rest and elevation.
            c) may do daily spinal taps to decrease CSF pressure.
            d) administer antibiotics as ordered to prevent meningitis.
4. Provide client teaching and discharge planning concerning
    a. Hormone therapy
        1) if gland is completely removed, client will have permanent diabetes insipidus (see below)
        2) cortisone and thyroid hormone replacement
        3) replacement of sex hormones
            a) testosterone: may be given for impotence in men
            b) estrogen: may be given for atropy of the vaginal mucosa in women
            c) human pituitary gonadotropins: may restore fertility in some women
    b. Need for lifelong follow-up and hormone replacement
    c. Need to wear Medic-Alert bracelet
    d. If transphenoidal approach was used
        1) avoid bending and straining at stool for 2 months post-op
        2) no toothbrushing until sutures are removed and incision heals (about 10 days)

Diabetes Insipidus

A. General information
    1. Hypofunction of the posterior pituitary gland resulting in deficiency of ADH
    2. Characterized by excessive thirst and urination
    3. Caused by tumor, trauma, inflammation, pituitary surgery
B. Assessment findings
    1. Polydipsia (excessive thirst) and severe polyuria with low specific gravity
    2. Fatigue, muscle weakness, irritability, weight loss, signs of dehydration
    3. Tachycardia, eventual shock if fluids not replaced
    4. Diagnostic tests
        a. Urine specific gravity less than 1.004
        b. Water deprivation test reveals inability to concentrate urine
C. Nursing interventions
    1. Maintain fluid and electrolyte balance.
        a. Keep accurate I&O.
        b. Weigh daily.
        c. Administer IV/oral fluids as ordered to replace fluid losses.
    2. Monitor vital signs and observe for signs of dehydration and hypovolemia.

3. Administer hormone replacement as ordered.
    a. Vasopressin (Pitressin) and vasopressin tannate (Pitressin tannate in oil); given by IM injection
        1) warm to body temperature before giving.
        2) shake tannate suspension to ensure uniform dispersion.
    b. Lypressin (Diapid): nasal spray
4. Provide client teaching and discharge planning concerning
    a. Lifelong hormone replacement; lypressin as needed to control polyuria and polydipsia
    b. Need to wear Medic-Alert bracelet

Syndrome of Inappropriate Antidiuretic Hormone Secretion (SIADH)

A. General information
   1. Hypersection of ADH from the posterior pituitary gland even when the client has abnormal serum osmolality.
   2. SIADH may occur in persons with bronchogenic carcinoma or other nonendocrine conditions.

B. Medical management
   1. Treat underlying cause if possible
   2. Diuretics and fluid restriction

C. Assessment findings
   1. Persons with SIADH cannot excrete a dilute urine
   2. Fluid retention and sodium deficiency.

D. Nursing interventions
   1. Administer diuretics (furosemide [Lasix]) as ordered.
   2. Restrict fluids to promote fluid loss and gradual increase in serum sodium.
   3. Monitor serum electrolytes and blood chemistries carefully.
   4. Careful intake and output, daily weight.
   5. Monitor neurologic status.

Disorders of the Adrenal Gland

Addison's Disease

A. General information
   1. Primary adrenocortical insufficiency; hypofunction of the adrenal cortex causes decreased secretion of the mineralocorticoids, glucocorticoids, and sex hormones
   2. Relatively rare disease caused by
       a. Idiopathic atrophy of the adrenal cortex possibly due to an autoimmune process
       b. Destruction of the gland secondary to tuberculosis or fungal infection

B. Assessment findings
   1. Fatigue, muscle weakness
   2. Anorexia, nausea, vomiting, abdominal pain, weight loss

3. History of frequent hypoglycemic reactions
4. Hypotension, weak pulse
5. Bronzelike pigmentation of the skin
6. Decreased capacity to deal with stress
7. Diagnostic tests: low cortisol levels, hyponatremia, hyperkalemia, hypoglycemia

C. Nursing interventions
1. Administer hormone replacement therapy as ordered.
   a. Glucocorticoids (cortisone, hydrocortisone): to stimulate diurnal rhythm of cortisol release, give $^2/_3$ of dose in early morning and $^1/_3$ of dose in afternoon
   b. Mineralocorticoids: fludrocortisone acetate (Florinef)
2. Monitor vital signs.
3. Decrease stress in the environment.
4. Prevent exposure to infection.
5. Provide rest periods; prevent fatigue.
6. Monitor I&O.
7. Weigh daily.
8. Provide small, frequent feedings of diet high in carbohydrates, sodium, and protein to prevent hypoglycemia and hyponatremia and provide proper nutrition.
9. Provide client teaching and discharge planning concerning
   a. Disease process; signs of adrenal insufficiency
   b. Use of prescribed medications for lifelong replacement therapy; never omit medications
   c. Need to avoid stress, trauma, and infections, and to notify physician if these occur as medication dosage may need to be adjusted
   d. Stress management techniques
   e. Diet modification (high in protein, carbohydrates, and sodium)
   f. Use of salt tablets (if prescribed) or ingestion of salty foods (potato chips) if experiencing increased sweating
   g. Importance of alternating regular exercise with rest periods
   h. Avoidance of strenuous exercise especially in hot weather

Addisonian Crisis

A. General information
1. Severe exacerbation of Addison's disease caused by acute adrenal insufficiency
2. Precipitating factors
   a. Strenuous activity, infection, trauma, stess, failure to take prescribed medications
   b. Iatrogenic: surgery on pituitary or adrenal glands, rapid withdrawal of exogenous steroids in a client on long-term steroid therapy

B. Assessment findings: severe generalized muscle weakness, severe hypotension, hypovolemia, shock (vascular collapse)

C. Nursing interventions

1. Administer IV fluids (5% dextrose in saline, plasma) as ordered to treat vascular collapse.
2. Administer IV glucocorticoids (hydrocortisone [Solu-Cortef]) and vasopressors as ordered.
3. If crisis precipitated by infection, administer antibiotics as ordered.
4. Maintain strict bed rest and eliminate all forms of stressful stimuli.
5. Monitor vital signs, I&O, daily weights.
6. Protect client from infection.
7. Provide client teaching and discharge planning: same as for Addison's disease.

Cushing's Syndrome

A. General information

1. Condition resulting from excessive secretion of corticosteroids, particularly the glucocorticoid cortisol
2. Occurs most frequently in females between ages 30–60
3. Primary Cushing's syndrome caused by adrenocortical tumors or hyperplasia
4. Secondary Cushing's syndrome (also called Cushing's disease): caused by functioning pituitary or nonpituitary neoplasm secreting ACTH, causing increased secretion of glucocorticoids
5. Iatrogenic: caused by prolonged use of corticosteroids

B. Assessment findings

1. Muscle weakness, fatigue, obese trunk with thin arms and legs, muscle wasting
2. Irritability, depression, frequent mood swings
3. Moon face, buffalo hump, pendulous abdomen
4. Purple striae on trunk, acne, thin skin
5. Signs of masculinization in women; menstrual dysfunction, decreased libido
6. Osteoporosis, decreased resistance to infection
7. Hypertension, edema
8. Diagnostic tests: cortisol levels increased, slight hypernatremia, hypokalemia, hyperglycemia

C. Nursing interventions

1. Maintain muscle tone.
   a. Provide ROM exercises.
   b. Assist with ambulation.
2. Prevent accidents or falls and provide adequate rest.
3. Protect client from exposure to infection.
4. Maintain skin integrity.

NURSING ALERT

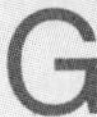
Glucocorticoid administration the morning of a surgery can help prevent acute adrenal insufficiency during surgery.

  a. Provide meticulous skin care.
  b. Prevent tearing of skin: use paper tape if necessary.
5. Minimize stress in the environment.
6. Monitor vital signs; observe for hypertension, edema.
7. Measure I&O and daily weights.
8. Provide diet low in calories and sodium and high in protein, potassium, calcium, and vitamin D.
9. Monitor urine for glucose and acetone; administer insulin if ordered.
10. Provide psychologic support and acceptance.
11. Prepare client for hypophysectomy or radiation if condition is caused by a pituitary tumor.
12. Prepare client for an adrenalectomy if condition is caused by an adrenal
tumor or hyperplasia.
13. Provide client teaching and discharge planning concerning
    a. Diet modifications
    b. Importance of adequate rest
    c. Need to avoid stress and infection
    d. Change in medication regimen (alternate day therapy or reduced dosage) if cause of the condition is prolonged corticosteroid therapy

Primary Aldosteronism (Conn's Syndrome)

A. General information
  1. Excessive aldosterone secretion from the adrenal cortex
  2. Seen more frequently in women, usually between ages 30–50
  3. Caused by tumor or hyperplasia of adrenal gland

B. Assessment findings
  1. Headache, hypertension
  2. Muscle weakness, polyuria, polydipsia, metabolic alkalosis, cardiac arrhythmias (due to hypokalemia)
  3. Diagnostic tests
     a. Serum potassium decreased, alkalosis
     b. Urinary aldosterone levels elevated

C. Nursing interventions
  1. Monitor vital signs, I&O, daily weights.
  2. Maintain sodium restriction as ordered.

3. Administer spironolactone (Aldactone) and potassium supplements as ordered.
4. Prepare the client for an adrenelectomy if indicated.
5. Provide client teaching and discharge planning concerning
   a. Use and side effects of medication if the client is being maintained on spironolactone therapy
   b. Signs of symptoms of hypo/hyperaldosteronism
   c. Need for frequent blood pressure checks and follow-up care

Pheochromocytoma

A. General information
   1. Functioning tumor of the adrenal medulla that secretes excessive amounts of epinephrine and norepinephrine
   2. Occurs most commonly between ages 25 and 50
   3. May be hereditary in some cases
B. Assessment findings
   1. Severe headache, apprehension, palpitations, profuse sweating, nausea
   2. Hypertension, tachycardia, vomiting, hyperglycemia, dilation of pupils, cold extremities
   3. Diagnostic tests
      a. Increased plasma levels of catecholamines; elevated blood sugar; glycosuria
      b. Elevated urinary catecholamines and urinary vanillylmandelic acid (VMA) levels
      c. Presence of tumor on X-ray
C. Nursing interventions
   1. Monitor vital signs, especially blood pressure.
   2. Administer medications as ordered to control hypertension.
   3. Promote rest; decrease stressful stimuli.
   4. Monitor urine tests for glucose and acetone.
   5. Provide high-calorie, well-balanced diet; avoid stimulants such as coffee, tea.
   6. Provide care for the client with an adrenalectomy (see below) as ordered; observe postadrenelectomy client carefully for shock due to drastic drop in catecholamine level.
   7. Provide client teaching and discharge planning: same as for adrenalectomy.

Adrenalectomy

A. General information
   1. Removal of one or both adrenal glands
   2. Indications
      a. Tumors of adrenal cortex (Cushing's syndrome, hyperaldosteronism) or medulla (pheochromocytoma)
      b. Metastatic cancer of the breast or prostate

NURSING ALERT

Monitor the patient who has undergone adrenalectomy closely the first 24–48 hours postoperatively. Their vital signs may fluctuate sharply. IV fluids are essential to counteract shock.

B. Nursing interventions: preoperative
  1. Provide routine pre-op care.
  2. Correct metabolic/cardiovascular problems.
     a. Pheochromocytoma: stabilize blood pressure.
     b. Cushing's syndrome: treat hyperglycemia and protein deficits.
     c. rimary hyperaldosteronism: treat hypertension and hypokalemia.
  3. Administer glucocorticoid preparation on the morning of surgery as ordered to prevent acute adrenal insufficiency.

C. Nursing interventions: postoperative
  1. Provide routine post-op care.
  2. Observe for hemorrhage and shock.
     a. Monitor vital signs, I&O.
     b. Administer IV therapy and vasopressors as ordered.
  3. Prevent infections (suppression of immune system makes clients especially susceptible).
     a. Encourage coughing and deep breathing to prevent respiratory infection.
     b. Use meticulous aseptic technique during dressing changes.
  4. Administer cortisone or hydrocortisone as ordered to maintain cortisol levels.
  5. Provide general care for the client with abdominal surgery.

D. Provide client teaching and discharge planning concerning
  1. Self-administration of replacement hormones
     a. Bilateral adrenalectomy: lifelong replacement of glucocorticoids and mineralocorticoids
     b. Unilateral adrenalectomy: replacement therapy for 6–12 months until the remaining adrenal gland begins to function normally
  2. Signs and symptoms of adrenal insufficiency
  3. Importance of follow-up care

Specific Disorders of the Thyroid Gland

Simple Goiter

A. General information
  1. Enlargement of the thyroid gland not caused by inflammation or neoplasm

2. Types
   a. Endemic: caused by nutritional iodine deficiency, most common in the "goiter belt" (midwest, northwest, and Great Lakes regions), areas where soil and water are deficient in iodine; occurs most frequently during adolescence and pregnancy
   b. Sporadic: caused by
      1) ingestion of large amounts of goitrogenic foods (contain agents that decrease thyroxine production): e.g., cabbage, soybeans, rutabagas, peanuts, peaches, peas, strawberries, spinach, radishes
      2) use of goitrogenic drugs: propylthiouracil, large doses of iodine, phenylbutazone, para-amino salicylic acid, cobalt, lithium
      3) genetic defects that prevent synthesis of thyroid hormone
3. Low levels of thyroid hormone stimulate increased secretion of TSH by pituitary; under TSH stimulation the thyroid increases in size to compensate and produces more thyroid hormone.

B. Medical management
1. Drug therapy
   a. Hormone replacement with levothyroxine (Synthroid) (T_4), dessicated thyroid, or liothyronine (Cytomel) (T_3)
   b. Small doses of iodine (Lugol's or potassium iodide solution) for goiter resulting from iodine deficiency
2. Avoidance of goitrogenic foods or drugs in sporadic goiter
3. Surgery: subtotal thyroidectomy (if goiter is large) to relieve pressure symptoms and for cosmetic reasons

C. Assessment findings
1. Dysphagia, enlarged thyroid, respiratory distress
2. Diagnostic tests
   a. Serum T_4 level low-normal or normal
   b. RAIU uptake normal or increased

D. Nursing interventions
1. Administer replacement therapy as ordered.
2. Provide care for client with subtotal thyroidectomy if indicated.
3. Provide client teaching and discharge planning concerning
   a. Use of iodized salt in preventing and treating endemic goiter
   b. Thyroid hormone replacement

Hypothyroidism (Myxedema)

A. General information
1. Slowing of metabolic processes caused by hypofunction of the thyroid gland with decreased thyroid hormone secretion; causes myxedema in adults and cretinism in children.

2. Occurs more often in women between ages 30 and 60
3. Primary hypothyroidism: atrophy of the gland possibly caused by an autoimmune process
4. Secondary hypothyroidism: caused by decreased stimulation from pituitary TSH
5. Iatrogenic: surgical removal of the gland or overtreatment of hyperthyroidism with drugs or radioactive iodine
6. In severe or untreated cases, *myxedema coma* may occur
   a. Characterized by intensification of signs and symptoms of hypothyroidism and neurologic impairment leading to coma
   b. Mortality rate high; prompt recognition and treatment essential
   c. Precipitating factors: failure to take prescribed medications; infection; trauma, exposure to cold; use of sedatives, narcotics, or anesthetics

B. Medical management
1. Drug therapy: levothyroxine (Synthroid), thyroglobulin (Proloid), dessicated thyroid, liothyronine (Cytomel)
2. Myxedema coma is a medical emergency
   a. IV thyroid hormones
   b. Correction of hypothermia
   c. Maintenance of vital functions
   d. Treatment of precipitating causes

C. Assessment findings
1. Fatigue; lethargy; slowed mental processes; dull look; slow, clumsy movements
2. Anorexia, weight gain, constipation
3. Intolerance to cold; dry, scaly skin; dry, sparse hair; brittle nails
4. Menstrual irregularities; generalized interstitial nonpitting edema
5. Bradycardia, cardiac complications (CAD, angina pectoris, MI, CHF)
6. Increased sensitivity to sedatives, narcotics, and anesthetics
7. Exaggeration of these findings in myxedema coma: weakness, lethargy, syncope, bradycardia, hypotension, hypoventilation, subnormal body temperature
8. Diagnostic tests
   a. Serum T_3 and T_4 level low
   b. Serum cholesterol level elevated
   c. RAIU decreased

D. Nursing interventions
1. Monitor vital signs, I&O, daily weights; observe for edema and signs of cardiovascular complications.
2. Administer thyroid hormone replacement therapy as ordered and monitor effects.
   a. Observe for signs of thyrotoxicosis (tachycardia, palpitations, nausea, vomiting, diarrhea, sweating, tremors, agitation, dyspnea).
   b. Increase dosage gradually, especially in clients with cardiac complications.

3. Provide a comfortable, warm environment.
4. Provide a low-calorie diet.
5. Avoid the use of sedatives; reduce the dose of any sedative, narcotic, or anesthetic agent by half as ordered.
6. Institute measures to prevent skin breakdown.
7. Provide increased fluids and foods high in fiber to prevent constipation; administer stool softeners as ordered.
8. Observe for signs of myxedema coma; provide appropriate nursing care.
   a. Administer medications as ordered.
   b. Maintain vital functions: correct hypothermia, maintain adequate ventilation.
9. Provide client teaching and discharge planning concerning
   a. Thyroid hormone replacement
      1) take daily dose in the morning to prevent insomnia.
      2) self-monitor for signs of thyrotoxicosis.
   b. Importance of regular follow-up care
   c. Need for additional protection in cold weather
   d. Measures to prevent constipation

Hyperthyroidism (Graves' Disease)

A. General information
   1. Secretion of excessive amounts of thyroid hormone in the blood causes an increase in metabolic processes
   2. Overactivity and changes in the thyroid gland may be present
   3. Most often seen in women between ages 30 and 50
   4. Cause unknown, but may be an autoimmune process
   5. Symptomatic hyperthyroidism may also be called thyrotoxicosis
B. Medical management
   1. Drug therapy
      a. Antithyroid drugs (propylthiouracil and methimazole ([Tapazole]): block synthesis of thyroid hormone; toxic effects include agranulocytosis
      b. Adrenergic blocking agents (commonly propranolol [Inderal]): used to decrease sympathetic activity and alleviate symptoms such as tachycardia
   2. Radioactive iodine therapy
      a. Radioactive isotope of iodine (e.g., ^{131}I) given to destroy the thyroid gland, thereby decreasing production of thyroid hormone
      b. Used in middle-aged or older clients who are resistant to, or develop toxicity from, drug therapy
      c. Hypothyroidism is a potential complication
   3. Surgery: thyroidectomy performed in younger clients for whom drug therapy has not been effective

C. Assessment findings
   1. Irritability, agitation, restlessness, hyperactive movements, tremor, sweating, insomnia
   2. Increased appetite, hyperphagia, weight loss, diarrhea, intolerance to heat
   3. Exophthalmos (protrusion of the eyeballs), goiter
   4. Warm, smooth skin; fine, soft hair; pliable nails
   5. Tachycardia, increased systolic blood pressure, palpitations
   6. Diagnostic tests
      a. Serum T_3 and T_4 levels elevated
      b. RAIU increased

D. Nursing interventions
   1. Monitor vital signs, daily weights.
   2. Administer antithyroid medications as ordered.
   3. Provide for periods of uninterrupted rest.
      a. Assign to a private room away from excessive activity.
      b. Administer medications to promote sleep as ordered.
   4. Provide a cool environment.
   5. Minimize stress in the environment.
   6. Encourage quiet, relaxing diversional activities.
   7. Provide a diet high in carbohydrates, protein, calories, vitamins, and minerals with supplemental feedings between meals and at bedtime; omit stimulants.
   8. Observe for and prevent complications.
      a. Exophthalmos: protect eyes with dark glasses and artificial tears as ordered.
      b. Thyroid storm: see below.
   9. Provide client teaching and discharge planning concerning
      a. Need to recognize and report signs and symptoms of agranulocytosis (fever, sore throat, skin rash) if taking antithyroid drugs
      b. Signs and symptoms of hyper/hypothyroidism

Thyroid Storm

A. General information
   1. Uncontrolled and potentially life-threatening hyperthyroidism caused by sudden and excessive release of thyroid hormone into the bloodstream
   2. Precipitating factors: stress, infection, unprepared thyroid surgery
   3. Now quite rare

B. Assessment findings
   1. Apprehension, restlessness
   2. Extremely high temperature (up to 106°F [40.7°C]), tachycardia, HF, respiratory distress, delirium, coma

C. Nursing interventions
   1. Maintain a patent airway and adequate ventilation; administer oxygen as ordered.

2. Administer IV therapy as ordered.
3. Administer medications as ordered: antithyroid drugs, corticosteroids, sedatives, cardiac drugs.

Thyroidectomy

A. General information
   1. Partial or total removal of the thyroid gland
   2. Indications
      a. Subtotal thyroidectomy: hyperthyroidism
      b. Total thyroidectomy: thyroid cancer
B. Nursing interventions: preoperative
   1. Ensure that the client is adequately prepared for surgery.
      a. Cardiac status is stable.
      b. Weight and nutritional status are normal.
   2. Administer antithyroid drugs as ordered to suppress the production and secretion of thyroid hormone and to prevent thyroid storm.
   3. Administer iodine preparations (Lugol's or potassium iodide solution) to reduce the size and vascularity of the gland and prevent hemorrhage.
C. Nursing interventions: postoperative
   1. Monitor vital signs and I&O.
   2. Check dressings for signs of hemorrhage; check for wetness behind neck.
   3. Place client in semi-Fowler's position and support head with pillows.
   4. Observe for respiratory distress secondary to hemorrhage, edema of the glottis, laryngeal nerve damage, or tetany; keep tracheostomy set, oxygen, and suction nearby.
   5. Assess for signs of tetany due to hypocalcemia secondary to accidental removal of parathyroid glands; keep calcium gluconate available (see Hypoparathyroidism, below).
   6. Encourage the client to rest voice.
      a. Some hoarseness is common.
      b. Check every 30–60 minutes for extreme hoarseness or any accompanying respiratory distress.
   7. Observe for thyroid storm due to release of excessive amounts of thyroid hormone during surgery.
   8. Administer IV fluids as ordered until the client is tolerating fluids by mouth.
   9. Administer analgesics as ordered for incisional pain.
   10. Relieve discomfort from sore throat.
       a. Cool mist humidifier to thin secretions.
       b. Administer analgesic throat lozenges before meals and prn as ordered.
       c. Encourage fluids.
   11. Encourage coughing and deep breathing every hour.

12. Assist the client with ambulation: instruct the client to place hands behind neck to decrease stress on suture line if added support necessary.
13. Provide client teaching and discharge planning concerning
    a. Signs and symptoms of hypo/hyperthyroidism
    b. Self-administration of thyroid hormones if total thyroidectomy performed
    c. Application of lubricant to the incision once sutures are removed
    d. Performance of ROM neck exercises 3–4 times a day
    e. Importance of regular follow-up care

Specific Disorders of the Parathyroid Glands

Hypoparathyroidism

A. General information
   1. Disorder characterized by hypocalcemia resulting from a deficiency of parathormone (PTH) production
   2. May be hereditary, idiopathic, or caused by accidental damage to or removal of parathyroid glands during surgery, e.g., thyroidectomy

B. Assessment findings
   1. Acute hypocalcemia (tetany)
      a. Tingling of fingers and around lips, painful muscle spasms, dysphagia, laryngospasm, seizures, cardiac arrhythmias
      b. Chvostek's sign: sharp tapping over facial nerve causes twitching of mouth, nose, and eye
      c. Trousseau's sign: carpopedal spasm induced by application of blood pressure cuff for 3 minutes
   2. Chronic hypocalcemia
      a. Fatigue, weakness, muscle cramps
      b. Personality changes, irritability, memory impairment
      c. Dry, scaly skin; hair loss; loss of tooth enamel
      d. Tremor, cardiac arrhythmias, cataract formation
      e. Diagnostic tests
         1) serum calcium levels decreased
         2) serum phosphate levels elevated
         3) skeletal X-rays reveal increased bone density

C. Nursing interventions
   1. Administer calcium gluconate by slow IV drip as ordered for acute hypocalcemia.
   2. Administer medications for chronic hypocalcemia.
      a. Oral calcium preparations: calcium gluconate, lactate, carbonate (Os-Cal)
      b. Large doses of vitamin D (Calciferol) to help absorption of calcium
      c. Aluminum hydroxide gel (Amphogel) or aluminum carbonate gel, basic (Basaljel) to decrease phosphate levels

3. Institute seizure and safety precautions.
4. Provide quiet environment free from excessive stimuli.
5. Monitor for signs of hoarseness or stridor; check for Chvostek's and Trousseau's signs.
6. Keep emergency equipment (tracheostomy set, injectable calcium gluconate) at bedside.
7. For tetany or generalized muscle cramps, may use rebreathing bag to produce mild respiratory acidosis.
8. Monitor serum calcium and phosphate levels.
9. Provide high-calcium, low-phosphorus diet.
10. Provide client teaching and discharge planning concerning
    a. Medication regimen; oral calcium preparations and vitamin D to be taken with meals to increase absorption
    b. Need to recognize and report signs and symptoms of hypo/hypercalcemia
    c. Importance of follow-up care with periodic serum calcium levels

Hyperparathyroidism

A. General information
   1. Increased secretion of PTH that results in an altered state of calcium, phosphate, and bone metabolism
   2. Most commonly affects women between ages 35 and 65
   3. Primary hyperparathyroidism: caused by tumor or hyperplasia of parathyroid glands
   4. Secondary hyperparathyroidism: caused by compensatory oversecretion of PTH in response to hypocalcemia from chronic renal disease, rickets, malabsorption syndrome, osteomalacia

B. Assessment findings
   1. Bone pain (especially at back), bone demineralization, pathologic fractures
   2. Renal colic, kidney stones, polyuria, polydipsia
   3. Anorexia, nausea, vomiting, gastric ulcers, constipation
   4. Muscle weakness, fatigue
   5. Irritability, personality changes, depression
   6. Cardiac arrhythmias, hypertension
   7. Diagnostic tests
      a. Serum calcium levels elevated
      b. Serum phosphate levels decreased
      c. Skeletal X-rays reveal bone demineralization

C. Nursing interventions
   1. Administer IV infusions of normal saline solution and give diuretics as ordered; monitor I&O and observe for fluid overload and electrolyte imbalances.

2. Assist client with self-care: provide careful handling, moving, and ambulation to prevent pathologic fractures.
3. Monitor vital signs; report irregularities.
4. Force fluids; provide acid-ash juices, e.g., cranberry juice.
5. Strain urine for stones.
6. Provide low-calcium, high-phosphorus diet.
7. Provide care for the client undergoing parathyroidectomy.
8. Provide client teaching and discharge planning concerning
   a. Need to engage in progressive ambulatory activities
   b. Increased intake of fluids
   c. Use of calcium preparations and importance of high-calcium diet following a parathyroidectomy

Specific Disorders of the Pancreas

Diabetes Mellitus

A. General information
   1. Diabetes mellitus represents a heterogenous group of chronic disorders characterized by hyperglycemia.
   2. Hyperglycemia is due to total or partial insulin deficiency or insensitivity of the cells to insulin.
   3. Characterized by disorders in the metabolism of carbohydrate, fat, and protein, as well as changes in the structure and function of blood vessels.
   4. Most common endocrine problem; affects over 11 million people in the United States.
   5. Exact etiology unknown; causative factors may include
      a. genetics, viruses, and/or autoimmune response in Type I
      b. genetics and obesity in Type II
   6. Types
      a. Type I (insulin-dependent diabetes mellitus [IDDM])
         1) secondary to destruction of beta cells in the islets of Langerhans in the pancreas resulting in little or no insulin production; requires insulin injections.
         2) usually occurs in children or in nonobese adults
      b. Type II (non-insulin-dependent diabetes mellitus [NIDDM])
         1) may result from a partial deficiency of insulin production and/or an insensitivity of the cells to insulin.
         2) usually occurs in obese adults over 40.
      c. Diabetes associated with other conditions or syndromes, e.g., pancreatic disease, Cushing's syndrome, use of certain drugs (steroids, thiazide diuretics, oral contraceptives).
   7. Pathophysiology
      a. Lack of insulin causes hyperglycemia (insulin is necessary for the transport of glucose across the cell membrane).

b. Hyperglycemia leads to osmotic diuresis as large amounts of glucose pass through the kidney; results in polyuria and glycosuria.
c. Diuresis leads to cellular dehydration and fluid and electrolyte depletion causing polydipsia (excessive thirst).
d. Polyphagia (hunger and increased appetite) results from cellular starvation.
e. The body turns to fats and protein for energy; but in the absence of glucose in the cell, fats cannot be completely metabolized and ketones (intermediate products of fat metabolism) are produced.
f. This leads to ketonemia, ketonuria (contributes to osmotic diuresis), and metabolic acidosis (ketones are acid bodies).
g. Ketones act as CNS depressants and can cause coma.
h. Excess loss of fluids and electrolytes leads to hypovolemia, hypotension, renal failure, and decreased blood flow to the brain resulting in coma and death unless treated.

8. Acute complications of diabetes include diabetic ketoacidosis, insulin reaction, hyperglycemic hyperosmolar nonketotic coma.

B. Medical management

1. Type I: insulin, diet, exercise
2. Type II: ideally managed by diet and exercise; may need oral hypoglycemics or occasionally insulin if diet and exercise are not effective in controlling hyperglycemia; insulin needed for acute stresses, e.g., surgery, infection
3. Diet
   a. Type I: consistency is imperative to avoid hypoglycemia
   b. Type II: weight loss is important since it decreases insulin resistance
   c. High-fiber, low-fat diet also recommended
4. Drug therapy
   a. Insulin: used for Type I diabetes (also occasionally used in Type II diabetes)
      1) types (Table 12-2)
         a) short acting: used in treating ketoacidosis; during surgery, infection, trauma; management of poorly controlled diabetes; to supplement longer-acting insulins
         b) intermediate: used for maintenance therapy
         c) long acting: used for maintenance therapy in clients who experience hyperglycemia during the night with intermediate-acting insulin
      2) various preparations of short-, intermediate-, and long-acting insulins are available (see Table 12-2)
      3) insulin preparations can consist of a mixture of beef and pork insulin, pure beef, pure pork, or human insulin. Human insulin is the purest insulin and has the lowest antigenic effect.

TABLE 12-1 Characteristics of Insulin Preparations

Drug	Synonym	Appearance	Action in Hours			Compatible Mixed with
			Onset	Peak	Duration	
Rapid acting						
Insulin injection	Regular insulin	Clear	½–1	2–4	6–8	All insulin preparations except lente
Insulin, zinc suspension, prompt	Semilente insulin	Cloudy	½–1	4–6	12–16	Lente preparations
Intermediate acting						
Isophane insulin injection	NPH insulin	Cloudy	1–1½	8–12	18–24	Regular insulin injection
Insulin zinc suspension	Lente insulin	Cloudy	1–1½	8–12	18–24	Regular insulin and semilente preparations
Long acting						
Insulin zinc suspension, extended	Ultralente insulin	Cloudy	4–8	16–20	30–36	Regular insulin and semilente preparations

4) human insulin is recommended for all newly diagnosed Type I diabetics, Type II diabetics who need short-term insulin therapy, the pregnant client, and diabetic clients with insulin allergy or severe insulin resistance.
5) insulin pumps are small, externally worn devices that closely mimic normal pancreatic functioning. Insulin pumps contain a 3 ml syringe attached to a long (42-inch), narrow-lumen tube with a needle or Teflon catheter at the end. The needle or Teflon catheter is inserted into the subcutaneous tissue (usually on the abdomen) and secured with tape or a transparent dressing.
6) The needle or catheter is changed at least every 3 days. The pump is worn either on a belt or in a pocket (see Figure 12-2). The pump uses only regular insulin. Insulin can be administered via the basal rate (usually 0.5–2.0 units/hr) and by a bolus dose (which is activated by a series of button pushes) prior to each meal.

b. Oral hypoglycemic agents (Table 12-3)
1) used for Type II diabetics who are not controlled by diet and exercise
2) increase the ability of islet cells of the pancreas to secrete insulin; may have some effect on cell receptors to decrease resistance to insulin

5. Exercise: helpful adjunct to therapy as exercise decreases the body's need for insulin.

C. Assessment findings
1. All types: polyuria, polydipsia, polyphagia, fatigue, blurred vision, susceptibility to infection
2. Type I: anorexia, nausea, vomiting, weight loss
3. Type II: obesity; frequently no other symptoms
4. Diagnostic tests
a. Fasting blood sugar
1) a level of 140 mg/dl or greater on at least two occasions confirms diabetes mellitus
2) may be normal in Type II diabetes
b. Postprandial blood sugar: elevated
c. Oral glucose tolerance test (most sensitive test): elevated
d. Glycosolated hemoglobin (hemoglobin A_{1c}) elevated

D. Nursing interventions
1. Administer insulin or oral hypoglycemic agents as ordered; monitor for hypoglycemia, especially during period of drug's peak action.
2. Provide special diet as ordered.
a. Ensure that the client is eating all meals.
b. If all food is not ingested, provide appropriate substitutes according to the exchange lists or give measured amount of

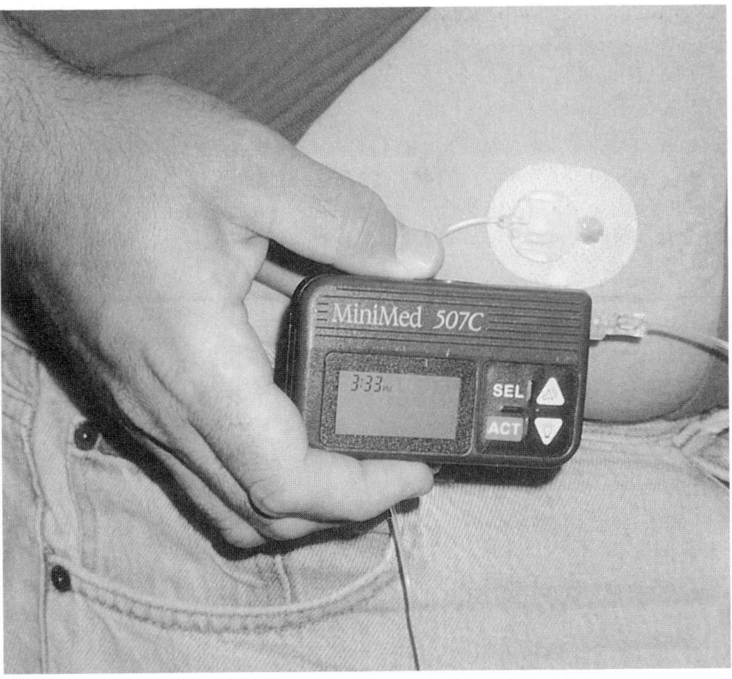

FIGURE 12-2 Insulin infusion pump

orange juice to substitute for leftover food; provide snack later in the day.

3. Monitor urine sugar and acetone (freshly voided specimen).
4. Perform finger sticks to monitor blood glucose levels as ordered (more accurate than urine tests).
5. Observe for signs of hypo/hyperglycemia.
6. Provide meticulous skin care and prevent injury.
7. Maintain I&O; weigh daily.
8. Provide emotional support; assist client in adapting to change in lifestyle and body image.
9. Observe for chronic complications and plan care accordingly.
   - **a.** Atherosclerosis: leads to coronary artery disease, MI, CVA, and peripheral vascular disease.
   - **b.** Microangiopathy: most commonly affects eyes and kidneys.
   - **c.** Kidney disease
     - **1)** recurrent pyelonephritis
     - **2)** diabetic nephropathy
   - **d.** Ocular disorders
     - **1)** premature cataracts
     - **2)** diabetic retinopathy

TABLE 12-3 Oral Hypoglycemic Agents

Drug	Onset of Action (hrs)	Peak Action (hrs)	Duration of Action (hrs)	Comments
Oral Sulfonylureas				
Acetohexamide (Dymelor)	1	4-6	12-24	
Chlorpropamide (Diabinase)	1	4-6	40-60	
Glyburide (Micronase, Diabeta)	15 min-1 hr	2-8	10-24	
Oral Biguanides				
Metformin (Glucophage)	2-2.5		10-16	Decreases glucose production in liver; decreases intestinal absorption of glucose and improves insulin sensitivity.
Oral Alpha-glucosidose Inhibitor				
Acarbose (Precose)	Unknown	1	Unknown	Delay glucose absorption and digestion of carbohydrates, lowering blood sugar.
Miglitol (Glyset)		2-3		
Troglitazone (Rezulin)	Rapid	2-3	Unknown	Reduces plasma glucose and insulin. Exact mechanism is unknown. Potentiates action of insulin in skeletal muscle and decreases glucose production in liver.

DELEGATION TIP

Properly trained ancillary personnel may measure and record blood glucose levels. Ancillary personnel must be trained to know what blood glucose levels are reportable to the RN.

- **e.** Peripheral neuropathy
  - **1)** affects peripheral and autonomic nervous systems
  - **2)** causes diarrhea, constipation, neurogenic bladder, impotence, decreased sweating

10. Provide client teaching and discharge planning concerning
- **a.** Disease process
- **b.** Diet
  - **1)** client should be able to plan meals using exchange lists before discharge
  - **2)** emphasize importance of regularity of meals; never skip meals
- **c.** Insulin
  - **1)** how to draw up into syringe
    - **a)** use insulin at room temperature.
    - **b)** gently roll vial between palms of hands.
    - **c)** draw up insulin using sterile technique.
    - **d)** if mixing insulins, draw up clear insulin before cloudy insulin.
  - **2)** injection technique
    - **a)** systematically rotate sites to prevent lipodystrophy (hypertrophy or atrophy of tissue).
    - **b)** insert needle at a 45° or 90° angle depending on amount of adipose tissue.
  - **3)** may store current vial of insulin at room temperature; refrigerate extra supplies.
  - **4)** provide many opportunities for return demonstration.
- **d.** Oral hypoglycemic agents
  - **1)** stress importance of taking the drug regularly.
  - **2)** avoid alcohol intake while on medication.
- **e.** Urine testing (not very accurate reflection of blood glucose level)
  - **1)** may be satisfactory for Type II diabetics since they are more stable.
  - **2)** use Clinitest, Tes-tape, Diastix for glucose testing.
  - **3)** perform tests before meals and at bedtime.
  - **4)** use freshly voided specimen.
  - **5)** be consistent in brand of urine test used.

6) report results in percentages.
7) report results to physician if results are greater than 1%, especially if experiencing symptoms of hyperglycemia.
8) urine testing for ketones should be done by Type I diabetic clients when there is persistent glycosuria, increased blood glucose levels, or if the client is not feeling well (Acetest, Ketostix).

f. Blood glucose monitoring
1) use for Type I diabetic clients since it gives exact blood glucose level and also detects hypoglycemia.
2) instruct client in finger-stick technique, use of monitor device (if used), and recording and utilization of test results.

g. General care
1) perform good oral hygiene and have regular dental exams.
2) have regular eye exams.
3) care for "sick days" (e.g., cold or flu)
    a) do not omit insulin or oral hypoglycemic agents since infection causes increased blood sugar.
    b) notify physician.
    c) monitor urine or blood glucose levels and urine ketones frequently.
    d) if nausea and/or vomiting occurs, sip on clear liquids with simple sugars.

h. Foot care
1) wash feet with mild soap and water and pat dry.
2) apply lanolin to feet to prevent drying and cracking.
3) cut toenails straight across.
4) avoid constricting garments such as garters.
5) wear clean, absorbent socks (cotton or wool).
6) purchase properly fitting shoes and break new shoes in gradually.
7) never go barefoot.
8) inspect feet daily and notify physician if cuts, blisters, or breaks in skin occur.

i. Exercise
1) undertake regular exercise; avoid sporadic, vigorous exercise.
2) food intake may need to be increased before exercising.
3) exercise is best performed after meals when the blood sugar is rising.

j. Complications
1) learn to recognize signs and symptoms of hypo/hyperglycemia.
2) eat candy or drink orange juice with sugar added for insulin reaction (hypoglycemia).

k. Need to wear a Medic-Alert bracelet.

Ketoacidosis (DKA)

A. General information
  1. Acute complication of diabetes mellitus characterized by hyperglycemia and accumulation of ketones in the body; causes metabolic acidosis
  2. Occurs in insulin-dependent diabetic clients
  3. Precipitating factors: undiagnosed diabetes, neglect of treatment; infection, cardiovascular disorder; other physical or emotional stress
  4. Onset slow, may be hours to days

B. Assessment findings
  1. Polydipsia, polyphagia, polyuria
  2. Nausea, vomiting, abdominal pain
  3. Skin warm, dry, and flushed
  4. Dry mucous membranes; soft eyeballs
  5. Kussmaul's respirations or tachypnea; acetone breath
  6. Alterations in LOC
  7. Hypotension, tachycardia
  8. Diagnostic tests
    a. Serum glucose and ketones elevated
    b. BUN, creatinine, hct elevated (due to dehydration)
    c. Serum sodium decreased, potassium (may be normal or elevated at first)
    d. ABGs: metabolic acidosis with compensatory respiratory alkalosis

C. Nursing interventions
  1. Maintain a patent airway.
  2. Maintain fluid and electrolyte balance.
    a. Administer IV therapy as ordered.
      1) normal saline (0.9% NaCl), then hypotonic (0.45% NaCl) sodium chloride
      2) when blood sugar drops to 250 mg/dl, may add 5% dextrose to IV.
      3) potassium will be added when the urine output is adequate.
    b. Observe for fluid and electrolyte imbalances, especially fluid overload, hypokalemia, and hyperkalemia.
  3. Administer insulin as ordered.
    a. Regular insulin IV (drip or push) and/or subcutaneously (SC).
    b. If given IV drip, give with small amounts of albumin since insulin adheres to IV tubing.
    c. Monitor blood glucose levels frequently.
  4. Check urine output every hour.
  5. Monitor vital signs.
  6. Assist client with self-care.
  7. Provide care for the unconscious client if in a coma.
  8. Discuss with client the reasons ketosis developed and provide additional diabetic teaching if indicated.

CLIENT TEACHING CHECKLIST

Teach the hypoglycemic client to use sources of glucose which contain very little fat, as fat will slow absorption of the sugars.

For mild hypoglycemia, readily available sources of glucose are:

- Apple juice, orange juice, and cola 4–6 oz.
- One tablespoon honey or grape jelly.
- 5–6 pieces of hard candy.

Insulin Reaction/Hypoglycemia

A. General information
   1. Abnormally low blood sugar, usually below 50 mg/dl
   2. Usually caused by insulin overdosage, too little food, nutritional and fluid imbalances from nausea and vomiting, excessive exercise
   3. Onset rapid; may develop in minutes to hours

B. Assessment findings
   1. Headache, dizziness, difficulty with problem solving, restlessness, hunger, visual disturbances
   2. Slurred speech; alterations in gait; decreasing LOC; pallor, cold, clammy skin; diaphoresis
   3. Diagnostic test: serum glucose level 50-60 mg/dl or lower

C. Nursing interventions
   1. Administer oral sugar in the form of candy or orange juice with sugar added if the client is alert.
   2. If the client is unconscious, administer 20-50 ml 50% dextrose IV push, or 1 mg glucagon IM, IV, or SC, as ordered.
   3. Explore with client reasons for hypoglycemia and provide additional diabetic teaching as indicated.

Hyperglycemic Hyperosmolar Nonketotic Coma (HHNK)

A. General information
   1. Complication of diabetes, characterized by hyperglycemia and a hyperosmolar state without ketosis
   2. Occurs in non-insulin-dependent diabetics or nondiabetic persons (typically elderly clients)
   3. Precipitating factors: undiagnosed diabetes; infections or other stress; certain medications (e.g., Dilantin, thiazide diuretics); dialysis; hyperalimentation; major burns; pancreatic disease

B. Assessment findings

 1. Similar to ketoacidosis but without Kussmaul respirations and acetone breath

 2. Laboratory tests

  a. Blood glucose level extremely elevated

  b. BUN, creatine, hct elevated (due to dehydration)

  c. Urine positive for glucose

C. Nursing interventions: treatment and nursing care is similar to DKA, excluding measures to treat ketosis and metabolic acidosis.

REVIEW QUESTIONS

1. A 57-year-old woman was admitted to the hospital for uncontrolled diabetes. Lab studies reveal a fasting blood sugar of 310. Her admission diagnosis is Type I diabetes mellitus. The client needs to understand that the type of diabetes that she has

 1. is associated with the destruction of beta cells.

 2. usually causes complete fat metabolism.

 3. often occurs in obese individuals.

 4. is rarely controlled.

2. A diabetic client who is taking regular and NPH insulin asks why she must mix the two insulins. The nurse explains that regular and NPH insulins are mixed to ensure

 1. immediate onset of the regular insulin.

 2. onset of the regular insulin within 2 hours.

 3. a peak action of the NPH insulin at 2 hours.

 4. a total duration of action of 24 hours.

3. A 45-year-old has a simple goiter. She is being seen by the community health nurse for teaching and follow-up regarding nutritional deficiencies related to her goiter. The client's problems are most likely associated with which nutritional deficiency?

 1. Calcium.

 2. Iodine.

 3. Iron.

 4. Sodium.

4. The nurse is teaching a woman who has a simple goiter. The nurse teaches the client that to enhance glandular function, she should eliminate which of the following foods?

1. Corn.
2. Milk.
3. Turnips.
4. Watermelon.

5. A 45-year-old is admitted to the hospital with Addison's disease. He has a respiratory infection. When the client's vital signs are assessed, his blood pressure is 90/40. The nurse should notify the physician immediately because

1. blood gases need to be drawn.
2. seizure activity is imminent.
3. shock may be developing.
4. the reading is atypical.

6. A client who is diagnosed with Addison's disease is admitted to the hospital. Which of the following would the nurse expect to find when assessing the client?

1. Acne.
2. Hyperpigmentation.
3. Moon face.
4. Supraclavicular fat pads.

7. A client who is diagnosed as having Addison's disease is receiving teaching about his disease from the nurse. Which statement the client makes indicates to the nurse that he understands the teaching?

1. "I should avoid strenuous exercise during hot weather."
2. "I should not eat salty foods."
3. "I need to take medication only when I am having symptoms."
4. "I should eat foods such as bananas and oranges several times daily."

8. The nurse is teaching a person who has Addison's disease about drug therapy for his condition. In evaluating the effectiveness of teaching regarding drug therapy, the nurse should expect him to be able to verbalize the need

1. to avoid antibiotics.
2. for lifelong therapy.
3. to taper the steroid dose.
4. to receive alternate-day therapy.

9. A 34-year-old is newly diagnosed with Type I diabetes. She is hospitalized for insulin dose stabilization and is being taught insulin administration and self-monitoring of blood glucose (SMBG) levels. The nurse tells the client that the major benefit of self-monitoring of blood glucose levels is

1. blood glucose is maintained at close to normal levels.
2. materials and laboratory expenses are cost efficient.
3. dependence on the health care system is reduced.
4. larger but fewer doses of insulin are required.

10. The nurse is teaching an adult client who has Type I diabetes mellitus about ketoacidosis. The nurse explains that the primary cause of the development of ketoacidosis is

1. a GI disturbance.
2. an insulin overdosage.
3. omitted meals.
4. not taking insulin regularly.

11. A client is to have the following diagnostic procedures: serum $T_3$and T_4, carotid arteriogram, and thyroid scan. In what order should the nurse schedule the tests?

1. Arteriogram, serum $T_3$and T_4, scan.
2. Serum $T_3$and T_4, scan, arteriogram.
3. Arteriogram, scan, serum $T_3$and T_4.
4. Serum $T_3$and T_4, arteriogram, scan.

12. After reading about the procedure for his upcoming thyroid scan, a client expresses concern about the dangers of being "radioactive" after the test. Which understanding about the test should guide the nurse's response?

1. There is no danger since the thyroid scan no longer involves the use of a radioactive isotope.
2. The radioactive isotope is only a tracer dose, which is not harmful to the client or others close to him.
3. The client must avoid close contact with others for five days following the test.
4. Wearing a lead shield during the test will protect the client from radioactivity.

13. The nurse is explaining to a client about a radioactive iodine uptake test. Which of the following over-the-counter medications should the nurse advise the client to avoid prior to the test?

1. Antiflatulents.
2. Poison ivy remedies.
3. Cough syrups.
4. Antifungal agents.

14. Select the most accurate explanation by the nurse to a client who is to have an oral glucose tolerance test and needs to understand the procedure.
    1. "You will go to the laboratory and your blood will be drawn."
    2. "After you drink a concentrated glucose solution, you cannot eat or drink anything until your blood is drawn."
    3. "You will eat a large meal and your blood will be drawn 2 hours later."
    4. "Your blood will be drawn, you will drink a concentrated glucose solution, and your blood will be drawn again."
15. An adult is suffering from adrenocortical insufficiency and is placed on glucocorticoid therapy. The nurse plans to include which of the following administration directions?
    1. "You will need to take the large dose of the medication at bedtime and the smaller dose in the morning until the prescription is finished."
    2. "You will need to take the medication at bedtime for life."
    3. "You will need to take the medication in the morning until the prescription is finished."
    4. "You will need to take the large dose of the medication in the morning and the smaller dose in the afternoon for life."
16. Which assessment is most important for the nurse to make when monitoring a client with a pituitary tumor that secretes ACTH?
    1. Height.
    2. Blood pressure.
    3. Pulse rate.
    4. Output.
17. The nurse is caring for a client who underwent surgical hypophysectomy. Which of the following assessments is most essential for the nurse to make immediately post-op?
    1. Blood pressure.
    2. Serum calcium levels.
    3. Breath sounds.
    4. Bowel sounds.
18. An adult has had a hypophysectomy with a complete removal of the pituitary gland. Which of the following statements represents to the nurse the most complete understanding of follow-up care?
    1. "I will need to wear a Medic-Alert bracelet."
    2. "I will need to take hormone replacements for the next 2 months."

3. "I will need to wear a Medic-Alert bracelet and take hormone replacements for the next year."
4. "I will need to have lifelong follow-up, to take hormone replacement therapy for the rest of my life, and to wear a Medic-Alert bracelet."

19. A 62-year-old female is admitted with a posterior pituitary tumor and is experiencing diabetes insipidus, a complication of that tumor. The nursing diagnosis most appropriate for this client is

1. fluid volume excess.
2. deficient fluid volume.
3. bowel incontinence.
4. diarrhea.

20. A client who has been taking prednisone to treat lupus erythematosus has discontinued the medication because of lack of funds to buy the drug. When the nurse becomes aware of the situation, which assessment is most important for the nurse to make first?

1. Breath sounds.
2. Capillary refill.
3. Blood pressure.
4. Skin integrity.

21. An adult is readmitted to the medical/surgical care unit in addisonian crisis. He is exhibiting signs of tachycardia, dehydration, hyponatremia, hyperkalemia, and hypoglycemia. The nurse should expect that the initial orders for this client will include

1. administration of oxygen via 100% nonrebreathing mask.
2. starting an IV solution of saline and dextrose.
3. administering potassium chloride.
4. preparing for an emergency tracheostomy.

22. A 29-year-old female is suffering from Cushing's syndrome. She is constantly lashing out at her coworkers and family. Her husband informs the nurse of this behavior. The nurse's best interpretation of this behavior is

1. mineralocorticoid excess.
2. glucocorticoid excess.
3. activity intolerance.
4. sensory-perceptual alterations.

23. A nurse at a weight loss center assesses a client who has a large abdomen and a rounded face. Which additional assessment finding would lead the nurse to suspect that the client has Cushing's syndrome rather than obesity from imbalance of food intake and body need?

1. Large thighs and upper arms.
2. Pendulous abdomen and large hips.
3. Abdominal striae and ankle enlargement.
4. Posterior neck fat pad and thin extremities.

24. A client has primary aldosteronism. Which assessment findings would the nurse expect to find initially?
    1. Decreased serum sodium and potassium.
    2. Decreased blood glucose and elevated temperature.
    3. Tachycardia and albuminuria.
    4. Hypertension and decreased serum potassium.
25. A client who is suspected of having a pheochromocytoma complains of sweating, palpitations, and headache. Which assessment is essential for the nurse to make first?
    1. Pupil reaction.
    2. Hand grips.
    3. Blood pressure.
    4. Blood glucose.
26. An adult is to have an adrenalectomy. The nurse is performing preoperative teaching. The client asks the nurse "What will I look like and behave like after surgery?" The nurse's best response is,
    1. "Don't worry about that now. You need to concentrate on the surgery."
    2. "You will only have a small incision."
    3. "I know you are worried, maybe we should resume the education session later."
    4. "After surgery you may not respond to any stressors, so we will do our best to help decrease stimuli and help you through it. Your appearance will not change immediately after the surgery."
27. An adult has undergone a bilateral adrenalectomy. Which of the following demonstrates to the nurse the best understanding of long-term care needs?
    1. When I run out of the medication the doctor gave me, I can stop taking the hormones.
    2. I can take the steroid replacement therapy once every three days.
    3. I need to take the steroid replacement therapy every day. I should not alter the dose or stop taking it.
    4. I can take the dose of the medication I feel I need.
28. An adult is admitted to the hospital for removal of a simple goiter. The nurse understands that a simple goiter is caused by

1. low intake of fat-free foods.
2. excessive thyroid-stimulating hormone (TSH) stimulation.
3. excessive adrenocorticotropic hormone (ACTH) stimulation.
4. low intake of goitrogenic foods.

29. An adult is currently being treated at the clinic for Graves' disease. It is essential for the nurse to assess for which of the following signs immediately?

1. Goiter.
2. Tachycardia.
3. Constipation.
4. Hypothermia.

30. A 35-year-old female visits her managed care physician for an annual physical examination. Routine laboratory studies reveal thyroxine (T_4) and triiodothyronine (T_3) levels are elevated, whereas the thyroid-stimulating hormone (TSH) level was undetectable. The nurse's understanding of these diagnostic tests is the client is experiencing

1. hypothyroidism.
2. addisonian crisis.
3. hypoparathyroidism.
4. hyperthyroidism.

31. An adult who is newly diagnosed with Graves' disease asks the nurse "Why do I need to take propranolol (Inderal)?" Based on the nurse's understanding of the medication and Graves' disease, the best response would be,

1. "The medication will limit thyroid hormone secretion."
2. "The medication will inhibit synthesis of thyroid hormones."
3. "The medication will relieve the symptoms of Graves' disease."
4. "The medication will increase the synthesis of thyroid hormones."

32. The nurse is preparing a room to receive a client immediately post-thyroidectomy. The nurse should be sure that which of the following equipment is available at the bedside?

1. Nasogastric tray.
2. Central venous tray set-up.
3. Tracheostomy tray.
4. Lumbar puncture tray.

33. An adult had a total thyroidectomy. Which statement by the client demonstrates to the nurse an adequate understanding of long-term care?

1. "I will need to take replacement hormones for the rest of my life."
2. "I should try to avoid stress and be alert for signs of recurrent hyperthyroidism."
3. "Thank goodness this is over, I will never have to worry about thyroid problems again!"
4. "I should increase my caloric intake to replace what I lost during the surgery."

34. The nurse is caring for a client who is status post-thyroidectomy. The client is exhibiting hyperreflexia, muscle twitching, and spasms. The first action the nurse should perform is to

1. assess for additional signs of tetany.
2. prepare to send a blood sample to the laboratory for a calcium level.
3. place the client in semi-Fowler's position.
4. administer post-op pain medication.

35. An adult who has Graves' disease just received a dose of sodium ^{131}I. Which of the following statements made to the nurse best demonstrates an understanding of immediate care needs?

1. "I should be able to go home after about 2 hours if I don't have any vomiting."
2. "I have my belongings with me to stay in the isolation room for the next 24 hours."
3. "My daughter is pregnant, so I told her I will not be able to see her for the next month."
4. "I brought my antithyroid drug with me so I will not miss a dose."

36. An adult has had hypoparathyroidism for 20 years. The client has come in to the center for a check-up. The nurse should assess the client for

1. hypothermia.
2. hyperthermia.
3. tetany.
4. hypertension.

37. A 45-year-old newly diagnosed type I diabetic asks the nurse "Why can't I take a pill for my diabetes like my 62-year-old neighbor?" The nurse understands that the primary difference between Type I diabetes and Type II diabetes is

1. that Type I diabetes and Type II diabetes can be controlled with injections of antibodies.
2. that Type I diabetes is the result of autoimmune destruction of beta cell function in the pancreas, whereas Type II diabetes is the result of the lack of responsiveness of beta cells to insulin.

3. that Type I diabetes insulin production is a circadian function, whereas in Type II diabetes, insulin production depends on serum glucose levels.
4. that Type I diabetes has a complication known as hyperglycemic hyperosmolar nonketosis, whereas Type II diabetes has a complication known as diabetic ketoacidosis.

38. The nurse administers the client's morning dose of regular insulin at 7:30 A.M. The nurse should anticipate to observe the client for a hypoglycemic reaction at which of the following times?

1. Immediately.
2. 10:00 A.M.
3. 1:00 P.M.
4. 7:30 P.M.

39. The nurse is planning an education session for a newly diagnosed diabetic. Which concept is essential to include when developing the plan of care?

1. All diabetic teaching needs to be accomplished within 20 hours before discharge.
2. Insulin injection sites should be cleaned with iodine prior to injection.
3. Snacks should be ingested prior to physical exercise.
4. Urine sugar levels should be checked prior to insulin administration.

40. The nurse is attending a bridal shower for a friend when another guest starts to tremble and complains of dizziness. The nurse notices a medical alert bracelet for diabetes. The best action for the nurse to take is to

1. encourage the guest to eat some baked ziti.
2. call the guest's personal physician.
3. offer the guest a peppermint.
4. give the guest a glass of orange juice.

41. A woman usually administers her NPH insulin at 6:00 A.M. but she plans to attend a banquet and fashion show next week, at which lunch will be served at 2:00 P.M. rather than noon when she usually eats lunch. Which of the following statements demonstrates to the nurse an understanding of peak action of NPH and risk for hypoglycemia?

1. "I will administer the insulin at my regular time, it is important to adhere to my schedule."
2. "I will take the insulin at 8:00 A.M. that day, as the insulin peaks in 6–12 hours."
3. "I will not take any insulin until they serve the lunch at the banquet."

4. "I will take the insulin at 10:00 A.M. that day as the peak action of NPH is four hours after administered."

42. A man is hospitalized for an infected foot ulcer. At 11:00 A.M. his blood glucose is 460 mg/dl and he has been up to the bathroom seven times this morning to urinate. The best action for the nurse to take is to

1. administer regular insulin according to the physician's sliding scale order.
2. administer NPH insulin according to the physician's sliding scale order.
3. notify the physician.
4. make sure the client's urinal is close to the bed so he does not have to keep getting up.

43. A 35-year-old diabetic is displaying signs of irritability and irrational behavior during an office visit. The nurse observes visible tremors in the client's hands. Based on the client's history and the nurse's understanding of diabetes mellitus, the nurse interprets these findings to be signs of

1. hyperglycemia.
2. diabetic ketoacidosis (DKA).
3. hyperglycemic hyperosmolar nonketosis (HHNK).
4. hypoglycemia.

44. Which statement by a woman newly diagnosed with NIDDM demonstrates to the nurse an adequate understanding of dietary needs?

1. "I need to stick to the meal plan the dietician explained to me."
2. "I usually have two to three drinks with dinner and I understand its okay to continue doing this."
3. "I should only buy foods that are labeled 'dietetic' from now on."
4. "It is okay to skip lunch on my shopping days as I never have time to eat."

45. The client came to the diabetic clinic for follow-up teaching on the complications of diabetes. The nurse explains that neuropathy is the result of

1. microangiopathies or metabolic defects that cause by-products to accumulate in the nerve tissues.
2. microvascular damage to the retina.
3. macroangiopathy in the extremities.
4. end-stage renal disease.

46. The nurse is teaching a Type II, non-insulin-dependent diabetic about the acute metabolic complications. The primary reason a Type II diabetic does not usually develop diabetic ketoacidosis is

1. that there is no insulin available for the state of hyperglycemia.
2. that the Type II diabetic has no protein or fat reserves.

3. that there is sufficient insulin to prevent the breakdown of protein and fatty acid for metabolic needs.
4. that there is insufficient serum glucose concentrations.

47. The primary caretaker for a man who was recently started on an oral hypoglycemic agent is his wife. The wife should know to watch for which of the following symptoms of hypoglycemia?

1. High blood sugar readings (greater than 250 mg/dl).
2. Presence of ketones in the urine.
3. Significant increase in urine output.
4. Cold sweats, weakness, and trembling.

48. Which of the following statements by a person who has diabetes mellitus shows the nurse that he has an adequate understanding of special foot care needs?

1. "I am looking forward to the summer when I can go barefoot in my house and at the beach."
2. "I like to use a heating pad at night as I always have cold feet."
3. "I used to take a shower every other night but now I am going to wash and examine my feet every night."
4. "I have a corn on my left foot, so I am going to go to the pharmacy to get something for it right away."

49. A client took her usual NPH insulin dose at 6:00 A.M., her lunch is delayed until 1:00 P.M., and she begins to feel weak. Which of the following actions demonstrates to the nurse an adequate understanding? The client

1. administers an extra 4 units of regular insulin.
2. administers an additional 4 units of NPH insulin.
3. goes and takes a nap.
4. drinks a cup of milk and then eats her lunch.

50. The nurse is teaching a client about diabetic management. The client asks the nurse "What is a hemoglobin A1c test?" The most appropriate answer for the nurse to give is,

1. "The hemoglobin A1c is a blood test that evaluates glycemic control over a 3-month time period by measuring the glucose attached to hemoglobin."
2. "The hemoglobin A1c is a blood test that measures the glucose attached to hemoglobin molecule over the last 7 days."
3. "The hemoglobin A1c test is a blood test that measures protein to evaluate glucose control over the last 7 days."

4. "The hemoglobin A1c test is a urine test that measures protein to evaluate glucose control over the last few months."

ANSWERS AND RATIONALES

1. 1. Type I diabetes mellitus, also know as insulin-dependent diabetes, occurs in individuals in whom the beta islet cells of the pancreas do not make insulin.
2. 4. NPH insulin is an intermediate-acting insulin. Regular insulin is a rapid-acting insulin. Mixing the two gives insulin over a 24-hour period, requiring fewer injections for the client.
3. 2. Lack of iodine in the diet is a primary contributor to the development of simple goiter.
4. 3. Turnips belong to a classification of foods called exogenous goitrogens. Goitrogens are thyroid-inhibiting substances and therefore should be avoided. Other goitrogens include rutabagas, cabbage, soybeans, peanuts, peaches, peas, strawberries, spinach, and radishes.
5. 3. Any emotional or physical stress, such as infection, may precipitate acute adrenal crisis with vascular collapse and shock.
6. 2. Addison's disease is characterized by bilateral hypofunction of the adrenal cortex, resulting in insufficient production of adrenal steroids including cortisol and aldosterone. There is increased production of melanocyte stimulating hormone (MSH), which stimulates production of melanin, a dark pigment. Persons with Addison's disease note that their skin is darker.
7. 1. If the person with Addison's perspires heavily he will lose sodium and fluid and become hyponatremic and hypovolemic. He should avoid strenuous exercise during hot weather.
8. 2. Addison's disease cannot be cured but it is controlled with lifelong hormone replacement.
9. 1. Self-monitoring of blood glucose has become an important part of diabetes management. Maintaining good control of blood sugar reduces complications. This is the best method to keep close control.
10. 4. In order to meet metabolic demand insulin must be taken on a regular basis. Ketoacidosis occurs when there is a lack of insulin in relation to metabolic demands.
11. 2. The blood work can be done quickly without preparation, while the remaining tests must be scheduled in advance. The scan must precede the arteriogram, since the arteriogram dye contains iodine that will interfere with the scan.

12. 2. The tracer dose used is much smaller than a therapeutic dose and is not harmful. The client can resume contact with others immediately following the test.

13. 3. Many cough syrups contain iodine, which interferes with the test. Other over-the-counter drugs to be avoided include salicylates, multivitamins, and some iodine-containing preparations found in health food stores.

14. 4. A fasting blood glucose is drawn before Glucola is administered. The client can drink only water as blood samples are obtained at designated intervals.

15. 4. Adrenal insufficiency requires lifelong gluco-corticoid replacement therapy. Glucocorticoids are given in divided doses, two-thirds in the morning and one-third in the afternoon to reflect the body's own circadian rhythm, which decreases the side effects of therapy.

16. 2. ACTH-secreting tumors can cause Cushing's syndrome, which can elevate the blood pressure to dangerously high levels.

17. 1. Hypophysectomy (removal of the pituitary gland) interferes with the secretion of both glucocorticoids and antidiuretic hormone, both of which are essential to maintain fluid balance and blood pressure. Careful monitoring of blood pressure is essential to ensure that hormone replacement therapy is adequate.

18. 4. Hormone replacement and follow-up care are needed for the rest of the client's life because the pituitary gland has been removed. This is the master gland that secretes trophic hormones that stimulate target glands to produce their hormones. A Medic-Alert bracelet is needed to alert others of the client's condition.

19. 2. Diabetes insipidus is characterized by polydipsia and polyuria. It occurs with lesions of the hypothalamus and pituitary. Because antidiuretic hormone synthesis is affected, the client is at high risk for dehydration, which is life-threatening.

20. 3. Withdrawal from glucocorticoid therapy can precipitate addisonian crisis, which is characterized by circulatory collapse and shock. Hypotension is a major manifestation of addisonian crisis and must be treated vigorously.

21. 2. Management of addisonian crisis includes glucocorticoid management. Intravenous replacement of sodium and dextrose is also necessary.

22. 1. Cushing's syndrome is caused by excessive corticosteroids. Excessive mineralocorticoid produces hypertension, acne, changes in secondary sex characteristics, and mood disturbances such as irritability, anxiety, euphoria, insomnia, irrationality, and psychosis.

23. 4. Clients with Cushing's syndrome exhibit central obesity, with a ''buffalo hump,'' a heavy trunk, and thin extremities. The accumulation of fat on the cheeks makes the face moon-shaped, or rounded.
24. 4. Hypertension and hyperkalemia are the classic manifestations of primary aldosteronism, in which the adrenal cortex secretes excessive mineralocorticoid.
25. 3. Clients with pheochromocytoma can experience episodes of life-threatening hypertension when the adrenal tumor secretes catecholamines that stimulate the sympathetic nervous system. These attacks are often accompanied by sweating, palpitations, and headache.
26. 4. The client cannot cope with stress because the client cannot produce corticosteroids.
27. 3. Without adrenal glands there is a lifelong need for a constant dose for replacement therapy daily.
28. 2. A simple goiter is an enlargement of the thyroid gland caused by excess thyroid-stimulating hormone (TSH) stimulation, growth-stimulating hormones, or excessive intake of goitrogenic foods.
29. 2. The client with Graves' disease is at risk for tachycardia, shock, hyperthermia, weight loss, and nervousness.
30. 4. Thyroxine and triiodothyronine levels are usually elevated and thyroid-stimulating hormone levels may be normal or undetectable in hyperthyroidism.
31. 3. Propranolol (Inderal) is a beta-adrenergic blocker that will relieve the symptoms of Graves' disease caused by increased circulating thyroid hormone. The symptoms are heat intolerance, palpitations, nervousness, tachycardia, and tremors.
32. 3. Oxygen, suction equipment, and a tracheostomy tray should be available in case airway obstruction occurs.
33. 1. The administration of thyroid hormone is needed after surgery because there is no thyroid gland to perform the usual functions.
34. 2. During a thyroidectomy it is possible for the parathyroid glands to be removed or damaged. If the parathyroid glands are disturbed, hypocalcemia may result.
35. 1. The client remains in the outpatient department for about 2 hours to be monitored for vomiting.
36. 3. The signs and symptoms of hypoparathyroidism are due to low serum calcium levels. A decrease in serum calcium may produce tetany. Tetany

produces tingling in lips, fingers, and feet. Severe tetany is associated with muscle spasms.

37. 2. Type I diabetes arises from the destruction of the beta cells, which results in little or no insulin production. Type II diabetes is the result of tissues being unresponsive to insulin, which eventually exhausts the production of insulin. Type II diabetics tend to be older than 35 years and overweight.

38. 2. The peak action for regular insulin occurs in 2 to 4 hours after administration. If regular insulin is administered at 7:30 A.M., then the client should be observed for hypoglycemia between 9:30 A.M. and 11:30 A.M.

39. 3. Snacks should be eaten prior to any exercise so glucose is readily available for the body's use.

40. 4. A conscious client experiencing hypoglycemia needs 5–20 grams of simple carbohydrates immediately. A 4–6 oz glass of orange juice would provide enough glucose to counteract hypoglycemia.

41. 2. The peak action for NPH is 6 hours after administration; therefore, delaying the administration 2 hours in the morning will allow the client to safely eat lunch at 2:00 P.M.

42. 1. At the first sign of diabetic ketoacidosis (elevated blood glucose and frequent urination) the nurse should administer insulin per physician's order to stabilize the blood glucose level.

43. 4. Hypoglycemia or low blood glucose occurs when there is more insulin than glucose in the serum or when blood glucose levels drop too rapidly. The signs of hypoglycemia include irritability, irrational behavior, dizziness, tremors, or loss of consciousness.

44. 1. The client needs to adhere to the meal plan that has been prescribed, as this is individualized according to the dietary needs.

45. 1. Neuropathy is one of the most common complications of diabetes caused by microangiopathies or metabolic defects that cause waste to build up in the nerves, resulting in demyelinization.

46. 3. A Type II diabetic is more likely to have hyperglycemic hyperosmolar nonketosis because there is sufficient insulin to prevent the metabolism of protein and fats for basic energy needs.

47. 4. The cardinal signs of hypoglycemia are cold sweats, weakness, and trembling. Additional signs include nervousness, irritability, pallor, increased heart rate, confusion, and fatigue.

48. 3. The diabetic client should wash the feet daily and examine for cuts, blisters, swelling, and any red, tender spots.

49. 4. The client is experiencing low blood sugar or hypoglycemia; ingesting a quick-acting carbohydrate source is the best action.

50. 1. Glycosylated hemoglobin, also known as the hemoglobin A_{1c} test, is used to determine glycemic control over time. Glucose attaches to hemoglobin and remains there for the life of the blood cell (120 days); therefore, the test indicates the overall glucose level of 120 days.

13

The Integumentary System

OVERVIEW OF ANATOMY AND PHYSIOLOGY

The integumentary system consists of the skin and its appendages, such as hair, nails, and various glands. The integumentary system not only provides a barrier against the external environment, it also plays a role in maintenance of the body's internal environment.

CHAPTER OUTLINE

Skin

A. Functions
   1. Protection: barrier to noxious agents (microorganisms, parasites, chemical substances) and to loss of water and electrolytes
   2. Thermoregulation: radiant cooling, evaporation
   3. Sensory perception: touch, temperature, pressure, pain
   4. Metabolism: excretion of water and sodium, production of vitamin D, wound repair

B. Layers (see Figure 13-1)
   1. *Epidermis*
      a. The avascular outermost layer
      b. Stratified into several layers
      c. Composed mainly of keratinocytes and melanocytes
         1) keratinocytes produce *keratin*, responsible for formation of hair and nails
         2) melanocytes produce *melanin*, a pigment that gives color to skin and hair
      d. Appendages (hair and nails, eccrine sweat glands, sebaceous glands, apocrine sweat glands) all derived from epidermis
   2. *Dermis:* layer beneath the epidermis composed of connective tissue that contains lymphatics, nerves, and blood vessels; elasticity of skin results from presence of collagen, elastin, and reticular fibers in the dermis, which also nourish the epidermis

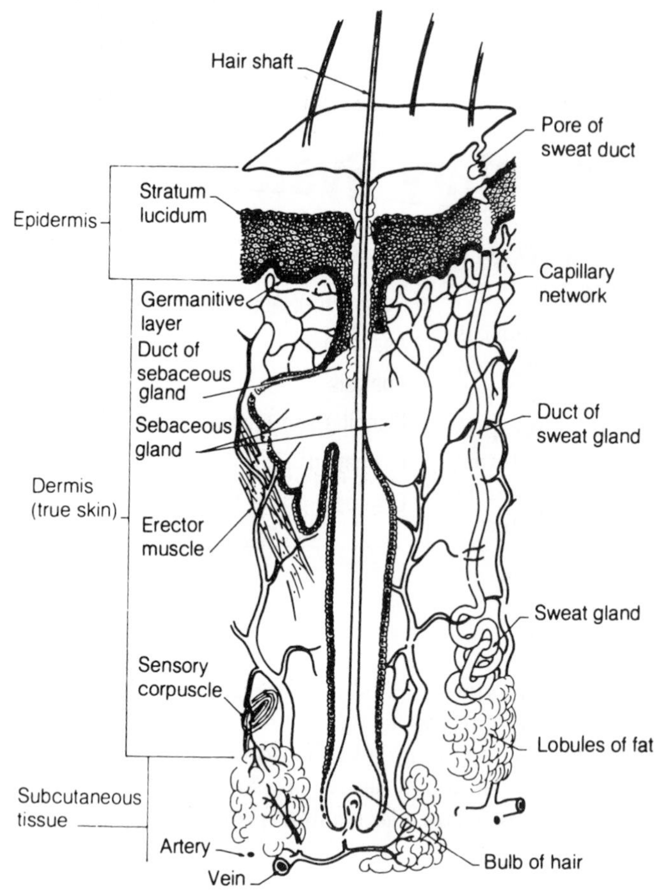

FIGURE 13-1 Cross section of skin: observe the skin layers and note the location of the glands in the dermal layer.

3. *Subcutaneous layer:* layer beneath the dermis composed of loose connective tissue and fat cells; stores fat; important in temperature regulation

Hair

A. Covers most of the body surface (except palms of hands, soles of feet, lips, nipples, and parts of external genitalia).
B. *Hair follicles:* tube-like structures, derived from epidermis, from which hair grows.
C. Hair functions as protection from external elements and from trauma.

DELEGATION TIP

Ancillary personnel may have many opportunities for skin inspection. Be specific about what observations are necessary to report.

D. Hair growth is controlled by hormonal influences and by blood supply.
E. Loss of body hair is called *alopecia*.

Nails

A. Dense layer of flat, dead cells; filled with keratin
B. Systemic illnesses may be reflected by changes in the nail or its bed; common changes include
   1. *Clubbing:* enlargement of fingers and toes, nail becomes convex; caused by chronic pulmonary or cardiovascular disease
   2. *Beau's line:* transverse groove caused by temporary halt in nail growth because of systemic disorder

Glands

A. *Eccrine sweat glands:* located all over the body; participate in heat regulation
B. *Apocrine sweat glands:* odiferous glands, found primarily in axillary, nipple, anal, and pubic areas; bacterial decomposition of excretions causes body odor
C. *Sebaceous glands:* oil glands, located all over the body except for palms of hands and soles of feet (abundant on face, scalp, upper chest, and back); produce *sebum*

ASSESSMENT

Health History

A. Presenting problem: symptoms may include changes in color or texture of skin, hair, nails; pruritus; infections; tumors; lesions; dermatitis; ecchymoses; rashes; dryness
B. Lifestyle: hygienic practices (skin-cleansing measures, use of cosmetics [type, brand names]); skin exposure (duration of exposure to sun, irritants [occupational], cold weather)
C. Nutrition/diet: intake of vitamins, essential nutrients, water; food allergies
D. Use of medications: steroids, vitamin use, hormones, antibiotics, chemotherapeutic agents
E. Past medical history: renal, hepatic, or collagen diseases; trauma or surgery; food, drug, or contact allergies
F. Family history: diabetes mellitus, allergic disorders, blood dyscrasias, specific dermatologic problems, cancer

Physical Examination

A. Color: note areas of uniform color; pigmentation; redness, jaundice, cyanosis.

B. Vascular changes

   1. Purpuric lesions: note ecchymoses, petechiae.

   2. Vascular lesions: note angiomas, hemangiomas, venous stars.

C. Lesions: note color, type, size, distribution, location, consistency, grouping (annular, circular, linear, or clustered).

D. Edema: differentiate pitting from nonpitting.

E. Moisture content: note dryness, clamminess.

F. Temperature: note whether increased or decreased, distribution of temperature changes.

G. Texture: note smoothness, coarseness.

H. Mobility/turgor: note whether increased or decreased.

Laboratory/Diagnostic Studies

A. Blood chemistry/electrolytes: calcium, chloride, magnesium, potassium, sodium

B. Hematologic studies: Hbg, hct, RBC, WBC

C. Biopsy

   1. Removal of a small piece of skin for examination to determine diagnosis

   2. Nursing care: instruct client to keep biopsied area dry until healing occurs

D. Skin testing

   1. Administration of allergens or antigens on the surface of or into the dermis to determine hypersensitivity

   2. Three types: patch, scratch, and intradermal

■ ANALYSIS

Nursing diagnoses for clients with a disorder of the integumentary system may include

A. Impaired skin integrity

B. Pain

C. Disturbed body image

D. Risk for infection

E. Ineffective airway clearance

F. Ineffective peripheral tissue perfusion

■ PLANNING AND IMPLEMENTATION

Goals

A. Restoration of skin integrity.

B. Client will experience absence of pain.

C. Client will adapt to changes in appearance.

D. Client will be free from infection.
E. Maintenance of effective airway clearance.
F. Maintenance of adequate peripheral tissue perfusion.

Interventions

Skin Grafts

A. Replacement of damaged skin with healthy skin to provide protection of underlying structures or to reconstruct areas for cosmetic or functional purposes
B. Graft sources
   1. *Autograft:* client's own skin
   2. *Isograft:* skin from a genetically identical person (identical twin)
   3. *Homograft or allograft:* cadaver of same species
   4. *Heterograft or xenograft:* skin from another species (such as a porcine graft)
   5. *Human amniotic membrane*
C. Nursing care: preoperative
   1. Donor site: cleanse with antiseptic soap the night before and morning of surgery as ordered.
   2. Recipient site: apply warm compresses and topical antibiotics as ordered.
D. Nursing care: postoperative
   1. Donor site
      a. Keep area covered for 24–48 hours.
      b. Use bed cradle to prevent pressure and provide greater air circulation
      c. Outer dressing may be removed 24–72 hours postsurgery; maintain fine mesh gauze (innermost dressing) until it falls off spontaneously.
      d. Trim loose edges of gauze as it loosens with healing.
      e. Administer analgesics as ordered (more painful than recipient site).
   2. Recipient site
      a. Elevate site when possible.
      b. Protect from pressure (use bed cradle).
      c. Apply warm compresses as ordered.
      d. Assess for hematoma, fluid accumulation under graft.
      e. Monitor circulation distal to graft.
   3. Provide emotional support and monitor behavioral adjustments; refer for counseling if needed.
E. Provide client teaching and discharge planning concerning
   1. Applying lubricating lotion to maintain moisture on surfaces of healed graft for at least 6–12 months
   2. Protecting grafted skin from direct sunlight for at least 6 months

3. Protecting graft from physical injury
4. Need to report changes in graft (fluid accumulation, pain, hematoma)
5. Possible alteration in pigmentation and hair growth; ability to sweat lost in most grafts
6. Sensations may or may not return

EVALUATION

A. Healing of burned areas; absence of drainage, edema, and pain over graft sites.
B. Relaxed facial expression/body posture; achieves effective rest patterns; participates in daily activities without pain.
C. Incorporates changes into self-concept without negating self-esteem; verbalizes about changes that occurred; demonstrates interest in physical appearance.
D. Achieves wound healing; vital signs within normal range; lungs clear; laboratory studies within normal range.
E. Lungs clear to auscultation; respiratory rate and depth within normal limits; free of dyspnea.
F. Palpable peripheral pulses of equal quality; adequate capillary refill; skin color normal in uninjured areas.

DISORDERS OF THE INTEGUMENTARY SYSTEM

Primary Lesions of the Skin

A. *Macule:* a flat, circumscribed area of color change in the skin without surface elevation, up to 2 cm in diameter
B. *Papule:* a circumscribed solid and elevated lesion, up to 1 cm in size
C. *Nodule:* a solid, elevated lesion extending deeper into the dermis, 1–2 cm in diameter
D. *Wheal:* a slightly irregular, transient superficial elevation of the skin with a palpable margin (e.g., hive)
E. *Vesicle:* circumscribed elevated lesion filled with serous fluid, less than 1 cm in diameter
F. *Bulla:* a vesicle larger than 1 cm in diameter
G. *Pustule:* a vesicle or bulla containing purulent exudate

Contact Dermatitis

A. General information
   1. An irritation of the skin from a specific substance or from a hypersensitivity immune reaction from contact with a specific antigen
   2. Caused by irritants (mechanical, chemical, biologic); allergens
B. Assessment findings
   1. Pruritus
   2. Erythema: localized edema; vesicles (oozing, crusting, and scaling [later])
   3. Diagnostic test: skin testing reveals hypersensitivity to specific antigen

C. Nursing interventions
   1. Apply wet dressings of Burrow's solution for 20 minutes 4 times a day to help clear oozing lesions.
   2. Provide relief from pruritus.
   3. Administer topical steroids and antibiotics as ordered.
   4. Provide client teaching and discharge planning concerning
      a. Avoidance of causative agent
      b. Preventing skin dryness
         1) use mild soaps (Ivory).
         2) soak in plain water for 20–30 minutes.
         3) apply prescribed steroid cream immediately after bath.
         4) avoid extremes of heat and cold.
      c. Allowing crusts and scales to drop off skin naturally as healing occurs
      d. Avoidance of wool, nylon, or fur fibers on sensitive skin
      e. Need to use gloves if handling irritant or allergenic substances

Psoriasis

A. General information
   1. Chronic type of dermatitis that involves accelerated turnover rate of the epidermal cells
   2. Predisposing factors include stress, trauma, infection; changes in climate may produce exacerbations; familial predisposition to the disease
B. Medical management
   1. Topical corticosteroids
   2. Coal tar preparations
   3. Ultraviolet light
   4. Antimetabolites (methotrexate)
C. Assessment findings
   1. Mild pruritus
   2. Sharply circumscribed scaling placques that are mostly present on the scalp, elbows, and knees; yellow discoloration of nails
D. Nursing interventions
   1. Apply occlusive wraps over prescribed topical steroids.
   2. Protect areas treated with coal tar preparations from direct sunlight for 24 hours.
   3. Administer methotrexate as ordered, assess for side effects.
   4. Provide client teaching and discharge planning concerning
      a. Feelings about changes in appearance of skin (encourage client to cover arms and legs with clothing if sensitive about appearance)
      b. Importance of adhering to prescribed treatment and avoidance of commercially advertised products

NURSING ALERT

Signs of malignant melanoma are changes in moles' appearance showing asymmetry; border notching; color variation with black, brown, red, or white hue; and diameter greater than 6 mm.

Skin Cancer

A. General information

1. Types of skin cancers

a. *Basal cell epithelioma:* most common type of skin cancer; locally invasive and rarely metastasizes; most frequently located between the hairline and upper lip

b. *Squamous cell carcinoma (epidermoid):* grows more rapidly than basal cell carcinoma and can metastasize; frequently seen on mucous membranes, lower lip, neck, and dorsum of the hands

c. *Malignant melanoma:* least frequent of skin cancers, but most serious; capable of invasion and metastasis to other organs

2. Precancerous lesions

a. *Leukoplakia:* white, shiny patches in the mouth and on the lip

b. *Nevi (moles):* junctional nevus may become malignant (signs include a color change to black, bleeding, and irritation); compound and dermal nevi unlikely to become cancerous

c. *Senile keratoses:* brown, scalelike spots on older individuals

3. Contributing factors include hereditary predisposition (fair, blue-eyed people; redheads and blondes); irritation (chemicals or ultraviolet rays)

4. Occurs more often in those with outdoor occupations who are exposed to more sunlight

B. Medical management: varies depending on type of cancer; surgical excision with or without radiation therapy most common; chemotherapy and immunotherapy for melanoma

C. Assessment findings: characteristics depend on specific type of lesion; biopsy reveals malignant cells

D. Nursing interventions: provide client teaching concerning

1. Limitation of contact with chemical irritants

2. Protection against ultraviolet radiation from sun

a. Wear thin layer of clothing.

b. Use sun block or lotion containing para-amino benzoic acid (PABA).

3. Need to report lesions that change characteristics and/or those that do not heal.

CLIENT TEACHING CHECKLIST

Clients with shingles/oral lesions should:

- Use soft toothbrush
- Eat soft foods
- Use a saline or H_2CO_3-based mouthwash.
- Use oral anesthetics to decrease discomfort.

Herpes Zoster (Shingles)

A. General information
  1. Acute viral infection of the nervous system
  2. The virus causes an inflammatory reaction in isolated spinal and cranial sensory ganglia and the posterior gray matter of the spinal cord
  3. Contagious to anyone who has not had varicella or who is immunosuppressed
  4. Caused by activation of latent varicella-zoster virus

B. Medical management
  1. Analgesics
  2. Corticosteroids
  3. Acetic acid compresses
  4. Acyclovir (Zovirax)

C. Assessment findings
  1. Neuralgic pain, malaise, itching, burning
  2. Cluster of skin vesicles along course of peripheral sensory nerves, usually unilateral and primarily on trunk, thorax, or face

D. Nursing interventions
  1. Apply acetic acid compresses or white petrolatum to lesions.
  2. Administer medications as ordered.
    a. Analgesics for pain.
    b. Systemic corticosteroids: monitor for side effects of steroid therapy.
    c. Acyclovir (Zovivax): antivalagent reduces severity when given early in illness.

Herpes Simplex Virus, Type I

A. General information
  1. Causes cold sores or fever blisters, canker sores, and herpetic whitlow
  2. Common disorder, frequently seen in women

   3. Primary infection occurs in children, recurrences in adults
   4. Self-limiting virus
- **B.** Assessment findings: clusters of vesicles, may ulcerate or crust; burning, itching, tingling; usually appears on lip or cheek
- **C.** Nursing interventions: keep lesions dry; apply topical antibiotics or anesthetic as ordered.

Burns

- **A.** Types
   1. Thermal: most common type; caused by flame, flash, scalding, and contact (hot metals, grease)
   2. Smoke inhalation: occurs when smoke (particular products of a fire, gases, and superheated air) causes respiratory tissue damage
   3. Chemical: caused by tissue contact, ingestion or inhalation of acids, alkalies, or vesicants
   4. Electrical: injury occurs from direct damage to nerves and vessels when an electric current passes through the body.
- **B.** Classification
   1. *Partial thickness*
      - **a.** Superficial partial-thickness (first degree)
         1) depth: epidermis only
         2) causes: sunburn, splashes of hot liquid
         3) sensation: painful
         4) characteristics: erythema, blanching on pressure, no vesicles
      - **b.** Deep partial thickness (second degree)
         1) depth: epidermis and dermis
         2) causes: flash, scalding, or flame burn
         3) sensation: very painful
         4) characteristics: fluid-filled vesicles; red, shiny, wet after vesicles rupture
   2. *Full thickness* (third and fourth degree)
      - **a.** Depth: all skin layers and nerve endings; may involve muscles, tendons, and bones
      - **b.** Causes: flame, chemicals, scalding, electric current
      - **c.** Sensation: little or no pain
      - **d.** Characteristics: wound is dry, white, leathery, or hard
- **C.** Medical management
   1. Supportive therapy: fluid management (IVs), catheterization
   2. Wound care: hydrotherapy, debridement (enzymatic or surgical)
   3. Drug therapy
      - **a.** Topical antibiotics: mafenide (Sulfamylon), silver sulfadiazine (Silvadene), silver nitrate, povidone-iodine (Betadine) solution
      - **b.** Systemic antibiotics: gentamicin

   c. Tetanus toxoid or hyperimmune human tetanus globulin (burn wound good medium for anaerobic growth)
   d. Analgesics
4. Surgery: excision and grafting

D. Assessment
1. Extent of burn injury by rule of nines: head and neck (9%); each arm (9%), each leg (18%), trunk (36%), genitalia (1%) (see Figure 13-2)
2. Lund and Browder method determines the extent of the burn injury by using client's age in proportion to relative body-part size.
3. Severity of burn
   a. Major: partial thickness greater than 25%; full thickness greater than or equal to 10%
   b. Moderate: partial thickness 15–25%, full thickness less than 10%
   c. Minor: partial thickness less than 15%; full thickness less than 2%

E. Stages
1. *Emergent phase*
   a. Remove person from source of burn.
      1) thermal: smother burn beginning with the head.
      2) smoke inhalation: ensure patent airway.

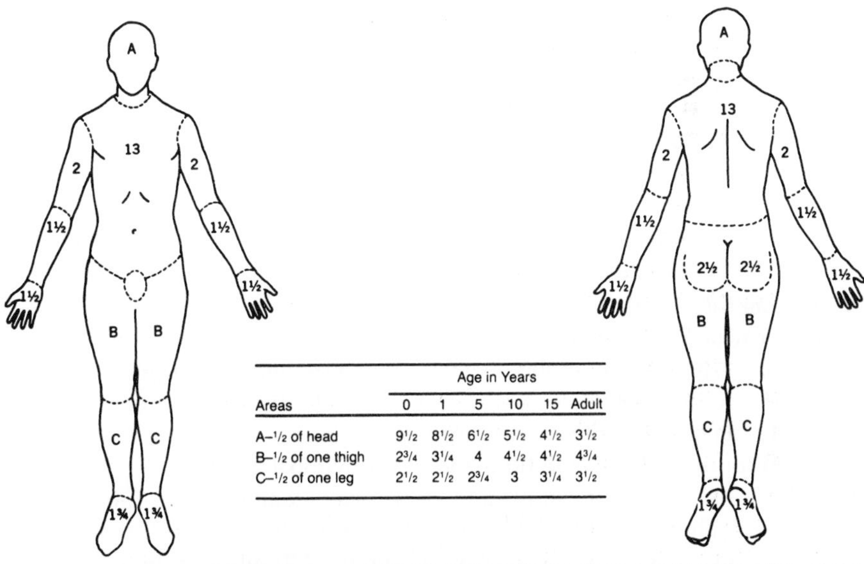

Areas	Age in Years 0	1	5	10	15	Adult
A–½ of head	9½	8½	6½	5½	4½	3½
B–½ of one thigh	2¾	3¼	4	4½	4½	4¾
C–½ of one leg	2½	2½	2¾	3	3¼	3½

FIGURE 13-2 Body proportions change with growth. Shown here, in percentage, is the relationship of thse body area to the whole body surface area at various ages. This method of determining the extent of the burned area is attributed to Lund and Browder.

3) chemical: remove clothing that contains chemical; lavage area with copious amounts of water.
4) electrical: note victim position, identify entry/exit routes, maintain airway.

b. Wrap in dry, clean sheet or blanket to prevent further contamination of wound and provide warmth.
c. Assess how and when burn occurred.
d. Provide IV route if possible.
e. Transport immediately.

2. *Shock phase* (first 24–48 hours)
   a. Plasma to interstitial fluid shift causing hypovolemia; fluid also moves to areas that normally have little or no fluid (third-spacing).
   b. Assessment findings
      1) dehydration, decreased blood pressure, elevated pulse, decreased urine output, thirst
      2) diagnostic tests: hyperkalemia, hyponatremia, elevated hct, metabolic acidosis
3. *Fluid remobilization or diuretic phase* (2–5 days postburn)
   a. Interstitial fluid returns to the vascular compartment.
   b. Assessment findings
      1) elevated blood pressure, increased urine output
      2) diagnostic tests: hypokalemia, hyponatremia, metabolic acidosis
4. *Convalescent (rehabilitation) phase*
   a. Starts when diuresis is completed and wound healing and coverage begin.
   b. Assessment findings
      1) dry, waxy-white appearance of full thickness burn changing to dark brown; wet, shiny, and serous exudate in partial thickness
      2) diagnostic test: hyponatremia

F. Nursing interventions

1. Provide relief/control of pain
   a. Administer morphine sulfate IV and monitor vital signs closely.
   b. Administer analgesics/narcotics 30 minutes before wound care.
   c. Position burned areas in proper alignment.
2. Monitor alterations in fluid and electrolyte balance.
   a. Assess for fluid shifts and electrolyte alterations (see Table 13-5).
   b. Administer IV fluids as ordered (see Table 13-1).
   c. Monitor Foley catheter output hourly (30 ml/hour desired).
   d. Weigh daily.
   e. Monitor circulation status regularly.
   f. Administer/monitor crystalloids/colloids/H_2O solutions.
3. Promote maximal nutritional status
   a. Monitor tube feedings/TPN if ordered.

TABLE 13-1 Guidelines and Formulas for Fluid Replacement for Burns

Consensus Formula	Evans Formula	Brooke Army Formula	Parkland/ Baxter Formula
Lactated Ringer's: 2-4 ml × wt. in kg × % body surface area (BSA) burned. Half to be given in first 8 hr after burn; remaining fluid to be given over next 16 hr.	1. Colloids: 1 ml × wt. kg × % BSA burned 2. Electrolytes (saline): 1 ml × wt. kg × % BSA burned 3. Glucose (5% in water): 2000 ml for insensible loss Day 1: Half to be given in first 8 hr; remaining half over next 16 hr. Day 2: Half of previous day's colloids and electrolytes; all of insensible fluid replacement. Maximum of 10,000 ml over 24 hr. Second- and third-degree burns exceeding 50% BSA calculated on basis of 50% BSA	1. Colloids: 0.5 ml × wt, kg × % BSA burned 2. Electrolytes (lactated Ringer's): 1.5 ml × wt, kg × % BSA burned 3. Glucose (5% in water): 2000 ml for insensible loss Day 1: Half to be given in first 8 hr; remaining half over next 16 hr. Day 2: Half of colloids, half of electrolytes, all of insensible fluid replacement. Second- and third-degree burns exceeding 50% BSA calculated on basis of 50% BSA.	Lactated Ringer's: 4 ml × wt, kg × % BSA burned. Day 1: Half to be given in first 8 hr; half to be given over next 16 hr. Day 2: Varies; colloid is added.

   b. When oral intake permitted, provide high-calorie, high-protein, high-carbohydrate diet with vitamin and mineral supplements.
   c. Serve small portions.
   d. Schedule wound care and other treatments at least 1 hour before meals.

4. Prevent wound infection.
   a. Place client in controlled sterile environment.

NURSING ALERT

Monitor burn clients for edema hoarseness, difficulty swallowing, stridor, and copious secretions as indications of respiratory injury.

- **b.** Use hydrotherapy for no more than 30 minutes to prevent electrolyte loss.
- **c.** Observe wound for separation of eschar and cellulitis.
- **d.** Apply mafenide (Sulfamylon) as ordered.
  - **1)** administer analgesics 30 minutes before application.
  - **2)** monitor acid-base status and renal function studies.
  - **3)** provide daily tubbing for removal of previously applied cream.
- **e.** Apply silver sulfadiazine (Silvadene) as ordered.
  - **1)** administer analgesics 30 minutes before application.
  - **2)** observe for and report hypersensitivity reactions (rash, itching, burning sensation in unburned areas).
  - **3)** store drug away from heat.
- **f.** Apply silver nitrate as ordered.
  - **1)** handle carefully; solution leaves a gray or black stain on skin, clothing, and utensils.
  - **2)** administer analgesic before application.
  - **3)** keep dressings wet with solution; dryness increases the concentration and causes precipitation of silver salts in the wound.
- **g.** Apply povidone-iodine (Betadine) solution as ordered.
  - **1)** administer analgesics before application.
  - **2)** assess for metabolic acidosis/renal function studies.
- **h.** Administer gentamicin as ordered: assess vestibular/auditory and renal functions at regular intervals.

5. Prevent GI complications.

- **a.** Assess for signs and symptoms of paralytic ileus.
- **b.** Assist with insertion of NG tube to prevent/control Curling's/stress ulcer; monitor patency/drainage.
- **c.** Administer prophylactic antacids through NG tube and/or IV cimetidine (Tagamet) or ranitidine (Zantac) (to prevent gastric pH of less than 5).
- **d.** Monitor bowel sounds.
- **e.** Test stools for occult blood.

6. Provide client teaching and discharge planning concerning

- **a.** Care of healed burn wound

1) assess daily for changes.
2) wash hands frequently during dressing change.
3) wash area with prescribed solution or
4) mild soap and rinse well with H_2O; dry with clean towel. apply sterile dressing.

b. Prevention of injury to burn wound
1) avoid trauma to area.
2) avoid use of fabric softeners or harsh detergents (might cause irritation).
3) avoid constrictive clothing over burn wound.

c. Adherence to prescribed diet

d. Importance of reporting formation of blisters, opening of healed area, increased or foul-smelling drainage from wound, other signs of infection

e. Methods of coping and resocialization

14

Complementary and Alternative Medicine (CAM)

OVERVIEW

CHAPTER OUTLINE

A. Definitions

1. Alternative medicine is a holistic approach to health and focuses on balancing the body to achieve optimal wellness.
2. Alternative medical systems are built upon a complex system of theory and practice and have often evolved apart from, and earlier than, the conventional medicine that is practiced in the United States.
3. Modalities that are generally not taught widely in Western medical schools nor generally available in hospitals in the United States or other Western societies (see Table 14-1).

B. Patterns of CAM use in the United States

1. Most clients do not tell their physician they are using CAM unless specifically asked.
2. Estimates that one in three adults aged 35 to 49 years is using at least one CAM therapy.
3. Higher incidence in incomes over $50,000 (48% vs. 43%).
4. 42% of CAM use is for treatment of a specific disease or illness, while 58% of use is, at least in part, to prevent future illness from occurring or to maintain health and vitality.

CLIENT TEACHING CHECKLIST

- Instruct clients to stop herbal supplements 2–3 weeks prior to surgery.
- Instruct client to discuss with health care provider when supplements may be restarted.

TABLE 14-1 Complementary and Alternative Modalities

Modality	What It Is	Common Uses
Ayurvedic Medicine	Ayurvedic tradition believes that all illnesses, physical or mental, are a state of disharmony or imbalance in the body's systems. Diagnosis is made by feeling the pulse and looking for indicators of disharmony on the tongue. Utilizes a wide variety of modalities such as medication, herbals, and massage. Nutrition and food groups play a key role in balancing the body systems. Practiced in India for more than 5,000 years.	Acute and chronic illness, promotion of health and wellness
Aromatherapy	The use of essential oils, distilled from plants, aromatherapy treats. Oils are massaged into the skin in diluted form, inhaled, or placed in water for diffusion. Aromatherapy is often used in conjunction with massage therapy, acupuncture, reflexology, herbology, chiropractic, and other holistic treatments.	Abdominal pain, stress and anxiety, insomnia, as an antiseptic, skin conditions
Massage	Manipulation of muscles and other soft tissue. Improves circulation, muscle fatigue, and promotes well-being. Multiple techniques including deep tissue, vibration, effleurage, percussion. Developed in both Western and Eastern cultures.	Back and neck pain, stress, insomnia, headache, promotion of well-being

Continued

Table 14-1 Continued

Modality	What It Is	Common Uses
Chiropractic	Manipulation of the spine to promote balance and health. Misalignments of the spine thought to cause pressure on the spinal nerve roots. Pressure from trauma or poor posture leads to decreased function and wellness. Adjustment or manipulation of the spine corrects the misalignment and results in a more balanced state of health.	Back and neck pain, stress, insomnia, headache
Acupuncture	Based on the concept of chi, or life-force energy. Very fine needles are placed along energy lines to disperse congestion, increase energy flow, and allow the body to heal and balance.	Pain relief, smoking cessation, treatment of acute and chronic illness; also used extensively with pets
Biofeedback	Use of a sensor unit (TENS) allows individuals to monitor their own bodies' response to stimuli. Usually a light and sound device. A method of monitoring minute metabolic changes in one's own body with the aid of sensitive machines. Individuals use imagery, breathing techniques, and visualization to control their heart rate, breathing, and thought process. These changes are audible and visible on the biofeedback unit.	Stress-related conditions such as asthma, migraines, insomnia, and high blood pressure

Hypnosis	A method of focusing on the unconscious mind and accessing the subconscious to access repressed emotions, forgotten events, and memories that may assist the client to heal. Trained hypnotherapist creates a calm, safe environment for the client. Client remains aware but focused on the subconscious mind rather than the present.	Anxiety, weight loss, pain relief, phobias, chronic pain
Homeopathy	A healing system that uses minute amounts of natural substances, called remedies, to stimulate the individual's immune system. These substances, given in larger dose, mimic the symptoms the client is experiencing. Based on the philosophy "like cures like."	Arthritis, abdominal complaints, allergies, fatigue, menstrual irregularities
Herbal Medicine	The use of plant products for treatment of a wide range of chronic and acute illnesses. Plants, and their derivatives, are used in a variety of forms, including dried, distilled, tincture, pills, caplets, elixirs, and topical preparations. One of the oldest complementary therapies, it is used widely throughout the world today as the primary source of medicinal products. Not regulated by the FDA in the United States.	Acute and chronic illness including, but not limited to, asthma, arthritis, abdominal pain, menstrual irregularities, cuts and bruises; used to enhance the functioning of the body's systems

Continued

Table 14-1 Continued

Modality	What It Is	Common Uses
Reflexology	Designed to stimulate chi, or life-force energy, in the body by applying pressure to meridians, or contact points, on the feet and hands. Pressure on the reflexology points stimulates flow of chi, allowing the client to restore balance in the body and promote healing. The practitioner uses the fingers to apply pressure to the reflexology points.	Respiratory symptoms, stress, headache, fatigue, pain
Reiki	Use of the practitioner's hands to "channel" the universal life-force energy to the client to promote healing. Tibetan healing system. Hands may hover above the client or lightly touch. Use light hand placements to channel healing energies to the recipient.	Pain, digestive problems, stress and stress-related disorders; assist the recipient in achieving spiritual focus and clarity
Therapeutic Touch	Practitioner "senses" client's energy field through auditory-visual-kinetic or intuitive systems. Using the hands, the practitioner facilitates a symmetrical and rhythmical flow of energy and redirects it, allowing the individual's energy to flow freely. Treatment is complete when the practitioner senses a symmetrical state and rhythmic order.	Headache, musculoskeletal pain, emotional distress

NURSING ALERT

Supplements which should not be consumed prior to surgery include echinacea, ephedra, garlic, ginkgo, ginseng, kava, Saint John's wort, and valerian.

REVIEW QUESTIONS

1. A 37-year-old man is seen in the outpatient clinic for treatment of psoriasis. The nurse should anticipate which of the following findings in this man?

1. Intense pain.

2. Discolored nails.

3. Abdominal lesions.

4. Hyperpigmented skin.

2. The physician prescribes coal tar preparations as part of the treatment plan for a man who has psoriasis. The nurse should include which statement in the teaching plan for this client?

1. Avoid sunlight immediately after the treatment.

2. Ingest the coal tar with liberal amounts of water.

3. Eat a high-carbohydrate diet.

4. Restrict activity for 24 hours.

3. An adult's shirt catches on fire and is now in flames. He panics and runs into his neighbor's yard. Which of the following interventions is appropriate? Select all that apply.

1. ______ Dousing the flames with water.

2. ______ Removing his burned clothing.

3. ______ Removing his jewelry.

4. ______ Rolling him on the ground.

4. The nurse is caring for a man admitted with severe burns sustained when his clothing caught fire while he was burning leaves. During the acute burn phase, the nurse explains to the man that his nursing care plan is directed toward all of the following except

1. strict aseptic technique.

2. proper alignment of all joints.

3. maintenance of fluid and electrolyte balance.

4. frequent and routine administration of narcotics.

5. The nurse is planning care for an adult man who is admitted with severe flame burns. Nursing care planning is based on the knowledge that the first 24–48 hours post-burn are characterized by

1. an increase in the total volume of intravascular plasma.

2. excessive renal perfusion with diuresis.

3. fluid shift from interstitial spaces to plasma.

4. fluid shift from plasma to interstitial spaces.

6. The nurse is caring for an adult who was admitted following severe burns sustained in a house fire. The nurse understands that an acceptable range for hourly urine output during the first 2 days post-burn is

1. 20 ml.

2. 30–50 ml.

3. 100–150 ml.

4. 150–200 ml.

7. The nurse is to perform a scratch test for allergy. Which statement best describes this procedure?

1. The antigen is directly applied to the skin and covered with a gauze dressing.

2. The allergen is applied superficially to a small cut of the outer layer of skin.

3. A small amount of allergen is injected into the intradermal layer of skin.

4. Suspected food allergy items are scratched from the diet, one at a time, until all allergy symptoms are no longer present.

8. An adult has undergone a skin graft from his left buttock to his right upper thigh. When caring for the recipient site, the nurse can expect to

1. apply silver sulfadiazine to promote rapid healing.

2. assess for bleeding and large amounts of fluid accumulation beneath the graft.

3. encourage the client to ambulate and do leg lifts on return from the OR.

4. encourage the client to take frequent soaking baths to relieve his soreness and discomfort.

9. A client with a skin graft has undergone a full-thickness skin graft from her right upper thigh to her upper chest area. The most appropriate nursing action in caring for her *donor* site is to

1. keep the fine mesh gauze dressing on her chest soaked with normal saline.

2. completely immobilize her right upper thigh area.

3. maintain the compression bandage on her right upper thigh for several days.
4. remove the nylon fabric adhered to the donor site no later than two to three days after grafting has taken place.

10. A client has undergone a skin graft. Which finding most likely indicates that complications with the recipient site may exist?

1. Small amounts of blood beneath the graft.
2. Small amounts of serum beneath the graft.
3. A meshed pattern in the graft.
4. Continuous bleeding beneath the graft.

11. A 42-year-old homemaker has been diagnosed with atopic dermatitis. She has severe pruritis. Which interventions are most appropriate to include in the plan of care?

1. Soak in a hot water bath at least once a day for 15–20 minutes.
2. Avoid use of air conditioning when possible.
3. When symptoms are worse, decrease bathing.
4. Use superfatted soaps or soap for sensitive skin.

12. The nurse is developing a teaching plan for a client with psoriasis. What information would the nurse need to know when developing the teaching plan?

1. It is a chronic disorder resulting in the development of blisters; an autoimmune disorder caused by circulating IgG antibodies. Management includes steroids and immunosuppressives. Nursing management focuses on self-concept and pain management.
2. It is a superficial inflammatory dermatitis occurring when two skin surfaces rub together, causing erythema, maceration, itching, and burning. Management includes liberal application of talc, or cellulose-containing powder, or corticosteroids.
3. It is a chronic recurrent, erythematous, inflammatory disorder involving keratin synthesis. Severe scaling and itching occurs. Management includes sunlight, tar preparation, and use of anthralin. Nursing management includes teaching clients about UV light therapy, and assisting with altered self-concept.
4. It is an area of very dry skin. Sometimes shallow ulcers occur. Itching, brown stained skin may occur. Management includes elevation of affected extremity, lotion, and support hose.

13. The nurse has been giving instructions to a 35-year-old white female about preventing skin cancer. Which statement best indicates understanding of skin cancer risk factors?

1. "I guess because I am dark complected I will be more prone to developing skin cancer."
2. "I used to lie in the sun all the time—now I just go to the tanning bed."
3. "My father was treated for melanoma, but my mom says not to worry."
4. "I really need to use sunscreen—even in winter."

14. A 60-year-old farmer presents with a diagnosis of basal cell epithelioma. The lesion would most likely be described as

1. dome shaped, shiny, with a well-defined border.
2. poorly marginated, flat red area.
3. red, dark blue, or purple macules.
4. erythema, edema, and blisters.

15. While providing a nursing history, a client with suspected malignant melanoma will most often relate which of the following?

1. A history of intense sunlight exposure.
2. Complaints of frequently occurring irregularly shaped, flat macules with overlying hard scale.
3. Consistent use of sunscreen agents.
4. Complaints of several lesions with a raised border and flattened center.

16. An adult presents with the following symptoms: clusters of vesicles on her right flank, constant pain, burning, itching, and discomfort in her flank area. She ranks her pain as a 5, with 5 being most severe. Which of the following diagnoses would be a priority when developing a plan of care for the client?

1. Pain, related to herpes simplex.
2. Pain, related to herpes zoster.
3. Pain, related to herpetic whitlow.
4. Pain, related to staphylococcal cellulitis.

17. When planning care for a client with herpes zoster, the nurse should include

1. teaching the client to avoid sexual contact during outbreaks.
2. administering analgesics and evaluating the efficacy.
3. informing the client that people who have not had chickenpox will not develop them from exposure to the client.
4. scheduling several diagnostic tests to confirm the presence of herpes zoster.

18. Which client statement best indicates the client understands how herpes simplex is transmitted?

1. "It is okay to share towels as long as it is a family member."
2. "I really don't need to use a condom, unless I have a sore."
3. "Once I'm over this spell, I won't need to worry about it again."
4. "I shouldn't have sex if some of those sores are around."

19. A 78-year-old man is admitted with severe flame burns resulting from smoking in bed. The nurse can expect his room environment to include

1. strict isolation techniques and policies.
2. a semi-private room.
3. liberal unrestricted visiting.
4. equipment shared between the client and the other burn client in the unit.

20. A 23-year-old factory worker was burned severely in an industrial accident. He has second-degree burns on his right leg and arm and on his back. He has third-degree burns on his left arm. The triage nurse, using the rule of nines, estimates the extent of the client's burns as ________________ %.

21. An adult was burned in a house fire 16 hours ago. She suffered second- and third-degree burns over 65% of her body. She is receiving lactated Ringer's at 200 ml/h. Which intervention is a *priority* at this time?

1. Monitoring hourly urine output.
2. Assessing for signs and symptoms of infection.
3. Performing range of motion q 1–2 h.
4. Meeting the high caloric needs of the client.

22. A nurse is providing care for a severely burned client during the shock phase of the burn injury. Which assessment findings would indicate that the client is receiving adequate fluid volume replacement?

1. Urine output 20 ml/h, CVP 3, weak pulses, K^+ level of 5.3.
2. Urine output 50 ml/h, BP 100/60, oriented to person and place.
3. Weak thready pulses, BP 70/40, pulse 130, Hct 52%.
4. Restlessness, confusion, urine output 15 ml/h, rapidly increasing weight.

23. A client with severe burns is receiving IV Zantac. Which statement best explains the reason for administration of this medication in this situation?

1. The client was treated for gastritis several years ago.
2. The medication will reduce hypoxemia in burn clients.
3. The medication is an H_2 receptor antagonist and will decrease acid secretion.
4. The medication will aid in removal of pulmonary secretions.

24. An 18-year-old was burned 6 weeks ago. She is now ready for discharge. Select the statement best reflecting understanding of discharge care.

   1. "I will be so glad to get home so that I don't have to wear this pressure thing anymore."

   2. "I will need to call my doctor if my temperature goes up or this burn area starts draining and oozing."

   3. "I really need to stick to a low-calorie, low-protein diet."

   4. "To prevent that area of new skin from feeling so tight, I can rub ice and baby oil on it."

25. A client has suffered a chemical burn. The best initial action is to

   1. roll the client in a blanket.

   2. secure lead-lined gloves and move the client away from the chemical.

   3. flush the area with copious amounts of water or normal saline.

   4. if the chemical is an acid, neutralize with a base.

26. A 25-year-old electrical worker has come in contact with a live power line. He is unconscious and is lying across the power line.The best initial action is to

   1. move the person away from the power line using a wooden pole.

   2. cover the person with a blanket.

   3. grab the person and pull him away from the power lines.

   4. flush the wound with copious amounts of water.

ANSWERS AND RATIONALES

1. 2. A yellow discoloration of the nails is frequently seen in psoriasis.

2. 1. Sunlight should be avoided after a coal tar treatment.

3. Dousing the flames should be selected. This is an appropriate way to smother the flames.
Removing his jewelry should be selected. Hot metal jewelry could increase burning. Rings should be removed before edema occurs.
Rolling him on the ground should be selected because it will smother flames.

4. 4. Narcotics should be given only after careful assessment in this phase due to the danger of shock and respiratory depression.

5. 4. The initial fluid alteration following a severe burn is a plasma-to-interstitial fluid and electrolyte balance, which is a nursing priority.

6. 2. A safe range for the hourly urine output post-burn is 30–50 ml. Less than this amount would indicate severely decreased renal arterial perfusion.

7. 2. The allergen is applied to a small superficial scratch that cuts the outer layer of the skin.

8. 2. Bleeding and large amounts of fluid accumulation beneath the graft may prevent successful adherence of the graft.

9. 3. Compression bandages are often applied in the operating room on top of a synthetic, semipermeable polyurethane film. This dressing allows the polyurethane film to adhere to the donor site, reducing accumulation of fluid.

10. 4. Continuous bleeding beneath a graft may prevent adherence of the graft.

11. 4. If a drying soap is used it will increase the pruritis. Superfatted soaps are less alkaline, therefore less drying.

12. 3. This is information the nurse would need prior to developing the teaching plan.

13. 4. Almost all cases of basal and squamous cell skin cancer diagnosed each year in the United States are considered to be sun-related.

14. 1. The most common presentation of BSE is a nodular lesion that is dome-shaped papules with well-defined borders. The lesions can have a pearly or shiny appearance because it does not keratinize.

15. 1. The majority of malignant melanoma appears to be associated with the intensity of sunlight exposure rather than the duration.

16. 2. Pain is a significant problem with herpes zoster. Topical solutions, cooling soaks, and use of analgesics are usually incorporated into the plan of care.

17. 2. Pain is usually present and can be quite severe. It is important to help the client obtain relief. Cool compresses, analgesics, and topical antipruritic preparations may be used.

18. 4. Sexual contact should be avoided during the initial and recurring infections. The client should also avoid touching the infected area, as it may be transferred to the eyes or face. Good handwashing is vital.

19. 1. Isolation is thought by some clinicians to reduce the incidence of cross contamination significantly. However, methods vary drastically from one center to another. The single most effective technique to prevent transmission of infection is handwashing!

20. The rule of nines is a quick assessment scale used to estimate the extent of burn injury. The basis of the rule is to divide the body into areas each representing 9% or a multiple of 9% of the total body surface area. This client's injuries were assigned the following percentages: R arm 9%, L arm 9%, R leg 18%, back 18%, total 54%.

21. 1. Urine output is the most readily available and reliable indicator for determining the adequacy of fluid resuscitation. Urine output should be monitored every hour and maintained between 30 and 50 ml/h.

22. 2. 50 ml/h of urine is adequate, BP is stable, clear sensorium is another positive sign that adequate fluid volume replacement is occurring. Pulses should also be easily palpable.

23. 3. Burn clients are very susceptible to development of stress ulcers. Routinely they receive Zantac to help prevent this complication.

24. 2. This statement demonstrates that the client realizes she must be alert to the signs and symptoms of infection and notify her physician if they do occur.

25. 3. Water will neutralize most chemicals while decreasing the heat reaction.

26. 1. Emergency treatment starts with separating the client from the power source. It is important to use nonconductive implements such as wooden poles to prevent injury to the rescuer.

Appendices Table of Contents

Appendix A: Standard Precautions

STANDARD PRECAUTIONS

FOR INFECTION CONTROL

Wash Hands (Plain soap)
Wash after touching **blood**, **body fluids**, **secretions**, **excretions**, and **contaminated items**.
Wash immediately **after gloves are removed** and **between patient contacts**.
Avoid transfer of microorganisms to other patients or environments.

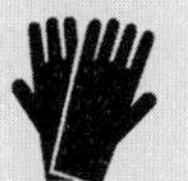

Wear Gloves
Wear when touching **blood**, **body fluids**, **secretions**, **excretions**, and **contaminated items**.
Put on **clean** gloves just **before touching mucous membranes** and **nonintact skin**.
Change gloves between tasks and procedures on the same patient after contact with material that may contain high concentrations of microorganisms. Remove gloves promptly after use, before touching noncontaminated items and environmental surfaces, and before going to another patient, and wash hands immediately to avoid transfer of microorganisms to other patients or environments.

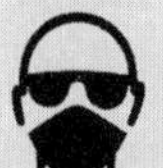

Wear Mask and Eye Protection or Face Shield
Protect mucous membranes of the eyes, nose and mouth during procedures and patient–care activities that are likely to generate **splashes** or **sprays** of **blood**, **body fluids**, **secretions**, or **excretions**.

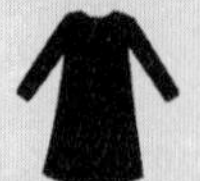

Wear Gown
Protect skin and prevent soiling of clothing during procedures that are likely to generate **splashes** or **sprays** of **blood**, **body fluids**, **secretions**, or **excretions**. Remove a soiled gown as promptly as possible and wash hands to avoid transfer of microorganisms to other patients or environments.

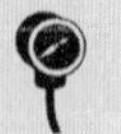

Patient-Care Equipment
Handle used patient–care equipment soiled with **blood**, **body fluids**, **secretions**, or **excretions** in a manner that prevents skin and mucous membrane exposures, contamination of clothing, and transfer of microorganisms to other patients and environments. Ensure that reusable equipment is not used for the care of another patient until it has been appropriately cleaned and reprocessed and single use items are properly discarded.

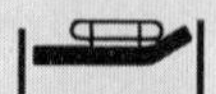

Environmental Control
Follow hospital procedures for routine care, cleaning, and disinfection of environmental surfaces, beds, bedrails, bedside equipment and other frequently touched surfaces.

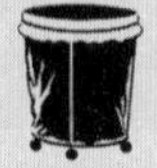

Linen
Handle, transport, and process used linen soiled with **blood**, **body fluids**, **secretions**, or **excretions** in a manner that prevents exposures and contamination of clothing, and avoids transfer of microorganisms to other patients and environments.

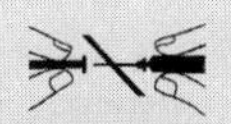
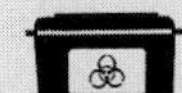
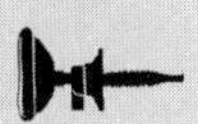

Occupational Health and Bloodborne Pathogens

Prevent injuries when using needles, scalpels, and other sharp instruments or devices; when handling sharp instruments after procedures; when cleaning used instruments; and when disposing of used needles.

Never recap used needles using both hands or any other technique that involves directing the point of a needle toward any part of the body; rather, use either a one-handed "scoop" technique or a mechanical device designed for holding the needle sheath.

Do not remove used needles from disposable syringes by hand, and do not bend, break, or otherwise manipulate used needles by hand. Place used disposable syringes and needles, scalpel blades, and other sharp items in puncture–resistant sharps containers located as close as practical to the area in which the items were used, and place reusable syringes and needles in a puncture–resistant container for transport to the reprocessing area.

Use **resuscitation devices** as an alternative to mouth–to–mouth resuscitation.

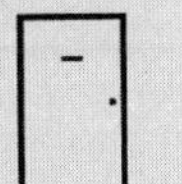

Patient Placement

Use a **private room** for a patient who contaminates the environment or who does not (or cannot be expected to) assist in maintaining appropriate hygiene or environmental control. Consult Infection Control if a private room is not available.

The information on this sign is abbreviated from the HICPAC Recommendations for Isolation Precautions in Hospitals.

Form No. **SPR** BREVIS CORP., 3310 S 2700 E, SLC, UT 84109

Appendix B: Nanda Nursing Diagnoses 2005–2006

Activity Intolerance

Risk for **A**ctivity Intolerance

Impaired **A**djustment

Ineffective **A**irway Clearance

Latex **A**llergy Response

Risk for Latex **A**llergy Response

Anxiety

Death **A**nxiety

Risk for **A**spiration

Risk for Impaired Parent/Infant/Child **A**ttachment

Autonomic Dysreflexia

Risk for **A**utonomic Dysreflexia

Disturbed **B**ody Image

Risk for Imbalanced **B**ody Temperature

Bowel Incontinence

Effective **B**reastfeeding

Ineffective **B**reastfeeding

Interrupted **B**reastfeeding

Ineffective **B**reathing Pattern

Decreased **C**ardiac Output

Caregiver Role Strain

Risk for **C**aregiver Role Strain

Impaired Verbal **C**ommunication

Readiness for Enhanced **C**ommunication

Decisional **C**onflict (Specify)

Parental Role **C**onflict

Acute **C**onfusion

Chronic **C**onfusion

Constipation

Perceived **C**onstipation

Risk for **C**onstipation

Defensive **C**oping

Ineffective **C**oping

Readiness for Enhanced **C**oping

Ineffective Community **C**oping

Readiness for Enhanced Community **C**oping

Compromised Family **C**oping

Disabled Family **C**oping

Readiness for Enhanced Family **C**oping

Risk for Sudden Infant **D**eath Syndrome

Ineffective **D**enial

Impaired **D**entition

Risk for Delayed **D**evelopment
Diarrhea
Risk for **D**isuse Syndrome
Deficient **D**iversional Activity
Energy Field Disturbance
Impaired **E**nvironmental Interpretation Syndrome
Adult **F**ailure to Thrive
Risk for **F**alls
Dysfunctional **F**amily Processes: Alcoholism
Interrupted **F**amily Processes
Readiness for Enhanced **F**amily Processes
Fatigue
Fear
Readiness for Enhanced **F**luid Balance
Deficient **F**luid Volume
Excess **F**luid Volume
Risk for Deficient **F**luid Volume
Risk for Imbalanced **F**luid Volume
Impaired **G**as Exchange
Anticipatory **G**rieving
Dysfunctional **G**rieving
Risk for Dysfunctional **G**rieving
Delayed **G**rowth and Development
Risk for Disproportionate **G**rowth
Ineffective **H**ealth Maintenance
Health-Seeking Behaviors (Specify)
Impaired **H**ome Maintenance
Hopelessness
Hyperthermia
Hypothermia
Disturbed Personal **I**dentity
Functional Urinary **I**ncontinence
Reflex Urinary **I**ncontinence
Stress Urinary **I**ncontinence
Total Urinary **I**ncontinence
Urge Urinary **I**ncontinence
Risk for Urge Urinary **I**ncontinence
Disorganized **I**nfant Behavior
Risk for Disorganized **I**nfant Behavior
Readiness for Enhanced Organized **I**nfant Behavior
Ineffective **I**nfant Feeding Pattern
Risk for **I**nfection
Risk for **I**njury
Risk for Perioperative-Positioning **I**njury
Decreased **I**ntracranial Adaptive Capacity
Deficient **K**nowledge
Readiness for Enhanced **K**nowledge (Specify)
Risk for **L**oneliness
Impaired **M**emory
Impaired Bed **M**obility
Impaired Physical **M**obility
Impaired Wheelchair **M**obility
Nausea
Unilateral **N**eglect
Noncompliance
Imbalanced **N**utrition: Less than Body Requirements
Imbalanced **N**utrition: More than Body Requirements
Readiness for Enhanced **N**utrition
Risk for Imbalanced **N**utrition: More than Body Requirements
Impaired **O**ral Mucous Membrane
Acute **P**ain
Chronic **P**ain
Readiness for Enhanced **P**arenting

Impaired **P**arenting

Risk for Impaired **P**arenting

Risk for **P**eripheral Neurovascular Dysfunction

Risk for **P**oisoning

Post-Trauma Syndrome

Risk for **P**ost-Trauma Syndrome

Powerlessness

Risk for **P**owerlessness

Ineffective **P**rotection

Rape-Trauma Syndrome

Rape-Trauma Syndrome: Compound Reaction

Rape-Trauma Syndrome: Silent Reaction

Impaired **R**eligiosity

Readiness for Enhanced **R**eligiosity

Risk for Impaired **R**eligiosity

Relocation Stress Syndrome

Risk for **R**elocation Stress Syndrome

Ineffective **R**ole Performance

Sedentary Life Style

Bathing/Hygiene **S**elf-Care Deficit

Dressing/Grooming **S**elf-Care Deficit

Feeding **S**elf-Care Deficit

Toileting **S**elf-Care Deficit

Readiness for Enhanced **S**elf-Concept

Chronic Low **S**elf-Esteem

Situational Low **S**elf-Esteem

Risk for Situational Low **S**elf-Esteem

Self-Mutilation

Risk for **S**elf-Mutilation

Disturbed **S**ensory Perception (Specify: Visual, Auditory, Kinesthetic, Gustatory, Tactile, Olfactory)

Sexual Dysfunction

Ineffective **S**exuality Patterns

Impaired **S**kin Integrity

Risk for Impaired **S**kin Integrity

Sleep Deprivation

Disturbed **S**leep Pattern

Readiness for Enhanced **S**leep

Impaired **S**ocial Interaction

Social Isolation

Chronic **S**orrow

Spiritual Distress

Risk for **S**piritual Distress

Readiness for Enhanced **S**piritual Well-Being

Risk for **S**uffocation

Risk for **S**uicide

Delayed **S**urgical Recovery

Impaired **S**wallowing

Effective **T**herapeutic Regimen Management

Ineffective **T**herapeutic Regimen Management

Readiness for Enhanced Management of **T**herapeutic Regimen

Ineffective Community **T**herapeutic Regimen Management

Ineffective Family **T**herapeutic Regimen Management

Ineffective **T**hermoregulation

Disturbed **T**hought Processes

Impaired **T**issue Integrity

Ineffective **T**issue Perfusion (Specify Type: Renal, Cerebral, Cardiopulmonary, Gastrointestinal, Peripheral)

Impaired **T**ransfer Ability

Risk for **T**rauma

Impaired **U**rinary Elimination

Readiness for Enhanced **U**rinary Elimination

Urinary Retention

Impaired Spontaneous **V**entilation

Dysfunctional **V**entilatory Weaning Response

Risk for Other-Directed **V**iolence

Risk for Self-Directed **V**iolence

Impaired **W**alking

Wandering

Appendix C: Ismp List of Error-Prone Abbreviations, Symbols, and Dose Designations

Abbreviations	Intended Meaning	Misinterpretation	Correction
μg	Microgram	Mistaken as "mg"	Use "mcg"
AD, AS, AU	Right ear, left ear, each ear	Mistaken as OD, OS, OU (right eye, left eye, each eye)	Use "right ear," "left ear," or "each ear"
OD, OS, OU	Right eye, left eye, each eye	Mistaken as AD, AS, AU (right ear, left ear, each ear)	Use "right eye," "left eye," or "each eye"
BT	Bedtime	Mistaken as "BID" (twice daily)	Use "bedtime"
cc	Cubic centimeters	Mistaken as "u" (units)	Use "mL"
D/C	Discharge or discontinue	Premature discontinuation of medications if D/C (intended to mean "discharge") has been misinterpreted	Use "discharge" and "discontinue"

		as "discontinued" when followed by a list of discharge medications	
IJ	Injection	Mistaken as "IV" or "intrajugular"	Use "injection"
IN	Intranasal	Mistaken as "IM" or "IV"	Use "intranasal" or "NAS"
HS	Half-strength	Mistaken as bedtime	Use "half-strength" or "bedtime"
hs	At bedtime, hours of sleep	Mistaken as half-strength	
IU**	International unit	Mistaken as IV (intravenous) or 10 (ten)	Use "units"
o.d. or OD	Once daily	Mistaken as "right eye" (OD-oculus dexter), leading to oral liquid medications administered in the eye	Use "daily"
OJ	Orange juice	Mistaken as OD or OS (right or left eye); drugs meant to be diluted in orange juice may be given in the eye	Use "orange juice"
Per os	By mouth, orally	The "os" can be mistaken as "left eye" (OS-oculus sinister)	Use "PO," "by mouth," or "orally"

Continued

Abbreviations	Intended Meaning	Misinterpretation	Correction
q.d. or QD**	Every day	Mistaken as q.i.d., especially if the period after the "q" or the tail of the "q" is misunderstood as an "i"	Use "daily"
qhs	At bedtime	Mistaken as "qhr" or every hour	Use "at bedtime"
qn	Nightly	Mistaken as "qh" (every hour)	Use "nightly"
q.o.d. or QOD**	Every other day	Mistaken as "q.d." (daily) or "q.i.d. (four times daily) if the "o" is poorly written	Use "every other day"
q1d	Daily	Mistaken as q.i.d. (four times daily)	Use "daily"
q6PM, etc.	Every evening at 6 PM	Mistaken as every 6 hours	Use "6 PM nightly" or "6 PM daily"
SC, SQ, sub q	Subcutaneous	SC mistaken as SL (sublingual); SQ mistaken as "5 every;" the "q" in "sub q" has been mistaken as "every" (e.g., a heparin dose ordered "sub q 2 hours before surgery" misunderstood as every 2 hours before surgery)	Use "subcut" or "subcutaneously"

ss	Sliding scale (insulin) or ½ (apothecary)	Mistaken as "55"	Spell out "sliding scale;" use "one-half" or "½"
SSRI	Sliding scale regular insulin	Mistaken as selective-serotonin reuptake inhibitor	Spell out "sliding scale (insulin)"
SSI	Sliding scale insulin	Mistaken as Strong Solution of Iodine (Lugol's)	
i/d	One daily	Mistaken as "tid"	Use "1 daily"
TIW or tiw	3 times a week	Mistaken as "3 times a day" or "twice in a week"	Use "3 times weekly"
U or u	Unit	Mistaken as the number 0 or 4, causing a 10-fold overdose or greater (e.g., 4U seen as "40" or 4u seen as "44"); mistaken as "cc" so dose given in volume instead of units (e.g., 4u seen as 4cc)	Use "unit"

Dose Designations and Other Information	Intended Meaning	Misinterpretation	Correction
Trailing zero after decimal point (e.g., 1.0 mg)**	1 mg	Mistaken as 10 mg if the decimal point is not seen	Do not use trailing zeros for doses expressed in whole numbers
No leading zero before a decimal dose (e.g., .5 mg)**	0.5 mg	Mistaken as 5 mg if the decimal point is not seen	Use zero before a decimal point when the dose is less than a whole unit

Continued

Dose Designations and Other Information	Intended Meaning	Misinterpretation	Correction
Drug name and dose run together (especially problematic for drug names that end in "L" such as Inderal40 mg; Tegretol300 mg)	Inderal 40 mg Tegretol 300 mg	Mistaken as Inderal 140 mg Mistaken as Tegretol 1300 mg	Place adequate space between the drug name, dose, and unit of measure
Numerical dose and uni of measure run together (e.g., 10mg, 100mL)	10 mg 100 mL	The "m" is sometimes mistaken as a zero or two zeros, risking a 10- to 100-fold overdose	Place adequate space between the dose and unit of measure
Abbreviations such as mg. or mL. with a period following the abbreviation	mg mL	The period is unnecessary and could be mistaken as the number 1 if written poorly	Use mg, mL, etc. without a terminal period
Large doses without properly placed commas (e.g., 100000 units; 1000000 units)	100,000 units 1,000,000 units	100000 has been mistaken as 10,000 or 1,000,000; 1000000 has been mistaken as 100,000	Use commas for dosing units at or above 1,000, or use words such as 100 "thousand" or 1 "million" to improve readability

Drug Name Abbreviations	Intended Meaning	Misinterpretation	Correction
ARA A	vidarabine	Mistaken as cytarabine (ARA C)	Use complete drug name
AZT	zidovudine (Retrovir)	Mistaken as azathioprine or aztreonam	Use complete drug name

CPZ	Compazine (prochlorperazine)	Mistaken as chlorpromazine	Use complete drug name
DPT	Demerol-Phenergan-Thorazine	Mistaken as diphtheria-pertussis-tetanus (vaccine)	Use complete drug name
DTO	Diluted tincture of opium, or deodorized tincture of opium (Paregoric)	Mistaken as tincture of opium	Use complete drug name
HCl	hydrochloric acid or hydrochloride	Mistaken as potassium chloride (The "H" is misinterpreted as "K")	Use complete drug name unless expressed as a salt of a drug
HCT	hydrocortisone	Mistaken as hydrochlorothiazide	Use complete drug name
HCTZ	hydrochlorothiazide	Mistaken as hydrocortisone (seen as HCT250 mg)	Use complete drug name
MgSO4**	magnesium sulfate	Mistaken as morphine sulfate	Use complete drug name
MS, MSO4**	morphine sulfate	Mistaken as magnesium sulfate	Use complete drug name
MTX	methotrexate	Mistaken as mitoxantrone	Use complete drug name

Continued

Drug Name Abbreviations	Intended Meaning	Misinterpretation	Correction
PCA	procainamide	Mistaken as Patient Controlled Analgesia	Use complete drug name
PTU	propylthiouracil	Mistaken as mercaptopurine	Use complete drug name
T3	Tylenol with codeine No. 3	Mistaken as liothyronine	Use complete drug name
TAC	triamcinolone	Mistaken as tetracaine, Adrenalin, cocaine	Use complete drug name
TNK	TNKase	Mistaken as "TPA"	Use complete drug name
ZnSO4	zinc sulfate	Mistaken as morphine sulfate	Use complete drug name

Stemmed Drug Names	Intended Meaning	Misinterpretation	Correction
"Nitro" drip	nitroglycerin infusion	Mistaken as sodium nitroprusside infusion	Use complete drug name
"Norflox"	norfloxacin	Mistaken as Norflex	Use complete drug name
"IV Vanc"	intravenous vancomycin	Mistaken as Invanz	Use complete drug name

Symbols	Intended Meaning	Misinterpretation	Correction
ʒ	Dram	Symbol for dram mistaken as "3"	Use the metric system
♏	Minim	Symbol for minim mistaken as "mL"	
x3d	For three days	Mistaken as "3 doses"	Use "for three days"
> and <	Greater than and less than	Mistaken as opposite of intended; mistakenly use incorrect symbol; "< 10" mistaken as "40"	Use "greater than" or "less than"
/ (slash mark)	Separates two doses or indicates "per"	Mistaken as the number 1 (e.g., "25 units/10 units" misread as "25 units and 110" units)	Use "per" rather than a slash mark to separate doses
@	At	Mistaken as "2"	Use "at"
&	And	Mistaken as "2"	Use "and"
+	Plus or and	Mistaken as "4"	Use "and"
°	Hour	Mistaken as a zero (e.g., q2° seen as q 20)	Use "hr," "h," or "hour"

**Abbreviations with a double asterisk are also included on the Joint Commission on Accreditation of Healthcare Organization's "minimum list" of dangerous abbreviations, acronyms, and symbols that must be included on an organization's "do not use" list effective January 1, 2004. An updated list of frequently asked questions about this JCAHO requirement can be found at www.jcaho.org.
Note: From *"ISMP List of Error-Prone Abbreviations, Symbols, and Dose Designations," 2003*, ISMP Medication Safety Alert! *8*(24), pp. 3–4.

Appendix D: Abbreviations

A, A, & O ×3	awake, alert, & oriented times three (to person, place & time)
$\bar{a}$	before
AB	abortion
abd	abdomen; abdominal
ABG	arterial blood gas
Abx	antibiotic
$\overline{ac}$	before meals
AC>BC	air conduction is greater than bone conduction
AC<BC	air conduction is less than bone conduction
ACL	anterior cruciate ligament
AD*	right ear
ADL	activities of daily living
AEB	as evidenced by
AFI	amniotic fluid index
AGA	appropriate for gestational age
AIDS	acquired immunodeficiency syndrome
AKA	above the knee amputation
ALS	amyotrophic lateral sclerosis
ant	anterior
AOM	acute otitis media
AP	apical pulse; anteroposterior
A&P	anterior & posterior; auscultation & percussion
AROM	active range of motion; artificial rupture of membranes
AS	aortic stenosis
AS*	left ear
ASA	acetylsalicylic acid
ASD	atrial septal defect

**The Institute for Safe Medication Practices (ISMP) considers these abbreviations dangerous because of possible misinterpretation. For additional information, see Appendix C: ISMP List of Error-Prone Abbreviations, Symbols, and Dose Designations.*

Atb	antibiotic
AU*	both ears
AV	arteriovenous
A-V	atrioventricular
A&W	alive & well
AWMI	anterior wall myocardial infarction
ax	axillary
BF	black female
bid	twice a day
bil	bilateral
BKA	below the knee amputation
BM	black male; breast milk; bowel movement
BP	blood pressure
BPH	benign prostatic hypertrophy
BPM	beats per minute
BS	bowel sounds; breath sounds
b/t	between
BSE	breast self-examination
BUN	blood urea nitrogen
bx	biopsy
C	Celsius, centigrade
$\bar{c}$	with
CA	cancer
CABG	coronary artery bypass graft
CAD	coronary artery disease
CBS	capillary blood sugar
CC	chief complaint
cc*	cubic centimeter
CCD	congenital cardiovascular defect
CHD	childhood diseases; congenital heart disease
CHF	congestive heart failure
CHI	closed head injury; creatinine height index
Cl	chloride
cm	centimeter
CMT	cervical motion tenderness
CMV	cytomegalovirus
CN I–XII	cranial nerves I–XII
CNS	central nervous system
c/o	complaining of; complaints of
CO_2	carbon dioxide
COA	coarctation of the aorta
COPD	chronic obstructive pulmonary disease
CP	chest pain; cerebral palsy
CPD	cephalopelvic disproportion
creat	creatinine

C/S	cesarean section delivery
CT	computerized tomography
CV	cardiovascular
CVA	costovertebral angle; cerebrovascular accident
CVP	central venous pressure
CVS	chorionic villi sampling
CXray	chest X ray
cx	cervix
d	day(s)
DBP	diastolic blood pressure
d/c*	discontinue; discharge
D&C	dilation & curettage
DDST II	Denver Developmental Screening Test II
DES	diethylstilbestrol
DM	diabetes mellitus
DOA	dead on arrival
DOB	date of birth
DOE	dyspnea on exertion
DTR	deep tendon reflex
DUB	dysfunctional uterine bleeding
DVT	deep vein thrombosis
DWM	divorced white male (DWF, DBM, DBF are variations of this)
dx	diagnosis
dz	disease
EAC	external auricular canal
EDC	expected date of confinement (delivery date)
EDD	estimated date of delivery
EEG	electroencephalogram
EENT	eyes, ears, nose, throat
EFM	electronic fetal monitoring
EKG	electrocardiogram
ENAP	examination, normal findings, abnormal findings, pathophysiology
EOM	extraocular muscle
ESR	erythrocyte sedimentation rate
ETOH	ethyl alcohol
F	Fahrenheit
FAS	fetal alcohol syndrome
Fe	iron
FHH	family health history
FHR	fetal heart rate
FHT	fetal heart tone
FLM	fetal lung maturity
FM	fetal movement
FOB	father of baby

FROM	full range of motion
FSH	follicle-stimulating hormone
FTT	failure to thrive
fx	fracture
Ⓖ	gallop
GC	gonorrhea and Chlamydia
GCS	Glasgow Coma Scale
GDM	gestational diabetes mellitus
GERD	gastroesophageal reflux disease
GI	gastrointestinal
GU	genitourinary
GYN	gynecologic
H/A	headache
HCG	human chorionic gonadotropin
HDL	high-density lipoprotein
HEENT	head, eyes, ears, nose, throat
HELLP	hemolysis, elevated liver enzymes, low platelets
H/H	hemoglobin & hematocrit
Hib	Haemophilus influenza b
HIV	human immunodeficiency virus
hl	health
HNP	herniated nucleus pulposus
h/o	history of
HOB	head of bed
HPI	history of present illness
HPV	human papillomavirus
HR	heart rate
hs*	at bedtime
HSV	herpes simplex virus
HT	height
HTN	hypertension
hx	history
IADL	instrumental activities of daily living
IBW	ideal body weight
ICP	intracranial pressure
ICS	intercostal space
IDDM	insulin-dependent diabetes mellitus
IDM	infant of diabetic mother
IICP	increased intracranial pressure
I&O	intake & output
IOP	intraocular pressure
IPPA	inspection, palpation, percussion, auscultation
IUD	intrauterine device
IUGR	intrauterine growth retardation
IUP	intrauterine pregnancy

IUPC	intrauterine pressure catheter
IV	intravenous
IWMI	inferior wall myocardial infarction
JVD	jugular venous distension
JVP	jugular venous pressure
K^+	potassium
kg	kilogram
KOH	potassium hydroxide
KUB	kidneys, ureters, bladder
L	liter
Ⓛ	left
LAD	left anterior descending (coronary artery)
lat	lateral
lbs	pounds
LBP	low back pain
LCM	left costal margin
LDL	low-density lipoprotein
LE	lower extremity
lg	large
LGA	large for gestational age
LH	leutinizing hormone
LLE	left lower extremity
LLL	left lower lobe (of lung)
LLQ	left lower quadrant (of abdomen)
LLSB	left lower sternal border
LMD	local medical doctor
LMP	last menstrual period
LOC	level of/loss of consciousness
LSB	left sternal border
LUE	left upper extremity
LUL	left upper lobe (of lung)
LUQ	left upper quadrant (of abdomen)
Ⓜ	murmur
MAC	mid-arm circumference
MAL	midaxillary line
MAMC	mid-arm muscle circumference
MCL	midclavicular line
MD	muscular dystrophy, doctor
Mec	meconium
MGR	murmur, gallop, rub
MI	myocardial infarction
MMR	measles, mumps, rubella
MMSE	Mini Mental State Exam
MN	midnight
MRI	magnetic resonance imaging

MS	multiple sclerosis
MSAFP	maternal serum alpha-fetal protein
MVA	motor vehicle accident
MVI	multivitamin
mets	metastasis of malignancy
ml	milliliter
mm Hg	millimeters of mercury
mo	month(s)
mod	moderate
mvt	movement
NA	not applicable
Na^+	sodium
NaCl	sodium chloride
NAD	no acute distress
NCP	nursing care plan
NGT	nasogastric tube
NIDDM	noninsulin dependent diabetes mellitus
NKA	no known allergies
NKDA	no known diagnosed or drug allergies
nl	normal
NPO	nothing by mouth
NS	normal saline
NSAID	nonsteroidal anti-inflammatory drug
NSR	normal sinus rhythm
NSVD	normal spontaneous vaginal delivery
N&V	nausea & vomiting
N, V, D	nausea, vomiting, diarrhea
O_2	oxygen
OB	obstetrics
OD*	right eye
OM	otitis media
OME	otitis media with effusion
OOB	out of bed
OPV	oral polio vaccine
OREF	open reduction with external fixation
ORIF	open reduction with internal fixation
OS*	left eye
OTC	over the counter (medications)
OU*	both eyes
Ø	no, none
Oz	ounce
$\overline{p}$	after
Pap	Papanicolaou
$\overline{pc}$	after meals
PDA	patent ductus arteriosus

PE	physical examination, pulmonary embolus
PERRLA	pupils equally round, reactive to light and accommodation
PFT	pulmonary function test
PHH	past health history
PID	pelvic inflammatory disease
PIH	pregnancy-induced hypertension
PLT	platelets
PMH	past medical history
PMI	point of maximal intensity or impulse
PMS	premenstrual syndrome
PND	paroxysmal nocturnal dyspnea
po	by mouth
post	posterior
PP	patient profile
PPD	purified protein derivative; packs per day
PPH	postpartum hemorrhage
prn	as necessary
PROM	passive range of motion; premature rupture of membranes
PS	pulmonic stenosis
PT	physical therapy
pt	patient
PTA	prior to admission (arrival)
PTV	prior to visit
PUD	peptic ulcer disease
PVC	premature ventricular complex (or contraction)
PVD	peripheral vascular disease
q	every
qd*	every day
qh	every hour
qid	four times a day
qod*	every other day
®	right; rectal
r	rectal
RCA	right coronary artery
RCM	right costal margin
RHD	rheumatic heart disease
RLE	right lower extremity
RLL	right lower lobe (of lung)
RLQ	right lower quadrant (of abdomen)
RML	right middle lobe (of lung)
ROM	range of motion
ROS	review of systems
RR	respiratory rate; red reflex

RSB	right sternal border
RT	related to, radiation therapy
RTC	return to clinic
RUE	right upper extremity
RUL	right upper lobe (of lung)
RUQ	right upper quadrant (of abdomen)
Rx	prescription drug
rx	reaction
$\bar{s}$	without
SAB	spontaneous abortion
SBE	subacute bacterial endocarditis
SBM	single black male (SBF, SWF, SWM are variations of this)
SBP	systolic blood pressure
SCA	sickle cell anemia
SDH	subdural hematoma
SEM	systolic ejection murmur
SEMI	subendocardial myocardial infarction
SGA	small for gestational age
SH	social history
SIDS	sudden infant death syndrome
sgy	surgery
sl	slight; slightly
SLE	systemic lupus erythematous
SOB	shortness of breath
s/p	status post
SQ*	subcutaneous
SROM	spontaneous rupture of membranes
SS#	social security number
s/s	signs & symptoms
SSCP	substernal chest pain
ST	sore throat
STD	sexually transmitted disease
sx	symptom
sz	seizure
T&A	tonsillectomy & adenoidectomy
TAB	therapeutic abortion
TAH	total abdominal hysterectomy
TB	tuberculosis
TENS	transcutaneous electrical nerve stimulation
THA	total hip arthoplasty
THR	total hip replacement
TIBC	total iron binding capacity
tid	three times a day
TKR	total knee replacement
TLC	total lymphocyte count

TM	tympanic membrane
TMJ	temporomandibular joint
TORCH	toxoplasmosis, other (syphilis, hepatitis B), rubella, cytomegalovirus, herpes simplex
TPR	temperature, pulse, respirations
tr	trace
TSE	testicular self-examination
TSF	triceps skin fold
TVH	total vaginal hysterectomy
tx	treatment
u/a	urinalysis
UC	uterine contraction
UCHD	usual childhood diseases
UE	upper extremity
URI	upper respiratory infection
U/S	ultrasound
UTI	urinary tract infection
UUN	urine urea nitrogen
VBAC	vaginal birth after cesarean
VE	vaginal examination
VS	vital signs
VSD	ventricular septal defect
VSS	vital signs stable
VTX	vertex
WBC	white blood cell
WD	well developed
WF	white female
wk	week
wkend	weekend
WM	white male
WN	well nourished
WNL	within normal limits
WT	weight
$\overline{x}$	except
X	times
yo	year old (age)
yr	year(s)

**The Institute for Safe Medication Practices (ISMP) considers these abbreviations dangerous because of possible misinterpretation. For additional information, see Appendix C: ISMP List of Error-Prone Abbreviations, Symbols, and Dose Designations*

SYMBOLS

~	similar
≅	approximately
@	at*
✔	check
Δ	change
↑	increased
↓	decreased
=	equals
#	pounds
>*	greater than
<*	less than
%	percentage
+ or ⊕*	positive
− or ⊖	negative
♀	female
♂	male
△1 △2 △3	trimester of pregnancy (one triangle for each trimester)
$\dot{\overline{\mathrm{I}}}$	one
2°	secondary

Appendix E: Preparation for NCLEX

The future belongs to those who believe in the beauty of their dreams. (Eleanor Roosevelt)

A new graduate from an educational program that prepares registered nurses will take the NCLEX, the national nursing licensure examination prepared under the supervision of the National Council of State Boards of Nursing. NCLEX is taken after graduation and prior to practice as a registered nurse. The examination is given across the United States. Graduates submit their credentials to the state board of nursing in the state in which licensure is desired. Once the state board accepts the graduate's credentials, the graduate can schedule the examination. This examination ensures a basic level of safe registered nursing practice to the public. The examination follows a test plan formulated on four categories of client needs that registered nurses commonly encounter. The concepts of the nursing process, caring, communication, cultural awareness, documentation, self-care, and teaching/learning are integrated throughout the four major categories of client needs (Table E-1).

TOTAL NUMBER OF QUESTIONS ON NCLEX

Graduates may receive anywhere from 75 to 265 questions on the NCLEX examination during their testing session. Fifteen of the questions are questions that are being piloted to determine their validity for use in future NCLEX examinations. Students cannot determine whether they passed or failed the NCLEX examination from the number of questions they receive during their session. There is no time limit for each question, and the maximum time for the examination is 5 hours. A 10-minute break is mandatory after 2 hours of testing. An optional 10-minute break may be taken after another 90 minutes of testing.

TABLE E-1 NCLEX Test Plan: Client Needs

Client Needs Tested	Percent of Test Questions
Safe, effective care environment:	
Management of care	7–13%
Safety and infection control	5–11%
Physiologic integrity:	
Basic care and comfort	7–13%
Pharmacological and parenteral therapies	5–11%
Reduction of risk potential	12–18%
Physiological adaptation	12–18%
Psychosocial integrity:	
Coping and adaptation	5–11%
Psychosocial adaptation	5–11%
Health promotion and maintenance:	
Growth and development through the life span	7–13%
Prevention and early detection of disease	5–11%

Each test question has a test item and four possible answers. If the student answers the question correctly, a slightly more difficult item will follow, and the level of difficulty will increase with each item until the candidate misses an item. If the student misses an item, a slightly less difficult item will follow, and the level of difficulty will decrease with each item until the student has answered an item correctly. This process continues until the student has achieved a definite passing or definite failing score. The least number of questions a student can take to complete the exam is 75. Fifteen of these questions will be pilot questions, and they will not count toward the student's score. The other 60 questions will determine the student's score on the NCLEX.

RISK FACTORS FOR NCLEX PERFORMANCE

Several factors have been identified as being associated with performance on the NCLEX examination. Some of these factors are identified in Table E-2.

TABLE E-2 Factors Associated with NCLEX Performance

- HESI Exit Exam
- Mosby Assesstest
- NLN Comprehensive Achievement test
- NLN achievement tests taken at end of each nursing course
- Verbal SAT score
- ACT score
- High school rank and GPA
- Undergraduate nursing program GPA
- GPA in science and nursing theory courses
- Competency in American English language
- Reasonable family responsibilities or demands
- Absence of emotional distress
- Critical thinking competency

REVIEW BOOKS AND COURSES

In preparing to take the NCLEX, the new graduate may find it useful to review several of the many NCLEX review books on the market. These review books often include a review of nursing content, or sample test questions, or both. They frequently include computer software disks with test questions for review. The test questions may be arranged in the review book by clinical content area, or they may be presented in one or more comprehensive examinations covering all areas of the NCLEX. Listings of these review books are available at *www.amazon.com*. It is helpful to use several of these books and computer software when reviewing for the NCLEX.

NCLEX review courses are also available. Brochures advertising these programs are often sent to schools and are available in many sites nationwide. The quality of these programs can vary, and students may want to ask former nursing graduates and faculty for recommendations.

THE NLN EXAMINATION AND THE HESI EXIT EXAM

Many nursing programs administer an examination to students at the completion of their nursing program. Two of these exams are the NLN Achievement test and the HESI Exit Exam. New graduates will want to review their performance on any of these exams because these results will help identify their weaknesses and help focus their review sessions.

Students who examine their feedback from the NLN examination or the HESI Exit Exam have important information that can help them focus their review for the NCLEX. A strategy for examining this feedback and organizing this review is outlined in the following section.

TABLE E-3 Preparation for the NCLEX Test

Name: ______________________________

Strengths: ______________________________

Weak content areas identified on NLN examination or HESI Exit Exam:

____

____

____

Weak content areas identified by yourself or others during formal nursing education pro-gram (include content areas in which you scored below a grade of B in class or any fac-tors from Table E-2):

____

____

____

Weak content areas identified in any area of the NCLEX test plan, including the following:

Safe, effective care environment

Physiological integrity

Psychosocial integrity

Health promotion and maintenance

Weak content areas identified in any of the top 10 patient diagnoses in each of the following:

Adult health

Women's health

Mental health nursing

Children's health

(Consider the 10 top medications, diagnostic tools and tests, treatments and procedures used for each of the ten diagnoses.)

Weak content areas identified in the following:

Therapeutic communication tools

Defense mechanisms

Growth and development

Other

TABLE E-4 Organizing Your NCLEX Study

Note your weaknesses identified in Table E-3.

Take a comprehensive exam from one of the review books and analyze your performance. Then, depending on this test performance and the weaknesses identified in Table E-3, your schedule could look like the following:

Day 1:	Practice adult health test questions. Score the test, analyze your performance, and review test question rationales and content weaknesses.
Day 2:	Practice women's health test questions. Repeat above process.
Day 3:	Practice children's health test questions. Repeat above process.
Day 4:	Practice mental health test questions. Repeat above process.
Day 5:	Continue with other weak content areas. Continue this process until you are doing well in all areas of the test.

■ ORGANIZING YOUR REVIEW

In preparing for NCLEX, identify your strengths and weaknesses. If you have taken the NLN examination or the HESI Exit Exam, note any content strength and weakness areas. Additionally, note any nursing program course or clinical content areas in which you scored below a grade of B. Purchase one or more of the NCLEX review books. It is useful to review questions developed by different authors. Review content in the review books in any of your weak content areas. Take a comprehensive exam in the review book or on the computer software disk and analyze your performance. Try to answer as many questions correctly as you can. Be sure to actually practice taking the examinations. Do not just jump ahead to look at the section on correct answers and rationales before answering the questions if you want to improve your examination performance.

Next, once you have completed the comprehensive examination, review the answers and rationales for any weak content areas and take another comprehensive exam. Repeat this process until you are doing well in all clinical content areas and in all areas of the NCLEX examination plan.

Finally, do a general review of the top 10 patient diseases, medications, diagnostic tests, and nursing procedures in each major nursing content area, as well as defense mechanisms, communication tips, and growth and development. Practice visualization and relaxation techniques as needed. These strategies will assist you in conquering the three areas necessary for successful test taking—anxiety control, content review, and test question practice. Table E-3 will help organize your study.

■ WHEN TO STUDY

Identify your personal best time. Are you a day person? Are you a night person? Study when you are fresh. Arrange to study 1 or more hours daily. Use Table E-4 to organize your study if you have 1 month to go.

Students who use this technique should increase their confidence in their ability to do well on the NCLEX.

Glossary

Abduction To move a body part away from the midline.

Abrasion Surface wounds involving loss of the epidermis and possibly part of the dermis that are caused by "dragging" of epidermal surface against another surface such as pavement, dirt, or gravel.

Absorption Process by which the end products of digestion pass through the epithelial membranes in the small and large intestines into the blood or lymph system; passage of a drug from the site of administration into the bloodstream.

Abstract Summary statement of a research article that identifies the purpose, methodology, findings, and conclusions.

Accommodation Component of cognitive development that allows for readjustment of the cognitive structure (mind-set) in order to take in new information.

Accountability Process that mandates that individuals are answerable for their actions and have an obligation (or duty) to act.

Accreditation Process by which a voluntary, nongovernmental agency or organization appraises and grants accredited status to institutions, programs, and services that meet predetermined structure, process, and outcome criteria.

Acculturation Process that consists of learning norms, beliefs, and behavioral expectations of a group through which people of a subculture assume the characteristics of the dominant culture.

Acid A molecule or an ion that can function as a hydrogen ion donor.

Acid-Base Balance Regulation of hydrogen ion concentration.

Acid-Base Buffer System A solution containing two or more chemical compounds that prevent marked changes in the hydrogen ion concentration when either an acid or a base is added to the solution.

Acidosis A condition that occurs when there is an excessive number of hydrogen ions in a solution.

Acquired Immunity Formation of antibodies (memory B cells) to protect against future invasions of an already experienced antigen.

Active-Assistive Range of Motion Range-of-motion exercises performed by the client with the assistance of the nurse.

Active Euthanasia Process of taking deliberate action that will hasten the client's death.

Active Immunity The development within the body of antibodies that neutralize or destroy the infective agent.

Active Listening Listening that focuses on the feelings of the individual who is speaking.

Active Range-of-Motion Range-of-motion exercises performed independently by the client.

Activities of Daily Living Activities of self-care related to bathing, hygiene, dressing, grooming, toileting, and eating.

Actual Nursing Diagnosis Nursing diagnosis that indicates that a problem exists; composed of the diagnostic label, related factors, and signs and symptoms.

Actual Social Support Social support that is given by others regardless of the recipient's perception of the support.

Acuity A patient classification based on amount of skilled nursing care needed; amount of independence versus dependence in self-care activities.

Acupressure The use of finger pressure applied to specific points (energy pathways) on the body to promote healing.

Acupuncture The use of needles inserted at specific points on the body (energy pathways) to promote healing.

Acute Care Short-term hospital care provided to patients with conditions of short duration requiring stays of, on average, less than 30 days.

Acute Illness Disruption (usually reversible) in functional ability characterized by a rapid onset, intense manifestations, and a relatively short duration.

Acute Pain Discomfort identified by sudden onset and relatively short duration, mild to severe intensity, and a steady decrease in intensity over several days or weeks.

Acute Wound Wound that is incurred suddenly and that heals in an orderly and predictable cascade of overlapping events.

Adaptation Component of cognitive development that refers to the changes that occur as a result of assimilation and accommodation; ongoing process by which an individual adjusts to stressors in order to achieve homeostasis.

Addiction Physiological and psychological dependence upon a substance.

Adduction To move a body part toward the midline.

Adherence Remaining faithful to a program of instruction or activity.

Adjuvant Medication Drugs used to enhance the analgesic efficacy of opioids, treat concurrent symptoms that exacerbate pain, and provide independent analgesia for specific types of pain.

Administrative Controls Strategies that minimize hazard exposure by altering work practices, such as training and policies and procedures.

Administrative Law Laws developed by groups who are appointed to governmental administrative agencies and who are entrusted with enforcing the statutory laws passed by the legislature.

Adolescence Developmental stage from the ages of 12 to 20 years that begins with the appearance of the secondary sex characteristics (puberty).

Advance Care Medical Directive Document in which a client, in consultation with the physician, relatives, or other personal advisers, provides precise instructions for the type of health care the client wants or does not want in a number of scenarios (e.g., end-of-life decisions).

Advance Directive Written instruction for health care that is recognized under state law and is related to the provision of such care when the individual is incapacitated.

Advanced Practice Nursing Practice of nursing at a level requiring an expanded knowledge base and clinical expertise in a specialty area.

Adventitious Breath Sounds Superimposed sounds on the normal vesicular, bronchovesicular, and bronchial breath sounds.

Adverse Reaction Any drug effect other than what is therapeutically intended.

Advocate Taking action to achieve a goal on behalf of another.

Aerobic Metabolism Metabolism of nutrients in the presence of oxygen; a metabolic pathway that uses oxygen to convert glucose into cellular energy.

Affect Mood or feeling.

Affective Domain Area of learning that involves attitudes, beliefs, and emotions.

Afferent Nerve Pathway Ascending pathways that transmit sensory impulses to the brain.

Afferent Pain Pathway Ascending spinal cord.

Ageism Imposition of age stereotypes and discrimination.

Agent Entity capable of causing disease.

Agglutination Clumping together of red blood cells.

Agglutinin A specific kind of antibody whose interaction with antigens is manifested as agglutination.

Agglutinogen Any antigenic substance that causes agglutination by the production of agglutinin.

Agnostics Those who do not know if God exists or not. They generally state that the existence of God is unknowable.

Airborne Controls Protective actions taken to minimize disease exposure risk when disease is transmitted via an airborne route.

Airborne Precautions Caregiving measures used to prevent the spread of airborne contaminants.

Airborne Transmission Mode of transfer of disease through contact with droplet, nuclei, or dust particles suspended in the air.

Algorithm Graphical representation or flowchart describing a set of steps used in a particular clinical decision-making process.

Algor Mortis Lack of skin elasticity as a result of death.

Alkalosis Excessive removal of hydrogen ions from a solution.

Allen Test Assessment procedure that measures the collateral circulation to the radial artery.

Allodynia Pain caused by a stimulus that does not normally evoke pain.

Allopathic That which is recognized by a specific culture as being traditional, conventional, or mainstream (e.g., Western medicine).

Alternative Therapies Treatment approaches that are not accepted by mainstream medical practice.

Ambulation Assisted or unassisted walking.

Ambulatory Care Care that is delivered to individuals whose institutional episodes of care are less than 24 hours.

Amniocentesis Withdrawal of amniotic fluid to obtain a sample for specimen examination.

Anabolism Constructive phase of metabolism.

Anaerobic Metabolism Metabolism of nutrients in the absence of oxygen; a metabolic pathway that converts glucose into energy in the absence of oxygen.

Analysis Breaking the whole down into parts that can be examined.

Analyte A substance dissolved in a solution; also called solute.

Anemia Reduction in the amount of hemoglobin in the blood, thus decreasing the oxygen-carrying capacity of the blood.

Anesthesia Absence of pain.

Aneurysm Localized (aortic) abnormal dilation or weakness of a wall of a blood vessel.

Angina Pain in the chest, neck, or arm resulting from myocardial ischemia.

Angina Pectoris Pain caused by tissue ischemia in the heart.

Angiocatheter An intracatheter with a metal stylet.

Angiogenesis Formation of new blood vessels.

Angiography Visualization of the vascular structures through the use of fluoroscopy with contrast medium.

Anhedonia Loss of pleasure from previously pleasurable activities.

Anions Ions with a negative charge.

Anorexia Nervosa Self-imposed starvation that results in a 15% or more loss of body weight.

Anthropogenic Descriptor for transmission of microorganisms resulting from changes in the relationship between humans and the environment.

Anthropometric Measurements Measurement of the size, weight, and proportions of the body.

Antibody An immunoglobulin produced by the body in response to bacteria, viruses, or other antigenetic substances; counteracts and neutralizes the effects of antigens, and destroys bacteria and other cells. Agglutinin is one type of antibody.

Anticipatory Grief Occurrence of grief work before an expected loss.

Antigen A substance, usually a protein, that causes the formation of an antibody and reacts specifically with that antibody (e.g., agglutinogen).

Antioxidant An agent that prevents or inhibits oxidation.

Anxiety Subjective response that occurs when a person experiences a threat to well-being; it is a diverse feeling of dread or apprehension.

Aphasia Impairment or absence of language function that can result from an injury to the cortex.

Apnea Temporary cessation of breathing.

Apnea Monitor Machine with chest leads that monitors the movement of the chest.

Appetite Desire for specific foods instead of food in general (hunger); involves a psychological desire or craving.

Aromatherapy Therapeutic use of concentrated essences or essential oils that have been extracted from plants and flowers.

Arousal A component linked closely to the appearance of wakefulness and alertness.

Arterial Blood Gases (ABGs) Measurement of levels of oxygen and carbon dioxide, as well as pH and bicarbonate ion in arterial blood.

Arterial Ulcer Lower extremity ulcers caused by chronic arterial insufficiency, which in turn causes chronic ischemia and marked tissue vulnerability.

Arteriography Radiographic study of the vascular system following the injection of a radiopaque dye through a catheter.

Arthritis An inflammation of the joints that causes pain and swelling.

Arthroplasty Total hip replacement.

Artifact Specific type of nonverbal message that includes items in the client's environment, manner of grooming, or use of clothing and jewelry.

Artificial Immunity Immunity produced following a vaccine, which may not last a lifetime.

Ascites Accumulation of fluid in the abdomen.

Asepsis Absence of microorganisms.

Aseptic Technique Infection control practice used to prevent the transmission of pathogens.

Aspiration Procedure performed to withdraw fluid that has abnormally collected or to obtain a specimen.

Assault Intentional and unlawful offer to touch a person in an offensive, insulting, or physically intimidating manner.

Assessment First step in the nursing process; includes collection, verification, organization, interpretation, and documentation of data.

Assessment Model Framework that provides a systematic method for organizing data.

Assimilation Component of cognitive development that involves taking in new experiences or information.

Assisted Suicide Situation in which a health care professional provides a client with the means to end his own life.

Atelectasis Collapsed alveoli.

Atheists Those who do not believe in the existence of God in any form.

Atherosclerosis Disease characterized by narrowing and eventual occlusion of the lumen (opening of the arteries) by deposits of lipids, fibrin, and calcium on the interior walls of the arteries.

Atherosclerotic Plaque A thick, hard deposit on the walls of the inner arteries that can clog the arteries in the heart and the brain.

Atrophy Reduction in muscle size and shape, resulting in thin, flabby muscles.

Attending Behaviors A set of nonverbal listening skills that conveys interest in what the other person is saying.

Auditory Channel Transmission of messages through spoken words and by cues.

Auditory Learner An individual who learns by hearing.

Auscultation Physical examination technique that involves listening to sounds in the body that are created by movement of air or fluid.

Auscultatory Gap The temporary disappearance of sounds at the end of Korotkoff phase I and beginning of phase II.

Autoantigen Antigen that originates from the body's own proteins.

Autocratic Leadership Style Style of leadership in which the leader maintains strong control, makes the decisions, and solves all the problems.

Autoimmune Disorder Condition in which the specific immune defense inappropriately reacts to the host's own tissue.

Autonomy Being self-directed, taking initiative instead of waiting for direction from others; ethical principle that refers to the individual's right to choose for oneself and the ability to act on that choice.

Autopsy Postmortem examination to determine the cause of death.

Autoregulation Redistribution of blood flow to areas of greatest need.

Avoidance A method of conflict management where the difficult situation is avoided with the assumption that given enough time, the issue will resolve itself and just go away.

Awareness The capacity to perceive sensory impressions and react appropriately through thoughts and actions.

Ayurveda A healing system based on Hindu philosophy and Indian philosophy that embraces the concept of an energy force in the body that seeks to maintain balance or harmony.

Bacteremia Bacteria in the blood.

Bacteriuria Bacteria in the urine.

Balance Coordination and stability of the body in space; having a sense of inner peace.

Barium Chalky-white contrast medium.

Barium Enema Rectal infusion of barium sulfate used to visualize the colon.

Barium Swallow Fluoroscopic visualization of the esophagus following the ingestion of barium sulfate.

Barrier Precautions Physical precautions used to minimize the risk of exposure to blood and body fluids.

Barthel Index A formal tool that evaluates an individual's ability to safely and independently perform activities of daily living in 10 areas of functioning.

Basal Metabolic Rate (BMR) Energy needed to maintain essential physiological functions when a person is at complete rest both physically and mentally.

Base A molecule or an ion that will combine with hydrogen ions.

Baseline Values The norms against which subsequent vital sign measurements can be compared.

Base of Support Foundation on which a person or object rests.

Basic Human Need Need that must be met for survival.

Battery Touching another person without consent.

Behavior Observable response of an individual to external stimuli.

Benchmarking Process that evaluates products, services, and priorities against the performance of others.

Beneficence Ethical principle regarding the duty to promote good and prevent harm.

Bereavement Period of grieving following the death of a loved one.

Bioavailability Readiness to produce a drug effect.

Bioethics Application of general ethical principles to health care.

Biofeedback Measurement of physiological responses that yields information about the relationship between the mind and body and helps clients learn how to manipulate these responses through mental activity.

Biographical Method A form of qualitative research in which research is performed on a specific person's life.

Biological Agent Living organism that invades a host, causing disease.

Biological Clock Endogenous mechanism capable of measuring time in a living organism.

Biopsy Excision of a small amount of tissue.

Biotransformation The chemical alteration of a medication in the body, usually by enzymes, into a form that can be excreted; also known as metabolism of a medication.

Bisexual Having an equal or almost equal preference for sexual partners of either gender.

Black Wound Wound containing necrotic tissue.

Bladder Training A program with the goal of teaching the client to suppress the urge to void and thereby gradually increasing the intervals between voiding.

Blanching White color of the skin when pressure is applied.

Blended Families Families in which children live with one birth parent and one stepparent.

Blood Pressure Measurement of pressure pulsations exerted against the blood vessel walls during systole and diastole.

Body Alignment Position of body parts in relation to each other.

Body Image Individual's perception of physical self, including appearance, function, and ability.

Body Mass Index (BMI) Determines whether a person's weight is appropriate for height by dividing the weight in kilograms by the height in meters squared.

Body Mechanics Purposeful and coordinated use of body parts and positions during activity.

Bodymind Inseparable connection and operation of thoughts, feelings, and physiological functions.

Bonding Formation of attachment between parent and child.

Bradycardia A heart rate less than 60 beats per minute in an adult.

Bradypnea Respiratory rate of 10 or fewer breaths per minute.

Breast Clinical Exam (BCE) Systematic palpation of the breasts by health care practitioner trained to do breast examination for the purpose of finding potentially cancerous lumps; performed annually.

Breast Self-Exam (BSE) Systematic palpation of the breasts by a woman on herself for the purpose of finding potentially cancerous lumps; performed monthly.

Bronchial Sounds Loud and high-pitched sounds with a hollow quality heard longer on expiration than inspiration from air moving through the trachea.

Bronchography Radiographic study of the trachea and bronchi following the injection of a contrast agent through a catheter.

Bronchovesicular Sounds Medium-pitched and blowing sounds heard equally on inspiration and expiration from air moving through the large airways, posteriorly between the scapula and anteriorly over bronchioles lateral to the sternum and second intercostal spaces.

Bruits Blowing sounds that are heard when the blood flow becomes turbulent as it rushes past an obstruction.

Bruxism Teeth grinding during sleep.

Buccal Pertaining to the inside cheek.

Budget A plan that provides formal quantitative expression for acquiring and distributing funds over the ensuing time period.

Bulimia Insatiable appetite.

Bulimia Nervosa An eating disorder characterized by episodic binge eating followed by purging.

Burnout State of physical and emotional exhaustion that occurs when caregivers deplete their adaptive energy; characterized by fatigue, depersonalization, and decreased feelings of personal accomplishment.

Burns Tissue injuries resulting from thermal, chemical, or electrical trauma.

Butterfly Needles Winged-tipped needle.

Cachexia Weight loss marked by weakness and emaciation that usually occurs with a chronic illness such as tuberculosis or cancer.

Calorie Quantity of heat required to raise the temperature of 1 gram of water 1 °C.

Capitated Rate Preset fees based on membership, not services provided; payment system used in managed care.

Carbohydrate Organic compound composed of carbon, hydrogen, and oxygen.

Carcinogens Chemicals that cause cancer.

Cardiac Catheterization Radiographic study with the use of a contrast medium injected into a vascular catheter that is threaded into the heart, coronary, and/or pulmonary vessels.

Cardiac Conduction System Specialized cells in the heart that generate and conduct electrical impulses; consists of the sinoatrial node, internodal pathways, atrioventricular node, bundle of His, right and left bundle branches, and Purkinje fibers.

Cardiac Cycle Series of electrical and mechanical events resulting in a cycle of atrial and ventricular contraction and relaxation.

Cardiac Output Measurement of blood pumped by the heart in 1 minute; measured by multiplying the heart rate by the ventricle's stroke volume.

Cardiopulmonary Resuscitation (CPR) Technique of applying respiration and chest compressions to support oxygenation in the event of cardiac and respiratory arrest.

Care Map A plan of care that is based on standards, reflects optimal timing of sequential steps provided by all members of the health care team, and identifies expected

Case Management Methodology for organizing client care through an episode of illnesses to achieve specific clinical and financial outcomes within an allotted time frame.

Case Study Method A type of qualitative research in which research is performed on a specific individual (case), a group, or an institution.

Catabolism Destructive phase of metabolism.

Categorical Imperative Concept that states that one should act only if the action is based on a principle that is universal.

Catharsis Process of talking out one's feelings; "getting things off the chest" through verbalization.

Cations Ions with a positive charge.

Causation Breach of duty that must be legally proved to have caused an injury.

Cavities Dental caries.

Ceiling Effect Phenomenon in which increasing doses of a medication above a certain level does not result in increased analgesic effect.

Cell-Mediated Immunity (Cellular Immunity) An immune process initiated when the antigen stimulates the release of activated T cells.

Centering Process of bringing oneself to an inward focus of serenity that is done before beginning an energetic touch therapy treatment.

Central Line Venous catheter inserted into the superior vena cava through the subclavian, internal, or external jugular vein.

Certification Process by which a nongovernmental agency or association certifies that an individual licensed to practice a profession has met predetermined standards specified by that profession for specialty practice.

Certified Nurse Midwife Advanced practice nurse who is prepared in nursing and midwifery.

Certified Registered Nurse Anesthetist Advanced practice nurse who is prepared in the science of anesthesiology.

Chain of Infection Phenomena of developing an infectious process.

Chakra A concentrated area of energy that influences the physical body, emotions, mental patterns, and spiritual awareness.

Change Dynamic process in which an individual's response to a stressor leads to an alteration in behavior.

Change Agent Individual who intentionally creates and implements change.

Channel Medium through which a message is transmitted.

Chaotic Family Power An absence of power structure within a family structure.

Charting by Exception (CBE) Charting method that requires the nurse to document only deviations from preestablished norms.

Chemical Agent Substance that interacts with a host, causing disease.

Chemical Restraints Medications used to control the client's behavior.

Chest Physiotherapy (CPT) Technique of percussing or vibrating the chest wall in an effort to mobilize pulmonary secretions; usually accompanies postural drainage.

Chiropractic Promotion of healing through manipulation of the spinal column.

Cholangiography Roentgenographic visualization of the integrity of the biliary system by a radiopaque contrast medium.

Cholesterol Lipid that is produced by the body and used in the synthesis of steroid hormones. Cholesterol is excreted in bile.

Cholinesterase Enzyme manufactured in the liver that is responsible for the breakdown of acetylcholine and other choline esters.

Chronemics Study of the effects of time on the communication process.

Chronic Acute Pain Discomfort that occurs almost daily over a long period (months or years) and that has a high probability of ending; also known as progressive pain.

Chronic Illness Disruption in functional ability usually characterized by a gradual, insidious onset with lifelong changes that are usually irreversible.

Chronic Malignant Pain Chronic pain as a result of progressive tissue injury.

Chronic Nonmalignant Pain Discomfort that occurs almost daily, has been present for at least 6 months, and ranges in intensity from mild to severe; also known as chronic benign pain.

Chronic Obstructive Pulmonary Disease (COPD) Category of alterations in ventilation including emphysema, asthma, and chronic bronchitis.

Chronic Pain Discomfort that is persistent, nearly constant, and long-lasting (6 months or longer); or recurrent pain that produces significant negative changes in a person's life.

Chronic Wound Wound that is caused by a chronic condition or that fails to heal in an orderly manner.

Chronobiology Science of studying biorhythms.

Chronological Age Exact age of a person from birth.

Chylomicrons Lipoproteins synthesized in the intestines that transport triglycerides to the liver.

Circadian Rhythm Biorhythm that cycles on a daily basis.

Civil Law Law that deals with relations between individuals.

Clean-Contaminated Wound Intentional wound created by entry into the alimentary, respiratory, or genitourinary tract under controlled conditions.

Clean Object Object on which there are microorganisms that are not usually pathogenic.

Cleansing Removal of soil or organic material from instruments and equipment used in providing client care.

Clean Wound Intentional wound in which no inflammation was encountered and the respiratory, alimentary, and oropharyngeal tracts were not entered.

Client Advocate Person who speaks up or acts on behalf of the client.

Client Behavior Incidents Mishaps that occur when the client's behavior or actions precipitate the incident.

Clinical Guidelines Consensus statements that are systematically developed to assist practitioners in making patient management decisions related to special clinical circumstances.

Clinical Nurse Specialist Advanced practice nurse who is educated in a recognized nursing specialty area and is authorized to provide direct nursing care to a select population.

Clinical Practice Guidelines Evidence-based standards of nursing and medical care for clients with the same clinical problem.

Closed-Ended Question Interviewing technique that consists of questions that can be answered briefly with one-word responses.

Closed Family System Family system that is considered to be at risk for dysfunction because its ideas and values may be out of sync with the broader community and because its isolation limits available resources to the family and its members.

Closed Suction Drainage System Drain with a reservoir that when compressed creates negative pressure, or a vacuum, which draws exudate away from a wound.

Cluster Set of data cues in which relationships between and among cues are established to identify a specific health state or condition.

Cognition The intellectual ability to think.

Cognitive Domain Area of learning that involves intellectual understanding.

Cognitive Reframing Stress management technique in which the individual changes her own negative perception of a situation or event to a more positive, less threatening perspective.

Cohabitate To live together without being married.

Cohesiveness The bonding among members of a group.

Coitus Vaginal/penile intercourse.

Colic Acute abdominal pain.

Collaboration A partnership in which all parties are valued for their contribution.

Collaborative Problems Certain physiological complications that nurses monitor to detect onset of changes in status.

Collagen Protein responsible for tissue repair.

Collagen Synthesis The production of collagen, which is a strong, fibrous, insoluble protein found in connective tissue.

Collectivism A cultural form where there is dependence on the family and other related small groups for basic needs.

Colloid Nondiffusible substances.

Colonization Multiplication of microorganisms on or within a host that does not result in cellular injury.

Communicable Agent Infectious agent transmitted to a client by direct or indirect contact, vehicle or vector, or airborne route.

Communicable Disease Disease caused by a communicable agent.

Communication Dynamic, continuous, and multidimensional process for sharing information as determined by standards or policies.

Community A group of people engaged in multifaceted relationships, sharing a common culture with the capacity to act collectively over a period of time.

Community Development Society (CDS) An organization that identifies communities as the building blocks for society.

Community Health Information Networks (CHINs) A computer-connecting network between a variety of agencies (e.g., hospitals, suppliers, physicians, laboratories) that facilitates coordinating client care.

Community Health Nursing (CHN) The field of nursing that provides health care to a wide variety of populations (e.g., communities, groups).

Community Partnerships Health care providers that bring together a large number of community-based agencies, health care clinicians, educational institutions, and public organizations to address the health needs of a specific community.

Comorbidity Existence of simultaneous disease processes within an individual.

Competency Ability, qualities, and capacity to function in a particular way.

Complementary Family Power A dominion-submission dynamic process existing within the family structure.

Complementary Therapies Treatment approaches that can be used in conjunction with conventional medical therapies.

Compliance A client's agreement with and ability to follow through with a health care practitioner's therapeutic recommendations.

Complicated Grief Associated with traumatic death such as death by homicide, suicide, or an accident.

Comprehensive Assessment Type of assessment that provides baseline client data, including a complete health history and current needs assessment.

Compromised Host Person whose normal defense mechanisms are impaired.

Computed Tomography Radiologic scanning of the body with x-ray beams and radiation detectors that transmit data to a computer, which transcribes the data into quantitative measurement and multidimensional images of the internal structures.

Concept Vehicle of thought.

Conceptual Framework (Model) Structure that links global concepts together to form a unified whole.

Conceptualization Process of developing and refining abstract ideas.

Conditions of Participation (COPs) Medicare requirements for services and reimbursement that are based on the client being homebound and requiring skilled services on an intermittent basis.

Conduction Loss of heat to an object in contact with the body.

Connection The integration of all of the aspects of being human; these connections include the self, other people, the world around us, and for some people, a supreme being.

Conscious Sedation Minimally depressed level of consciousness during which the client retains the ability to maintain a continuously patent airway and to respond appropriately to physical stimulation or verbal commands.

Consciousness State of awareness of self, others, and the surrounding environment.

Consent Voluntary act by which a person agrees to allow someone else to do something.

Constipation Infrequent and difficult passage of hard stool.

Constitution Set of basic laws that defines and limits the powers of government.

Construct Abstraction or mental representation inferred from situations, events, or behaviors.

Consultation Method of soliciting help from a specialist in order to resolve diagnoses.

Consultative Leadership Style Leadership style that is based on the concepts of consultation. The leader carefully explains the rationale for a decision and its effect on followers so as to allow greater understanding and acceptance of the decision.

Contact Precautions Caregiving measures used to prevent the direct transmission of a communicable disease from the host.

Contact Transmission Mode of transfer of disease through direct contact.

Contaminated Wound Open, traumatic wound or intentional wound with acute nonpurulent inflammation.

Continuous Passive Motion Device (CPM) Device that increases range of motion and stimulates healing of the articular cartilage by decreasing swelling and the formation of adhesions.

Continuous Quality Improvement Approach to quality management in which scientific, data-driven approaches are used to study work processes that lead to long-term system improvements.

Contraction Mobilization of wound edges to reduce the size of the tissue defect.

Contract Law Enforcement of agreements among private individuals.

Contrast Medium Radiopaque substance that facilitates roentgen imaging of the body's internal structures.

Controlled Substance The Comprehensive Drug Abuse Prevention and Control Act of 1971 established five classes (called schedules) of drugs that require detailed records of distribution and use (most of these drugs are CNS stimulants or depressants, which have high risk for abuse or addiction).

Contusion Disruption of blood vessels in the soft tissue caused by blunt trauma and resulting in bruising with no disruption of the skin surface.

Convalescent Stage Period of time in which acute symptoms of an infection begin to disappear until the client returns to the previous state of health.

Convection Movement of heat away from the body's surface.

Coping A complex of behavioral, cognitive, and physiological responses that aim to prevent or minimize unpleasant or harmful experiences that challenge one's personal resources.

Correlational Designs Methods of data analysis that investigate the correlation (relationship) of one variable with another variable or multiple variables.

Corrosives Health hazard classification; substances that will erode or damage skin on contact.

Costal (Thoracic) Breathing Occurs when the external intercostal muscles are used to move the chest upward and outward.

Counterstimulation Technique used to achieve relaxation by activating the endogenous opioid and monoamine analgesia systems.

Crackle An audible breath sound heard on inspiration over the base of the lungs. May be either a dry, high-pitched popping of short duration or a moist, low-pitched gurgling of long duration.

Creative Problem Solving Goal-directed thinking that leads to achievement by using a new idea or method.

Credibility The quality or power of inspiring beliefs.

Crepitus Grating or crackling sensation caused by two rough surfaces rubbing together, as in subcutaneous emphysema.

Criminal Law Acts or offenses against the welfare or safety of the public.

Crisis Acute state of disorganization that occurs when the individual's usual coping mechanisms are no longer effective.

Crisis Intervention Specific technique used to assist clients in regaining equilibrium.

Criteria Standards that are used to evaluate whether the behavior demonstrated indicates accomplishment of the goal.

Critical Pathway Abbreviated summary of key elements from the case management plan.

Critical Period Time of the most rapid growth or development in a particular stage of the life cycle in which an individual is most vulnerable to stressors of any type.

Critical Social Theory A theory that is directed toward making social changes to alter health-damaging conditions.

Critical Thinking Disciplined, deliberate method of thinking used to search for meaning; employs strategies such as asking questions, evaluating evidence, identifying assumptions, examining alternatives, and seeking to understand various points of view.

Cross-Functional Team Interdepartmental, multidisci-plinary group that is assigned to study an organization-wide process.

Cross-Section Studies Studies involving data collection at one specific measurement point in time.

Crystallized Intelligence The application of life experiences and learned skills to solve problems.

Crystalloid Electrolyte solution with the potential to form crystals.

Cues Small amounts of data that are applied to the decision-making process.

Cullen's Sign Bluish discoloration around the umbilicus in postoperative clients; can indicate intra-abdominal or perineal bleeding.

Cultural Assimilation Process by which individuals from a minority group are absorbed by the dominant culture and take on the characteristics of the dominant culture.

Cultural Competence Process through which the nurse provides care that is appropriate to the client's cultural context.

Cultural Diversity Individual differences among people that result from racial, ethnic, and cultural variables.

Culture Dynamic and integrated structures of knowledge, beliefs, behaviors, ideas, attitudes, values, habits, customs, languages, symbols, rituals, ceremonies, and practices that are unique to a particular group of people; growing microorganisms to identify a pathogen.

Customer Anyone who uses the products, services, or processes provided by an organization.

Cutaneous Pain Discomfort caused by stimulation of the cutaneous nerve endings in the skin.

Cyanosis Blue or gray discoloration of the skin, resulting from reduced oxygen levels in the arterial blood.

Cystocele Bladder hernia that protrudes through the vagina.

Cystography Radiographic study used to visualize the excretory function by instilling an aqueous iodine contrast agent into the bladder through a urinary catheter.

Cytology Study of cells.

Cytomegalovirus (CMV) DNA virus that causes intranuclear and intracytoplasmic changes in infected cells.

Data Clustering Process of grouping significant cues together according to a specific assessment model to establish a nursing diagnosis.

Data Interpretation Recognition of patterns in data to determine nursing diagnoses.

Data Verification Process through which data are validated as being complete and accurate.

Deadspace Condition in which lung tissue is well ventilated but poorly perfused.

Deamination Removal of the amino groups from the amino acids.

Debridement Removal of necrotic tissue.

Decision Making The consideration and selection of interventions that facilitate the achievement of a desired outcome.

Declarative Knowledge Specific facts or information and an understanding of the nature of that knowledge.

Defamation Act that occurs when information that damages an individual's reputation is communicated to a third party either in writing (libel) or verbally (slander).

Defecation Evacuation of feces from the rectum.

Defendant Person being sued in a lawsuit.

Defense Mechanisms Unconscious operations that protect the mind from anxiety.

Defining Characteristics Collected data that are also known as signs and symptoms, subjective and objective data, or clinical manifestations.

Deglutition Swallowing of food.

Degree Unit that measures the heat of the body.

Dehiscence Partial or complete separation of the wound edges and the layers below the skin.

Delegation Process of transferring a selected nursing task in a situation to an individual who is competent to perform that task.

Democratic Leadership Style Style of leadership (also called participative leadership) that is based on the belief that every group member should have input into the development of goals and problem solving.

Deontology Ethical theory that considers the intrinsic moral significance of an act itself as the criterion for determination of good.

Dependence Reliance on or need to take a drug.

Dependent Nursing Intervention Nursing action that requires an order from a physician or other health care professional.

Dependent Variable Outcome variable of interest.

Depersonalization Treating an individual as an object rather than as a person.

Dermal-Epidermal Junction Anatomical point at which epidermis connects with dermis, characterized by interdigitating connections.

Dermatome Map Cutaneous area whose sensory receptors and axons feed into a single dorsal root of the spinal cord.

Dermis Innermost layer of skin.

Descriptive Studies Those studies that describe a phenomenon of interest.

Detrusor Muscle Smooth muscle of the bladder wall.

Development Behavioral changes in functional abilities and skills.

Developmental Tasks Certain goals that must be achieved during each developmental stage of the life cycle.

Diabetes Mellitus A disease in which the pancreas fails to secrete adequate levels of insulin to accommodate blood glucose levels.

Diagnosis Science and art of identifying problems or conditions.

Dialectic Process Process involving a transaction that the changing person has with the changing world.

Diaphoresis Profuse perspiration.

Diaphragmatic (Abdominal) Breathing Occurs when the diaphragm contracts and relaxes as observed by the movement of the abdomen.

Diarrhea Passage of liquified stool (increased frequency and consistency of stool sufficient to represent a change in bowel habits).

Diastole Process of cardiac chamber filling.

Dietary Fiber The part of food that body enzymes cannot digest and absorb.

Diffusion Movement of molecules in a solution or a gas from an area of high concentration to one of low concentration.

Diffusion Defect Decrease in efficiency of gas diffusion from the alveolar space into the pulmonary capillary blood.

Digestion Mechanical and chemical processes that convert nutrients into a physically absorbable state.

Digital Subtraction Angiography Computerized imaging of the vasculature with visualization on a monitor screen following the intravenous injection of iodine through a catheter.

Direct Contact Transmission of a communicable disease from the host.

Direct Expenses Those expenditures that are directly attributable to the department and will include both labor and nonlabor components.

Dirty and Infected Wound Traumatic wound with retained dead tissue, or intentional wound created when purulent drainage was present.

Dirty Object Object on which there is a high number of microorganisms, including some that are potentially pathogenic.

Disability A lack of ability to perform an activity a normal person can perform.

Disaccharide Double sugar.

Discharge Planning Planning that involves critical anticipation and consideration for the client's needs after discharge; the client begins to resume self-care activities before leaving the health care environment.

Discipline Field of study.

Disease Prevention/Health Protection Behavior motivated by a desire to actively avoid illness, detect it early, or maintain functioning within the constraints of an illness.

Disenfranchised Grief Grief experienced in situations where grief is discouraged and social supports are absent.

Disinfectant Chemical solution used to clean inanimate objects.

Disinfection Elimination of pathogens, with the exception of spores, from inanimate objects.

Disorientation A mentally confused state in which the person's awareness of time, place, self, and/or situation is impaired.

Disseminated Intravascular Coagulation (DIC) An acquired hemorrhagic syndrome characterized by uncontrollable formation and deposition of thrombi.

Dissolution Rate at which a drug becomes a solution.

Distance Learning Educational courses designed in formats that allow the educators and the students to be in different geographic locations.

Distraction Technique of focusing attention on stimuli other than pain.

Distress Experienced when stressors evoke an ineffective response.

Distribution Movement of drugs from the blood into various body fluids and tissues.

Documentation Written evidence of the interactions between and among health care professionals, clients and their families, and health care organizations; the administration of tests, procedures, treatments, and client education; the result or client's response to these diagnostic tests and interventions.

Dominant Culture Group whose values prevail within a society.

Doppler Handheld transducer.

Droplet Precautions Methods of care used for suspected or confirmed diagnosis of infectious disease transmitted via attachment to large droplets of moisture during exhalation.

Drug Any substance that, when taken into a living organism, may modify one or more of its functions.

Drug Allergy Hypersensitivity to a drug.

Drug Incompatibility Undesired chemical or physical reaction between a drug and a solution, between two drugs, or between a drug and the container or tubing.

Drug Tolerance Reaction that occurs when the body becomes accustomed to a specific drug and requires larger doses of the drug to produce the desired therapeutic effect.

Dullness A high-pitched sound of short duration.

Durable Power of Attorney Document or legal status that enables any competent individual to name someone to exercise health-related decision-making authority, under specific circumstances, on the client's behalf when the client is incapable of making own decisions.

Duration The time period that a medication has its action.

Duty Obligation created either by law or contract, or by any voluntary action.

Dysfunctional Grief Failure to progress through the stages of overwhelming emotions associated with grief; or failure to demonstrate any behaviors commonly associated with grief.

Dyspnea Difficulty in breathing as observed by labored or forced respirations through the use of accessory muscles in the chest and neck to breathe.

Dysrhythmia Irregular heartbeat.

Dysuria Painful urination.

Echocardiography Ultrasonic procedure used to reveal abnormal structure or motion of the heart wall and thrombi.

Ecomap A graphic representation of the family within the social network.

Edema Detectable accumulation of increased interstitial fluid.

Efferent Nerve Pathway Descending pathways that send sensory impulses from the brain.

Efferent Pain Pathway Descending spinal cord.

Effleurage Massage technique consisting of long, smooth strokes used at the beginning and end of treatment and between other movements.

Electrocardiogram (ECG or EKG) Graphic recording of the heart's electrical activity.

Electrochemical Gradient Sum of all the diffusion forces acting on the membrane.

Electroencephalogram (EEG) Graphic recording of the brain's electrical activity.

Electrolyte Element or compound that when dissolved in water or another solvent dissociates (separates) into ions (electrically charged particles) and provides for cellular reactions.

Electronic Health Record (EHR) Methodof documentation where all information related to the client is recorded electronically rather than on a traditional paper record. It is sometimes referred to as a computerized patient/client record.

Electronic Mail (e-mail) Method of transmitting data or text files from one computer to another over an intranet or the Internet.

Embryonic Stage Developmental stage that occurs during the first 2 to 8 weeks after fertilization of a human egg.

Emergency Assessment A rapid assessment of a client who is experiencing a life-threatening problem or crisis.

Emollients Products that penetrate the epidermis to restore lost skin oils that keep the skin soft and supple.

Emotional Intelligence (EI) Leadership effectiveness that focuses on emotional considerations of the persons in the group.

Empathy Understanding another person's perception of a situation.

Empowerment Process of enabling others to do for themselves.

Encoding Use of language and other specific signs and symbols for sending messages.

Endorphins Group of opiate-like substances produced naturally by the brain; these substances raise the pain threshold, produce sedation and euphoria, and promote a sense of well-being.

Endoscopy Visualization of a body organ or cavity through a scope.

Energetic-Touch Therapies Techniques in which the hands are used to direct or redirect the flow of the body's energy fields to enhance balance within the fields.

Engineering Controls Strategies that eliminate or minimize the hazard exposure through substitution, mechanical devices, or a process change.

Enteral Instillation Administration of drugs through a gastrointestinal tube.

Enteral Nutrition The nonvolitional delivery of nutrients through a gastrointestinal tube.

Environment Place or community where care is provided.

Environment of Care The organizational safety program as defined by JCAHO, developed to provide a safe environment for clients, visitors, and staff; encompasses management of seven specific areas: safety, security, utilities, medical equipment, emergency, hazardous materials and waste, and fire prevention.

Enzyme Protein produced in the body that catalyzes chemical reactions in organic matter.

Epidemiology The study of the cause and distribution of diseases, disability, and death among populations.

Epidermis Outermost layer of skin.

Epithelialization Growth of epithelial tissue.

Equipment Incidents Accidents resulting from the malfunction or improper use of medical equipment.

Equity Process that acts in accordance with the spirit, not the letter, of the law.

Erectile Dysfunction Inability of a man to achieve or maintain an erection.

Ergonomic Stressors Working conditions such as repetitive tasks and manual client lifting that have the potential to lead to work-related injury.

Erythema Increased blood flow to an inflamed area.

Erythrocytes Red blood cells.

Erythrocyte Sedimentation Rate (ESR) The rate with which the RBCs settle in saline or plasma over a specified time period.

Eschar Necrotic (dead) tissue that is brown or black and usually dry.

Essential Amino Acids Amino acids that are required for growth and development and must be obtained from food.

Ethical Dilemma Situation that occurs when there is a conflict between two or more ethical principles.

Ethical Principles Tenets that direct or govern actions.

Ethical Reasoning Process of thinking through what one ought to do in an orderly, systematic manner in order to provide justification of actions based on principles.

Ethics Branch of philosophy concerned with determining right from wrong on the basis of a body of knowledge.

Ethnicity Cultural group's perception of themselves (group identity) and others' perception of them.

Ethnocentrism Assumption of cultural superiority and an inability to accept other cultures' ways of organizing reality.

Ethnography A type of qualitative research whose approach involves anthropology, in which a person's culture is examined by studying the meanings of the actions and events of the culture's members.

Ethnomethodology A type of qualitative methodology in which interpretations of ethnography are made in a particular social world.

Etiology Related cause of or contributor to a problem.

Eupnea Easy respirations with a normal breath rate of breaths per minute that are age-specific.

Eustress Type of stress that results in positive outcomes.

Euthanasia Intentional action or lack of action causing the merciful death of someone suffering from a terminal illness or incurable condition; derived from the Greek word *euthanatos,* which literally means "good or gentle death."

Evaluation Fifth step in the nursing process; involves determining whether client goals have been met, partially met, or not met.

Evaporation Continuous insensible heat loss from the skin and lungs when water is converted from a liquid to a gas.

Evidenced-Based Nursing A decision-making approach based on integrating clinical expertise with the best available evidence from systematic research.

Evidenced-Based (Nursing) Practice The application of the best available empirical evidence, including recent research findings, to clinical practice in order to aid clinical decision making.

Evisceration Protrusion of the internal viscera through a disrupted wound.

Exclusive Provider Organization Organizationin which care must be delivered by the plan in order for clients to receive reimbursement for health care services.

Excretion Elimination of drugs from the body.

Existentialism Movement that is centered on individual existence in an incomprehensible world and the role that free will plays in it.

Expected Outcome Detailed, specific statement that describes the methods through which a goal will be achieved and includes aspects such as direct nursing care, client teaching, and continuity of care.

Experimental Design A method of statistical analysis in which an independent variable is tested against a dependent variable.

Expert Systems Decision-making support systems.

Expert Witness Person called by parties in a malpractice suit who is a member of the same profession as the party being sued and who is qualified to testify to the expected behaviors usually employed by members of the profession when in a similar situation.

Expiration (Exhalation) Movement of gases from the lungs to the atmosphere.

Exploratory Studies Those studies that describe in detail the nature of phenomena and try to identify contributing factors.

Expressed Contract Conditions and terms of a contract given in writing by the concerned parties.

Expressive Aphasia The ability to understand communication, but inability to speak clearly back to the sender of a message.

Extended Family Family members from previous generations, such as grandparents, uncles, and aunts.

Extension Straightening of a joint.

External Customer An individual who is not employed by the organization, and who uses the services the organization provides.

External Respiration See *Oxygen Uptake*.

External Stimuli Elements that generate messages from outside the person in the environment and include sensations, sights, sounds, touch, taste, and smells.

Extinction Ability to discriminate the points of distance when two body parts are simultaneously touched.

Extraurethral Incontinence Uncontrolled loss of urine caused when the sphincter mechanism has been bypassed.

Extubation Removal of an endotracheal tube.

Exudate Material and cells discharged from blood vessels.

Facilitator A person who assists others in making decisions or developing a plan of action.

False Imprisonment Situation that occurs when clients are made to wrongfully believe they cannot leave a place.

Family Process The way a family is organized to address functional needs.

Fascia Thin layer of connective tissue covering the muscle.

Fat-Soluble Vitamins Vitamins that require the presence of fats for their absorption from the gastrointestinal tract and for cellular metabolism.

Fatty Acids Basic structural units of most lipids that contain carbon chains and hydrogen.

Fecal Incontinence Involuntary loss of stool of sufficient duration and volume to create a social or hygienic problem.

Feedback Information the sender receives about the receiver's reaction to a message.

Fee-for-Service Where health care recipient directly pays the provider for services as they are provided.

Felony Crime of a serious nature usually punishable by imprisonment in a state penitentiary or by death.

Female Genital Mutilation (FGM) Ritualistic removal of clitoris; often culturally based to control female sexual drive.

Fetal Alcohol Syndrome Condition in which fetal development is impaired by maternal consumption of alcohol.

Fetal Stage Intrauterine developmental period from 8 weeks to birth.

Fibroblast Any cell from which connective tissue is developed.

Fidelity Ethical concept that means faithfulness and keeping promises.

Fight-or-Flight Response State in which the body becomes physiologically ready to respond to a stressor by either fighting or running away from the danger (which may be actual or perceived).

Firewall A protective mechanism that establishes limited access into a computer system.

Fixation Inadequate mastery or failure to achieve a developmental task that inhibits healthy progression through subsequent stages.

Flashback Rush of blood back into intravenous tubing when a negative pressure is created on the tubing.

Flatulence Discharge of gas from the rectum.

Flexion To bend a joint.

Flora Vegetation of microorganisms on the human body.

Flow Rate Volume of fluid to infuse over a set period of time.

Fluency Ability to talk in a steady manner.

Fluid Intelligence Ability to acquire new concepts and adapt to unfamiliar situations; mental activities based on organizing information.

Fluoroscopy Immediate, serial images of the body's structure or function.

Focus Charting Documentation method using a columnar format to chart data, action, and response.

Focused Assessment Type of assessment that is limited in scope in order to focus on a particular need or health care problem or potential health care risks.

Focused Questions Questions asked to obtain information that is more specific about a problem or condition.

FOCUS PDCA An acronym describing the Shewhart/Deming model for quality improvement.

Fomite Object that has become contaminated with a microorganism.

Formal Contract Written contract that cannot be changed legally by an oral agreement.

Fowler's Stages of Spiritual Development Six categories of spiritual development across the life span purported by James Fowler in 1981.

Fraud Wrong that results from a deliberate deception intended to produce unlawful gain.

Free Radicals A molecule containing an odd number of electrons; free radicals are released during times of ischemic injury.

Friction Force of two surfaces moving against one another; massage technique whereby the heels of the hands or the thumb pads are used to apply deep, penetrating pressure on knotted muscles.

Frigidity A women's lack of desire for sex or inability to achieve orgasm.

Full Disclosure Communication of complete information to potential research subjects regarding the nature of the study, the subjects' right to refuse participation, and the likely risks and benefits that will be incurred.

Full-Thickness Wound Wound involving the entire epidermis and dermis.

Functional Ability Physical, cognitive, and psychological skills needed to carry out activities of daily living, mobility, work, and family roles.

Functional Assessment Assessment of the client's ability to perform activities of daily living.

Functional Health Patterns A systematic holistic approach to evaluate all areas of human needs, recognizing that the needs are interdependent.

Functional Incontinence Loss of urine caused by altered mobility or dexterity, access to the toilet, or changes in mentation.

Functional Independence Measurement (FIM) A formal tool that evaluates an individual's ability to safely and independently perform activities of daily living specific to self-care, sphincter control, transfers, locomotion, communication, and social cognition.

Functional Team Departmental or unit-specific group whose scope is limited to departmental or work area processes.

Gait or Transfer Belt Two-inch-wide webbed belt worn by the client for the purpose of stabilization during transfers and ambulation.

Gallop Extra heart sounds.

Gate Control Pain Theory Theory proposing that the cognitive, sensory, emotional, and physiological components of the body can act together to block an individual's perception of pain.

Gay Male who has affectional and sexual tendencies for males; more holistic term than *homosexual* when it includes women who have affectional tendencies for females.

Gender (Biologic Sex) Biologic structure of a person's genitals that designate them as male, female, or intersexed.

Gender Bender A person who dresses as opposite gender or androgynously, challenging societally prescribed gender behaviors, especially dress.

Gender Identity View of one's self as male or female in relationship to others.

Gender Role Masculine or feminine role adopted by a person; often culturally and socially determined.

General Adaptation Syndrome Physiological response that occurs when a person experiences a stressor.

General Anesthesia Anesthesia that causes the client to lose all sensation and consciousness; used for major surgical procedures.

Generalized Spiritual Assessment An assessment that includes the four elements of spirituality: transcendence, connection, balance, and purpose.

Generativity A sense that one is making a contribution to society.

Genogram A graphic representation of the family form.

Genome The DNA contained in an organism or a cell, which includes both the chromosomes within the nucleus and the DNA in the mitochondria.

Germicide Chemical that can be applied to both animate and inanimate objects to kill pathogens.

Germinal Stage Developmental stage that begins with conception and lasts approximately 10 to 14 days.

Gingivitis Inflammation of the gums.

Glasgow Coma Scale (GCS) An international scale used in grading neurologic responses to determine the client's level of consciousness.

Global Migration An ongoing trend of people crossing regions, countries, and international boundaries to reside and maintain themselves in new and unfamiliar places.

Gluconeogenesis Conversion of amino acids into glucose or glycogen.

Glucose 6-Phosphate Dehydrogenace (G6PD) An enzyme in RBCs that metabolizes glucose.

Glycolysis Breakdown of glucose by enzymes located inside the cell's cytoplasm.

Glycosylated Hemoglobin A_1(Hb A_1) A form of hemoglobin (hemoglobin A_1) in the red blood cells; it combines strongly with glucose in the process called glycosylation.

Goal Aim, intent, or end.

Goniometer A protractor with two movable arms used to measure the angles of skeletal joint during range of motion.

Good Samaritan Acts Laws that provide protection to health care providers by ensuring immunity from civil liability when the caregiver provides assistance at the scene of an emergency and does not intentionally or recklessly cause the client injury.

Grand Theory Theory composed of concepts representing global and complex phenomena.

Granulation Tissue Tissue consisting of newly formed blood vessels and newly synthesized connective tissue.

Graphesthesia Ability to identify numbers, letters, or shapes when drawn on the skin.

Grief Series of intense physical and psychological responses that occur following a loss.

Grief Work Phrase coined from Lindemann, it describes the process experienced by the bereaved. It consists of freedom from attachment to the deceased, becoming reoriented to the environment in which the deceased is no longer present, and establishing new relationships.

Grounded Theory A type of qualitative research in which field research seeks to explore and describe the phenomena in naturalistic settings.

Group Communication A complex level of communication that occurs when three or more people meet in face-to-face encounters or through another communication medium, such as a conference call.

Group Dynamics Study of the events that take place during small-group interaction and the development of subgroups.

Groupthink Going along with the majority opinion while personally having another viewpoint.

Growth Quantitative (measurable) changes in the physical size of the body and its parts.

Growth Factors Polypeptides released during clot breakdown and synthesized by a number of cells that serve as primary regulators of wound repair.

Guided Imagery A process in which the person uses all the senses to experience the sensation of relaxation.

Half-Life Time it takes the body to eliminate half of the blood concentration level of the original drug dose.

Halitosis Bad breath.

Hallucination A sensory perception that occurs in the absence of external stimuli and is not based on reality.

Handicap Inability to perform one's roles in society.

Handwashing Rubbing together of all surfaces and crevices of the hands using a soap or chemical and water.

Hardiness The ability to survive stress.

Hazardous Condition A situation (aside from the disease for which treatment is provided) that increases the risk of a serious adverse outcome.

Healing Process of recovery from illness, accident, or disability.

Healing Touch Energy-based therapeutic modality that alters the energy fields through the use of touch, thereby affecting physical, mental, emotional, and spiritual health.

Health Process through which the person seeks to maintain an equilibrium that promotes stability and comfort; includes physiological, psychological, sociocultural, intellectual, and spiritual well-being.

Health Care Delivery System Mechanism for providing services that meet the health-related needs of individuals.

Health History Review of the client's functional health patterns prior to the current contact with a health care agency.

Health Maintenance Behavior directed toward maintaining a current level of health.

Health Maintenance Activities The activities and behaviors an individual performs to maintain or improve a current level of health.

Health Maintenance Organization (HMO) Prepaid health plan that provides primary health care services for a preset fee and focuses on cost-effective treatment methods.

Health Policies Written decisions directing or influencing the actions or decisions of others.

Health-Promoting Behaviors Actions that increase well-being or quality of life.

Health Promotion Process undertaken to increase levels of wellness in individuals, families, and communities.

Health-Seeking Behaviors Activities that are directed toward attaining and maintaining a state of well-being.

Heart Failure Inability of the heart to pump enough blood to meet the metabolic needs of the body; often accompanied by a backup of blood in the venous circuits (congestive heart failure).

Heaves Lifting of the cardiac area secondary to an increased workload and force of left ventricular contraction.

Heimlich Maneuver Application of sharp, upward thrusts to the abdomen in order to remove an airway obstruction.

Hematoma Localized collection of blood underneath the tissue.

Hematuria Blood in the urine; *microscopic hematuria* is the presence of blood noted on microscopic examination of the urine; *gross hematuria* is the presence of blood visible to the naked eye.

Hemoconcentration Reduced volume of plasma water and the increased concentration of blood cells, plasma proteins, and protein-bound constituents; occurs with increased capillary hydrostatic pressure, which causes water to shift from the intravascular into the interstitial space.

Hemodynamic Regulation Physiological function of blood circulating to maintain an appropriate environment in tissue fluids.

Hemoglobin Electrophoresis A laboratory test that uses an electromagnetic field to identify various types of hemolytic anemia.

Hemolysis A breakdown of red cells and the release of hemoglobin.

Hemorrhage Persistent bleeding.

Hemorrhagic Exudate Discharge with a large component of red blood cells; present with severe inflammation.

Hemorrhoids Perianal varicosity of the hemorrhoidal veins.

Hemostasis Cessation of bleeding.

Heterosexism Perspective of assumption that people are heterosexual.

Heterosexual Describes sexual activity between a man and a woman.

High-Biological-Value Proteins (Complete Proteins) Proteins that contain all of the essential amino acids.

High-Level Wellness State in which individuals function at their maximum health potential while remaining in balance with the environment.

High-Risk Sexual Behavior Behavior that leads to increased risk of contracting STIs (e.g., unprotected sex, multiple sexual partners, sexual activity that involves blood or exposure to blood).

Historical Research A type of research in which data relating to past events is systematically collected.

History Study of the past, including events, situations, and individuals.

Holism The belief that individuals function as complete units that cannot be reduced to the sum of their parts.

Home Health Agencies Organizations that provide services using health professionals in an individual's place of residence.

Home Health Care An organized, nonphysician health service provided by professionals to clients in their homes.

Home Health Care Nursing A subspecialty of community health nursing and can be offered to a variety of clients throughout the age spectrum.

Homeopathy The treatment of disease with minute drug dosages.

Homeostasis Equilibrium (balance) between physiological, psychological, sociocultural, intellectual, and spiritual needs.

Homosexuality Sexual activity between two members of the same sex.

Hospice Type of care for the terminally ill founded on the concept of allowing individuals to die with dignity and surrounded by those who love them.

Host Simple or complex organism that can be affected by an agent.

Human Genome Project An international research proj ect to map each human gene and to completely sequence human DNA.

Humectants Products that attract and hold water in the epidermal layer.

Humoral Immune Response An immune response initi ated when an antigen is recognized and B lymphocytes are activated.

Humoral Immunity Stimulation of B cells and antibody production.

Hydrostatic Pressure Pressure that a liquid exerts on the sides of the container that holds it; also called filtration force.

Hygiene Science of health.

Hyperalgesia Extreme sensitivity to pain.

Hypercalcemia Excess in the extracellular level of calcium

Hypercapnia Elevation of carbon dioxide levels in the blood indicating inadequate alveolar ventilation.

Hyperchloremia Excess in the extracellular level of chlo ride.

Hyperglycemia Condition characterized by a blood glucose level greater than 110 mg/dl.

Hyperkalemia Excess in the extracellular level of potassium.

Hypermagnesemia Excess in the extracellular level of magnesium.

Hypernatremia Excess in the extracellular level of sodium

Hyperphosphatemia Excess in the extracellular level of phosphorus.

Hypersomnia Alteration in sleep pattern characterized excessive sleep, especially in the daytime.

Hypertension Refers to a persistent systolic pressure greater than 135–140 mm Hg and a diastolic pressure greater than 90 mm Hg.

Hyperthyroidism Increased secretion of thyroid hormones, which increases the rate of metabolism.

Hypertonic Solution with more solutes in proportion to the volume of body water; also called a hyperosmolar solution

Hypertonicity Increased muscle tone.

Hypertrophy Refers to an increase in muscle size and shape due to an increase in muscle fiber.

Hyperventilation Characterized by deep, rapid ventilations.

Hypervolemia Increased circulating fluid volume.

Hypnagogic Hallucinations Lifelike dreams and hallucinations that often incorporate elements of the environment and are experienced during the hypnagogic state.

Hypnagogic State Condition experienced when one is between sleep and wake.

Hypnosis State of heightened awareness and focused concentration.

Hypocalcemia Deficit in the extracellular level of calcium.

Hypochloremia Deficit in the extracellular level of chloride.

Hypodermis Tissue layer underlying the dermis, composed of adipose tissue and connective tissue (also known as subcutaneous tissue).

Hypoglycemia Condition characterized by a blood glucose level less than 80 mg/dl.

Hypokalemia Deficit in the extracellular level of potassium.

Hypomagnesemia Deficit in the extracellular level of magnesium.

Hyponatremia Deficit in the extracellular level of sodium.

Hypophosphatemia Deficit in the extracellular level of phosphorus.

Hypotension A systolic blood pressure less than 90 mm Hg or 20–30 mm Hg below the client's normal blood pressure.

Hypothesis Statement of an asserted relationship between dependent variables.

Hypothyroidism Decreased secretion of thyroid hormones, which decreases the metabolic rate.

Hypotonic Solution with less solute in proportion to the volume of water; also called a hypo-osmolar solution.

Hypotonicity A flabby muscle with poor tone.

Hypoventilation Characterized by shallow respirations.

Hypoxemia Decreased oxygen level in the blood.

Hypoxia Oxygen deprivation of the body's cells.

Identity What sets one person apart as a unique individual; it may include a person's name, gender, ethnic identity, family status, occupation, and various roles.

Idiopathic Insomnia Sleeplessness with an unknown origin.

Idiosyncratic Reaction Reaction of overresponse, under-response, or an atypical response.

Illness Inability of an individual's adaptive responses to maintain physical and emotional balance that subsequently results in an impairment in functional abilities.

Illness Stage Time interval when client is presenting or manifesting specific signs and symptoms of an infectious agent.

Illusion An inaccurate perception or misinterpretation of sensory stimuli.

Imagery Relaxation technique in which the individual uses the imagination to visualize a pleasant, soothing image.

Immediate Memory The retention of information for a specified and usually short period of time.

Immunity A specific defense mechanism used to combat infection.

Immunoglobulins Plasma protein cells that produce large amounts of antibodies in five different classes (IgM, IgG, IgA, IgD, and IgE).

Impaction Hard bolus of stool that obstructs the fecal stream.

Impaired Nurse Nurse who is habitually intemperate or is addicted to the use of alcohol or habit-forming drugs.

Impairment Loss of function at the organ level.

Implantable Port Device with a radiopaque silicone catheter and a plastic or stainless steel injection port with a self-sealing silicone-rubber septum.

Implementation Fourth step in the nursing process; involves the execution of the nursing plan of care formulated during the planning phase of the nursing process.

Implied Contract Contract that recognizes a relationship between parties for services.

Impotence Male's inability to have or sustain an erection.

Incentive Spirometers Breathing devices that measure the client's ventilatory volumes.

Incidence Refers to the prevalence of a disease in a population or community. The predictive value of the same test can be different when applied to people of differing ages, genders, and geographic locations.

Incident Report Documentation of an unusual occurrence or an accident in delivery of client care.

Incontinence Loss of the ability to initiate, control, or inhibit elimination.

Incubation Period Time interval between the entry of an infectious agent in the host and the onset of symptoms.

Independent Nursing Intervention - Nursing action initiated by the nurse that does not require direction or an order from another health care professional.

Independent Variable Variable that is believed to cause or influence the dependent variable.

Indirect Contact Transmission of a communicable disease by any medium.

Indirect Expenses Those costs that are allocated from the operation of the larger organization to the various service units.

Individualism A predominant cultural type that focuses on an independent lifestyle that flourishes in urban settings.

Infancy Developmental stage from the first month to the first year of life.

Infarction Death (necrosis) of an area of tissue caused by oxygen deprivation.

Infection Actual invasion and multiplication of microor-ganisms in body tissue with cellular injury.

Infection Chain A process of elements that when linked together result in an infection.

Infectious Agent Microorganism that causes infections.

Infertility Inability to conceive.

Infiltration See page of foreign substances into the interstitial tissue.

Inflammation Nonspecific cellular response to tissue injury or infection; involves increased blood flow in the affected area.

Inflammatory Phase Initial phase of wound repair, characterized by vessel dilatation, migration of white blood cells to wound bed, and clinical signs of erythema, edema, and exudate production.

Information Technology The use of computers to gather, organize, process, and communicate information.

Informed Consent Client understands the reason for the proposed intervention, its benefits, and risks, and agrees to the treatment by signing a consent form.

Ingestion Route of exposure whereby exposure to chemical or microorganism is via gastrointestinal tract.

Inhalation Route of exposure whereby exposure to chemical or microorganism is via respiratory tract.

Initial Planning Planning that involves development of an initial plan of care by the nurse who performs the admission assessment and gathers the comprehensive admission assessment data.

Injection Route of exposure whereby exposure to chemical or microorganism is via percutaneous exposure or compromised skin.

Injury Physical, financial, or emotional harm.

Insensible Heat Loss Heat that is lost through the continuous, unnoticed water loss that occurs with vaporation.

Insomnia Chronic inability to sleep, or inadequate quality of sleep.

Inspection Physical examination technique that involves careful visual observation.

Inspiration (Inhalation) Intake of air into the lungs.

Insulin Pancreatic hormone that aids in the diffusion of glucose into the liver and muscle cells and the synthesis of glycogen.

Integrative Therapy A clinical approach that combines Western technological medicine with techniques from Eastern medicine.

Integumentary System Skin, hair, scalp, and nails; provides the body with external protection, regulates temperature, and is a sensory organ for pain, temperature, and touch.

Intentional Wound Wound acquired during treatment (such as surgery) or therapy (such as venipuncture).

Interdependent Nursing Intervention Nursing action that is implemented in a collaborative manner with other health care professionals.

Intermittent Claudication Ischemia to the extremities usually brought on by activity and relieved by rest.

Internal Customer An individual employed by the organization who must depend on the efficiency and productivity of other employees to do his work.

Internal Respiration Process of gas exchange between capillary blood and the body's cells, in which the cells receive oxygen and carbon dioxide is removed.

Internal Stimuli Those elements that generate messages and are found within the person, including such things as hunger, fatigue, and myriad cognitive experiences (e.g., thoughts, fantasies).

Interpersonal Communication Process that occurs between two people in face-to-face encounters, over the telephone, or through other communication media.

Intersexed Person born with both sets or ambiguous genitalia.

Interstate Nursing Practice An agreement among states to mutually recognize each other's licenses.

Interview Therapeutic interaction that has a specific purpose.

Intracath Plastic tube for insertion into a vein.

Intractable Pain Pain that is resistant to all pain-relieving therapies.

Intradermal (ID) Injection into the dermis.

Intramuscular (IM) Injection into the muscle.

Intraoperative (during surgery) Phase that begins when the client is transferred to the operating room and ends when the client is transferred to a postanesthesia care unit.

Intrapersonal Communication Messages one sends to oneself, including "self-talk," or communication with oneself.

Intrapsychic Theory Theory that focuses on an individual's unconscious processes. Feelings, needs, conflicts, and drives are considered to be motivators of behavior.

Intravenous (IV) Injection into a vein.

Intravenous Pyelogram A series of x-rays of the kidneys, ureters, and bladder following the administration of an intravenous iodine preparation.

Intravenous (IV) Therapy Administration of nutrients, fluids, electrolytes, or medications by the venous route.

Intubation Insertion of an endotracheal tube into the bronchus through the nose or mouth to ensure an airway.

Invasive Accessing the body tissues, organs, or cavities through some type of instrumentation procedure.

Ischemia Oxygen deprivation, usually caused by poor perfusion, that is usually temporary and localized.

Ischemic Pain Discomfort resulting when the blood supply of an area is restricted or obstructed.

Isotonic Solution with body water and solutes (sodium) in equal amounts; also called an isosmolar solution.

Jargon Technical language that is often specific to a discipline.

Joint Commission on Accreditation of Healthcare Organizations (JCAHO) An independent, non-profit health care accrediting body, charged with setting health care quality standards.

Judgment The ability to compare or evaluate alternatives to life situations and arrive at an appropriate course of action.

Judicial Decisions Authoritative decisions based on the interpretation of laws; made by a judge.

Jurisprudence Body of judge-made law.

Justice Ethical principle based on the concept of fairness that is extended to each individual.

Kardex Summary worksheet reference of basic client care information.

Keloid Scar tissue that extends beyond the boundaries of the original wound.

Ketogenesis Conversion of amino acids into keto acids or fatty acids.

Ketones Products of incomplete fat metabolism.

Ketonuria Abnormally high concentration of ketones in the urine.

Kilocalorie Equivalent to 1,000 calories.

Kinesthetic Channel Transmission of messages through sensation of touch.

Kinesthetic Learner A person who processes information by experiencing the information or by touching and feeling.

Laceration Cuts to skin and soft tissues.

Laissez-Faire Leadership Style Style of leadership in which the leader assumes a passive, nondirective, and inactive style.

Lancinating Type of pain that is typically described as piercing or stabbing.

Laser Plume Product of combustion when laser is applied to living human tissue; may contain pathogens.

Late Potentials Electrical activity that occurs after normal depolarization of the ventricles.

Law That which is laid down or fixed.

Leadership Interpersonal process that involves motivating and guiding others to achieve goals.

Leadership Theory Conceptual support framework for leadership.

Learning Process of assimilating information with a resultant change in behavior.

Learning Plateau Peak in effectiveness of teaching and depth of learning.

Learning Style Way in which an individual incorporates new information.

Legal Regulation Process by which the state attests to the public that the individual licensed to practice is competent to do so.

Lentigo Senilis Benign, brown pigmented areas on the face, hands, and arms of older people.

Lesbian Female who has affectional and sexual tendencies toward females.

Leukocytes White blood cells.

Level of Evidence A categorization of research support (with four levels) generated to support a particular strategy of care.

Liability Obligation one has incurred or might incur through any act or failure to act.

Libido Level of desire for sexual activity.

Licensure Method by which a state holds the nurse accountable for safe practice to citizens of that state.

Licensure by Endorsement Process by which an individual who is duly licensed as a registered nurse under the laws of one state or country has her credentials accepted and approved by another state or country.

Licensure by Examination Process by which an individual who has completed an approved program of studies leading to registered nurse licensure seeks initial licensure by successfully passing a standardized competency examination.

Line of Gravity Vertical line passing through the center of gravity.

Lipids Organic compounds that are insoluble in water but soluble in organic solvents such as ether and alcohol; also known as fats.

Lipoproteins Blood lipids bound to protein.

Literature Review The part of the research process that involves reviewing the published and unpublished sources of information used in a given study.

Liver Mortis Bluish purple discoloration that is a byproduct of red blood cell destruction.

Living Will Document prepared by a competent adult that provides direction regarding medical care should the person become incapacitated or otherwise unable to make decisions personally.

Local Adaptation Syndrome Physiological response to a stressor (e.g., trauma, illness) affecting a specific part of the body.

Local Anesthesia Anesthesia that causes the client to lose sensation to a localized body part (e.g., spraying the back of the throat with lidocaine decreases the gag reflex).

Localized Infection Infection limited to a defined area or single organ.

Lock-Out Interval Minimum time allowed between doses for the client to self-medicate; feature found in infusion pumps used for patient-controlled analgesia.

Locus of Control A person's perception of the source of control over events and situations affecting the person's life.

Logrolling A technique for moving a client whose body must remain in straight alignment.

Longitudinal Studies Studies that involve data collection over time in a particular research sample.

Long-Term Acute Care Care arenas provided in acute facilities to clients with conditions of longer duration than acute care clients.

Long-Term Outcome Statement written in objective format demonstrating an expectation to be achieved in resolution of the nursing diagnosis over a long period of time, usually over weeks or months.

Loss Any situation in which a valued object is changed or is no longer accessible to an individual.

Low-Biological-Value Proteins (Incomplete Proteins) Proteins lacking in one or more of the essential amino acids.

Lumbar Puncture Aspiration of cerebrospinal fluid from the subarachnoid space.

Lymphangiography Radiographic study of the lymphatic system following a catheter injection of an oil-based dye.

Lymphokine Mediator substance released by lymphocytes.

Maceration Overhydration of skin secondary to diaphore-sis or to prolonged exposure to exogenous moisture.

Macrophages Immunologically active cells that phagocytize pathogens and break down necrotic tissue; they also secrete growth factors to regulate wound repair.

Magnetic Resonance Imaging (MRI) An imaging technique that uses radiowaves and a strong magnetic field to make continuous cross-sectional images of the body.

Maladaptation Process of ineffective coping with stressors.

Malignant Hyperthermia (MH) A potentially lethal syndrome caused by a hypermetabolic state that is precipitated by the administration of certain anesthetic agents.

Malnutrition Nutritional alterations related to inadequate intake, disorders of digestion or absorption, or overeating.

Malpractice Professional person's wrongful conduct, improper discharge of professional duties, or failure to meet the standards of acceptable care that results in harm to another person.

Mammography A low-dose radiographic study of the breast tissue.

Managed Care System of providing and monitoring care in which access, cost, and quality are controlled before or during delivery of services. These networks "manage" or control costs in many ways (e.g., by limiting referrals to costly specialists). HMOs are a common form of managed care.

Management Accomplishment of tasks either by oneself or by directing others.

Mandatory Licensure Laws Legislation that prohibits any individual from practicing as a registered nurse without a current license.

Mandatory Overtime Work hours imposed on a nurse over an agreed-upon, predetermined work schedule.

Mastication Chewing into fine particles and then mixing the food with enzymes in saliva.

Material Principle of Justice Rationale for determining when there can be unequal allocation of scarce resources.

Material Safety Data Sheet (MSDS) Reference sheet supplied by the manufacturer and kept on file by the employer; contains safety information on hazardous chemicals in the workplace.

Maturation Process of becoming fully grown and developed; involves physiological and behavioral aspects.

Maturation Phase Third phase of full-thickness wound repair, during which the scar tissue is remodeled via the simultaneous processes of collagen lysis and collagen synthesis.

Maturational Loss Adolescent that loses the younger child's freedom from responsibility.

Medical Asepsis Practices that reduce the number, growth, and spread of microorganisms.

Medical Diagnosis Clinical judgment by the physician that identifies or determines a specific disease, condition, or pathological state.

Medical Model Traditional approach to health care in which the focus is on treatment and cure of disease.

Medicare Certified A process that requires an agency to have inspections (e.g., reviews of charts, policies/ procedures, billing practices, qualifications of care providers) from Medicare representatives in order to receive funding from the Medicare program.

Medication A medicinal substance.

Medication Interaction The effects caused when multiple medications are administered together.

Medicine A drug or remedy.

Meditation Quieting the mind by focusing one's attention.

Melanocyte A melanin-forming cell.

Menarche Onset of the first menstrual period.

Message Stimulus produced by a sender and responded to by a receiver.

Metabolic Rate Rate of heat liberated during chemical reactions.

Metabolism Aggregate of all chemical reactions in every body cell.

Metacommunication Relationship aspect of communication, which refers to the message about the message.

Metaparadigm Unifying force in a discipline that names the phenomena of concern to that discipline.

Micro-Range Theory Theory that explains a specific phenomenon of concern to a discipline.

Middle Adulthood Developmental stage from the ages of 40 to 65 years.

Middle-Range Theory Theory that addresses more concrete and more narrowly defined phenomena than a grand theory but does not cover the full range of phenomena of concern to a discipline.

Mid-Upper-Arm Circumference Measures skeletal muscle mass and serves as an indicator of protein reserve.

Migrants Laborers who move from one location to another in pursuit of work.

Minerals Inorganic elements.

Minority Group Group of people who constitute less than a numerical majority of the population and who, because of their cultural or physical characteristics, are labeled and treated differently from others in the society.

Misdemeanor Offense less serious than a felony that may be punished by a fine or sentence to a local prison for less than 1 year.

Mixed Agonist-Antagonist Compound that blocks opi-oid effects on one receptor type while producing opioid effects on a second receptor type.

Mobility Ability to engage in activity and free movement.

Modeling The process the nurse uses in developing an image and understanding within the client's framework and from the client's perspective.

Mode of Transmission Process that bridges the gap between the portal of exit of the biological agent from the reservoir and the portal of entry of the susceptible "new" host.

Monosaccharides Simple sugars.

Monounsaturated Fatty Acids Fatty acids with one double or triple bond.

Morality Behavior in accordance with custom or tradition that usually reflects personal or religious beliefs.

Moral Maturity Ability to decide for oneself what is right.

Motivation The internal drive or externally arising stimulus to action or thought.

Mourning Period of time during which grief is expressed and resolution and integration of the loss occur.

Moxibustion Type of acupuncture that involves the application of heat from certain burning substances, such as herbs, at acupuncture points on the body.

Murmur Swishing or blowing sounds of long duration heard in the heart during the systolic and diastolic phases, created by turbulent blood flow through a valve.

Muscle Tissue composed of contractile fibers that control position and movement.

Muscle Layer A type of tissue layer composed of contractile cells or fibers that affects the movement of an organ or a part of the body.

Muscle Tone Normal state of balanced tension present in the body that allows muscles to respond quickly to stimuli.

Musculoskeletal Disorders Soft tissue injuries related to repeated trauma or other ergonomic stressors.

Music-Thanatology Holistic and palliative method for use of music with dying clients; solely concerned with dissipating any obstacle to a peaceful passage.

Myelography Study of the spinal cord and its surrounding subarachnoid spaces through the use of radiography and pantopaque, a contrast agent.

Myocardial Infarction Necrosis of the heart muscle.

Myofascial Pain Syndromes Group of muscle disorders characterized by pain, muscle spasm, tenderness, stiffness, and limited motion.

Myoneuronal Junction Point at which nerve endings come in contact with muscle cells.

N-95 Particulate Filtering Respirator A filter device commonly used in health care for protection against diseases transmitted by tiny particles of virus or bacteria remaining suspended in the air for long periods of time.

Narcolepsy Sleep alteration characterized by sudden uncontrollable urges to fall asleep.

Narrative Charting A story format of documentation that describes the client's status, interventions and treatments, and the response to treatments.

Natural Immunity The genetically determined response of protection within a specific species.

Near Miss A deviation from a process that does not actually harm the client, but could place the client at risk if it were to occur again.

Necrosis Tissue death as the result of disease or injury.

Necrotizing Fasciitis Severe and rapidly progressing infectious process caused by beta-hemolytic strep; spreads along fascial planes.

Need Anything that is absolutely essential for existence.

Negative Nitrogen Balance Condition that exists when nitrogen output exceeds intake or protein catabolism exceeds anabolism.

Negligence Failure of an individual to provide the care in a situation that a reasonable person would ordinarily provide in a similar circumstance.

Negotiation A method of conflict management whereby the parties decide what they must retain and what they are willing to give up in order to reach a compromise position.

Neonatal Period First 28 days of life following birth.

Networking Process of building connections with others.

Neuralgia Paroxysmal pain that extends along the course of one or more nerves.

Neuropathic Pain Discomfort from damage to portions of the peripheral or central nervous system.

Neuropathic Ulcer Ulcers caused by painless repetitive trauma in clients with reduced sensory awareness due to neurologic lesions or disease processes.

Neuropeptides Amino acids produced in the brain and other sites in the body that act as chemical communicators.

Neurotransmitters Chemical substances produced by the body that facilitate nerve impulse transmission.

New Age Spirituality A spiritual philosophy that incorporates various religions into a personal spiritual ethic; these concepts include such ideas as everything is God, and therefore God is within the self; religion is universal; and people should live in balance with nature.

Nitrogen Balance Net result of intake and loss of nitrogen that measures protein anabolism and catabolism.

Nociception Process by which an individual becomes aware of pain.

Nociceptor Receptive neuron for painful sensations.

Nocturia Awakening from sleep to urinate.

Nonblanching Erythema Redness of the skin that cannot be dissipated with direct pressure; usually reflects vascular injury and extravasation of blood out into the tissues.

Nonessential Amino Acids Amino acids that can be synthesized in the adult body.

Noninvasive Body is *not* entered with any type of instrument.

Nonmaleficence Ethical principle that means the duty to cause no harm to others.

Nonprofit Agencies Those agencies that have a tax-exempt status.

Nonverbal Message Message communicated without words.

Nosocomial Infection Infection acquired in the hospital that was not present or incubating at the time of the client's admission.

Nuclear Dyads Married heterosexual couples without children, either by choice or situation.

Nuclear Family A married heterosexual man and woman and their biologic children.

Nurse-Client Relationship One-to-one interactive process between client and nurse that is directed at improving the client's health status or assisting in problem solving.

Nurse Epidemiologist A direct care provider role in which the nurse studies illnesses, their causes, and the illnesses distribution in groups of people.

Nurse Practice Act Law determined by each state governing the practice of nursing.

Nurse Practitioner Advanced practice nurse educated in a specified area of care who is authorized to provide primary care to individuals, families, and other groups in a variety of settings.

Nursing An art and a science that assists individuals to learn to care for themselves whenever possible; it also involves caring for others when they are unable to meet their own needs.

Nursing Audit Process of collecting and analyzing data to evaluate the effectiveness of nursing interventions.

Nursing Diagnosis Second step in the nursing process; a clinical judgment about individual, family, or community (aggregate) responses to actual, possible, or risk (potential) health problems, wellness states, or syndromes.

Nursing Informatics The use of information technologies by nurses.

Nursing Intervention Action performed by a nurse that helps the client achieve the results specified by the expected outcomes.

Nursing Intervention Classification (NIC) Standardized language for nursing interventions.

Nursing Leadership Interpersonal process in nursing that involves motivating and guiding others to achieve goals.

Nursing Minimum Data Set (NMDS) Elements contained in clinical records and abstracted for studies on the effectiveness and costs of nursing care.

Nursing Order Statement written by the nurse that is within the scope of nursing practice to plan and initiate.

Nursing Process Systematic method of providing care to clients; consists of five steps: (1) assessment, (2) diagnosis, (3) outcome identification and planning, (4) implementation, and (5) evaluation.

Nursing Research Systematic application of formalized methods for generating valid and dependable information about the phenomena of concern to the discipline of nursing.

Nursing Sensitive Outcome Changes in client health status that reflect direct influence of nursing interventions.

Nutraceuticals Natural substances found in plant or animal foods that act as protective or healing agents.

Nutrition Process by which the body metabolizes and uses nutrients.

Nystagmus Involuntary, rhythmical oscillation of the eyes.

Obesity Weight that is 20% or more above the ideal body weight.

Objective Data Observable and measurable data that are obtained through both standard assessment techniques performed during the physical examination, and laboratory and diagnostic tests.

Obligatory Loss of Proteins Degradation of the body's own proteins into amino acids in response to inadequate protein intake.

Observation Skill of watching carefully and attentively.

Obstructive Pulmonary Disease Category of lung diseases characterized by obstruction of the airways and trapping of air distal to the obstruction.

Occult Blood in the stool that can be detected only through a microscope or by chemical means.

Older Adulthood Developmental stage occurring from the age of 65 and beyond.

Oliguria Diminished production of urine (typically less than 400 ml/24 hours).

Ongoing Assessment Type of assessment that includes systematic monitoring and observation related to specific problems.

Ongoing Planning Planning that entails continuous updating of the client's plan of care.

Onset of Action Time it takes the body to respond to a drug after administration.

Open-Ended Questions Interview technique that encourages the client to elaborate about a particular concern or problem.

Open Family System A family system that interacts with the environment and in doing so maintains growth and balance.

Operational Decisions Similar to rules and regulations, having the same authority, but less permanent.

Operative Knowledge An understanding of the nature of knowledge (knowing the "how" or "why").

Opposition One body part being across from another part at nearly 180 degrees.

Oppression Condition in which the rules, modes, and ideals of one group are imposed on another group.

Oral Cholecystography Visualization of the gallbladder and presence of stones through the administration of radiopaque iodine tablets.

Organization Means by which members of a profession join together to promote and protect the profession as a valuable service to society.

Organizational Culture Commonly held beliefs, values, norms, and expectations that drive the workforce.

Orientation Perception of self in relation to the surrounding environment.

Orientation Phase First stage of the therapeutic relationship in which the nurse and client become acquainted, establish trust, and determine the expectations of each other.

Orthostatic Hypotension (Postural Hypotension) Refers to a sudden drop of 25 mm Hg in systolic pressure and 10 mm Hg in diastolic pressure when the client moves from a lying to a sitting or a sitting to a standing position.

Osmolality Measurement of the total concentration of dissolved particles (solutes) per kilogram of water.

Osmolarity Concentration of solutes per liter of cellular fluid.

Osmole Unit of measure of osmotic pressure.

Osmosis Process caused by a concentration difference of water.

Osmotic Pressure Force that develops when two solutions of different strengths are separated by a selectively permeable membrane.

Osteoarthritis The most common type of degenerative arthritis in which the joints become stiff and tender to touch.

Osteoporosis Process in which reabsorption exceeds accretion of bone.

Outcome A domain in Donabedian's quality assurance model, which evaluates health and disability consequences, positive and negative, related to health care delivery.

Outcome and Assessment Information Set (OASIS) A method to collect needed information on all Medicare home health beneficiaries. Data is collected electronically from all Medicare-certified agencies and is used to provide a foundation for OBQI.

Outcome Based Quality Improvement (OBQI) A process to increase quality care and determine those services that are contributing (or not contributing) to the outcomes of care.

Outcome Evaluation Process of comparing the client's current status with the expected outcomes.

Output The response from the family to throughput.

Oxygen Uptake Process of oxygen diffusing from the alveolar space into the pulmonary capillary blood; also called external respiration.

Oxyhemoglobin Dissociation Curve Graphic representation of the relationship between partial pressure of oxygen and oxygen saturation.

Pain State in which an individual experiences and reports the presence of physical discomfort; may range in intensity from uncomfortable sensation to severe discomfort.

Pain Threshold Level of intensity at which pain becomes appreciable or perceptible.

Pain Tolerance Level of intensity or duration of pain that a person is willing to endure.

Palliative Care Control of the symptoms rather than cure.

Palpation Physical examination technique that uses the sense of touch to assess texture, temperature, moisture, organ location and size, vibrations and pulsations, swelling, masses, and tenderness.

Pansexual Crosses all sexual proclivities.

Papanicolaou Test Smear method of examining stained exfoliative cells.

Paracentesis Aspiration of fluid from the abdominal cavity.

Paradigm Pattern, model, or mind-set that strongly influences one's decisions and behaviors.

Paradigm Revolution Turmoil experienced by a discipline when a competing paradigm gains acceptance over the dominant, prevailing paradigm.

Paradigm Shift Acceptance of a competing paradigm over the prevailing paradigm.

Parasomnia Sleep alteration resulting from activation of physiological systems at inappropriate times during the sleep-wake cycle.

Paraverbal Communication The way in which a person speaks, including voice tone, pitch, and inflection.

Paraverbal Cue Verbal message accompanied by cues, such as tone and pitch of voice, speed, inflection, volume, and other nonlanguage vocalizations.

Parenteral Denoting any medication route other than the alimentary canal (e.g., intravenous, subcutaneous, intramuscular).

Parenteral Nutrition Nutrients bypass the small intestine and enter the blood directly.

Paresthesia Abnormal sensation such as burning, prickling, or tingling.

Parish Nursing An organization whereby a religious or health care system coordinates registered nurses in providing nursing care to members of a church congregation.

Paroxysmal Nocturnal Dyspnea Episode of sudden shortness of breath occurring during sleep.

Partial Thickness Wound Wound involving the epidermis and part of the dermis.

Participative Leadership Style Leadership style where every person's viewpoints are considered as valuable and have equal voice in making decisions.

Passive Euthanasia Process of cooperating with the client's dying process.

Passive Immunity Immunity that is acquired by the introduction of preformed antibodies.

Passive Range of Motion Range-of-motion exercises performed by the nurse for the dependent client.

Patency Openness of tube lock or bodily passageway.

Paternalism Practice by which health care providers decide what is "best" for clients and then attempt to coerce clients to act against their own choices.

Pathogen Microorganism that causes disease.

Pathogenicity Ability of a microorganism to cause disease.

Patient-Controlled Analgesia (PCA) Device that allows the client to control the delivery of intravenous or subcutaneous pain medication in a safe, effective manner through a programmable pump.

Patient-Focused Care Specific approach to care delivery that involves the decentralization of services, physical redesign of units, and cross-training of employees to bring client care and services to the client in order to minimize contacts with large numbers of staff and to increase overall client satisfaction.

Peak Plasma Level Achievement of the highest blood concentration of a single drug dose until the elimination rate equals the rate of absorption.

Peer Evaluation Process by which professionals provide critical performance appraisal and feedback that is geared toward corrective action.

Peer Review Chart review by a peer to assess appropriateness of physician treatment and interventions.

Penrose Drain Flexible drain that functions by gravity.

Perceived Social Support Social support that is perceived by the recipient of the support.

Perception Person's sense and understanding of the world.

Percussion Physical examination technique that uses short, tapping strokes on the surface of the skin to create vibrations of underlying organs.

Percutaneous When an action is effected through the layers of the skin.

Performance Improvement Activities and behaviors that each individual does to meet customers' expectations.

Perineal Care Cleansing of the external genitalia, perineum, and surrounding area.

Perioperative Refers to the management and treatment of the surgical client during the three phases of surgery: preop-erative, intraoperative, and postoperative.

Peripherally Inserted Central Catheters (PICC) Large-bore catheters inserted into large vessels and are used for (1) specific types of prolonged IV therapy or (2) to administer fluids that are damaging to the vessels (e.g., chemotherapy).

Peristalsis Coordinated, rhythmic, serial contraction of the smooth muscles of the gastrointestinal tract.

Permeability Capability of a substance, molecule, or ion to diffuse through a membrane.

Person One of the four metaparadigm concepts in nursing that refers to the individual, family, or group who are the interest of nursing.

Personal Digital Assistants (PDA) Handheld wireless computer devices.

Personal Protective Equipment Clothing and equipment worn to provide a barrier between the hazard and an individual.

Petrissage Massage technique using squeezing, kneading, and rolling movements to release muscle tension and stimulate circulation.

Phagocytosis Process by which certain cells engulf and dispose of foreign bodies.

Phantom Limb Pain Neuropathic pain in which pain sensations are referred to an area from which an extremity has been amputated.

Pharmacodynamics Effects that the medication causes at the site of action in the body; includes biochemical changes, functional changes, and therapeutic and nontherapeutic effects.

Pharmacokinetics Study of the absorption, distribution, metabolism, and excretion of drugs.

Phenomenon Observable fact or event that can be perceived through the senses and is susceptible to description and explanation.

Phenomenology A type of philosophy used in qualitative research whereby the approach (methods) to research is considered.

Phenylketonuria (PKU) Genetic disorder that can lead to impaired intellectual functioning if untreated.

Philosophy Statement of beliefs that is the foundation for one's thoughts and actions.

Phlebitis Inflammation of a vein.

Phlebotomist Individual who performs venipuncture.

Phospholipids Composed of one or more fatty acid molecules and one phosphoric acid radical, and usually contain a nitrogenous base.

Physical Agent Factor in the environment capable of causing disease in a host.

Physical Dependence Reaction of the body to abrupt discontinuation of a medication; also known as withdrawal syndrome.

Physical Restraints Manual methods or physical equipment attached to the client to reduce the client's movement.

Phytonutrients Chemical found in plants.

PIE Charting Documentation method using problem, intervention, evaluation (PIE) format.

Piggybacked Addition of an intravenous solution to infuse concurrently with another infusion.

Piloerection Hairs standing on end as a result of the body's decrease in body temperature.

Plaintiff Party who initiates a lawsuit that seeks damages or other relief.

Planning Third step of the nursing process; includes the formulation of guidelines that establish the proposed course of nursing action in the resolution of nursing diagnoses and the development of the client's plan of care.

Plan of Care Written guide that organizes data about a client's care into a formal statement of the strategies that will be implemented to help the client achieve optimal health.

Plateau Level at which a drug's blood concentration is maintained.

Pleura Lining of the chest cavity.

Pleural Friction Rub Heard on either inspiration or expiration over anterior lateral lungs as a continuous creaking, grating sound.

Pneumatic Compression Device Device that provides intermittent compression cycles to the veins of the extremities to promote circulation.

Pneumothorax Collection of air or gas in the pleural space, causing the lungs to collapse.

Point-of-Care Charting Documentation system that allows health care providers to gain immediate access to client information at the bedside.

Poison Any substance that causes an alteration such as injury or death in the client's health when inhaled, injected, ingested, or absorbed by the body.

Political Action Teams Often developed within professional organizations to analyze or address a particular policy issue of concern.

Politics Way in which people try to influence decision making, especially decisions about the use of resources.

Polyp A small, abnormal growth of tissue.

Polypharmacy Concurrent use of several different medications.

Polysaccharide Complex sugar.

Polyunsaturated Fatty Acids Fatty acids that have many carbons unbonded to hydrogen atoms.

Port-a-Cath A port that has been implanted under the skin with a catheter inserted into the superior vena cava or right atrium through the subclavian or internal jugular vein.

Portal of Entry Pathway by which infectious agents gain access to the body.

Portal of Exit Pathway by which pathogens leave the body of a host.

Positive Nitrogen Balance Condition that exists when nitrogen intake exceeds output and protein anabolism exceeds catabolism.

Possible Nursing Diagnosis Nursing diagnosis that indicates a situation exists in which a problem could arise unless preventive action is taken; or a "hunch" or intuition by the nurse that cannot be confirmed or eliminated until more data have been collected. It is composed of the diagnostic label and related factors.

Postoperative (after surgery) Begins when the client leaves the operating room and is taken to a postanesthesia care unit; this phase continues until the client is discharged from the care of the surgeon.

Postural Drainage A technique of positioning that promotes gravity drainage of specific lung lobes.

Power Ability to do or act, resulting in the achievement of desired results.

Prana The flow of life energy referred to in the practice of yoga.

Preadolescence Developmental stage from the ages of approximately 10 to 12 years.

Pre-Albumin Precursor of albumin.

Precapillary Sphincters Smooth muscles surrounding the smallest arterioles that control blood flow through the capillary beds.

Predictive Value The ability of screening test results to correctly identify the disease state, such as a true-positive correctly identifies persons who actually have the disease, whereas a true-negative correctly identifies persons who do not actually have the disease.

Preferred Provider Organization (PPO) Type of managed care model in which member choice is limited to providers within the system.

Prenatal Period Developmental stage beginning with conception and ending with birth.

Preoperative (Before surgery) Refers to the time interval that begins when the decision is made for surgery until the client is transferred to the operating room.

Presbycusis Hearing loss associated with old age.

Presbyopia The inability of the lens to change shape causing the farsightedness of the middle years.

Preschool Stage Developmental stage from the ages of 3 to 6 years.

Prescriptive Authority Legal recognition of the ability to prescribe medications.

Presence The process of "just being" with another; a thera peutic nursing intervention.

Pressing A conflict resolution approach where there is an exchange for support or acquiescence relative to the decision in question.

Pressure/Shear Force Deep wounds caused by prolonged pressure and exposure to sliding force.

Pressure Ulcer Localized area of tissue necrosis that develops when soft tissue is compressed between a bony prominence and an external surface for a prolonged period of time; also known as bedsore or decubitus ulcer.

Primary Care Provider Health care provider whom a client sees first for health care; typically, a family practitioner (physician/nurse), internist, or pediatrician.

Primary Health Care Client's point of entry into the health care system; includes assessment, diagnosis, treatment, coordination of care, education, preventive services, and surveillance.

Primary Intention Healing Healing process of a wound with minimal tissue loss and well-approximated edges; occurs with minimal granulation tissue and scarring.

Primary Source Major provider of information about client; research article written by one or more researchers.

prn (As Necessary) Orders Prescribed actions that are implemented according to circumstances.

Proactive Initiating change rather than responding to change imposed by others.

Problem-Oriented Medical Record (POMR) Documentation focused on the client's problem with a structured, logical format to narrative charting called

SOAP (subjective and objective data, assessment, plan).

Procedures Specific step-by-step evidence-based directions on how to perform a specific clinical activity or technical skill.

Process Series of steps or acts that lead to accomplishment of a goal or purpose.

Process Evaluation Measurement of nursing actions by examination of each phase of the nursing process.

Process Improvement Process that examines the flow of client care between departments in order to ensure that the processes work as they were designed and that acceptable levels of performance are achieved.

Prodromal Stage Time interval from the onset of non-specific symptoms until specific symptoms of the infectious agent begin to manifest themselves.

Profession Group (vocational or occupational) that requires specialized education and intellectual knowledge.

Professional Organizations Members engaged in the same professional pursuit, often with similar goals and concerns.

Professional Regulation Process by which nursing ensures that its members act in the public interest by providing a unique service that society has entrusted to them.

Professional Standards Authoritative statements developed by the profession by which quality of practice, service, and/or education can be judged.

Progressive Muscle Relaxation - Stress management technique involving tensing and relaxing muscles.

Proliferative Phase Second phase of wound healing in which there is rapid regeneration of new tissue cells.

Proposition Statement that proposes a relationship between concepts.

Proprietary Agencies Private organizations that were not tax-exempt, and their profits did not have to be reinvested into the agency but could be used to reward investors.

Proprioception Awareness of posture, movement, and changes in equilibrium and the knowledge of position, weight, and resistance of objects in relation to the body.

Prosody Melody of speech that conveys meaning through changes in the tempo, rhythm, and intonation.

Prospective Payment System (PPS) Reimbursement for client care according to the client's diagnosis.

Prospective Study A study that actively follows subjects over the period of the study and does not rely on data collected retrospectively, except as background information.

Proteins Organic compounds of amino acid polymers connected by peptide bonds that contain carbon, hydrogen, oxygen, and nitrogen.

Protocol Series of standing orders or procedures that should be followed under certain specific conditions.

Proxemics Study of the distance between people and objects.

Psychomotor Domain Area of learning that involves performance of motor skills.

Psychoneuroimmunology Study of the complex relationship between the cognitive, affective, and physical aspects of humans.

Puberty Appearance of secondary sex characteristics that signals the beginning of adolescence.

Public Law Law that deals with an individual's relationship to the state.

Pulse Bounding of blood flow in an artery that is palpable at various points on the body.

Pulse Deficit Condition in which the apical pulse rate is greater than the radial pulse rate.

Pulse Oximeter Sensor device used to measure the oxygen saturation level of blood.

Pulse Oximetry The use of an oximeter to determine the oxygen saturation of blood.

Pulse Pressure Measurement of the ratio of stroke volume to compliance (total distensibility) of the arterial system.

Pulse Quality Refers to the "feel" of the pulse, its rhythm and forcefulness.

Pulse Rate Indirect measurement of cardiac output obtained by counting the number of apical or peripheral pulse waves over a pulse point.

Pulse Rhythm Regularity of the heartbeat.

Pulse Volume Measurement of the strength or amplitude of the force exerted by the ejected blood against the arterial wall with each contraction.

Purpose Having a sense of meaning and purpose in life.

Purulent Exudate Thick discharge composed of leuko-cytes, liquefied dead tissue debris, and dead and living bacteria; also known as pus.

Pyogenic Bacteria Bacteria that produce pus.

Pyorrhea Periodontal disease.

Pyrexia When heat production exceeds heat loss and body temperature rises above the normal range.

Pyrogens Bacteria, viruses, fungi, and some antigens.

Pyuria Pus (white blood cells) in the urine.

Qualitative Analysis Integration and synthesis of narrative, nonnumerical data.

Qualitative Research Systematic collection and analysis of subjective narrative materials, using procedures for which there tends to be a minimum of research-imposed control.

Quality Meeting or exceeding requirements of the client.

Quality Assurance Framework Traditional approach to quality management in which monitoring and evaluation focus on individual performance, deviation from standards, and problem solving.

Quality Improvement A process for change using a multidisciplinary approach to problem identification and resolution.

Quantitative Research Systematic collection of numerical information, often under conditions of considerable control.

Quasi-Experimental Design A method of statistical analysis that is a modified experiment where control or randomization is not possible, so that all subjects have some exposure to the independent variable.

Race Grouping of people based on biologic similarities such as physical characteristics.

Racism Discrimination directed toward individuals who are misperceived to be inferior because of biologic factors.

Radiation Loss of heat in the form of infrared rays.

Radiofrequency Ablation The delivery of low-voltage, high-frequency, alternating electrical current to cauterize the abnormal myocardial tissue.

Radiography Study of x-rays or gamma-ray-exposed film through the action of ionizing radiation.

Range of Motion (ROM) Extent to which a joint can move.

Rapid Relaxation Response (RRR) A useful coping method that is similar to transcendental meditation. The person selects a mantra, a word or phrase that can be used repetitively to help manage symptoms or unwanted emotions.

Rapport Bond or connection between two people that is based on mutual trust.

Rationale Explanation based on the theories and scientific principles of natural and behavioral sciences and the humanities.

Readiness for Learning Evidence of willingness to learn.

Receiver Person who intercepts the sender's message.

Recent Memory The result of events that have occurred over the past 24 hours.

Receptive Aphasia The ability to speak well, but the inability to understand the message that is spoken.

Recommended Dietary Allowances (RDA) Recommended allowances of essential nutrients established by the Food and Nutritional Academy of Sciences–National Research Council.

Recurrent Acute Pain Discomfort marked by cycles of repetitive pain episodes that alternate with pain-free intervals; this pain may recur over a prolonged period or throughout a person's lifetime.

Red Cell Indices Laboratory measurement of the size and hemoglobin content of the red cells.

Red Wound Wound in the proliferative phase of repair.

Referred Pain Discomfort from the internal organs that is felt in another area of the body.

Reflexology A system of massage in which the feet and hands are massaged in an attempt to favorably influence other body functions.

Reframing Technique of monitoring negative thoughts and replacing them with positive ones.

Regeneration Method of tissue repair in which lost tissue is replaced with no cosmetic or functional deficit.

Regional Anesthesia Anesthesia that causes the client to lose sensation in a particular area of the body (e.g., laparo-scope for a tubal sterilization).

Regurgitation Backward flow of blood through a diseased heart valve, also known as insuffiency.

Rehabilitate To restore to a normal, healthy, or highest level of functioning possible.

Reiki A form of energy work that was founded in the 1800s when Mikao Usui studied a tradition of using hands for healing by Buddhist monks.

Reincarnation A belief that one will be reborn in another form of life after own physical death.

Relaxation Response State of increased arousal of the parasympathetic nervous system that leads to a relaxed physiological state.

Relaxation Techniques Methods used to decrease anxiety and muscle tension.

Religion A system of beliefs and practices that usually involves a community of like-minded people.

Relocation Stress Syndrome A nursing diagnosis that applies when a client experiences physiological and psychological symptoms when moved to a different environment.

Remote Memory The retention of experiences that occurred during earlier periods of life.

Research Systematic method of exploring, describing, explaining, relating, or establishing the existence of a phenomenon, the factors that cause changes in the phenomenon, and how the phenomenon influences other phenomena.

Research Design Overall plan used to conduct research.

Reservoir (or Source) A place for an organism to live while awaiting a host.

Resident Flora Microorganisms that are always present, usually without altering the client's health.

Resident Infectious Agents Microorganisms that are always present on skin and can be reduced through hand-washing, but not totally removed.

Residual The amount of substance left during and after the organ's normal functioning (e.g., the amount of fluids remaining in the stomach during and after tube feeding).

Respiration The act of breathing.

Respirator Protective devices worn to protect the respiratory tract from exposure to inhalation hazards.

Rest State of relaxation and calmness, both mental and physical.

Restorative Nursing Care Nursing care provided to clients who have residual impairment as a result of disease or injury; seeks to increase the client's independence and ability to perform self-care.

Restraints Protective devices used to limit the physical activity of a client or to immobilize a client or extremity.

Restrictive Pulmonary Disease A category of lung diseases characterized by impaired mobility or elasticity of the lungs or chest wall.

Retrospective Studies Studies involving existing data usually found in medical records or client care records.

Review of Systems A brief account of any recent signs or symptoms related to any body system.

Rhonchi Heard predominantly on expiration over the trachea and bronchi as a continuous, low-pitched musical sound.

Rigor Mortis Stiffening of the body after death caused by contraction of the skeletal and smooth muscles.

Risk for Infection State in which an individual is at increased risk for being invaded by pathogenic organisms.

Risk Nursing Diagnosis Nursing diagnosis that indicates that a problem does not yet exist but specific risk factors are present; composed of the diagnostic label preceded by the phrase "Risk for" with the specific risk factors listed.

Role Set of expected behaviors associated with a person's status or position.

Role Competence The family member's ability to perform a role.

Role Conflict When the expectations of one role compete with the expectations of other roles.

Role Overload A form of role stress or strain that occurs when the family member lacks the time, resources, or energy to perform the role.

Role Strain A subjective personal response of psychological distress in which an individual anticipates or has an actual inability to satisfactorily perform a role.

Role Stress A condition of role expectations that is likely to contribute to family or individual dysfunction.

Role Transition Changes in role assignment for developmental, situational, or illness-related reasons.

Rolfing A form of deep tissue massage and manipulation to correct body posture.

Rounds Reporting method; care team members walk to clients' rooms and discuss care and progress with each other and with the clients.

Routes of Exposure Methods by which chemicals and other potentially hazardous substances are assimilated into the body (e.g., inhalation, ingestion, injection).

Rules and Regulations Provide specific guidance for implementation of a law.

Saccharides Sugar units.

Satiety Feeling of fulfillment from food.

Saturated Fatty Acids Glycerol esters of organic acids whose atoms are joined by a single-valence bond.

Scar Formation Method of repair involving replacement of lost tissue with connective tissue and an epithelial cover.

School-Age Period Developmental stage from the ages of 6 to 12 years.

Scope of Practice Legal boundaries of practice for health care providers as defined in state statutes.

Sebum Substance produced by the skin to kill bacteria.

Secondary Gain Outcomes of the sick role other than alleviation of anxiety (primary gain); examples include gaining attention and sympathy, avoiding responsibilities, and receiving financial compensation or reward.

Secondary Intention Healing Healing process of a wound that has extensive tissue loss and poorly approximated edges; occurs with gradual tissue replacement and scarring.

Secondary Source Source of data other than the client, family members, other health care providers, or medical records; article in which an author addresses the research of someone else.

Self-Care Learned behavior and a deliberate action in response to a need.

Self-Care Deficit State in which an individual is not able to perform one or more activities of daily living.

Self-Concept Individual's perception of self; includes self-esteem, body image, and ideal self.

Self-Efficacy Belief in one's ability to succeed; according to social cognitive theory of learning, this serves as an internal motivator for change.

Self-Esteem Individual's perception of self-worth; includes judgments about one's self and one's capabilities.

Self-Ideal The perception of behavior based on personal standards and self-expectations.

Semipermeable Selective permeability of membranes.

Sender Person who generates a message.

Sensation The ability to receive and process stimuli received through the sensory organs.

Sensitivity Determines the susceptibility of a pathogen to an antibiotic; the ability of a test to correctly identify those individuals who have the disease.

Sensitizer Chemical or substance that causes allergy in susceptible individuals.

Sensory Deficit A change in the perception of sensory stimuli.

Sensory Deprivation A state of reduced sensory input from the internal or external environment, manifested by alterations in sensory perceptions.

Sensory Overload Increased perception of the intensity of auditory and visual stimuli.

Sensory Perception The ability to receive sensory impressions and, through cortical association, relate the stimuli to past experiences to form an impression of the nature of the stimulus.

Sentinel Event Unexpected event involving client death or serious injury; includes near misses.

Serous Exudate Watery discharge composed primarily of serum, with a low protein count.

Servant Leadership Leadership that is based on the needs of others and on helping those served.

Sex Roles Culturally determined patterns associated with being male or female.

Sexual Dysfunction Physical inability to perform sexually, but can also be a psychological inability to perform sexually.

Sexual Health Ability to form mutually consensual, developmental-appropriate sexual relationships that are safe and respectful of self and others; includes emotional, physical, and psychological components.

Sexuality Human characteristic that refers not just to gender but to all the aspects of being male or female, including feelings, attitudes, beliefs, and behavior.

Sexually Transmitted Infections (STIs) Formerly known as sexually transmitted diseases (STDs); infections most notably transmitted via sexual activity, including any oral, anal, vaginal, or penile activity.

Sexual Orientation Individual's preference for ways of expressing sexual feelings.

Shaman Folk healer-priest who uses natural and supernatural forces to help others.

Shamanism Practice of entering altered states of consciousness with the intent of helping others.

Shear Force Forces exerted against the skin by movement or repositioning.

Shiatsu A combination of acupressure, massage, and joint manipulation.

Short-Term Outcome Statement written in objective format demonstrating an expectation to be achieved in resolution of the nursing diagnosis in a short period of time, usually a few hours or days.

Shunting Condition in which alveolar regions are well-perfused but not adequately ventilated.

Sick Role A set of social expectations met by an ill person, such as being exempt from the usual social role responsibilities and being obligated to get well and to seek competent help.

Side Effects Mild nontherapeutic drug effect.

Signal-Averaged Electrocardiography (SAECG) Surface ECG that amplifies late potentials.

Simultaneity Paradigm Nursing viewpoint that focuses on the quality of life from the client's perspective and conceptualizes the interaction between person and environment as mutual and simultaneous.

Single-Payer System Health care delivery model in which the government is the only entity to reimburse.

Single Point of Entry Entry into the health care system is required through a point designated by the plan.

Situational Leadership Style of leadership in which there is a blending of styles based on current circumstances and events.

Situational Loss Occurs in response to external events, usually beyond the individual's control (such as the death of a significant other).

Situational Role Transitions Changes that are made in role when families experience the addition or loss of a family member.

Skin Absorption Route of exposure whereby exposure to chemical or biologic substances occurs via passage through the skin barrier.

Skin Contact Route of exposure whereby exposure to chemical or biologic substances occurs via contact with skin.

Skinfold Measurement Measures the amount of body fat.

Skin Shear Result of dragging skin across a hard surface.

Skin Tear Superficial skin lesion that occurs when the superficial layers of the skin separate from the underlying tissues.

Skin Turgor Normal resiliency of the skin.

Sleep State of altered consciousness during which an individual experiences fluctuations in level of consciousness, minimal physical activity, and a general slowdown of the body's physiological processes.

Sleep Apnea A syndrome in which breathing periodically ceases during sleep, often associated with heavy snoring.

Sleep Cycle Sequence of sleep that begins with the four stages of no rapid eye movement (NREM) sleep, a return to stage 3, then stage 2, and then passage into the first rapid eye movement (REM) stage.

Sleep Deprivation Prolonged inadequate quality and quantity of sleep.

Sleep Paralysis Experience of waking from sleep and being unable to move, speak, or cry out.

Slough Necrotic (dead) tissue that is gray, yellow, or white and usually soft.

Small-Group Ecology Study of proxemics in small-group situations.

Smart Card A computerized disk that stores client information.

Snellen Chart A chart of graduating black letters that test visual acuity.

SOAP Charting Documentation method using subjective data, objective data, assessment, and plan.

Social Marketer A role that uses marketing techniques and skills to promote healthy living as well as health promotion programs.

Social Support Providing for people in a social network.

Solute A substance dissolved in a solution; also called analyte.

Solvent A liquid with a substance in solution.

Somatic Pain Nonlocalized discomfort originating in tendons, ligaments, and nerves.

Somnambulism Sleepwalking.

Source-Oriented (SO) Charting Narrative recording by each member (source) of the health care team on a separate record.

Spasticity Increase in muscle tension.

Specific Gravity Weight of urine compared with weight of distilled water; a specific gravity greater than 1.000 indicates solutes in the urine.

Specificity The ability of a test to correctly identify those individuals who do not have the disease.

Spherocytes Small, thick red cells.

Spiritual Distress The client's perception that his belief system, or his place within it, is threatened.

Spirituality Relationship with one's self, a sense of connection with others, and a relationship with a higher power or divine source.

Spores Single-celled microorganisms or microorganisms in the resting or inactive stage.

Sprain Trauma to ligaments, tendons, or bones around joint caused by twisting or pulling.

Stagnation A sense of nonmeaning in one's life.

Standard of Care Delineates the extent and character of the nurse's duty to the client; defined by organizational policy or professional standards of practice.

Standard Precautions Guidelines recommended by the Centers for Disease

Control and Prevention to reduce the risk of infection.

Standing Order Standardized intervention written, approved, and signed by a physician that is kept on file within health care agencies to be used in predictable situations or in circumstances requiring immediate attention.

Stat Order An order for a single dose of medication to be given immediately.

Statutory Law Laws enacted by legislative bodies.

Stenosis Narrowing or constriction of a blood vessel or valve.

Stereognosis Ability to identify objects by manipulation and touch.

Stereotyping Belief that all people within the same racial, ethnic, or cultural group act alike and share the same beliefs and attitudes.

Sterilization Total elimination of all microorganisms including spores.

Stock Supplied Medications dispensed and labeled in large quantities for storage in the medication room or nursing unit.

Stoma Surgically created opening.

Stomatitis Inflammation of the oral mucosa.

Stool Fecal material.

Straight Holistic term for a person who has sexual contact and engages in intimate relationships with people of the opposite gender.

Strain Stretch injury of muscles, tendons, or ligaments.

Stress Body's reaction to any stimulus.

Stressor Any stimulus encountered by an individual; leads to the need to adapt.

Stress Test Measures the client's cardiovascular response to exercise tolerance.

Stress Urinary Incontinence Uncontrolled loss of urine caused by physical exertion in the absence of a bladder contraction.

Striae Red or silver-white streaks over the breasts or axillae.

Stridor Heard predominantly on inspiration as a continuous crowing sound.

Stroke Volume Measurement of blood that enters the aorta with each ventricular contraction.

Structure A domain in Donabedian's quality assurance model encompassing the integrity of the infrastructure within the health care organization (e.g., physical environment, human resources).

Structure Evaluation Determination of the health care agency's ability to provide the services offered to its client population.

Subacute Care Short-term aggressive care that emphasizes restorative interventions before the client's reentry into the community.

Subculture Group of people with characteristic patterns of behavior that distinguish it from the larger culture or society.

Subcutaneous (SC/SQ) Injection into the subcutaneous tissue.

Subjective Data Data from the client's point of view, including feelings, perceptions, and concerns.

Sublingual Under the tongue.

Substitution Replacing a particular substance with a less hazardous alternative.

Superficial Wound Wound confined to the epidermis layer.

Supination Turning a body part upward.

Supplemental Recommendation Area of noncompli-ance is identified during a JCAHO survey, not as serious as a Type I; must be resolved in a timely fashion.

Suppository A substance specifically designed to insert into a bodily orifice other than the mouth (anus, vagina, urethra). The suppository is typically composed of a vehicle containing a medication.

Suppression Conscious defense mechanism whereby a person decides to avoid dealing with a stressor at the present time.

Suppuration Formation of pus, or purulent exudate.

Surfactant Phospholipid secreted by Type II alveolar cells that reduces the alveolar surface tension and thus helps prevent alveolar collapse.

Surgical Asepsis Practices that eliminate all microorgan-isms from an object or area.

Survey Method Those studies that involve surveying the subjects in a research study for responses to given questions or statements.

Susceptible Host Person who lacks resistance to an agent and is therefore vulnerable to disease.

Sustained Release Specially coated medication that allows for slow, controlled absorption over an extended period of time.

Suture Surgical means of closing a wound by sewing, wiring, or stapling.

Symmetrical (Egalitarian) Family Power Power that is shared between family members.

Synergy Combined power of many people.

Synthesis Putting data together in a new way.

Systemic Infection Infection that affects the entire body with involvement of multiple organs.

Systole Process of cardiac chamber emptying or ejecting blood.

Tachycardia A heart rate in excess of 100 beats per minute in an adult.

Tachypnea Respiratory rate greater than 24 breaths per minute.

Tactile Fremitus Vibrations created by sound waves.

Tao A spiritual belief system (with its roots in China) that is ascribed to the oneness of all things in nature.

Tapotement Massage technique using a light tapping of the fingers that stimulates movement in tired muscles.

Target Organ Chemicals Chemicals that have health effects on a particular organ.

Taxonomy of Nursing Diagnoses Type of classification where the diagnostic label is grouped according to which human response the client demonstrates to the actual or perceived stressor.

Teaching Active process in which one individual shares information with another as a means to facilitate behavioral changes.

Teaching-Learning Process Planned interaction promoting a behavioral change that is not a result of maturation or coincidence.

Teaching Strategies Techniques employed by the teacher to promote learning.

Team Group of individuals who work together to achieve a common goal.

Telecare Nursing care and community support to clients at a distance.

Telehealth Using telecommunication and information technology to provide health care at a distance from the care setting.

Telemedicine The delivery of medical care via computerized equipment.

Telenursing The delivery of nursing care via computerized equipment.

Teleology Ethical theory that states that the moral value of a situation is determined by its consequences.

Teratogen Anything that adversely affects normal cellular development in the embryo or fetus.

Teratogenic Substance Substance that can cross the placental barrier and impair normal growth and development.

Termination Phase Third and final stage of the therapeutic relationship; focuses on evaluation of goal achievement and effectiveness of treatment.

Tertiary Intention Healing Healing process of a wound in which primary closure of a wound is undesirable; occurs when circulation is poor or when infection is present.

Testicular Self-Exam (TSE) Systematic palpation of the testicles by a man on himself for the purpose of finding lumps that potentially may be cancerous; should be done monthly after a hot shower.

Testimony Written or verbal evidence given by a qualified expert in an area.

Thallium Radionuclide that is the physiological analogue of potassium.

Theory Set of concepts and propositions that provide an orderly way to view phenomena.

Therapeutic Describes actions that are beneficial to the client.

Therapeutic Communication Use of communication for the purpose of creating a beneficial outcome for the client.

Therapeutic Massage Application of pressure and motion by the hands with the intent of improving the recipient's well-being.

Therapeutic Procedure Incidents Accidents that occur during the delivery of medical or nursing interventions.

Therapeutic Range Achievement of a constant therapeutic blood level of a medication within a safe range.

Therapeutic Relationship Relationship that benefits the client's health status.

Therapeutic Touch Holistic technique that consists of assessing alterations in a person's energy fields and using the hands to direct energy to achieve a balanced state.

Therapeutic Use of Self Process in which nurses deliberately plan their actions and approach the relationship with a specific goal in mind before interacting with the client.

Thermoregulation Body's physiological function of heat regulation to maintain a constant internal body temperature.

Thoracentesis The aspiration of fluids from the pleural cavity.

Thrills Vibrations that feel similar to a purring cat.

Thrombus Blood clot.

Throughput Input from the community that is processed.

Toddler Developmental stage beginning at approximately 12 to 18 months of age, when a child begins to walk, and ending at approximately age 3.

Tolerance Phenomenon of requiring larger and larger doses of an analgesic to achieve the same level of pain relief.

Tort Civil wrong committed upon a person or property stemming from a direct invasion of some legal right of the person, the infraction of some public duty, or the violation of some private obligation by which damages accrue to the person.

Tort Law Enforcement of duties and rights among individuals independent of contractual agreements.

Totality Paradigm Nursing viewpoint that conceptualizes the interaction between person and environment as constant in order to accomplish goals and maintain balance.

Total Parenteral Nutrition Intravenous infusion of a solution containing dextrose, amino acids, fats, essential fatty acids, vitamins, and minerals.

Total Quality Management Method of management and system operation that is used to achieve continuous quality improvement.

Touch Means of perceiving or experiencing through tactile sensation.

Toxic Effect Reaction that occurs when the body cannot metabolize a drug, causing the drug to accumulate in the blood.

Tracheotomy A surgical procedure in which an opening (stoma) is made through the anterior neck into the trachea; an artificial airway (tracheostomy tube) is placed into the stoma.

Transcendence Finding meaning larger than the person's individual self and life.

Transcultural Nursing Formal area of study and practice focused on comparative analysis of different cultures and subcultures with respect to cultural care, health and illness beliefs, and values and practices, with the goal of providing health care within the context of the client's culture.

Transcutaneous Electrical Nerve Stimulation (TENS) Method of applying minute amounts of electrical stimulation to large-diameter nerve fibers via electrodes placed on the skin to block the passage of pain to the dorsal spinal root.

Transdermal Absorption through the skin into the systemic circulation.

Transducer Instrument that converts electrical energy to sound waves.

Transferrin (nonheme iron) Combination of a blood protein and iron.

Transformational Leadership Leadership that promotes the end values of justice, equality, and human rights, as well as endorses the modal values of honesty, loyalty, and fairness.

Transgender Person who dresses and engages in roles of the person of the opposite gender.

Transient Flora Microorganisms that attach to the skin for a brief period of time but do not continuously live on the skin.

Transient Infectious Agents Those microorganisms that are picked up by the skin from another person or object.

Transmission-Based Precautions Precautions designed for clients documented or suspected to be infected with highly transmissible pathogens for which additional precautions beyond Standard Precautions are needed.

Transsexual Belief that one is psychologically of the sex opposite own anatomical gender.

Transvestite Person who dresses as the opposite gender than birth gender.

Trigger Point Hypersensitive point in a muscle, ligament, fascia, or joint capsule that when stimulated causes a local twitch or jump response.

Triglycerides Lipid compounds consisting of three fatty acids and a glycerol molecule.

Trocar Large-bored abdominal paracentesis needle.

Troponin Cardiac-specific proteins involved in muscle contraction.

Trough A groove or channel in which substances may travel through.

T-Tube Artificial drain placed in the common bile duct during surgery.

Tunneling Areas of soft tissue destruction underlying intact skin that extend in one direction (usually at right angles) from the primary ulcer bed.

Tympany A low-pitched sound of long duration.

Type and Crossmatch Laboratory test that identifies the client's blood type (e.g., A or B) and determines the compatibility of the blood between potential donor and recipient.

Type I Recommendation Typically the most serious finding during JCAHO survey process; requires resolution of deficiency within a specified time frame.

Ultrasound Use of high-frequency sound waves instead of x-ray film to visualize deep body structures; also called an echogram.

Uncomplicated Grief A fairly predictable grief reaction following a significant loss, ending with the relinquishing of the lost object and resumption of the previous life.

Understaffing Failure of a facility to provide a sufficient number of professional staff to meet the needs of their clients.

Unified Nursing Language System (UNLS) A language system developed by the American Nurses Association in 1991 that encompasses common nursing terms from a variety of vocabularies that can be used interchangeably as synonyms for the same concept.

Unintentional Wound Wound resulting from trauma or accident.

Unit Dose Form System of packaging and labeling each dose of medication, usually for a 24-hour period.

Unprofessional Conduct Conduct that could adversely affect the health and welfare of the public.

Unsaturated Fatty Acids Glycerol esters of organic acids whose atoms are joined by double or triple valence bonds.

Urgency Timely intervention of surgery.

Urge Urinary Incontinence Uncontrolled discharge of urine caused by hyperactive (unstable) contractions of the detrusor muscle.

Urinalysis Laboratory analysis of the urine.

Urinary Incontinence Uncontrolled loss of urine of sufficient duration and volume to create a social or hygienic problem.

Urinary Retention Inability to completely evacuate the bladder.

Urobilinogen Derived from the normal bacterial action of intestinal flora on bilirubin.

Urodynamics A set of tests that measure bladder and surrounding abdominal pressures.

Utility Ethical principle that states that an act must result in the greatest amount of good for the greatest number of people involved in a situation.

Vaccination Inoculation with a vaccine to produce immunity against specific diseases.

Value Variation of the variable.

Values Principles that influence the development of beliefs and attitudes.

Values Clarification Process of analyzing one's own values to better understand what is truly important to oneself.

Variable Anything that may differ from the norm.

Variations Goals not met or interventions not performed according to the time frame; also called variance.

Vasoconstriction The narrowing of the vessels, usually leading to reduced blood flow.

Vasodilation The widening of the vessels, usually leads to increased blood flow.

Vector-Borne Transmission Mode of transmission of disease through animate objects.

Vehicle Transmission Mode of transmission of disease through inanimate objects.

Venipuncture Puncturing of a vein with a needle to aspirate blood.

Venography Radiographic study of the venous system of the lower extremities following the injection of an iodine contrast agent.

Venous Access Devices (VAD) Venous catheters made of different types of materials and available in single, double, triple, or even quadruple lumens.

Venous Ulcers Lower extremity ulcers caused by chronic venous insufficiency and the resultant fragility of the tissues.

Ventilation Movement of air into and out of the lungs for the purpose of delivering fresh air to the alveoli.

Ventilation–Perfusion (V/Q) Mismatching Condition in which perfusion and ventilation of the lung areas are not adequately balanced.

Veracity Ethical principle that means that one should be truthful, neither lying nor deceiving others.

Verbal Message Message communicated through words or language, both spoken and written.

Vesicant Medication that causes blisters and tissue injury when it escapes into surrounding tissue.

Vesicular Sounds Soft, breezy, and low-pitched sounds heard longer on inspiration than expiration that result from air moving through the smaller airways over the lung's periphery, with the exception of the scapular area.

Vibration Massage technique using rapid movements that stimulate or relax muscles.

Virulence Degree of pathogenicity of an infectious microorganism (pathogen).

Visceral Pain Discomfort felt in the internal organs.

Visual Channel Transmission of messages through sight, observation, and perception.

Visual Learner A person who learns by processing information by seeing.

Vital Capacity Amount of air exhaled from the lungs after a minimal full inspiration.

Vital Signs Measurement of the client's body temperature (T), pulse (P) rate, respiratory (R) rate, and blood pressure (BP).

Vitamins Organic compounds.

Voiding Process of urine evacuation.

Walking Rounds Reporting method used when the members of the care team walk to each client's room and discuss care and progress with each other and the client.

Water-Soluble Vitamins Vitamins that require daily ingestion in normal quantities because they are not stored in the body.

Wellness Condition in which an individual functions at optimal levels.

Wellness Nursing Diagnosis Nursing diagnosis that indicates the client's expression of a desire to obtain a higher level of wellness in some area of function. It is composed of the diagnostic label preceded by the phrase "potential for enhanced."

Wheezes Heard predominantly on expiration all over the lungs as a continuous sonorous wheeze or sibilant wheeze.

Whistle-blowing Calling attention to the unethical, illegal, or incompetant actions of others.

Withdrawal Syndrome State in which symptoms occur after abrupt discontinuation of a narcotic.

Work of Breathing Amount of muscular energy (work) required to accomplish ventilation.

Working Phase Second stage of the therapeutic relationship in which problems are identified, goals are established, and problem-solving methods are selected.

Wound Disruption in the integrity of a body tissue.

Yellow Wound Wound with fibrinous slough or purulent exudate from bacteria.

Young Adulthood Developmental stage from the ages of 21 to approximately 40 years.

Z-Track Technique Method of intramuscular (IM) injection to seal the medication in the muscle, preventing the drug from irritating the subcutaneous tissue.

Code Legend

NP	**Phases of the Nursing Process**
As	Assessment
An	Analysis
Pl	Planning
Im	Implementation
Ev	Evaluation

CN	**Client Need**
Sa	Safe Effective Care Environment
Sa/1	Management of Care
Sa/2	Safety and Infection Control
He/3	Health Promotion and Maintenance
Ps/4	Psychosocial Integrity
Ph	Physiological Integrity
Ph/5	Basic Care and Comfort
Ph/6	Pharmacological and Parenteral Therapies
Ph/7	Reduction of Risk Potential
Ph/8	Physiological Adaptation

CL	**Cognitive Level**
K	Knowledge
Co	Comprehension
Ap	Application
An	Analysis

SA	**Subject Area**
1	Medical-Surgical
2	Psychiatric and Mental Health
3	Maternity and Women's Health
4	Pediatric
5	Pharmacologic
6	Gerontologic
7	Community Health
8	Legal and Ethical Issues

Practice Test 1

EYE, EAR, NOSE, AND THROAT DISORDERS - COMPREHENSIVE EXAM

1. When preparing a client for an annual eye exam that includes pupil dilation, the nurse should prepare for what drugs to be administered? ________________

2. Which of the following instructions should the nurse give a client following a tonometry?
   1. Wear an eye shield for 24 hours
   2. Take Tylenol every four hours to ease discomfort
   3. Be careful not to rub the eyes for about four hours after the exam
   4. Instill eye drops to protect the eye from light

3. The client is having difficulty removing a hard contact lens prior to an eye exam. When intervening in this situation, the nurse performs which of the following to remove the lens?
   1. Sliding the lens under the upper or lower lid
   2. Lifting an edge with a fingernail
   3. Pressing on the center of the lens
   4. Bringing the eyelid margins toward the edges of the lens

4. When caring for a client with bilateral eye patches, which of the following should the nurse include in this client's plan of care to decrease anxiety?
   1. Touch the client before speaking to him
   2. Explain the plan of care prior to beginning care
   3. Close the door to decrease the noise
   4. Leave the room lights on at all times

5. Which of the following directions should the nurse give when delegating walking a blind client to an unlicensed assistive personnel?
   1. "Let the client take your arm during ambulation."
   2. "Take the client's arm during ambulation."
   3. "Position the client in front and to your side with ambulation."
   4. "Allow the client to ambulate independently as you walk along."
6. After a trauma has occluded the client's vision, which of the following should the nurse implement to promote the client's independence at mealtime?
   1. Ask a volunteer to feed the client
   2. Ask a member of the family to assist with the client at mealtime
   3. Order foods that do not require utensils for cutting
   4. Assist the client to locate the food by comparing the arrangement to the numbers on a clock
7. Which of the following statements by the client indicates the client has bilateral cataracts?
   1. "I have had a gradually diminishing eyesight."
   2. "I have a fullness within the eye."
   3. "My eye hurts."
   4. "I frequently see flashes of light."
8. The nurse assesses which of the following in a client with closed-angle glaucoma?

   Select all that apply:

   [ ] 1. Colored halos around light
   [ ] 2. Blurred vision
   [ ] 3. Photophobia
   [ ] 4. Loss of central vision
   [ ] 5. Itching
   [ ] 6. Eye pain
9. Which of the following should receive priority in the plan of care for a client who had a scleral buckling procedure?
   1. Pain around the eye
   2. Nausea and vomiting
   3. Anxiety about the outcome of surgery
   4. Boredom with the facility routine

10. The nurse should question which of the following drug orders for a client who has glaucoma?
    1. Atropine sulfate
    2. Morphine sulfate
    3. Magnesium sulfate
    4. Ferrous sulfate
11. The client states, "Please bring me something so I can clean my ears." The best response by the nurse would be
    1. "It is best to use the corner of a soapy washcloth."
    2. "Do you prefer a short or long cotton applicator?"
    3. "Have you ever tried removing wax with a hairpin?"
    4. "I can refer you to the physician who will clean them."
12. The nurse should ask a client who complains of ringing in the ears which of the following questions?
    1. "What childhood diseases have you had?"
    2. "Were you born prematurely?"
    3. "Do you eat a well-balanced diet?"
    4. "How much aspirin do you take?"
13. A client with a hearing aid complains of a shrill noise called feedback. The nurse performs which of the following to reduce this problem?
    1. Repositions the hearing aid within the ear
    2. Cleans the hearing aid with a soft cloth
    3. Replaces the battery in the hearing aid
    4. Decreases the volume in the hearing aid
14. The client is taking all of the following drugs and complains of a decrease in hearing.The nurse evaluates which of these drugs to be affecting the hearing?
    1. Acetaminophen (Tylenol)
    2. Propranolol (Inderal)
    3. Gentamicin (Garamycin)
    4. Cimetidine (Tagamet)
15. The nurse assesses the ear canal of a client to be red, swollen, and tender. Which additional assessment findings indicates an infection in the canal?
    1. There is a foul-smelling drainage present
    2. Neck pain
    3. Head hematoma
    4. Cerumen

16. The nurse assesses which of the following clinical manifestations to be present in a client who has an inner ear infection?Select all that apply:
   [ ] 1. Headaches in the morning
   [ ] 2. Sore throat with swallowing
   [ ] 3. Nasal congestion
   [ ] 4. Dizziness
   [ ] 5. Nausea
   [ ] 6. Nystagmus

17. After cataract surgery, a client complains of feeling nauseated. The priority nursing intervention for this client is to
   1. offer dry crackers to eat
   2. instruct the client to deep breathe until the nausea subsides
   3. administer an antiemetic drug
   4. explain that this is a normal occurrence after surgery

18. A client asks the nurse what a hordeolum is. The appropriate response by the nurse is ______________.

19. Before developing a plan of care for a client with a conductive hearing loss, the nurse should consider which of the following?
   1. A hearing aid is generally not necessary
   2. It is permanent and not correctable
   3. The damage occurs in the inner ear
   4. It occurs as a result of the aging process

20. Which of the following should the nurse include in the plan of care for a client with chlamydial conjunctivitis?
   1. Instruct the client on the sexual implications
   2. Administer antihistamines
   3. Administer topical steroids
   4. Instruct the client to use artificial tears

21. Which of the following should the nurse include in the plan of care for a client after a tympanoplasty?
   1. Instruct the client to cough or sneeze with the mouth open
   2. Eliminate the noise in the client's room
   3. Encourage the client to ambulate
   4. Turn down the lights in the client's room

22. A client is admitted with a hearing loss, fever, and a purulent, foul-smelling drainage from the ears. The nurse suspects what disorder? ______________

23. The nurse is reviewing the normal limits of a hearing assessment for a client who presents complaining of a decrease in hearing. Which of the following findings would indicate the need for additional investigation?
    1. Sound heard equally in both ears with the Weber test
    2. Bone conduction greater than air conduction with Rinne test
    3. 25 dB on audiogram
    4. Pearly, shiny, and semitransparent tympanic membrane with an otoscope

24. When obtaining a nursing history from a client who has primary open-angle glaucoma, the nurse expects to find which of the following clinical manifestations?
    1. Seeing floating specks
    2. Loss of peripheral vision
    3. Flashes of light
    4. Intolerance to light

25. When providing care to a client who has had a stapedectomy, the nurse should include which of the following instructions?
    1. "It is a normal reaction for you to feel depressed or angry after losing your hearing."
    2. . The doctor will prescribe a hearing aid for you to help you with the permanent hearing loss."
    3. "Expect a purulent drainage and fever in the post-op period."
    4. "You will experience a decrease in hearing post-op."

ANSWERS AND RATIONALES

1. **Mydriatics.** Mydriatics are drugs used during a routine eye examination to dilate the pupils of the eye. This makes it possible for the inner structures of the eye to be examined.
   NP = Pl
   CN = Ph/6
   CL = Ap
   SA = 5

2. **3.** Eye drops are used prior to tonometry to anesthetize the eye, making the eye more susceptible to injury. Because of this, the client should be

instructed to avoid rubbing the eye for four hours following the examination. There is no discomfort requiring Tylenol following tonometry. Eye drops do not protect the eye from light. An eye shield is not necessary with a tonometry.
NP = Pl
CN = Ph/7
CL = Ap
SA = 1

3. 4. Contact lenses remain in position as a result of the surface tension created by the moisture between the contact lens and the cornea. Techniques for removing a lens involve breaking the seal by allowing air beneath the edge of the lens. Fingernails should never be used because they could damage the cornea. Pressing on the center will not break the tension.
NP = Im
CN = Ph/5
CL = Ap
SA = 1

4. 2. An anxious client may feel threatened when in a strange environment and unable to see. Explaining the care prior to beginning prepares the client for what is planned and allows the client to give input. A client with limited vision should always be spoken to before being touched. Shutting the door would further isolate the client and could increase anxiety if help were needed. Lighting would assist the partially sighted client but not a client who cannot see.
NP = Pl
CN = Ph/8
CL = Ap
SA = 1

5. 1. A client who is blind feels safer and more secure by following the lead sighted person. Having the client who is blind slightly behind and to the side when grasping the sighted person's arm facilitates this. Safety is a higher priority in an unfamiliar environment than independence.
NP = Pl
CN = Sa/1
CL = An
SA = 8

6. 4. Using the example of the numbers on a clock can help the blind client to locate food and to be independent with feeding. Involving others to assist the client will decrease the client's sense of independence. Limiting foods that do not require cutting also may imply that the client has limited independence.

NP = Im
CN = Ph/5
CL = Ap
SA = 1

7. 1. The development of cataracts is a gradual and progressive loss of eyesight.Degeneration of the lens diminishes vision. Fullness or pain is more likely due to trauma or inflammation. Flashes of light are a symptom of a detached retina.
NP = Ev
CN = Ph/8
CL = An
SA = 1

8. 1, 2, 6. Clinical manifestations of closed-angle glaucoma include seeing colored halos around lights, blurred vision, frontal headaches, and eye pain. Itching and burning may indicate an allergic reaction. Loss of central vision is a clinical manifestation of macular degeneration.
NP = As
CN = Ph/8
CL = Ap
SA = 1

9. 2. Nausea and vomiting increase the intraocular pressure and should be treated immediately to prevent injury. Some pain may be expected and can be treated with analgesics. Pain will not affect the surgical outcome. Anxiety and boredom are not physiological problems so are a lower priority at this time.
NP = Pl
CN = Sa/1
CL = An
SA = 1

10. 1. Atropine sulfate and other anticholinergics cause pupil dilation. This blocks the outflow of the aqueous humor and increases the intraocular pressure, which can lead to blindness. Morphine sulfate is an analgesic. Magnesium sulfate is Epsom salts. Ferrous sulfate is an iron preparation. None of these are contraindicated in a client with glaucoma.
NP = An
CN = Ph/6
CL = An
SA = 5

11. 1. An accumulation of cerumen is best removed by washing the ears with soapy water and a soft washcloth. Sharp or hard objects can injure the ear canal or eardrum. A referral would be needed if the cerumen is impacted in the ear.

NP = An
CN = Ph/5
CL = An
SA = 1

12. 4. In addition to ringing in the ears, or tinnitus, being associated with a number of ear disorders, it is a common clinical manifestation of individuals taking repeated, high dosages of aspirin.
NP = Im
CN = Ph/8
CL = An
SA = 1

13. 1. Feedback occurs when a hearing aid is not positioned correctly in the ear. Cleaning, battery replacement, and volume control will not affect feedback.
NP = Im
CN = Ph/5
CL = Ap
SA = 1

14. 3. Aminoglycoside antibiotics (Garamycin) are considered ototoxic and nephrotoxic. Inderal may cause vertigo but does not affect auditory acuity. Neither cimetidine nor acetaminophen is known to be ototoxic.
NP = Ev
CN = Ph/6
CL = An
SA = 5

15. 1. Cerumen, or earwax, is the only normal substance found with inspection. Drainage suggests an inflammatory process. Because the drainage is foul smelling, an infection is suspected. Hearing can be decreased due to swelling. A head hematoma could be the result of a trauma, which could rupture the eardrum but not cause infection.
NP = As
CN = Ph/7
CL = An
SA = 1

16. 4, 5, 6. Dizziness, nausea, vomiting, and nystagmus are clinical manifestations of an inflammation of the labyrinth of the inner ear. Headaches may indicate meningeal involvement in the brain. An upper respiratory infection is more likely the cause of sore throat or nasal congestion.
NP = As
CN = Ph/8

CL = Ap
SA = 1

17. 3. Although offering a client dry crackers and instructing a client to deep breathe until the nausea subsides may be helpful in assisting to control nausea following cataract surgery, the priority intervention would be to administer an antiemetic drug.
NP = Im
CN = Sa/1
CL = Ap
SA = 1

18. **an infection of the sebaceous glands on the eyelash follicle.** A hordeolum is an infection of the sebaceous glands on the eyelash follicle.
NP = An
CN = Ph/8
CL = Co
SA = 1

19. 1. A conductive hearing loss occurs in the outer and middle ear and impairs the sound being conducted from the outer to the inner ear. It is caused by conditions interfering with air conduction, such as impacted cerumen, middle ear disease, otosclerosis, and atresia or stenosis of the external auditory canal. A hearing aid is usually not necessary due to the excellent results of treatment of the underlying problem.
NP = Pl
CN = Ph/8
CL = An
SA = 1

20. 1. Chlamydial conjunctivitis is the adult inclusion conjunctivitis caused by the oculogenital type of *Chlamydia trachomatis*. The treatment of choice is systemic antibiotics and education on the implications. Topical steroids are used in viral conjunctivitis and allergic conjunctivitis. Artificial tears and topical antihistamines are used in allergic conjunctivitis.
NP = Pl
CN = Ph/8
CL = Ap
SA = 1

21. 1. The client is instructed to avoid blowing the nose and to cough and sneeze with an open mouth as an increased pressure in the eustachian tube and middle ear cavity could dislodge the tympanum graft.
NP = Pl
CN = Ph/8
CL = Ap
SA = 1

22. **Chronic otitis media.** Chronic otitis media is an infection that generally presents in childhood. Fever and purulent drainage indicate infection and possibly a ruptured eardrum.
NP = An
CN = Ph/8
CL = Ap
SA = 1

23. 2. The Rinne test uses air conduction and bone conduction. The tuning fork is activated and held close to the auditory meatus until the client can no longer hear it. When that takes place, it is immediately placed to the mastoid bone. It is normal if the client cannot hear it. Sound is heard better by air conduction than bone conduction. It would be normal if sound is heard equally in both ears. The Weber test uses bone conduction. The base of a vibrating tuning fork is placed in the vertex of the skull, forehead, or on the front of the teeth. The client is asked if sound is heard better in one ear than the other. When bone conduction is greater than air conduction, this is abnormal and additional investigation is warranted. The normal hearing is in the 0 to 25 dB range on the audiogram. The tympanic membrane should be pearly, shiny, and semitransparent.
NP = An
CN = Ph/8
CL = An
SA = 1

24. 2. Primary open-angle glaucoma is the most common form of glaucoma. The early clinical manifestation may go unnoticed until severe irreversible vision loss is present. The first clinical manifestation is loss of peripheral vision. Clients experience a gradual visual field loss, which appears to look like "tunnel vision" in open-angle glaucoma. Floating specks are seen with aging. Flashes of light would indicate a detached retina. An intolerance to light might indicate a migraine.
NP = As
CN = Ph/8
CL = Ap
SA = 1

25. 4. A stapedectomy is the treatment of choice for otosclerosis. Otosclerosis is a "hardening of the ear." A decrease in hearing is normal in the normal post-op period. Most clients (90 to 95%) get their hearing back.
NP = Pl
CN = He/3
CL = Ap
SA = 1

RESPIRATORY DISORDERS - COMPREHENSIVE EXAM

1. The nurse assesses a client recovering from a severe fracture of the left leg to be dyspneic, restless, tachycardic, and covered with petechiae over the chest. The client is also hypotensive with a weak, rapid pulse and decreased breath sounds, with a pleural friction rub on auscultation. The client is complaining of chest pain. Based on the history and clinical manifestations, which of the following is most likely the cause of the client's distress?
   1. Spontaneous pneumothorax
   2. Pneumonia
   3. Myocardial infarction
   4. Pulmonary embolism
2. Which of the following should the nurse include in the discharge instructions on how to care for a client with long-standing restrictive lung disease during the winter months?
   1. Have periodic arterial blood gas (ABG) analysis to check pO_2 levels
   2. Take the influenza vaccine and broad-spectrum antibiotics as prescribed
   3. Smoke low-tar cigarettes
   4. Stay home until warm weather returns in the spring
3. A client admitted to the hospital following a motorcycle accident with multiple rib fractures and a pneumothorax has a right chest tube connected to water seal drainage with 20 cm suction. While getting out of bed, the client accidentally pulls the chest tube out. The first nursing action is to
   1. notify the physician.
   2. start oxygen at 4 L/min oxygen per mask.
   3. place client back in bed and elevate to semi-Fowler's position.
   4. apply a Vaseline or impermeable dressing over the insertion site.
4. A client is diagnosed with a right pneumothorax on the basis of chest x-ray and dyspnea. Which of the following indicates to the nurse that the client's condition is deteriorating?
   1. Tracheal deviation to the left
   2. Sibilant wheezes
   3. Hypertension
   4. Painful respirations

5. When planning the activity schedule for a client with pneumonia, the most appropriate time to take the client for a short walk is
   1. right after lunch.
   2. after a short nap.
   3. before getting scheduled arterial blood gases drawn.
   4. after using the metered-dose inhaler.
6. The nurse is caring for a client with lung cancer who is receiving pleurodesis therapy to treat repeated pleural effusions. Which of the following is the priority nursing action after the physician injects the agent through the client's chest tube?
   1. Turn the client to the affected side
   2. Turn the client to the unaffected side
   3. Clamp the chest tube for the prescribed time
   4. Ambulate the client
7. A client with acquired immunodeficiency syndrome (AIDS) develops *Pneumocystis carinii* pneumonia. The priority nursing diagnosis for this client is
   1. impaired gas exchange.
   2. altered nutrition: less than body requirements.
   3. risk for infection.
   4. activity intolerance.
8. The nurse is evaluating the arterial blood gas (ABG) results for a client with a long history of chronic obstructive pulmonary disease (COPD). The results are pH = 7.33, pCO_2 = 49 mm Hg, pO_2 = 78 mm Hg, HCO_3 = 28 mm Hg. The nurse concludes that the initiative to breathe in a client with emphysema is triggered by ______________.
9. A client with adult respiratory distress syndrome (ARDS) is intubated and placed on mechanical ventilation. Blood gas analysis (ABG) reflects PaO_2 of 60 mm Hg on 100% fraction of inspired oxygen (FIO_2). To improve the client's oxygenation, the nurse should place the client on which of the following prescribed treatments?
   1. Time-cycled ventilation
   2. Volume-cycled ventilation
   3. Positive end-expiratory pressure (PEEP)
   4. Pressure support
10. The nurse identifies which of the following assessment findings in a client who is experiencing respiratory failure?Select all that apply:

1. Hypoxemia
2. Hypercapnia
3. Hyperventilation
4. Bradycardia
5. Cyanosis
6. Hypotension

11. The nurse should monitor a client with bacterial pneumonia for which of the following clinical manifestations?Select all that apply:
    1. Hypertension
    2. Altered mental status
    3. Tachycardia
    4. Rapid, shallow respirations
    5. Edema
    6. Chest pain
12. The nurse is collecting a nursing history on a client admitted with intrinsic asthma. Which of the following questions should the nurse ask?
    1. "Have you had a recent upper respiratory infection?"
    2. "Have you gotten a new pet?"
    3. "Do you have allergies to molds and dust?"
    4. "Are you under a lot of emotional stress?"
13. The nurse is caring for a client with acute asthma who has a respiratory rate of 42 breaths/minute. Which of the following measures should receive priority in the client's plan of care?
    1. Apply a cardiac monitor to the client
    2. Administer a bronchodilator by nebulizer
    3. Obtain a full medical history
    4. Provide emotional support to the client and family
14. About 30 minutes after the nurse administers the initial dose of an antibiotic to a client with a urinary tract infection, the client complains of chest tightness and shortness of breath. The client appears restless and confused, and has a respiratory rate of 40 breaths/minute. The nurse should notify the physician of which of the following?
    1. Pulmonary embolism
    2. Cor pulmonale
    3. Respiratory failure
    4. Pulmonary hypertension

15. A client is admitted to the burn unit with a 12% total body surface burn injury and extensive smoke inhalation injury. Forty-eight hours after admission, the client develops severe hypoxemia, requiring intubation and mechanical ventilation on 100% FIO_2. The nurse evaluates that this client has developed ______________.

16. A client with a pulmonary embolism is being treated with ventilator support and positive end-expiratory pressure (PEEP). The client's PaO_2 is 68 mm Hg. Which of the following nursing actions is the priority for the nurse to perform to reduce oxygen demand?

1. Administer prescribed paralytic agents

2. Administer prescribed diuretics

3. Place the client in Trendelenburg position

4. Administer prescribed bronchodilators

17. Following a left pneumonectomy the client returns with no chest tube in the left side. The client's family asks why a chest tube is not in place. The appropriate response by the nurse is

1. "A chest tube will be inserted later at the bedside."

2. "A chest tube generally is not needed."

3. "The breath sounds on the left are shallow."

4. "Chest physiotherapy will be ordered for the left side."

18. A client's family asks the nurse what caused the client's pulmonary embolism. The nurse's response should be based on an understanding that pulmonary embolism is most commonly caused by

1. a venous thrombus.

2. a septic thrombus.

3. amniotic fluid.

4. a fat thrombus.

19. The nurse is evaluating the function of a closed system chest drainage set. The nurse notes that there is continuous rapid bubbling in the water-seal chamber.
The nurse evaluates this to mean

1. there is an air leak in the system.

2. the client's lungs have fully inflated.

3. the wall suction is too low.

4. the chest drainage tube is clotted.

20. A postoperative client is in the postanesthesia recovery area. Orders are to extubate the client when blood gases are within normal range and the client is awake. Prior to extubation, the nurse should assess the client for an ability to

1. Answer questions and wiggle the toes
2. Blink the eyes and use the hands
3. Raise the head off the pillow and follow commands
4. Nod the head yes or no

21. The nurse is doing preoperative teaching for a client and is discussing the incentive spirometer and its use after surgery. For the best results, the nurse includes which of the following in the teaching?Select all that apply:

1. Take a deep breath and blow out through pursed lips
2. Form a loose seal with lips around mouthpiece
3. Inhale slowly and deeply
4. Raise the cylinder as high as possible
5. Do 10 repetitions daily

22. The nurse is suctioning a client with a tracheostomy who is being treated for pneumonia. Using standard precautions, which of the following personal protective equipment would be appropriate during this procedure?Select all that apply:

[ ] **1.** Gloves
[ ] **2.** Mask
[ ] **3.** Goggles or shield
[ ] **4.** Gown
[ ] **5.** Shoe covers

23. Which of the following should the nurse assess in a client exhibiting signs of central cyanosis?

1. Buccal mucous membranes and lips
2. Nail beds
3. Fingers and toes
4. Pulse oximetry

24. A client is admitted with a suspected diagnosis of sarcoidosis. Which of the following assessment findings support this diagnosis?Select all that apply:

[ ] **1.** Productive cough
[ ] **2.** Chest discomfort
[ ] **3.** Dyspnea
[ ] **4.** Barrel chest

[ ] **5.** Night sweats

[ ] **6.** Hemoptysis

25. The nurse is assisting the physician with a therapeutic bronchoscopy for a client who is on a ventilator. During the procedure, which of the following is the priority for the nurse to report?

1. Pulse oximetry of 72%

2. Respiratory rate of 22

3. Occasional premature ventricular contractions on monitor

4. Blood pressure 160/88

26. A client with chronic obstructive pulmonary disease is receiving oxygen therapy by nasal cannula at a rate of 4 L/min. During the nurse's morning assessment, the client complains of an occipital headache on awakening, extreme drowsiness, and respirations of 10 breaths/minute and shallow. Which of the following actions should the nurse take?

1. Notify the physician and increase the oxygen flow rate to 6 L/min

2. Continue to monitor the client and encourage the client to relax

3. Notify the physician and decrease the oxygen flow rate to 1 L/min

4. Change the method of oxygen administration to an oxygen mask

27. The registered nurse appropriately assigns a licensed practical nurse (LPN) to perform which of the following tasks?

1. Assess a client with a chest tube for a possible air leak

2. Develop a teaching plan for a client with an incentive spirometer

3. Evaluate a client's readiness to be weaned off a ventilator

4. Walk a client with chronic obstructive pulmonary disease

28. The nurse is evaluating a client using an incentive inspirometer. Which of the following would indicate that the client needs further investigation?

1. Sitting upright during the procedure

2. Using a tight seal around the mouthpiece

3. Blowing forcefully into the mouthpiece

4. Coughing deeply after the treatment

29. The nurse is discharging a client with a respiratory disorder. Which of the following should the nurse include in the education on the appropriate use of cough medications?

1. Adjust the dose of the cough medicine based on the severity of the cough

2. Restrict fluids before and after taking a cough medicine

3. Read the medication label to see if it contains sugar if diabetic and avoid taking
4. Understand that adverse effects, such as an inability to sleep and anxiousness, are expected

30. Based on an understanding of postural drainage, the nurse should include which of the following?
    1. Schedule postural drainage 30 minutes after meals
    2. Use Trendelenburg position for the client experiencing dyspnea
    3. Maintain each position for one hour
    4. Administer nebulization therapy prior to postural drainage

31. The nurse is preparing to perform tactile fremitus. Which of the following should the nurse include in the procedure?
    1. After placing the ulnar aspect of an open hand on the client's right anterior apex, instruct the client to say "99"
    2. Place the thumbs of both hands on the costal margins and pointing toward the xiphoid process
    3. Position the finger pad of the index finger on the client's trachea and move laterally to the right
    4. With the client breathing normally, percuss the right lung from the apex to below the diaphragm

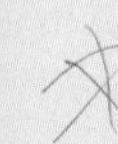

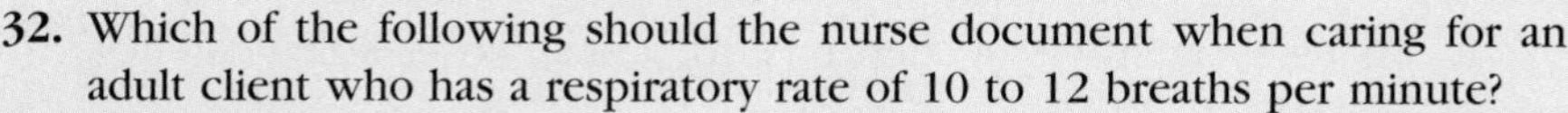

32. Which of the following should the nurse document when caring for an adult client who has a respiratory rate of 10 to 12 breaths per minute?
    1. Bradypnea
    2. Tachypnea
    3. Eupnea
    4. Apnea

33. Which of the following conditions does the nurse suspect in a client experiencing Kussmaul's respirations?
    1. Diabetic ketoacidosis
    2. Chronic obstructive pulmonary disease
    3. Central nervous system lesion
    4. Tuberculosis

34. The nurse is discharging a client with a respiratory disorder. Which of the following measures would be essential to include in the client's discharge instructions?
    1. Have the chimney cleaned once a year
    2. Change the furnace filter monthly

3. Check the smoke detector twice a year
4. Avoid regular exercise

35. The nurse is performing a physical assessment on an older adult client. Which of the following would be an anticipated respiratory finding in this client?
    1. Kyphosis and barrel chest
    2. Increased cough reflex
    3. Increased ciliary action
    4. Larger muscle mass

36. The nurse is instructing a client to cough and deep breathe. What position should the nurse instruct the client to assume to promote the most effective coughing? _______________

37. Guaifenesin (Robitussin) has been prescribed for a client who asks the nurse what it is for. Which of the following is the correct response by the nurse? "Guaifenesin (Robitussin) is
    1. a bronchodilator that will reduce bronchospasm."
    2. an expectorant that facilitates thinning secretions."
    3. a cough suppressant."
    4. a calcium channel blocker that prevents vasoconstriction."

38. The registered nurse is preparing the clinical assignments for the day. Which of the following would be appropriate to delegate to unlicensed assistive personnel?
    1. Assessment of the oral cavity
    2. Palpation of a radial pulse
    3. Auscultation of the lung sounds
    4. Inspection of the abdomen

39. The nurse is caring for a client with a history of chronic obstructive pulmonary disease who has recently been diagnosed with lung cancer. Which of the following assessment findings does the nurse evaluate as the result of a long-standing hypoxia?
    1. Clubbing of the nails
    2. Onychophagy
    3. Onychorrhexis
    4. Pterygium

40. The registered nurse is preparing the clinical assignments for a respiratory unit. Which of the following assignments should the nurse delegate to a licensed practical nurse?

1. Perform a respiratory assessment on an older adult client
2. Administer a prescribed bronchodilator to a client
3. Perform postural drainage on a client with pneumonia
4. Develop a teaching plan for a client with chronic obstructive pulmonary disease

ANSWERS AND RATIONALES

1. 4. Lower extremity fractures and surgery, as well as bed rest, place this client in a high-risk situation for pulmonary embolism. Classic clinical manifestations of pulmonary emboli include sudden onset, dyspnea, petechiae, and decreased breath sounds, usually with a pleural friction rub. Signs of circulatory collapse are also consistent with a diagnosis of pulmonary emboli. Pneumonia would be a slower onset with clinical manifestations more consistent with infection such as fever, chills, cough, and sputum production. Breath sounds may be diminished due to consolidation. Spontaneous pneumothorax would have a sudden onset but there would likely be no petechiae and the breath sounds would obviously be different with a possible deviation of the trachea from midline. Circulatory compromise would be obvious, similar to the pulmonary embolism. Myocardial infarction is a possibility, but this client is not a high risk for an MI when compared to a pulmonary embolism based on circumstances.
   NP = As
   CN = Ph/8
   CL = An
   SA = 1
2. 2. Broad-spectrum antibiotics are indicated under medical supervision as a prophylactic treatment for those prone to lung infections, particularly in the winter months. Individuals with chronic respiratory problems are encouraged to get annual influenza injections. Clients with lung disease are discouraged from smoking any substance in any form. ABGs are indicated only during exacerbation of lung disease. Clients with chronic respiratory disease are cautioned to avoid high concentrations of people in confined areas during active cold and pneumonia season (such as church, public transportation) but are not to socially isolate themselves.
   NP = Pl
   CN = He/3
   CL = Ap
   SA = 1

3. 4. The first action would be to prevent further air from entering the pleural cavity. A Vaseline, plastic, or other nonpermeable dressing must be securely placed over the site until the chest tube can be reinserted by the physician. The client is the first priority. Placing the client back in bed with the head of bed up will facilitate breathing. The physician must be called as soon as the priority client needs are met or it can be done by someone else while the nurse attends to the client. The use of oxygen and the delivery system (nasal cannula or mask) will be determined by the client's needs.
NP = Im
CN = Sa/1
CL = An
SA = 8

4. 1. A pneumothorax is characterized by chest pain, dyspnea, tachypnea, hypotension, tachycardia, and hyperresonant breath sounds over affected side. The client has asymmetric chest movement, is diaphoretic, and has subcutaneous emphysema and cyanosis, and with severe or progressive pneumothorax, a shift of the mediastinum and trachea is present (pushed to unaffected side). Hypotension occurs due to increased intrathoracic pressure and decreased cardiac output. Pain with respiration is characteristic of pneumothorax and is not an indication of severity.
NP = An
CN = Ph/8
CL = An
SA = 1

5. 4. The client will tolerate activities after receiving respiratory treatments of medications. After the administration of bronchodilators (often administered by metered-dose inhaler), the client will have the best oxygen exchange and will better tolerate activity. However, a good assessment of the client should be made before any activity by taking all things into consideration to evaluate tolerance. It is more appropriate to know what the ABG results are before activity for the client. The client may need to rest after a meal and before an activity. Taking a short nap before an activity may be appropriate but the most important consideration is the oxygenation of the client.
NP = Pl
CN = Sa/1
CL = An
SA = 1

6. 3. After the injection of the sclerosing agent through the chest tube, the tube must be clamped to prevent the agent from draining back out of the pleural space. Sometimes a repositioning schedule is prescribed to disperse

the agent but the usefulness of activity and positioning are controversial. Ambulation has no specific purpose in the immediate period after injecting a sclerosing agent.

NP = Pl
CN = Sa/1
CL = Ap
SA = 1

7. 1. Altered nutrition: less than body requirements, risk for infection, and activity tolerance are all appropriate nursing diagnoses for a client with AIDS, but the highest priority nursing diagnosis for a client with *Pneumocystis carinii* pneumonia is impaired gas exchange. Airway, breathing, and circulation, in that order, are priorities for any client.

NP = An
CN = Sa/1
CL = An
SA = 8

8. **low oxygen (O_2) levels.** Because of the long-standing chronic obstructive respiratory disease and hypercapnia, the client will have developed an alteration in the respiratory drive. The client's drive to breathe is triggered by low oxygen. That is why clients with COPD are restricted to low oxygen flow rates (2 to 3 L/min). For a client with normal respiratory drive, the initiative to breathe is triggered by increased CO_2 levels.

NP = Ev
CN = Ph/5
CL = An
SA = 1

9. 3. With the ventilator already at 100% FIO_2 more pressure at the level of the alveoli to promote gas exchange will be needed. PEEP is generally used at higher levels for clients with ARDS to improve gas exchange over the alveolar capillary membrane. Of the types of ventilation (time-cycled, volume-cycled, or pressure-cycled), the pressure-cycled ventilation mode is more likely to be used. Pressure support is used to override resistance of the tubing and equipment and is dependent on the client's respiratory effort. PEEP is an important component of ventilator support for the client with ARDS.

NP = Pl
CN = Ph/8
CL = An
SA = 1

10. 1, 2, 5. A client experiencing acute respiratory failure is at the point where the exchange of oxygen and carbon dioxide in the lungs cannot

match the rate of consumption and production at the cellular level and the client demonstrates hypoxemia ($PaO_2 < 60$ mm Hg), with or without hypercapnia ($PaCO_2 > 50$ mm Hg). Alveolar hypoventilation occurs. Other signs or clinical manifestations include dyspnea, tachypnea, tachycardia, headache, cyanosis, restlessness, decreased or absent breath sounds, and adventitious breath sounds.
NP = As
CN = Ph/8
CL = Ap
SA = 1

11. 2, 3, 4, 5. Clinical manifestations of bacterial pneumonia include hypotension, altered mental status, tachycardia, hyperthermia, rapid, shallow respirations, dehydration, and chest pain. A client may be admitted to the hospital with dehydration and altered mental status. Vital signs may include a temperature of 39.2°C or 102.6°F, blood pressure of 100/62, pulse 104, and rapid, shallow respirations at 24 per minute. The client may complain of chest pain.
NP = As
CN = Ph/8
CL = Ap
SA = 1

12. 1. Extrinsic asthma is triggered by dust, molds, pets, or other easily identifiable allergens or inhaled particles. Stress or emotional response is also considered an extrinsic factor. These are all outside the respiratory tract. An intrinsic stimulus is related to physiological conditions within the respiratory tract such as inflammation or infection.
NP = As
CN = Ph/8
CL = An
SA = 1

13. 2. Nebulized bronchodilators open airways and increase the amount of oxygen delivered. Bronchodilators can increase the heart rate, but for a young client it may not be necessary to place the client on a cardiac monitor unless there is a past history of cardiac problems. Medical history and emotional support are important, but only after the first phase of the attack is resolved. Airway, breathing, and circulation are priorities. With information from the history, the nurse may be able to identify the cause of the attack and provide education on how to prevent further episodes.
NP = Pl
CN = Sa/1

CL = An
SA = 1

14. 3. With the recent ingestion of an antibiotic and the respiratory signs of impending failure, this most likely reflects an allergic response to the drug and impending anaphylaxis with eventual respiratory failure or arrest. Considering the circumstances and the information provided, the client is not at high risk for pulmonary emboli, nor does the client have the medical conditions that contribute to cor pulmonale or pulmonary hypertension.
NP = An
CN = Ph/8
CL = An
SA = 1

15. **adult respiratory distress syndrome (ARDS).** Clients with burn and inhalation injuries are at risk for the development of adult respiratory distress syndrome (ARDS).
NP = Ev
CN = Ph/8
CN = Ap
SA = 1

16. 1. Neuromuscular blockers cause skeletal muscle paralysis and reduce the cellular demand for oxygen. This should provide a better balance between oxygen supply and demand for the client. Bronchodilators may be used but are not typically the first choice unless there is bronchoconstriction. Diuretics may reduce pulmonary edema if present. The question asked about reducing oxygen demand, not improving oxygen delivery. The most effective position to improve oxygenation is semi-Fowler's to facilitate diaphragm movement.
NP = Pl
CN = Sa/1
CL = Ap
SA = 1

17. 2. A pneumonectomy is the removal of an entire lung. Serous fluid is allowed to fill the space and it will eventually consolidate, preventing extensive mediastinal shift of the heart and remaining lung; therefore, a chest tube is not needed. Tissue from the other lung can't cross the mediastinum, although a slight shift may be evident until the empty space is filled with fluid. There will be no breath sounds and no lung tissue to benefit from CPT therapy on the left. Remember a wedge resection is a very small area of tissue close to the surface of the lung that is removed; a segmental resection is the removal of a segment of the

lung; a lobectomy is the removal of a lobe, and a pneumonectomy is the removal of an entire lung.
NP = An
CN = Ph/8
CL = An
SA = 1

18. 1. Venous thrombi originating in the thigh and pelvis are the most common sources for pulmonary emboli. Immobility is a significant contributing factor. When dislodged, the clots are returned through the venous system and lodge in the pulmonary vasculature. Septic thrombi, amniotic fluid, or fat thrombi are all other possible sources for pulmonary emboli but not the most common.
NP = An
CN = Ph/8
CL = Ap
SA = 1

19. 1. Continuous rapid bubbling in the water-seal chamber indicates an air leak in the system. It is a priority to attempt to find and correct the leak. When the client's lungs have fully inflated, the fluctuation (tidaling) in the water-seal chamber will be minimal or absent. The suction is actually controlled at the collection device and is most commonly set at 20 cm water pressure. If wall suction is applied, it should be set at a moderate suction (80 to 120 mm Hg). Monitor for sudden changes in the amount of chest drainage and clinical manifestations of cardiac tamponade or respiratory distress. This will not be reflected in the water-seal chamber.
NP = Ev
CN = Ph/8
CL = An
SA = 1

20. 3. A client will be unable to speak when intubated but may be able to nod the head and wiggle fingers and toes. The nurse will want to assess both neurological status and respiratory function before extubation. If a client can raise the head off the pillow, this indicates that there is adequate diaphragmatic strength to breathe effectively once extubated. The ability to follow commands is important, but most important is the ability to ventilate adequately on one's own.
NP = As
CN = Ph/8
CL = Ap
SA = 1

21. 1, 3, 4. Proper use of incentive spirometry involves inspiratory effort. A loose seal will not be effective and the usual frequency is 10 repetitions every two to four hours. An incentive spirometry does not replace the need to cough and deep breathe after surgery, but sometimes it is the stimulant for that process and helps decrease atelectasis.

NP = Im
CN = He/3
CL = Ap
SA = 1

22. 1, 2, 3. Standard precautions require that the nurse take precautions to avoid becoming exposed to mucus during suctioning. The eyes and face should be protected during this procedure. Gloves are always worn. During the actual suctioning, sterile gloves would be required.

NP = Pl
CN = Sa/2
CL = Ap
SA = 1

23. 1. Central cyanosis reflects a decrease in oxygen saturation of hemoglobin in arterial blood. Peripheral cyanosis is caused by slow blood circulation to distal parts of the body. The buccal mucosa and lips (circumoral) cyanosis is more reflective of central cyanosis. Nail beds blanching and oxygen to fingers or toes are dependent upon circulation. Pulse oximetry is dependent upon blood flow and binding to hemoglobin.

NP = As
CN = Ph/8
CL = Ap
SA = 1

24. 2, 3. Sarcoidosis is an interstitial lung disease that causes fibrosis of the lung tissue. Clinical manifestations of sarcoidosis include a nonproductive cough, dyspnea, and chest discomfort. Barrel chest is seen in emphysema. Night sweats and hemoptysis occur in tuberculosis.

NP = As
CN = Ph/8
CL = Ap
SA = 1

25. 1. During a bronchoscopy, the most immediate concern is to maintain oxygenation for the client (airway, breathing, circulation). The occasional premature ventricular contractions (PVC) and elevated blood pressure are most likely a response to the hypoxia. The procedure should be stopped until the SaO_2 returns to $> 90\%$. A respiratory rate of 22 is not significant.

NP = An
CN = Sa/1
CL = An
SA = 1

26. 3. Clients with chronic obstructive pulmonary disease (COPD) have a tendency to hypoventilate and retain CO_2. Gradually the respiratory center loses its sensitivity to the elevated CO_2 level. When O_2 is administered in high concentrations, the hypoxia stimulus is eliminated and the rate and depth of respirations decrease. The appropriate nursing action is to monitor the vital signs, decrease the delivery rate of oxygen, and assess the client's status. Nasal cannula is the preferred method of administration for COPD clients because it allows for a low concentration delivery rate.
NP = Pl
CN = Ph/8
CL = Ap
SA = 1

27. 4. Only a registered nurse can assess, evaluate, and develop. An licensed practical nurse (LPN) would not have the critical thinking skills to assess, plan, or evaluate a client's care. It would be appropriate to assign an LPN to walk a client. This is a task within the job description of an LPN.
NP = Pl
CN = Sa/1
CL = Ap
SA = 8

28. 3. The client should be sitting upright when using an incentive inspirometer. The client should form a tight seal around the mouthpiece. Coughing should be encouraged after the treatment. Slow, deep breaths should be delivered into the mouthpiece.
NP = An
CN = Ph/8
CL = An
SA = 1

29. 3. Clients with diabetes mellitus should be instructed to read the label of cough medicines to see if they contain sugar. If they do, they should be instructed to avoid taking them. The dose of cough medicines should not be based on the severity of the cough. Fluids should not be restricted before and after taking the medicine. Cough medicine may cause drowsiness.
NP = Pl
CN = Ph/6
CL = An
SA = 5

30. 4. Nebulization therapy should be performed prior to postural drainage. Postural drainage should not be scheduled right after the client has eaten. Several hours should be waited after eating before performing postural drainage. Placing the client in the Trendelenburg position would result in dyspnea. Each position assumed during postural drainage should be maintained for 10 to 15 minutes.

NP = Pl
CN = Ph/8
CL = AP
SA = 1

31. 1. Tactile or vocal fremitus is a vibration of the chest wall that is palpable during a spoken word. It is assessed by placing the ulnar aspect of an open hand on the client's right anterior apex while instructing the client to say "99." Placing the thumbs of both hands on the costal margins and pointing toward the xiphoid process assesses thoracic expansion. The tracheal position is assessed by positioning the finger pad of the index finger on the client's trachea and moving laterally to the right. Diaphragmatic excursion is assessed when the client is breathing normally. The right lung from the apex to below the diaphragm should be assessed.

NP = Pl
CN = Ph/8
CL = An
SA = 1

32. 3. Eupnea is normal breathing with a respiratory rate of 10 to 12 breaths per minute. Bradypnea is a respiratory rate lower than 10 breaths per minute and may occur in a client who has sustained a head injury. Tachypnea is a respiratory rate of greater than 24 breaths per minute. It may be associated with a hypermetabolic and hypoxia state. Apnea is a lack of respirations for 10 or more seconds as a result of traumatic brain injury that caused a herniation of the brain stem.

NP = Im
CN = Ph/8
CL = Ap
SA = 1

33. 1. Kussmaul's respirations are characterized by respirations that are extreme in rate and depth. They are characteristic of diabetic ketoacidosis. Clients with chronic obstructive pulmonary disease have difficulty exhaling and air trapping. Sighing is characteristic of central nervous system lesions. A client with tuberculosis does not necessarily have difficulty with respirations.

NP = An
CN = Ph/8
CL = An
SA = 1

34. 2. Changing the furnace filter monthly should be included in the discharge instruction of a client with a respiratory disorder. The chimney should be cleaned four times a year. The smoke detector should be checked monthly. Regular exercise has no effect on a client with a respiratory disorder.
NP = P1
CN = Ph/7
CL = Ap
SA = 1

35. 1. Kyphosis is an excessive convexity of the thoracic spine sometimes known as "humpback." It and a barrel chest are anticipated assessment findings in an older adult client. Older adult clients would have both a decreased cough reflex and ciliary action. Their muscles would also become smaller and atrophy.
NP = Ev
CN = Ph/8
CL = Ap
SA = 1

36. **Sit upright with the feet flat on the floor.** The most effective position to enhance coughing and deep breathing is sitting upright with the feet flat on the floor.
NP = Pl
CN = Ph/8
CL = An
SA = 1

37. 2. Guaifenesin (Robitussin) is an expectorant that facilitates thinning secretions.
NP = An
CN = Ph/6
CL = Co
SA = 5

38. 2. Palpation of a radial pulse to unlicensed assistive personnel is an appropriate clinical assignment. Assessment of the oral cavity, auscultation of the lung sounds, and inspection of the abdomen are all assignments that require the skills of a nurse to perform.
NP = P1
CN = Sa/1
CL = An
SA = 8

39. 1. Clubbing of the nails occurs from long-standing hypoxia such as that which occurs in lung cancer or chronic obstructive pulmonary disease. Onychophagy is excessive biting of the nails. Onychorrhexis is a split in

the nail that is brittle with lengthwise ridges. It may result from trauma, toxic exposure to solvents, or harsh filing. Pterygium is an abnormal overgrowth of the cuticle that becomes attached to the nail. It occurs in Raynaud's disease.
NP = Ev
CN = Ph/8
CL = An
SA = 1

40. 2. A licensed practical nurse may administer a bronchodilator to a client. Performing a respiratory assessment, performing postural drainage, and developing a teaching plan are skills that require a registered nurse.
NP = Pl
CN = Sa/1
CL = An
SA = 8

CARDIOVASCULAR DISORDERS - COMPREHENSIVE EXAM

1. The nurse is reviewing the laboratory tests of an admitted client suspected of having a myocardial infarction. Which of the following, indicating cardiac muscle damage, should the nurse report?
   1. Elevated serum creatine kinase (myocardial bands) and troponin
   2. PT (prothrombin time), INR (international normalized ratio)
   3. A low HDL and a high LDL
   4. Low K+ (potassium) and Mg++ (magnesium)
2. Which of the following discharge instructions is the priority for a client following a coronary angioplasty?Select all that apply:
   [ ] 1. Return to primary clinic for follow-up appointment in one week
   [ ] 2. Learn more about risk factors to prevent heart disease
   [ ] 3. Take one acetaminophen (Tylenol) daily to prevent blood clots
   [ ] 4. If bleeding occurs at the angioplasty site, call immediately
   [ ] 5. Have someone hold firm pressure over it
   [ ] 6. Call 911
3. The nurse should monitor the client with a mitral valve prolapse as being at risk for developing which cardiac disease?
   1. First-degree heart block
   2. Bacterial endocarditis

3. Ventricular septal defect
4. Hypertension

4. The nurse is taking the history of a client with clinical manifestations of an acute myocardial infarction (MI) in the emergency room prior to beginning fibrinolytic (thrombolytic) therapy. Which of the following should the nurse notify the physician of?
   1. A recently developed second-degree A-V block
   2. A history of asthma
   3. A history of cerebral hemorrhage
   4. An allergy to aspirin

5. Prior to administering nitroglycerin to a client suspected of experiencing cardiac ischemic pain, the nurse should ask the client which of the following drugs have been taken in the last 24 hours?
   1. Digoxin (Lanoxin)
   2. Sildenafil (Viagra)
   3. Verapamil (Calan)
   4. Warfarin (Coumadin)

6. The nurse on the telemetry unit monitoring the client's rhythm notes that the PR interval is becoming consistently longer, and then a QRS is absent altogether. The nurse documents this rhythm as

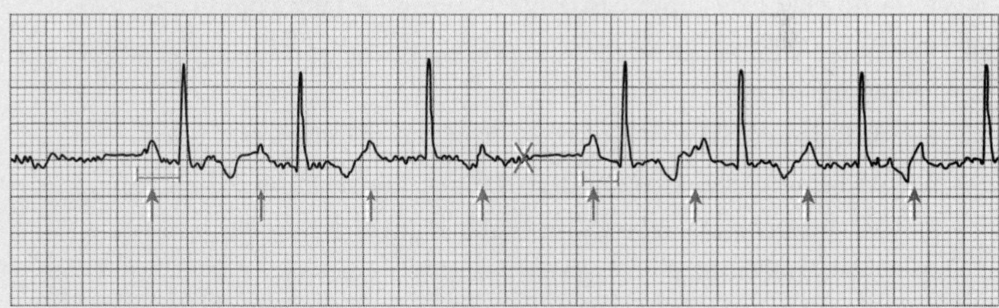

   1. First-degree A-V block
   2. Second-degree A-V block, type I (Wenckebach)
   3. Second-degree A-V block, type II (Mobitz II)
   4. Third-degree A-V block

7. The nurse is admitting a client from the physician's office who has reported clinical manifestations of dizziness and fatigue. The client's blood pressure is 88/46 and the heart monitor shows a third-degree heart block, with ventricular rate of 39 beats per minute. Which of the following is the priority intervention for this client?

1. Administer lidocaine (Xylocaine HCl)
2. Schedule the client for a coronary angiogram
3. Administer verapamil (Calan)
4. Assist with providing the client with a temporary pacemaker

8. While resting in bed, the client's rhythm suddenly shows ventricular tachycardia on the heart monitor. The nurse finds the client alert and having a pulse of 180 and a blood pressure of 110/60. Which of the following interventions should the nurse implement first?
   1. Synchronized electrical cardioversion
   2. Electrical defibrillation
   3. IV lidocaine (Xylocaine HCl)
   4. CPR

9. The staff nurse is explaining to a graduate nurse why a client with a heart rate of 40 beats per minute needs a permanent pacemaker. The nurse correctly describes the client's second-degree block, type II (Mobitz II) as follows:
   1. PR interval remains constant, but periodically a QRS complex is dropped
   2. PR interval gradually lengthens until a QRS complex is dropped
   3. P waves and QRS complexes function independently of each other
   4. The client has no measurable P waves or QRS complexes

10. The nurse should assess the functioning of the aortic valve in which of the following areas?
    1. 5th intercostal space to the left of the midclavicular line
    2. 2nd intercostal space to the right of the sternum
    3. 4th intercostal space to the right of the sternum
    4. 2nd intercostal space to the left of the sternum

11. In reviewing cardiac waveform strips for a hospitalized client, the nurse instructed a student nurse that the P wave represents:
    1. ventricular depolarization.
    2. ventricular repolarization.
    3. atrial depolarization.
    4. isoelectric line (the resting phase).

12. The nurse should implement which of the following interventions for the client with pyelonephritis who has a temperature of 38.3°C or 101°F, a blood pressure of 112/68, and sinus tachycardia with a ventricular rate of 118 beats per minute on the ECG monitor?Select all that apply:

[ ] **1.** Administer acetaminophen (Tylenol) PO

[ ] **2.** Perform immediate synchronized cardioversion

[ ] **3.** Administer atropine 1.0 mg IV push

[ ] **4.** Increase fluids

[ ] **5.** Apply oxygen

[ ] **6.** Administer digoxin (Lanoxin) 0.25 mg IV push

13. The clinic nurse has completed instructing a client newly diagnosed with atrial fibrillation. Which of the following statements shows the client has a proper understanding of the use of warfarin (Coumadin)?

1. "It helps to keep my heart from going too fast."

2. "It helps to prevent blood clots."

3. "I shouldn't eat foods high in potassium."

4. "It will dissolve any blood clots I might have."

14. A client on an ECG monitor demonstrating frequent premature ventricular contractions (PVCs) complains of dizziness and chest pain. Which of the following is the priority for the nurse to implement when the rhythm changes to ventricular tachycardia and the client becomes pulseless?

1. Immediate electrical defibrillation

2. Blood draw of arterial blood gases

3. Blood draw of the serum potassium level

4. Administration of IV digoxin (Lanoxin)

15. During the night shift, the nurse notes that the client's heart monitor drops to 50 beats per minute, demonstrating a sinus bradycardia. Upon being awakened for assessment, the client's blood pressure reads 104/70. At this time, the nurse may proceed with which of the following?

1. No immediate treatment is indicated

2. Administer atropine 0.5 to 1 mg IV push

3. Administer atenolol 50 mg p.o.

4. Apply a temporary pacemaker

16. A client has presented to the emergency department with complaints of dyspnea and a sudden onset of ripping pain between the shoulder blades radiating to the chest. The nurse notes a 12 point difference in blood pressures between the left and right arm. Which of the following tests or procedures does this nurse anticipate the client should undergo?

1. Coronary artery bypass surgery

2. CAT scan

3. Cardiac stress test
4. Thrombolytic therapy

17. Which of the following statements by the client demonstrates an understanding of the discharge teaching provided to a client who has chronic arterial vascular disease?
    1. "I will need to take four aspirin a day if my disease worsens."
    2. "I should sleep with a hot water bottle on my feet to increase blood flow."
    3. "I need to regularly take my medication to cure my disease."
    4. "I need to control my weight and eat a low-fat diet."

18. A client with no pertinent medical history is admitted to the medical unit with a deep vein thrombosis (DVT), a diagnosis new to the client. The client asks, "What will my initial treatment be?" The nurse's best response is based on an understanding that which of the following are standard treatments for a client with a deep vein thrombosis?Select all that apply:
    [ ] 1. Removal of the clot by a vascular surgeon
    [ ] 2. Immediate implantation of an intracaval filter by the interventional radiologist
    [ ] 3. Heparin
    [ ] 4. Elevation
    [ ] 5. A daily dose of warfarin (Coumadin)
    [ ] 6. Rest for the leg

19. An hour after receiving a client back from permanent pacemaker insertion, the nurse notes increasing frequency of ventricular tachycardia on the heart monitor. The nurse should consider which of the following before performing the next nursing action?
    1. This is a normal finding in the first few postoperative hours after placement
    2. The pacemaker lead may be dislodging and is stimulating the ventricle
    3. A permanent pacemaker may not be the right option for this client
    4. An international normalized ratio (INR) is necessary to evaluate the client's condition further

20. After reviewing four client records, the nurse evaluates which of the following clients as most likely to need an electrophysiology (EP) study?
    1. A client with dyspnea and orthopnea
    2. A client with suspected atrial thrombosis

3. A client with an elevated temperature after valve replacement
4. A client with frequent dysrhythmias on a Holter monitor

21. The nurse informs the client who has received a permanent pacemaker that which of the following tests will be ordered postoperatively?
    1. Angiogram
    2. Chest x-ray
    3. Transesophageal echocardiogram (TEE)
    4. Cardiac stress test

22. The nurse is teaching a class on heart failure. Which of the following statements about right-sided heart failure should the nurse include in the class?
    1. Increased fluid volumes are appropriate interventions
    2. Treatment of the underlying cause will not affect the disease
    3. Administration of albuterol (Proventil) metered dose inhalers may be effective
    4. Peripheral edema and a feeling of fullness are common clinical manifestations

23. A client who has diabetes mellitus and heart disease was found unresponsive, tachycardic, hypotensive, and with a blood glucose of 28. After administering D5W, which of the following drugs is the priority for the nurse to administer?
    1. Epinephrine
    2. Antibiotics
    3. Vasopressors
    4. Nitroglycerin

24. Which of the following meal selections should the nurse assist a client with heart failure to make?Select all that apply:
    [ ] 1. Baked potato
    [ ] 2. Baked ham
    [ ] 3. Cheese sandwich
    [ ] 4. French onion soup
    [ ] 5. Lean roast beef
    [ ] 6. Tomato juice

25. Which of the following interventions are the priority for a client who develops unstable angina?Select all that apply:
    [ ] 1. Provide for bed rest
    [ ] 2. Prepare the client for coronary artery bypass surgery

[ ] 3. Perform ECG monitoring

[ ] 4. Maintain the client's oxygen saturation level at 87%

[ ] 5. Administer systemic heparin

[ ] 6. Evaluate the serum cardiac markers (CK-MB, troponin) as positive

26. Postoperatively, a client who received a permanent pacemaker asks the nurse why a chest x-ray is necessary. The appropriate response by the nurse is
    1. "To rule out arterial disease."
    2. "To check for optimal pacemaker functioning."
    3. "To rule out a pneumothorax."
    4. "To check programming functions."

27. The nurse is instructing a group of student nurses on the normal conduction pathway through the heart. Describe the circuit by numbering the structures in their proper order in the conduction pathway through the heart.

    ________________ 1. A-V node

    ________________ 2. Purkinje fibers

    ________________ 3. Bundle of His

    ________________ 4. Sinoatrial (S-A) node

    ________________ 5. Bundle branches

    ________________ 6. Internodal tracts

28. The nurse describes the ECG monitor of a client with ischemic heart disease as having a progressively lengthening PR interval followed by a P wave without a QRS complex. The nurse reports this ECG pattern as

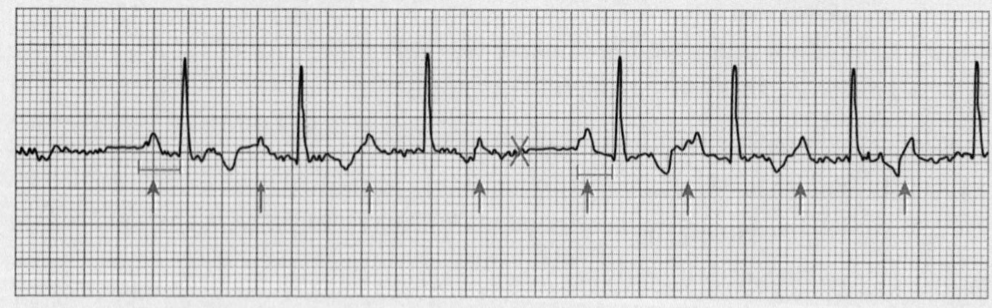

    1. second-degree A-V block type I (Mobitz I or Wenckebach).
    2. ventricular fibrillation.
    3. premature atrial contractions.
    4. atrial fibrillation.

29. The nurse is admitting a 78-year-old client following an acute myocardial infarction with a history of congestive heart failure. The nurse assesses the client to be experiencing visual changes, nausea, and vomiting. The nurse further assesses the serum potassium level to be 2.8 mEq. The nurse evaluates the following rhythm on the ECG monitor to be ________________.

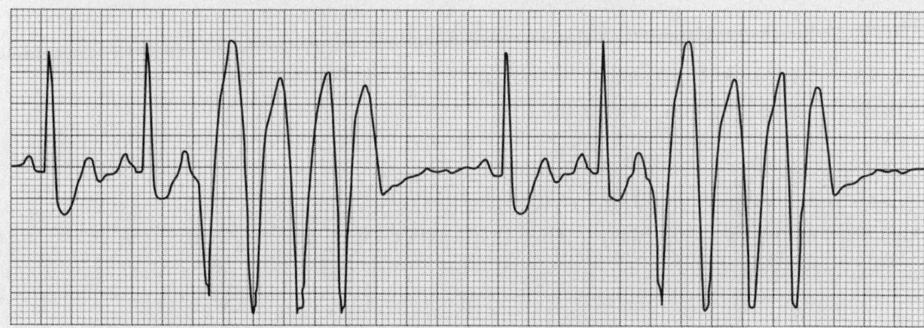

30. The nurse receives a report that which of the following clients would be the most appropriate candidate for a permanent pacemaker?

1. Prophylactically for a client after open heart surgery

2. A client experiencing bradycardia and A-V block after an acute inferior myocardial infarction

3. A client with a third-degree A-V block

4. A client who had an inferior myocardial infarction with a bundle branch block

31. The nurse is signing off orders on four clients. Which of the following orders should the nurse question?

1. Administer atropine to a client with sinus bradycardia

2. Administer lidocaine to a client with a second-degree A-V block type II (Mobitz II)

3. Discontinue epinephrine for a client with an accelerated junctional rhythm

4. Obtain a digoxin level for a client with a junctional rhythm

32. When preparing a client for a transcutaneous pacemaker, which of the following is a priority to inform the client?

1. A fever may be experienced within the first week after placement

2. Airplane travel is not possible because the pacemaker sets off airport security

3. Uncomfortable muscle contraction may be felt when a current passes through the chest wall
4. Microwave ovens are to be avoided because they will cause the pacemaker to malfunction

33. A nurse asks another nurse what the ST segment on the ECG represents. The appropriate response is that the ST segment represents
    1. depolarization of the atria and contraction of the atria.
    2. the period when the impulse spreads through the atria, A-V node, bundle of His, and Purkinje fibers.
    3. the period between ventricular depolarization and repolarization.
    4. the time it takes for depolarization of both ventricles.

34. The nurse is evaluating the ECG strip of a thoracotomy client which demonstrates a constant quivering pattern with no organized atrial activity and a rate of 350 beats per minute to be indicative of which of the following dysrhythmias?

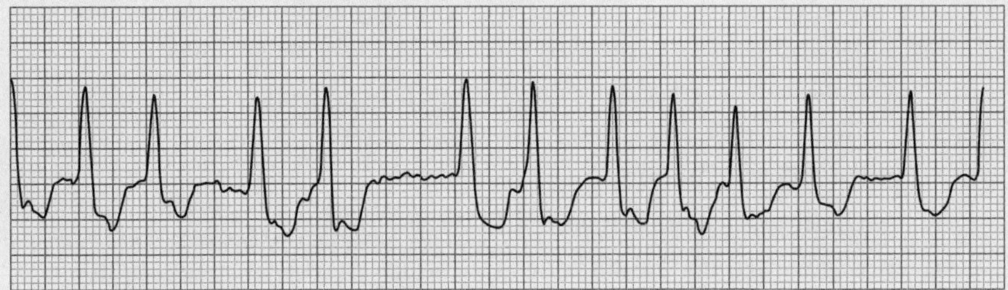

    1. Atrial flutter
    2. Ventricular tachycardia
    3. Idioventricular rhythm
    4. Atrial fibrillation

35. The nurse is caring for a client with premature ventricular contractions (PVCs). Which of the following would indicate to the nurse that the client's condition is deteriorating?
    1. Absence of a PR interval
    2. Six or more PVCs per minute
    3. Wide and bizarre QRS complex greater than 0.12 seconds
    4. Absence of a P wave

36. The nurse is admitting a client who had an ECG demonstrate a normal P wave, PR interval of 0.14 seconds, QRS of 0.06 seconds, but a heart rate of 140 beats per minute. The nurse evaluates this ECG pattern to be indicative of which of the following dysrhythmias?

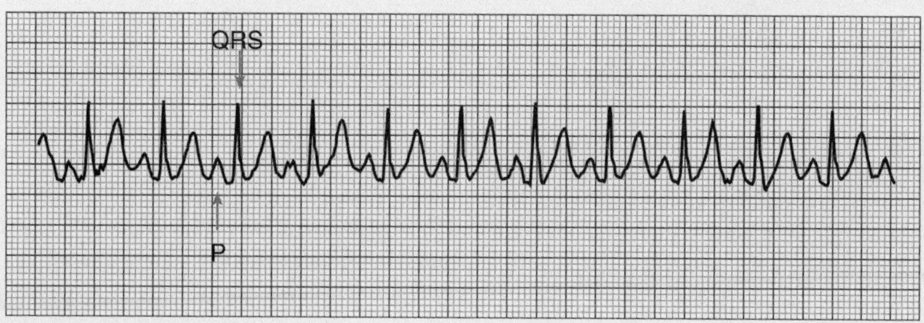

1. Sinus tachycardia
2. Ventricular tachycardia
3. Atrial flutter
4. Ventricular fibrillation

37. Which of the following assessments would provide the nurse with the most accurate information about a client's pacemaker that is failing to capture?
    1. The client has an elevated temperature
    2. There is a redness at the pacemaker insertion site
    3. A hematoma is present at the pacemaker insertion site
    4. The client is experiencing symptomatic bradycardia

38. The nurse is admitting a client who complains of a "flutter sensation in the chest" and extreme fatigue of a two-week duration. During the admission interview, the nurse discovers the client drinks excessive amounts of alcohol and caffeine. The client also smokes two packs of cigarettes per day. The nurse assesses the client to be experiencing what dysrhythmia?

    ____

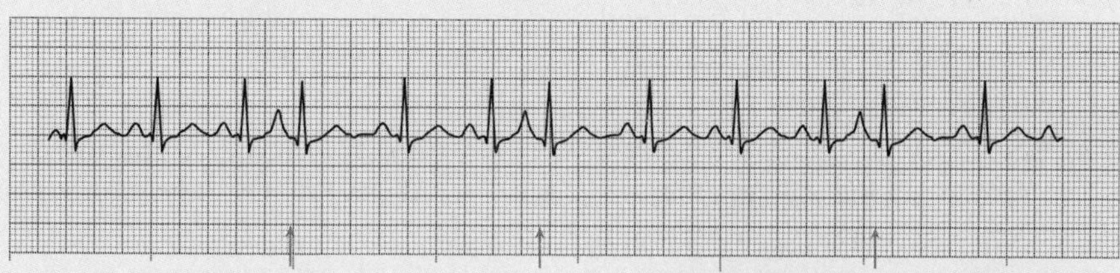

39. The nurse enters a client's room and assesses occasional wide and bizarre QRS complex on the ECG monitor but with no measurable rhythm or rate. What is the priority intervention? ______________

40. Which of the following may the registered nurse delegate to unlicensed assistive personnel?
    1. Evaluate a client with sinus bradycardia for clinical manifestations
    2. Assess a client's pacemaker insertion site for redness

3. Monitor the pulse of a client with a first-degree A-V heart block
4. Plan the diet for a client following an acute myocardial infarction

ANSWERS AND RATIONALES

1. 1. The myocardial bands of creatine kinase and troponin are serum markers for cardiac tissue damage. Prothrombin time (PT) and international normalized ratio (INR) are measurements for serum levels of warfarin (Coumadin) therapy. High-density lipoproteins (HDLs) transport lipids away from arteries to the liver for metabolism, so high levels are desirable. Low-density lipoproteins (LDLs) contain large amounts of cholesterol and tend to bind to arterial walls. Though both lipoproteins are risk factors at abnormal levels, neither is an indicator of heart damage. Abnormal levels of potassium (K+) or magnesium (Mg++) may put the client at risk for cardiac dysrhythmias, but are not used as direct indicators of myocardial damage. Creatine kinase myocardial bands (CK-MB) is an enzyme specific to the myocardial cell, which will begin to rise within four to six hours after a myocardial infarction. Troponin is a myocardial muscle protein that elevates also within four to six hours after heart damage, but can remain elevated for two weeks. Both can be referred to as serum cardiac markers, and are measured for a client with angina to rule out an MI.
   NP = An
   CN = Ph/8
   CL = An
   SA = 1
2. 4, 5, 6. The femoral or brachial arteries used for catheterization are large arteries with potential for bleeding complications, so the client should be instructed to call immediately if signs of bleeding occur.
   NP = Pl
   CN = Sa/1
   CL = Ap
   SA = 1
3. 2. The client with mitral valve prolapse is at risk for developing bacterial endocarditis. A first-degree heart block is often an adverse reaction to cardiac drugs. A ventricular septal defect is a congenital condition. Hypertension is not caused by mitral valve prolapse.
   NP = As
   CN = Ph/8
   CL = An
   SA = 1

4. 3. A second-degree A-V block is not a contraindication to receiving fibrinolytic (thrombolytic) therapy to dissolve clots in the coronary arteries. Asthma is a contraindication to receiving beta blockers. Aspirin-sensitive individuals should not be given aspirin in acute coronary syndrome events. The contraindication to receiving fibrinolytics listed here is cerebral hemorrhage because the client is at risk for a second bleed.
NP = An
CN = Ph/8
CL = An
SA = 1

5. 2. Daily digoxin for inotropic effect and slowing of the heart rate does not affect nitroglycerin use. Verapamil, used for chronic angina, hypertension, or dysrhythmias, also does not affect use of nitrates in a client suspected of cardiac ischemic pain. Although a client taking warfarin has many drugs that should not be taken concurrently, nitroglycerin is not one of them. It is essential to report the use of Viagra within 24 hours because the combination of nitroglycerin and Viagra causes profound hypotension.
NP = An
CN = Ph/6
CL = An
SA = 5

6. 2. A first-degree block involves a prolonged PR. A second-degree block, type II (Mobitz II) involves consistent PR intervals, but suddenly dropped QRS complexes. A third-degree block is seen when the P and QRS complexes occur independently of each other. The rhythm described here is a classic second-degree heart block, type I (Wenckebach). It may occur transiently after an MI, or be a precursor of a more severe block. Usually no treatment is needed. However, if the client is symptomatic, atropine may be given or a pacemaker may be indicated.
NP = An
CN = Ph/8
CL = An
SA = 1

7. 4. Lidocaine (Xylocaine) and verapamil (Calan) are not appropriate drug choices for a client with a third-degree block because each is for tachycardia and characteristic of a third-degree heart block is bradycardia. A coronary angiogram is often indicated for the client with angina in coronary artery disease. The priority here is the client's poor cardiac output due to low ventricular rate. The client is symptomatic, so the first intervention should be to apply a temporary pacemaker to increase cardiac output and raise the blood pressure.

NP = Pl
CN = Ph/8
CL = Ap
SA = 1

8. 3. Only if the client is hemodynamically unstable (BP less than 90 systolic, angina, dyspnea, decreased level of consciousness) would electrical cardioversion be appropriate. Electrical defibrillation and CPR are indicated for a client in ventricular tachycardia without any pulse, or in ventricular fibrillation. IV lidocaine is the correct intervention in this case, as the client is hemodynamically stable at this point. Lidocaine IV increases the electrical stimulation threshold of the ventricles in a client experiencing ventricular tachycardia, thereby stabilizing the cardiac membrane.
NP = Im
CN = Ph/8
CL = Ap
SA = 1

9. 1. A PR interval that gradually lengthens until a QRS is dropped describes a second-degree block, type I (Wenckebach). P waves and QRS complexes independent of each other may describe a third-degree heart block. Having no measurable P waves or QRS complexes describes ventricular fibrillation, which would require immediate defibrillation, CPR, and potentially implantation of an internal cardioverter defibrillator (ICD). The client's rhythm is a second-degree block, type II, which often leads to a higher heart block with clinical manifestations of fatigue, dizziness, and decreased blood pressure. The nurse should measure the ventricular rate alone (not the P waves) to get an accurate heart rate.
NP = An
CN = Ph/8
CL = An
SA = 1

10. 2. The 5th intercostal space to the left of the midclavicular line is best for auscultating the mitral valve (or apical pulse). The 4th intercostal space to the right of the sternum is best for listening to the functioning of the tricuspid valve. The pulmonic valve is less commonly problematic and is best heard at the 2nd intercostal space to the left of the sternum. The best placement of the stethoscope for the aortic valve is the 2nd intercostal space to the right of the sternum.
NP = As
CN = Ph/8
CL = Ap
SA = 1

11. 3. Ventricular depolarization is represented by the QRS wave, and ventricular repolarization by the QT interval. The isoelectric line is the flat baseline prior to the P wave. Atrial depolarization is represented by the P wave, which is generally positive in deflection, round, and uniform. The P wave represents atrial depolarization.
NP = Im
CN = Ph/8
CL = Ap
SA = 1

12. 1, 4. The blood pressure of a client with pyelonephritis of 112/68 is stable. The fever of 38.3°C or 101°F is likely the cause of a mildly elevated heart rate (118). Administration of acetaminophen (Tylenol) and increased fluids are the appropriate interventions. An immediate synchronized cardioversion is indicated for unstable ventricular tachycardia with a pulse, or for unstable atrial flutter or fibrillation. An unstable client is described as experiencing chest pain, dyspnea, loss of consciousness, and hypotension. If the nurse gave atropine, it would worsen the situation because atropine would stimulate the already high heart rate. Digoxin (Lanoxin) IV push may be appropriate for a client in a rapid atrial fibrillation or flutter because such a client is not unstable. To treat the underlying cause of the fast heart rate would be most appropriate for this client.
NP = Im
CN = Ph/8
CL = Ap
SA = 1

13. 2. Warfarin (Coumadin) is an anticoagulant used as a prophylaxis and in the treatment of atrial fibrillation that does not assist in keeping the heart rate from beating too fast. Digoxin (Lanoxin) would prevent the heart from going too fast. Avoiding high-potassium foods is important for the client in renal failure who is undergoing hemodialysis, not the client on warfarin. Warfarin therapy does not dissolve clots, but rather prevents them. The warfarin therapy needs to be monitored through laboratory levels of international normalized ratio (INR).
NP = Ev
NP = Ph/6
CL = An
SA = 5

14. 1. For pulseless ventricular defibrillation, immediate synchronized cardioversion is the priority intervention. CPR should be done until emergency responders arrive if cardioversion is not available or if the nurse is not trained in performing cardioversion. A blood draw for

potassium and arterial blood gases may be appropriate in this situation, but not as the first intervention. Digoxin (Lanoxin) is not indicated for ventricular tachycardia.
NP = Pl
CN = Sa/1
CL = Ap
SA = 1

15. 1. For the stable client in sinus bradycardia, further assessment may be performed, but no immediate treatment is needed. Further assessment may include oxygen saturation, 12-lead ECG, chest x-ray, and consideration of possible causes (e.g., cardiac drugs). If the client were to become hypotensive or experience chest pain or dyspnea, atropine IV may be given, as well as consideration of a temporary pacemaker. However, atenolol would be contraindicated at this point, due to its effect of lowering blood pressure and an already low heart rate.
NP = Im
CN = Ph/8
CL = Ap
SA = 1

16. 2. A CAT scan is the appropriate test because the client is showing signs of possible dissecting aneurysm. A cardiac stress test may be indicated for a client with angina clinical manifestations. The coronary artery bypass surgery would be indicated for a client who showed disease during an angiogram and was not a candidate for a percutaneous coronary intervention during the angiogram. Thrombolytic therapy is contraindicated for a potentially bleeding client because of its effect of exacerbating bleeding. Appropriate interventions may include serial hemoglobins, antihypertensive drugs, oxygen, pain relief, IV fluids, possible transfusions, and immediate surgical repair.
NP = An
CN = Ph/8
CL = An
SA = 1

17. 4. Taking several aspirin a day can actually reverse the antiplatelet effect of one aspirin in a client with chronic arterial vascular disease. Sleeping with a hot water bottle may be dangerous to an individual with vascular disease who may have reduced sensation due to nerve damage. Burns can occur without the warning sign of pain. While pentoxifylline (Trental) may reduce blood viscosity and increase erythrocyte flexibility to improve blood flow, there is no cure for chronic arterial vascular disease. Controlling risk factors does help prevent worsening of the disease, and

includes management of hypertension, diabetes, weight and lipid management, tobacco avoidance, and use of exercise regimes.
NP = Ev
CN = Ph/8
CL = Ap
SA = 1

18. 3, 4, 6. Immediate clot removal is not common for a deep vein thrombosis. Implantation of an intracaval filter in the inferior vena cava is usually done for the client who cannot take warfarin (Coumadin) or has had multiple clots. Daily warfarin may be prescribed to prevent clots, but it will not reach a therapeutic level the first day it is administered and so heparin IV or SQ is needed initially to prevent further clots while the body tries to lyse an acute clot. Heparin, elevation of the affected extremity, and bed rest until the client is anticoagulated on warfarin (Coumadin) are the commonly ordered interventions.
NP = An
CN = Ph/8
CL = An
SA = 1

19. 2. Ventricular tachycardia appearing on the heart monitor an hour after permanent pacemaker placement is not a normal finding. A chest x-ray should be done quickly to see if a lead has slipped, causing ventricular irritability and tachycardia. The client may need immediate return to have the cardiologist readjust lead placement. The international normalized ratio (INR) should have been drawn prior to surgery if the client was on warfarin to make sure the blood was not too thin, but too-thin blood would not be a cause of tachycardia.
NP = An
CN = Ph/8
CL = An
SA = 1

20. 4. An electrophysiology (EP) study is done to find the source of a dysrhythmia. The client with frequent dysrhythmias would be most likely to have the study done. The cardiologist may then use an electrode-tipped catheter to "burn" extra pathways that cause tachycardias.
NP = Ev
CN = Ph/8
CL = An
SA = 1

21. 2. While a stress test or coronary angiogram may be important diagnostic tests for coronary artery disease in a client with anginal clinical manifestations, neither is a standard procedure after a pacemaker

insertion. A transesophageal echocardiogram (TEE) is done to check for heart size, wall motion, valvular abnormalities, and possible thrombi, but not routinely after a pacemaker. The test routinely ordered after permanent pacemaker insertion is a chest x-ray, to check for lead placement and possible pneumothorax.
NP = Im
CN = Ph/7
CL = Ap
SA = 1

22. 4. Diuresis, not increased fluid volumes, is commonly indicated for a client with heart failure exacerbation. Treatment of the underlying cause may help reduce the disease severity. Albuterol is helpful for shortness of breath if it is caused by asthma, not heart failure. Peripheral edema and a feeling of fullness are characteristics of right-sided heart failure.
NP = Pl
CN = Ph/8
CL = An
SA = 1

23. 3. Following administration of D5W, it would be appropriate to administer vasopressors to a client with diabetes mellitus and heart failure who was found unresponsive, hypotensive, tachycardic, and had a blood glucose of 28. Hypoglycemia may be a cause of neurogenic shock, for which vasopressors would be indicated. Epinephrine would be appropriate for anaphylactic shock, and antibiotics for septic shock. Nitroglycerin may be given for the client in an acute myocardial infarction.
NP = An
CN = Ph/6
CL = An
SA = 5

24. 1, 5. The client with heart failure should have a low-sodium diet. Processed ham and cheese, as well as canned products such as tomato juice, are high in sodium. Baked potato and lean beef are the best low-sodium selections.
NP = Im
CN = Ph/5
CL = Ap
SA = 1

25. 1, 3, 5. Oxygen saturation level should be at least 90% for the client experiencing unstable angina. While serum cardiac markers may be positive in the subendocardial MI (non-Q wave) stage, they are not positive in the client with unstable angina. Immediate coronary bypass surgery is often the route only after coronary angiography shows that the client's left

main is occluded and the client is unstable. Priority interventions for a client experiencing unstable angina include rest, continuous ECG monitoring with serial ECGs and cardiac markers, as well as systemic heparin to prevent dislodged plaque from occluding a coronary artery.

NP = Pl

CN = Sa/1

CL = An

SA = 1

26. 3. A chest x-ray after pacemaker placement is taken to assure that a lead wire did not puncture the lung following placement of a permanent pacemaker. Arterial disease is ruled out by coronary angiogram. Pacemaker functioning can be assessed by ECG monitoring, and programming functions can be evaluated by computer interrogation.

NP = An

CN = Ph/8

CL = An

SA = 1

27. 4, 6, 1, 3, 5, 2. The normal conduction pathway through the heart starts in the sinoatrial (S-A) node followed by conduction through the internodal tracts, A-V node, bundle of His, bundle branches, and Purkinje fibers.

NP = Im

CN = Ph/8

CL = Co

SA = 1

28. 1. A second-degree A-V block type I (Mobitz I or Wenckebach) is a conduction delay that occurs at the level of the A-V node. The impulses that start in the sinoatrial (S-A) node take longer and longer to pass through the A-V node. This results in lengthening PR intervals. Eventually the sinus impulse becomes blocked and there is a P wave on the ECG monitor with no QRS after it (dropped beat). Ventricular fibrillation is a lethal rhythm in which there is a chaotic rhythm originating in the ventricles. It is an unorganized and uncoordinated pattern with rapid impulses that cause the heart to fibrillate rather than contract. This is a medical emergency. Premature atrial contractions originate outside the S-A node from an irritable focus within the atria. Atrial fibrillation is an extreme irritability of the atria. It is a constant, generalized quivering with no signs of organized atrial activity.

NP = Ev

CN = Ph/8

CL = An

SA = 1

29. Ventricular tachycardia. Ventricular tachycardia is a lethal rhythm that exists when three or more premature ventricular contractions (PVCs) occur in a row at a rate greater than 100 beats per minute.
NP = As
CN = Ph/8
CL = Ap
SA = 1

30. 3. A priority intervention for a client with a third-degree A-V block is a pacemaker. A permanent pacemaker would not be used after open heart surgery. An anterior myocardial infarction may lead to a third-degree A-V block.
NP = Ev
CN = Ph/8
CL = An
SA = 1

31. 2. The nurse should question an order for lidocaine to be administered to a client with a second-degree A-V block type II (Mobitz II). There may be a profound bradycardia that needs to be treated. Lidocaine is contraindicated because it would further slow the rate. A client with symptomatic sinus bradycardia is treated with atropine. It is appropriate to discontinue epinephrine for a client with an accelerated junctional rhythm because excessive administration of catecholamines such as epinephrine, norepinephrine, or dopamine may be the cause. Junctional rhythms may occur as a result of a digitalis toxicity, so obtaining a digoxin level is appropriate.
NP = An
CN = Sa/1
CL = An
SA = 1

32. 3. A transcutaneous pacemaker is an external pacemaker that may cause uncomfortable muscle contractions when a current passes through the chest wall. A fever is not an occurrence after external pacemaker insertion. It may be a complication of permanent pacemaker insertion. Airport travel does not need to be avoided. The small case of a pacemaker rarely sets off the airport security. Should that happen, the client may tell the airport security of the existence of a pacemaker or obtain a physician's note. Microwave ovens do not affect the functioning of the pacemaker.
NP = Im
CN = Sa/1

CL = An
SA = 1

33. 3. The ST segment is the period between ventricular depolarization and repolarization. The P wave is the first wave of the cardiac cycle that represents atrial depolarization. The PR interval is the period when the impulse spreads through the atria, A-V node, bundle of His, and Purkinje fibers. The QRS complex represents ventricular depolarization.
NP = An
CN = Ph/8
CL = Ap
SA = 1

34. 4. Atrial flutter is a dysrhythmia with very irritable atria. The atria discharge at approximately 250 to 350 beats per minute. The waveforms produced resemble the teeth of a saw. Ventricular tachycardia is a lethal rhythm with three or more premature ventricular contractions (PVCs) occurring in a sequence at a rate of greater than 100 beats per minute. Idioventricular rhythm (ventricular escape rhythm) is a lethal rhythm in which no impulses are conducted to the ventricles from above the bundle of His. Atrial fibrillation is a rhythm in which there is an extreme atrial irritability. There is a constant quivering with no sign of organized atrial activity.
NP = Ev
CN = Ph/8
CL = An
SA = 1

35. 2. Characteristics of premature ventricular contractions (PVCs) include a wide and bizarre QRS complex greater than 0.12 seconds. The P wave may be absent and, if present, is not premature. The rate is usually regular but does depend on the underlying rhythm. The PR interval is absent because the ectopic beat originates in the ventricles.
NP = An
CN = Ph/8
CL = An
SA = 1

36. 1. Sinus tachycardia is a dysrhythmia in which the sinoatrial (S-A) node discharges more than 100 beats per minute. The P wave is normal, the PR interval is between 0.12 and 0.20 seconds, and a QRS complex is less than 0.12 seconds. The atrial and ventricular depolarization remains normal. It may be a normal rate for infants or young children. Ventricular fibrillation is a lethal rhythm originating in the ventricles resulting in the heart fibrillating. Atrial flutter resembles the teeth of a saw in which the atria discharge at 250 to 350 beats per minute. Ventricular tachycardia is a lethal

rhythm in which there are three or more premature ventricular contractions (PVCs) in a row at a rate greater than 100 beats per minute.
NP = Ev
CN = Ph/8
CL = An
SA = 1

37. 4. A pacemaker that fails to capture may occur when the electrical current to the heart muscle is insufficient to produce atrial and ventricular contractions, resulting in symptomatic bradycardia. An elevated temperature and redness at the insertion area may indicate an infection. A hematoma at the pacemaker insertion site may indicate bleeding into the surrounding tissue.
NP = As
CN = Ph/8
CL = Ap
SA = 1

38. **Premature atrial contractions.** Premature atrial contractions are a dysrhythmia originating outside the S-A node resulting from an irritable focus within the atria. Contributing causes include alcohol, cigarettes, and caffeine. The client may feel fatigued as a result.
NP = As
CN = Ph/8
CL = An
SA = 1

39. **Call a code.** A dysrhythmia in which there is no measurable rhythm or rate and an occasional wide and bizarre QRS indicates the presence of an agonal rhythm. The priority intervention is to call a code followed by CPR. Epinephrine and atropine may be administered.
NP = Im
CN = Sa/1
CL = An
SA = 1

40. 3. A first-degree A-V is a dysrhythmia in which there is a consistent delay in the A-V conduction system. Usually no intervention is needed. The heart rate generally ranges between 60 and 100 beats per minute. Unlicensed assistive personnel (UAP) cannot assess, plan, or evaluate.
NP = Pl
CN = Sa/1
CL = An
SA = 8

GASTROINTESTINAL DISORDERS - COMPREHENSIVE EXAM

1. When preparing a client for an upper gastrointestinal series, it would be essential for the nurse to plan to explain which of the following aspects of the procedure?

1. The stools will be white until the barium is expelled

2. The test takes approximately 2 hours and it is important for the client to lie still

3. The nurse will monitor bowel sounds hourly for 24 hours

4. A mild sedative will be administered 30 minutes before the procedure

2. When preparing a client for a cholecystography, the nurse should

1. Administer a radiopaque dye and fat-free meal the evening before the procedure

2. Instruct the client on postprocedure coughing and deep breathing techniques

3. Administer enemas the evening before the procedure and the morning of the procedure

4. Position the client on the right side and encourage lying still during the procedure

3. A client's family member asks the nurse how the physician could diagnose the client on the results of a barium enema that showed a "string sign"? The nurse's response is based on the understanding that what disease is characterized by a "string sign" on a barium enema? ______________

4. The nurse is collecting a nursing history from a client admitted with atrophic gastritis. The nurse should question the client about a past medical history of

1. Cardiac disease

2. Chronic obstructive pulmonary disease

3. Intestinal parasites

4. Pernicious anemia

5. A client with diverticulitis is having difficulty marking the menu. The nurse assists the client to mark which of the following breakfast selections?Select all that apply:

[ ] **1.** Fried eggs

[ ] **2.** Bran cereal

[ ] 3. Hash brown potatoes

[ ] 4. Cream puff

[ ] 5. Whole wheat toast

[ ] 6. Pecan nut bread

6. A client has developed gastroesophageal reflux. Which of the following regimens does the nurse select as most effective for this client?
   1. Provide the client with a glass of milk at bedtime
   2. Encourage the client to lie down and rest after meals
   3. Elevate the head of the bed on four- to six-inch blocks
   4. Instruct the client on a high-calorie, high-fat diet

7. The priority goal of nursing care in the postoperative period following a Nissen repair of a sliding hiatal hernia is
   1. prevention of respiratory complications.
   2. return of peristalsis to normal.
   3. promotion of wound healing.
   4. independence in activities of daily living.

8. A nurse is caring for a client with a peptic ulcer. Which of the following measures is essential to include in the client's discharge instructions?
   1. Instruct the client to avoid straining at stool for four to six weeks
   2. Encourage the client to drink 2500 ml/day to prevent complications
   3. Instruct the client to eat three balanced meals a day and to avoid alcohol and smoking
   4. Encourage the client to take Motrin (ibuprofen) or aspirin (acetylsalicylic acid) for pain

9. The nurse is admitting a client with a peptic ulcer who is experiencing a sudden sharp pain in the abdomen. The client becomes anxious and assumes a fetal position. The nurse suspects the client's ulcer has perforated. Which of the following clinical manifestations support the nurse's assessment?
   Select all that apply:

[ ] 1. Rigid, boardlike abdomen

[ ] 2. Slow, deep respirations

[ ] 3. Hyperactive bowel sounds

[ ] 4. Anxiety

[ ] 5. Bradycardia

[ ] 6. Weakness

10. The nurse understands that which of the following organs is most likely to be involved in confined perforation of a peptic ulcer?

1. Pancreas

2. Liver

3. Gallbladder

4. Small intestine

11. The nurse is preparing to insert a nasogastric (NG) tube. Which of the following nursing measures facilitates insertion of a nasogastric tube?

1. Place the NG tube in warm water prior to insertion

2. Apply gentle pressure to push the tube past any resistance

3. Ask the client to swallow as the tube is being advanced

4. Have the client lie supine when passing the tube

12. The nurse informs the client to follow which of the following diets to reduce the likelihood of developing dumping syndrome?Select all that apply:

[ ] **1.** Low calorie with fluids at meals

[ ] **2.** Low carbohydrate

[ ] **3.** Moderate fat

[ ] **4.** High fiber

[ ] **5.** Moderate protein

[ ] **6.** Low residue

13. The nurse should implement which of the following activity orders for a client with acute hepatitis?

1. Encourage ambulation

2. Sit up in chair

3. Bedrest

4. No specific activity orders

14. The nurse is caring for a client beginning the posticteric phase of hepatitis. Which of the following would indicate to the nurse that a client's condition is deteriorating?

1. Jaundice

2. Malaise

3. Fatigue

4. Hepatomegaly

15. A female client with hepatitis A asks the nurse how she got the disease. Based on an understanding of the spread of the disease, which of the following is the most appropriate response?

 1. Fecal-oral contamination
 2. Diseased animals
 3. Unprotected sexual contact
 4. Infected serum

16. The physician orders a low-fat diet for a client after cholecystectomy. The nurse assists the client to select which of the following foods for mealtime?Select all that apply:

 [ ] 1. Cheese omelet
 [ ] 2. Roast beef sandwich
 [ ] 3. Chocolate pudding
 [ ] 4. Applesauce
 [ ] 5. Ham salad
 [ ] 6. Bacon, lettuce, tomato sandwich

17. A client who had a cholecystectomy is ready to be discharged and the dietitian instructs the client to remain on a low-fat diet for several more weeks. The client asks the nurse, "Will I have to stay away from fat for the rest of my life?" Which of the following responses would be most appropriate?

 1. "You'll have to remain on a fat-free diet from now on to avoid problems."
 2. "After you have fully recovered from surgery, you'll probably be able to eat a normal diet, avoiding excessive fat."
 3. "It's too early to say. Later, when we see whether the operation is successful, we'll know the answer."
 4. "Only your doctor can answer that. Why don't you ask your physician before you are discharged from the hospital?"

18. The nurse is caring for a client with cirrhosis who has developed ascites. Which of the following is the priority treatment goal?

 1. Provide good skin care to decrease pruritus
 2. Restrict fats and sodium in the diet
 3. Maintain a normal body weight
 4. Return fluid to the vascular bed

19. The nurse is caring for a client with hepatic encephalopathy. Which of the following nursing interventions is appropriate?

1. Encourage the client to assume a side-lying position with legs drawn up
2. Provide a high-calorie, high-carbohydrate, and low-protein diet
3. Instruct the client to avoid heavy lifting, pushing, and pulling for 6 weeks
4. Administer pain medication every 4 hours as ordered for severe pain

20. The nurse is assessing a client in the icteric phase of hepatitis. Which of the following would the nurse expect to be the major assessment findings?Select all that apply:

[ ] **1.** Malaise
[ ] **2.** Jaundice
[ ] **3.** Dark-colored urine
[ ] **4.** Fatigue
[ ] **5.** Right upper abdominal pain
[ ] **6.** Clay-colored stools

21. A nurse is discharging a client with hepatitis. Which of the following nursing measures would be essential to include in the client's plan of care?

1. Instruct the client to follow a low-carbohydrate diet
2. Instruct the client to take acetaminophen (Tylenol) for pain
3. Encourage the medical follow-up for one year
4. Encourage resuming normal activities upon discharge

22. The nurse is admitting a client who is vomiting and experiencing right upper quadrant pain that radiates to the right scapula. The nurse suspects what disease? _______________

23. The nurse identifies which of the following clients to be at greatest risk for developing cholecystitis?

1. A 42-year-old female who has three children
2. A 55-year-old male who has a history of chronic alcoholism
3. A 28-year-old female who is taking oral contraceptives
4. A 75-year-old male who has a history of congestive heart failure

24. The nurse assesses a client with hepatic encephalopathy for apraxia by

1. assessing the client's breath for a musty, sweet odor.
2. asking the client to draw a simple figure and noting any deterioration.
3. reviewing the bilirubin and alkaline phosphate levels.
4. asking the client to extend an arm, dorsiflex the wrist, and extend the fingers.

25. A client is admitted with hepatitis B of unknown etiology. Which of the following would be an appropriate question for the nurse to ask?
   1. "Have you recently traveled abroad?"
   2. "Have you recently used substances considered caustic without wearing rubber gloves?"
   3. "Have you recently received a tattoo, manicure, or pedicure from a salon?"
   4. "Have you recently been camping or been gardening?"
26. The registered nurse is preparing the client assignments for the day. Which of the following clients would be most appropriate to delegate to a licensed practical nurse?
   1. A client with fulminant hepatitis
   2. A client with a pleural effusion as a result of pancreatitis
   3. A client with cholecystitis who is scheduled to have an oral cholecystogram
   4. A client with a peptic ulcer requiring preoperative teaching for a Billroth I
27. Which of the following four clients is most appropriate for the registered nurse to delegate to a licensed practical nurse to care for?
   1. A client with a perforated peptic ulcer scheduled for surgery
   2. A client with gastroenteritis who has an order for IV therapy
   3. A client with cholecystitis and colic pain ordered to receive Demerol IM
   4. A client with diverticulitis ordered to have high-fiber diet planning and teaching
28. The nurse gives a client which of the following instructions when collecting a stool specimen?
   1. Cleanse from the urinary meatus to the anus
   2. Defecate into the toilet bowl
   3. Void first before defecating
   4. Place toilet tissue into the bedpan
29. The nurse observes another staff member irrigating a nasogastric tube with 30 ml water. Which of the following statements by the nurse is most appropriate?
   1. "Irrigate with normal saline because hypotonic solutions such as water cause an electrolyte loss."
   2. "Try irrigating with 60 ml of water to enhance a more rapid return."

3. "You correctly irrigated the nasogastric tube."
4. "Make sure you record the 30 ml water used for irrigating on the intake and output."

30. Which of the following changes during the nurse's assessment of a client is reported as a critical sign of intestinal obstruction?

1. Diarrhea
2. Steatorrhea
3. Dysphagia
4. Abdominal distention

31. The nurse assesses which of the following to be characteristic of a client with ulcerative colitis?

1. Left lower abdominal pain and tenderness
2. Persistent periumbilical pain that shifts to the right lower quadrant
3. 15 to 20 stools per day with blood or mucus
4. 3 to 5 steatorrhea stools per day

32. Which of the following menu selections does the nurse assist a client with ulcerative colitis to make?Select all that apply:

[ ] **1.** Raisin bran cereal
[ ] **2.** Whole grain bread
[ ] **3.** Baked chicken
[ ] **4.** Milk
[ ] **5.** Mashed potatoes
[ ] **6.** Applesauce

33. The nurse is caring for a client with ulcerative colitis who states, "I have a greater risk of getting colon cancer." The most appropriate response by the nurse is

1. "There is no increased risk of colon cancer."
2. "Follow-up is essential with periodic colonoscopy."
3. "The incidence of cancer is slightly decreased with surgery."
4. "Colon cancer occurs most frequently in early stages."

34. The nurse is preparing for a herniorrhaphy. Which of the following aspects of the post-op care should the nurse to explain to the client?

1. A heating pad will be applied to the incision
2. A low-residue diet will be prescribed
3. Coughing is encouraged every two hours
4. Intake and output will be accurately measured

35. The nurse is teaching a client that had a hemorrhoidectomy to prevent hemorrhoids in the future. Which of the following would the nurse be correct to include in the teaching?

  1. Low-residue diet
  2. Test stools for occult blood weekly
  3. Use of stool softeners
  4. Sit for longer periods of time

36. A client with a stoma is experiencing diarrhea and asks the nurse if there are any foods that are contributing. Which of the following foods should the nurse inform him or her to avoid?Select all that apply:

  [ ] 1. Eggs
  [ ] 2. Cabbage
  [ ] 3. Spinach
  [ ] 4. Strong cheese
  [ ] 5. Alcohol
  [ ] 6. Green beans

37. The nurse is irrigating a client's colostomy and the client begins to experience cramping. The most appropriate nursing action would be

  1. Insert the irrigation catheter farther
  2. Clamp the irrigation for a few seconds
  3. Raise the level of the irrigation bag
  4. Discontinue the irrigation

38. When preparing a client for a liver biopsy, the nurse explains which of the following aspects of the procedure?

  1. Nothing by mouth will be permitted for 8 hours prior to the procedure
  2. A laxative will be administered the evening before the procedure
  3. Ambulation is important postprocedure to promote peristalsis
  4. Lying on the right side is maintained for two hours postprocedure

39. A client admitted for a gastrointestinal work-up is experiencing frequent loose stools. The priority goal for the nurse is to

  1. Assist with self-care activities for the client
  2. Ensure fluid and electrolyte replacement
  3. Instruct the client on correct medical asepsis
  4. Restrict food and fluids to decrease peristalsis

40. The nurse is collecting a nursing history from a client suspected to have an obstruction of the alimentary canal. Which of the following questions should the nurse ask first to elicit the most accurate assessment?

1. "Are you frequently awakened during the middle of the night because of pain?"
2. "Have you recently lost a lot of weight?"
3. "Do you have difficulty swallowing foods or liquids?"
4. "Have you experienced any bleeding?"

41. When preparing a client to collect a stool specimen, it would be essential for the nurse to explain which of the following aspects of the procedure?

1. No medication or food restrictions prior to the collection
2. The specimen may be stored at room temperature before being taken to the lab
3. Urine may be included with the stool specimen in the container
4. Avoid placing toilet paper with the specimen

42. Based on an understanding of bleeding that can occur in the gastrointestinal tract, bleeding that occurs in the upper gastrointestinal tract results in what color stool? ________

ANSWERS AND RATIONALES

1. 1. An upper gastrointestinal series or barium swallow is an x-ray study with fluoroscopy and a contrast medium. It diagnoses conditions of the esophagus, stomach, and upper duodenum. It takes approximately 30 minutes for the test to be performed. There is no sedation prior to positioning. The only discomfort may involve assuming various positions on the x-ray table. The stools may be white for up to 72 hours postprocedure. Fluids are to be encouraged to prevent constipation.
NP = Pl
CN = Ph/7
CL = Ap
SA = 1

2. 1. A cholecystography is a radiography test in which a radiopaque dye and fat-free meal are administered the evening before the procedure. There is no need to perform coughing and deep breathing exercises postprocedure. No enemas are given before the procedure. The client does not lie on the right side during the procedure.

NP = Pl
CN = Ph/7
CL = Ap
SA = 1

3. **Crohn's disease.** Crohn's disease is an inflammatory process of part of the gastrointestinal tract. It often affects the terminal ileum, jejunum, and colon. A classic finding on a barium enema is a "string sign."
NP = An
CN = Ph/8
CL = Co
SA = 1

4. **4.** A client with atrophic gastritis has an increased incidence of gastric cancer and may have a history of pernicious anemia. It would be important to question the client about a history of pernicious anemia.
NP = An
CN = Ph/8
CL = An
SA = 1

5. **2, 5.** Diverticulitis is an inflammation of the diverticula most commonly in the sigmoid colon. A high-fiber diet is recommended. Bran cereal and whole wheat bread would be appropriate food choices.
NP = Im
CN = Ph/5
CL = Ap
SA = 1

6. **3.** Gastroesophageal reflux is a disorder in which gastric acid refluxes back into the lower esophagus generally from an incompetent lower esophageal sphincter (LES). Appropriate nursing interventions include elevating the head of the bed on four- to six-inch blocks and a high-protein, low-fat diet. It is helpful to elevate the head of the client's bed and for the client to avoid lying down after meals.
NP = Ev
CN = Ph/8
CL = Ap
SA = 1

7. **1.** The priority goal for a client following a Nissen repair of a sliding hiatal hernia is to prevent respiratory complications from regurgitation of gastric contents into the trachea.There may be a high incidence of hospitalization due to respiratory complications.
NP = Ev
CN = Ph/7

CL = An
SA = 1

8. 3. A client who has peptic ulcer disease should be instructed to eat three well-balanced meals a day and avoid alcohol and smoking. Smoking is an irritant to the gastric mucosa. It delays healing of the mucosa and increases gastric motility. Nonsteroid anti-inflammatories and aspirin are to be discontinued because they are irritating to the gastric mucosa and may result in bleeding. Straining at stool and encouraging fluids have no bearing on the peptic ulcer.
NP = Pl
CN = Ph/8
CL = Ap
SA = 1

9. 1, 4. Clinical manifestations of a perforated peptic ulcer include severe upper abdominal pain. The abdomen becomes rigid and boardlike. The respirations become rapid and shallow. The client experiences nausea and vomiting and has accompanying anxiety. The bowel sounds are also absent.
NP = Ev
CN = Ph/8
CL = An
SA = 1

10. 1. The most common organ to be involved in a perforated peptic ulcer is the pancreas because of its close proximity to the ulcer.
NP = Ev
CN = Ph/7
CL = An
SA = 1

11. 3. The client should be sitting with the head of the bed elevated 30 to 45 degrees to prevent aspiration. The client should swallow as the tube is being advanced. The end of the tube is placed in water prior to insertion to activate the lubricant jelly. Never advance the tube when resistance is felt.
NP = Pl
CN = Ph/7
CL = Ap
SA = 1

12. 2, 3, 5. The diet of choice for dumping syndrome is low carbohydrate, moderate fat, and moderate protein. Fluids are to be avoided during meals, but should be taken between meals.
NP = Im
CN = Ph/5

CL = Ap
SA = 1

13. 3. The activity order for a client with acute hepatitis is bedrest to allow for the liver cells to regenerate and heal.
NP = Im
CN = Ph/5
CL = Ap
SA = 1

14. 1. The posticteric phase of hepatitis is considered the convalescent phase of hepatitis. It starts with the disappearance of jaundice and can last two to four months. Relapses may occur. If jaundice reappears, it may indicate the client's condition is deteriorating.
NP = An
CN = Ph/8
CL = An
SA = 1

15. 1. Hepatitis A is spread through fecal-oral contamination. Hepatitis B and C are spread through exposure to blood products, sexual contact, and perinatal transmission. Hepatitis D routes of transmission are similar to hepatitis B. Hepatitis E is also spread by fecal-oral contamination.
NP = An
CN = Ph/8
CL = An
SA = 1

16. 2, 4. Cheese omelet, chocolate pudding, ham salad, and bacon, lettuce, tomato sandwich are high-fat foods. Roast beef sandwich and applesauce are lower fat food choices.
NP = Pl
CN = Ph/5
CL = Ap
SA = 1

17. 2. The client may be instructed to avoid excess fat for 4 to 6 weeks postoperatively but then may eat well-balanced meals avoiding excessive fat.
NP = An
CN = Ph/5
CL = An
SA = 1

18. 4. The priority goal for a client with cirrhosis who has developed ascites is to return the fluid to the vascular bed.
NP = Pl
CN = Sa/1

CL = Ap
SA = 1

19. 2. Hepatic encephalopathy is a neuropsychiatric manifestation of the damage sustained to the liver resulting in coma. The goal of the interventions should be to reduce the formation of ammonia. The client should be placed on a high-carbohydrate and low- or no-protein diet. A high-carbohydrate diet is given because the liver does not synthesize or store glucose. Instructing a client to avoid heavy lifting, pushing, or pulling and administering pain medications are appropriate interventions after abdominal surgery.
NP = Pl
CN = Ph/8
CL = Ap
SA = 1

20. 2, 3, 6. Clinical manifestations for the icteric phase of hepatitis include jaundice, dark-colored urine, and clay-colored stools. Malaise and fatigue are clinical manifestations that occur in the posticteric phase. Right upper abdominal pain is associated with the preicteric phase.
NP = As
CN = Ph/8
CL = Ap
SA = 1

21. 3. Because relapses are common with hepatitis, medical follow-up for one year is recommended. Rest is essential to allow the liver to regenerate. Small, frequent meals may be tolerated best if there is any associated nausea.
NP = Pl
CN = Ph/8
CL = Ap
SA = 1

22. **Cholecystitis.** Cholecystitis is characterized by right upper quadrant pain that radiates to the right scapula. Vomiting is also a frequent manifestation.
NP = An
CN = Ph/8
CL = Ap
SA = 1

23. 1. The classic picture of a client with cholecystitis is a woman over 40 years old and multiparous.
NP = Ev
CN = Ph/7

CL = An
SA = 1

24. 2. Apraxia is the inability to construct simple figures. Asterixis is commonly known as the liver flap or flapping tremors. This is a clinical manifestation of impending coma found in hepatic encephalopathy. Asterixis starts by affecting the hands and arms. It can be assessed by asking the client to extend an arm, dorsiflex the wrist, and extend the fingers. Fector hepaticus is a musty, sweet odor of the client's breath.
NP = As
CN = Ph/7
CL = Ap
SA = 1

25. 3. Hepatitis B may be transmitted percutaneously or through permucosal exposure. The client may have been infected through a contaminated needle while obtaining a tattoo or during a manicure or pedicure.
NP = An
CN = Sa/2
CL = An
SA = 1

26. 3. A client with fulminant hepatitis is in a crisis state. Fulminant hepatitis is a rare, severe, life-threatening form of hepatitis resulting in necrosis and liver failure. A pleural effusion is a systemic complication of pancreatitis. The client would be critically ill and would require the critical thinking only a registered nurse may offer. A client who has a peptic ulcer and is scheduled for a Billroth I or gastroduodenostomy requiring preoperative teaching should be cared for by a registered nurse. The most appropriate client assignment for a licensed practical nurse is a client with cholecystitis who is scheduled to have an oral cholecystogram. It is within the job description of the licensed practical nurse to administer the preparative measures for the oral cholecystogram.
NP = An
CN = Sa/1
CL = An
SA = 8

27. 3. A licensed practical nurse may administer prescribed Demerol IM to a client experiencing colic pain with cholecystitis. A client admitted with a perforated peptic ulcer is in an emergency state. When the peptic ulcer perforates, peritonitis may occur causing sepsis, shock, and possible death. Surgery, insertion of a nasogastric tube, and IV fluids is the usual treatment plan. Because it is an emergency situation involving critical thinking and acute assessment skills, a registered nurse should care for this client. A client with gastroenteritis ordered to have IV fluids should have a

registered nurse care for him or her because administering IV fluids is a job function reserved for the registered nurse. A client with diverticulitis ordered to have high-fiber diet planning and teaching is a function of the registered nurse. A licensed practical nurse cannot plan the original teaching plan. A licensed practical nurse may only reinforce already planned teaching.
NP = An
CN = Sa/1
CL = An
SA = 8

28. 3. A client should void prior to defecating for a stool specimen so the stool is urine free. Toilet paper should not be placed in the container because it would contaminate the specimen. Cleansing from the urinary meatus to the anus is not necessary with a stool specimen. It is a step in obtaining a midstream catch. The client should be instructed to void into a dry, clean container and not the toilet bowl to avoid contamination.
NP = Im
CN = Ph/7
CL = Ap
SA = 1

29. 1. The procedure for irrigating a nasogastric tube requires that normal saline be used because hypotonic solutions such as water cause an electrolyte loss.
NP = Ev
CN = Ph/7
CL = An
SA = 1

30. 4. A critical sign indicating an intestinal obstruction is abdominal distention. Diarrhea would be a manifestation of gastroenteritis. Steatorrhea is a clinical manifestation of pancreatitis. Dysphagia is a manifestation that occurs in many upper gastrointestinal disorders such as hiatal hernia.
NP = Ev
CN = Ph/8
CL = Ap
SA = 1

31. 3. Fifteen to 20 stools per day with blood or mucus is characteristic of ulcerative colitis.Left lower abdominal pain and tenderness is characteristic of diverticulitis. Persistent periumbilical pain that shifts to the right lower quadrant is found in appendicitis. Three to five steatorrhea stools per day may be found in chronic pancreatitis.
NP = As
CN = Ph/8

CL = Co
SA = 1

32. 3, 5, 6. The appropriate diet for ulcerative colitis should be high protein, high calorie, and low residue including foods such as baked chicken, mashed potatoes, and applesauce. Raisin bran cereal and whole grain bread are high-fiber foods. Milk is contraindicated with ulcerative colitis.
NP = Im
CN = Ph/5
CL = Ap
SA = 1

33. 2. Follow-up is essential with periodic colonoscopy for a client with ulcerative colitis to decrease the risk of colon cancer developing.
NP = An
CN = Ph/7
CL = An
SA = 1

34. 4. Post-op care for a client following a herniorrhaphy includes applying an ice pack to the area and measuring the intake and output. Difficulty voiding frequently requires catheterization. Coughing is to be discouraged. A high-fiber diet will prevent constipation.
NP = Pl
CN = Ph/8
CL = Ap
SA = 1

35. 3. Post-op teaching following a hemorrhoidectomy includes a high-fiber diet and use of stool softeners.
NP = Pl
CN = Ph/8
CL = Ap
SA = 1

36. 2, 3, 5, 6. Diarrhea-producing foods include cabbage, alcohol, coffee, spinach, green beans, raw fruits, and spicy foods. Strong cheese is a gas-forming food. Eggs are odor producing.
NP = Pl
CN = Ph/5
CL = Ap
SA = 1

37. 2. If a client experiences cramping during a colostomy irrigation, the irrigation tubing should be clamped for a few seconds. The irrigation tubing would not be inserted farther unless it is not inserted sufficiently

enough, causing leakage around the stoma. Raising the level of the irrigation bag would result in the irrigation fluid being introduced at a faster rate, causing a worsening of the cramping. It would not be necessary to discontinue the irrigation solution because of cramping. Clamping the tubing for a few seconds should allow the colon to rest and take care of the cramping.
NP = Im
CN = Ph/8
CL = Ap
SA = 1

38. 4. A client does not have to be NPO prior to a liver biopsy. There is no preparation before the procedure. The client should lie on the right side postprocedure to splint the incision.
NP = Im
CN = Ph/7
CL = Ap
SA = 1

39. 2. Ensuring fluid and electrolyte replacement is a nursing priority for a client who is experiencing frequent loose stools because of the risk of the client becoming dehydrated. Assisting with self-care activities or instructing on correct medical asepsis are not the priority interventions.
NP = Ev
CN = Ph/7
CL = An
SA = 1

40. 3. The first question to ask a client who is suspected of an obstruction of the alimentary canal is if there is any difficulty swallowing foods or liquids. Pain that occurs in the middle of the night and losing weight may be late clinical manifestations. Bleeding is not a manifestation of an obstruction.
NP = An
CN = Ph/8
CL = An
SA = 1

41. 4. A diet high in meat, poultry, fish, and green leafy vegetables may produce false-positive results. Drugs such as aspirin and anti-inflammatory drugs may also produce false-positive results. The stool specimen should be free of urine to avoid contaminating the results. Toilet paper should also not be placed with the specimen. The specimen should be taken to the lab immediately after collection.

NP = Pl
CN = Ph/7
CL = Ap
SA = 1

42. **Black.** Bleeding high in the gastrointestinal tract results in black stools. Bleeding low in the gastrointestinal tract results in red stools.
NP = An
CN = Ph/8
CL = Ap
SA = 1

Practice Test 2

GASTROINTESTINAL DISORDERS - COMPREHENSIVE EXAM

1. Which of the following abdominal findings should be reported as a critical sign of an abdominal aortic aneurysm?

1. Dull abdominal sounds heard over the liver
2. Pain experienced during the iliopsoas test
3. Positive ballottement test
4. Presence of a bruit over an abdominal vessel

2. The nurse is caring for an older adult client in a long-term care facility who is experiencing constipation. Which of the following interventions should the nurse implement?

1. Offer 2000 to 3000 ml of fluids daily
2. Administer a stimulant laxative to the client
3. Schedule a routine daily time for defecation at the evening meal
4. Assist the client to select a diet rich in pasta, eggs, and lean meats

3. The nurse should include which of the following when preparing to insert a nasogastric tube?

1. Ask the client to occlude one nostril and breathe through the other nostril
2. Position the client in a semi-Fowler's position
3. Place the tube in ice
4. Measure the tube from the client's earlobe to the nose to the sternum

ANSWERS AND RATIONALES

1. 4. The presence of a bruit over an abdominal vessel may suggest an abdominal aortic aneurysm. It is normal to percuss a dull sound over the liver. Ballottement test is a palpatory technique used to displace excess fluid in the abdominal cavity for the purpose of locating a mass or organ. The iliopsoas muscle test detects the presence of appendicitis. During the test, the client should not experience any pain.
   NP = An
   CN = Ph/7
   CL = An
   SA = 1

2. 1. Increasing fluid intake to 2000 to 3000 ml is an effective intervention in the management of constipation. Although administering a stimulant laxative may be an effective technique for constipation, it is not the most appropriate intervention because it may lead to a colon that becomes dependent on laxatives. Pasta, eggs, and lean meats are constipating foods. A diet rich in fruits and vegetables should be encouraged. For many clients, the best time for defecation is in the morning after breakfast.
   NP = Pl
   CN = Ph/8
   CL = Ap
   SA = 1

3. 1. When preparing to insert a nasogastric tube, the client should occlude one nostril and breathe through the other nostril. If the nare is occluded, it may cause trauma during insertion of the tube. The client should be placed in a high-Fowler's position. The tube should be measured from the tip of the nose to the earlobe to the xiphoid process.
   NP = Pl
   CN = Ph/8
   CL = Ap
   SA = 1

ENDOCRINE DISORDERS - COMPREHENSIVE EXAM

1. The nurse is caring for a client with an anterior pituitary disorder. Which of the following observations would indicate to the nurse a severe anterior pituitary deficiency?
   1. Intolerance to heat
   2. Increased sexual arousal

3. Frequent episodes of hypoglycemia
4. Increased pulse rate

2. A client has a transsphenoid total hypophysectomy. During the first 24-hour period postoperatively, which of the following is an anticipated finding?
   1. Blood pressure at 80/50
   2. Constant swallowing
   3. Urinary output of 150 ml in a two-hour period
   4. A runny nose
3. The nurse caring for a postoperative client who has had a transsphenoid hypophysectomy performs which of the following nursing interventions?
   1. Change the nasal packing
   2. Suction the nasal cavity
   3. Apply an ice collar to the neck
   4. Elevate the head of bed
4. The nurse admitting a client suspected of having diabetes insipidus anticipates finding which of the following clinical manifestations?
   1. Recent weight gain of 20 pounds
   2. Urine specific gravity of 1.005
   3. Urine output of 1500 ml per day
   4. Blood pressure of 150/90
5. Ongoing nursing care measures associated with a client who has hyperthyroidism should include
   1. providing high-energy snacks between meals.
   2. keeping the room temperature warm.
   3. limiting visitors to immediate family.
   4. forcing fluids to 3000 ml per day.
6. Planning the post-op care for a client who had a subtotal thyroidectomy should include which of the following interventions?
   1. Keep the head of the bed flat for the first 12 hours post-op
   2. Administer Synthroid 0.1 mg daily beginning in a.m.
   3. Begin range of motion exercises when fully awake
   4. Check for muscle tremors every two hours
7. Which of the following changes in the assessment of a client who has hyperthyroidism should the nurse report as a critical symptom of a thyroid crisis?
   Select all that apply:

[ ] **1.** Extreme elevation in body temperature

[ ] **2.** Apathetic response to stimuli

[ ] **3.** Decreased respirations

[ ] **4.** Tachycardia

[ ] **5.** Severe head and neck pain

[ ] **6.** Loss of skin turgor

8. Which of the following statements by the nurse should be included in the instructions for a client who is to receive ^{123}I for the treatment of hyperthyroidism?

1. "You should notice that your symptoms have disappeared several days after the treatment."

2. "You will need to observe special radioactive precautions with your urine after your treatment."

3. "You will need to watch for symptoms of an underactive thyroid gland for the next several years after treatment."

4. "You will only need one dose of the radioactive iodine to treat your thyroid condition."

9. Which of the following instructions is a priority for the nurse to include in the discharge plan for a client with hypothyroidism?

1. Take a daily laxative to prevent constipation

2. Eat a diet low in calories to promote weight reduction

3. Avoid extra clothing or blankets to keep the body from overheating

4. A sedative may be taken if there is difficulty sleeping

10. The nurse is collecting a nursing history for a client admitted with hyperparathyroidism. Which of the following questions should the nurse ask?

1. "Do you have any trouble breathing when you lie down?"

2. "Do you have any numbness or tingling in your extremities?"

3. "Have you hurt yourself in a fall recently or experienced bone pain?"

4. "Have you had any change in bowel habits recently?"

11. The nurse is caring for a client with hypoparathyroidism. Which of the following would indicate to the nurse that the client's condition is deteriorating?

1. Lack of strength in the upper muscle groups

2. Rigidity of the head and neck muscles

3. Loss of sensation in the hands and feet

4. Painful involuntary muscle spasms

12. In caring postoperatively for a client who had the parathyroid glands removed, the nurse should consider which of the following in goal planning?
    1. Prevention of pulmonary emboli
    2. Prevention of hemorrhage
    3. Maintenance of fluid and electrolyte balance
    4. Maintenance of cardiac stability
13. Which of the following should the nurse include in the discharge instructions of a client with Cushing's syndrome?
    1. Eat foods high in protein and potassium
    2. Take the prescribed prednisone once a day with meals
    3. Have hard candy readily available to treat hypoglycemia
    4. Increase fluid intake to at least 10 glasses per day
14. The nurse performs an assessment on a client diagnosed with primary aldosteronism.Which of the following assessment findings would be characteristic of this disorder?
    Select all that apply:
    [ ] 1. Leg cramps
    [ ] 2. Hypotension
    [ ] 3. Scanty urine output
    [ ] 4. Decreased thirst
    [ ] 5. Muscle weakness
    [ ] 6. Fatigue
15. The nurse is developing a teaching plan for a client with Addison's disease. Which of the following should the nurse include in the discharge instructions for a client with this disease?
    1. Increase the dosage of hormone replacement if you gain more than five pounds
    2. Increase salt intake in times of illness, very hot weather, and stress
    3. Monitor B/P frequently and decrease fluids if blood pressure drops when standing
    4. Inject Solu-Cortef subcutaneously when vomiting persists during an acute episode of gastroenteritis
16. The nurse is caring for a client suspected of having Addison's disease. Which of the following assessments would support this diagnosis?
    Select all that apply:
    [ ] 1. Bronze-like pigmentation of skin
    [ ] 2. Pedal edema

[ ] **3.** Hypertension

[ ] **4.** Headaches

[ ] **5.** Vomiting

[ ] **6.** Diarrhea

17. When observing for complications following an adrenalectomy for pheochromocytoma, the nurse should monitor for which of the following in the daily assessments of the client?

1. Hypertension

2. Respiratory obstruction

3. Hemorrhage

4. Paresthesia

18. The nurse conducts diabetes education classes for clients newly diagnosed with diabetes mellitus. Which of the following statements from a client with type 2 diabetes indicates an understanding of self-care management taught in class?

1. "I will need to take insulin for the rest of my life."

2. "If I lose weight, I'll be better able to control my blood sugar."

3. "I should check my blood sugar level after each meal to see if I need more insulin."

4. "I should expect to find ketones in my urine when I check it daily."

19. Which of the following should the nurse include in the diabetic nutritional management plan for a client who has diabetes mellitus?

1. Carbohydrate food sources are the only food sources that count toward foods that convert to glucose

2. Simple carbohydrates are preferred for the major percentage of carbohydrates

3. Protein and fat sources should provide the higher percentage of calories

4. Saturated fats should be limited to 10% of total calories

20. The nurse is caring for a client who has diabetes mellitus and is NPO for an x-ray at 0800. When preparing the client for the test, the nurse should

1. Reschedule the client's 0700 insulin for 1200 and feed the client after returning from the x-ray

2. Check with the physician to see if the 0700 insulin dose should be decreased

3. Withhold the 0700 insulin until the client returns to the room and the tray arrives on the unit
4. Give the insulin as ordered at 0700 followed by breakfast immediately after returning from x-ray

21. The nurse is performing an assessment on a client with diabetes mellitus. Which of the following findings should the nurse report as indicative of diabetic ketoacidosis?

1. Alcohol breath
2. Hypertension
3. Rapid, deep breathing
4. Cool, moist skin

22. A client's family member asks the nurse why the client developed diabetic ketoacidosis.The appropriate response from the nurse is that diabetic ketoacidosis results from

1. taking more than the prescribed insulin dose.
2. needing more insulin than what's available.
3. exercising after the morning dose of insulin.
4. skipping the noon meal.

23. A client's family member asks the nurse the purpose of performing hourly blood glucose readings on the client being treated for diabetic ketoacidosis. Which of the following is the appropriate response by the nurse?

1. "It provides an estimate of the amount of fluid retention."
2. "It identifies early symptoms of kidney damage."
3. "It serves as a guide for further insulin orders."
4. "It determines the severity of liver damage."

24. The nurse includes which of the following instructions in the teaching plan for a client with diabetes mellitus?

1. Perform blood glucose monitoring more frequently when ill
2. Avoid alcohol products
3. Eat the largest meal of the day before the peak action time of the insulin
4. Acetone in the urine indicates the need for less insulin

25. Which of the following should the nurse include in the instructions regarding proper foot care for a client newly diagnosed with diabetes mellitus?

1. Rub lotion on the feet and between the toes to prevent dryness
2. Wear shoes and socks at all times except when walking barefoot on the beach

3. Use a pumice stone to smooth corns and calluses
4. Examine the feet with a mirror three times a week

26. The registered nurse making out the client assignments may appropriately delegate which of the assignments to unlicensed assistive personnel?
    1. Bathe a client just admitted with diabetic ketoacidosis
    2. Monitor the blood pressure of a client in an Addisonian crisis
    3. Assist a client with Cushing's disease to mark a low-calorie, -carbohydrate, and -sodium diet
    4. Walk with a client who had the parathyroid gland removed three days ago

27. The nurse prioritizes the care of the following four clients. Prioritize the client who should be treated first, followed by the second, third, and fourth, based on the level of severity of their conditions (with fourth being the least severe).

    ________________ 1. A client with Cushing's syndrome
    ________________ 2. A client with hyperglycemic hyperosmolar nonketotic syndrome
    ________________ 3. A client with diabetic ketoacidosis
    ________________ 4. A client with myxedema

28. The nurse administers which prescribed drug on an emergency basis to a client with hypoparathyroidism who is experiencing tetany?

    ____

29. The family of a client in hyperglycemic hyperosmolar nonketotic syndrome asks the nurse what the usual treatment is. The most appropriate response by the nurse is that the usual treatment is
    1. to administer IV rapid-acting insulin.
    2. the same as diabetic ketoacidosis except insulin does not play a role because acidosis is not present.
    3. to reverse shock, restore blood circulation, and replace needed steroids.
    4. surgery to remove the pituitary tumor.

30. A client who has a blood glucose of 160 mg/dl asks the nurse, "Do I have type 1 diabetes mellitus?" The most appropriate response by the nurse is
    1. "I don't know. You will have to ask your doctor."
    2. "You will need to have a second blood glucose test to see if it is elevated before the diagnosis can be made."

3. "Any time the blood glucose exceeds 120 mg/dl, a diagnosis of diabetes mellitus is made."
4. "The diagnosis of diabetes mellitus can only be made when the blood glucose exceeds 180 mg/dL."

ANSWERS AND RATIONALES

1. 3. All hormones secreted by the anterior pituitary gland (ACTH, TSH, growth hormone, FSH, LH, and prolactin) are usually affected when there is anterior pituitary deficiency. Frequent episodes of hypoglycemia would occur with a deficiency in ACTH. Intolerance to heat would occur with an excess of TSH. Increased sexual arousal would occur with an excess of ACTH, and an increased pulse rate would occur with an excess of TSH.
NP = An
CN = Ph/8
CL = An
SA = 1

2. 3. Average urinary output is 1 to 2 liters in a 24-hour period; thus, an output of 150 ml in a two-hour period would be within the normal range. A blood pressure of 80/50 could be an indication of shock. Constant swallowing and a runny nose are postoperative complications of a transsphenoid hypophysectomy, not anticipated findings.
NP = Ev
CN = Ph/8
CL = An
SA = 1

3. 4. The surgical incision for a transsphenoid hypophysectomy is made beneath the upper lip to gain access into the nasal cavity. Postoperatively the head of the bed should be elevated to facilitate drainage from the operative site. The nasal packing may be reinforced but is not changed for 24 hours. Suctioning the nasal cavity would be contraindicated for this type of surgery. An ice collar applied to the neck would not be necessary for this type of surgery.
NP = Im
CN = Ph/8
CL = Ap
SA = 1

4. 2. Clients with diabetes insipidus excrete large volumes of dilute urine with a low specific gravity that ranges from 1.001 to 1.005. The client would lose weight rather than gain weight. A urine output of 1500 ml per day is within the lower normal range but a client with diabetes insipidus is

excreting larger volumes of urine. Fluid volume loss is characterized by hypotension.
NP = As
CN = Ph/8
CL = Ap
SA = 1

5. 1. Metabolism is greatly increased in hyperthyroidism, necessitating additional high-energy foods to meet the daily caloric requirements. Increased metabolism causes the client to feel warm, thus a cooler environment is needed. It is not necessary to limit visitors in states of increased metabolism and these clients do not need additional fluids because of their increased metabolism.
NP = Pl
CN = Ph/8
CL = Ap
SA = 1

6. 4. A postoperative complication of thyroidectomy surgery is the development of tetany. The nurse should check the client for muscle tremors every two hours. Because a thyroidectomy involves neck surgery, the head of the bed is elevated to facilitate breathing and drainage. Synthroid is not prescribed immediately postoperatively due to the presence of stored thyroid hormones, which are released into the circulation. Range-of-motion exercises to the neck are not begun until the suture line has healed.
NP = Pl
CN = Ph/8
CL = Ap
SA = 1

7. 1, 4. Thyroid crisis or storm is accelerated hyperthyroidism, which would result in extreme elevation in body temperature and a rapid pulse rate. An apathetic response to stimuli, decreased respirations, and loss of skin turgor are clinical manifestations of hypothyroidism.
NP = An
CN = Ph/8
CL = An
SA = 1

8. 3. There is a high incidence of hypothyroidism after a client is treated with ^{123}I so clients need to be observed for the symptoms of hypothyroidism for several years following treatment. The clinical manifestations of hyperthyroidism do not disappear until three to four weeks after treatment. Clients treated with ^{123}I are not considered to be radioactive

so radiation precautions do not need to be followed. Some clients need a second or third dose of ^{123}I before treatment is considered successful.
NP = Ev
CN = He/3
CL = An
SA = 1

9. 2. A diet low in calories is necessary for clients with hypothyroidism because they have a decreased metabolic rate, do not burn calories well, and may thus gain weight. These clients have constipation but a diet high in fiber is preferred to daily laxative use. Decreased metabolism causes the client to feel cold rather than warm. Sedatives are likely to cause respiratory depression when given to clients with hypothyroidism and are contraindicated.
NP = Pl
CN = He/3
CL = Ap
SA = 1

10. 3. In hyperparathyroidism, bone becomes decalcified, leading to fractures and bone pain. In this condition there is an overproduction of the hormone parathormone, but the gland does not enlarge, which causes difficulty in breathing. There is no alteration in bowel function. There is numbness and tingling in the extremities with hypoparathyroidism but not with hyperparathyroidism.
NP = As
CN = Ph/8
CL = Ap
SA = 1

11. 4. A major complication of hypoparathyroidism is tetany, which is a state of increased neuromuscular activity that progresses to painful involuntary muscle spasms. Lack of strength and loss of sensation are not present in neuromuscular irritability. Tetany is characterized by spasms of muscles rather than rigidity of muscles.
NP = An
CN = Ph/7
CL = An
SA = 1

12. 2. A major complication of a parathyroidectomy is postoperative hemorrhage. Clients having this surgery do not normally develop pulmonary emboli, fluid and electrolyte imbalance, or cardiac instability.
NP = Pl
CN = Ph/8

CL = An
SA = 1

13. 1. Clients with Cushing's syndrome have protein wasting and hypokalemia and should have a diet that is high in both protein and potassium. In Cushing's syndrome, there is an excessive production of glucocorticoids so prednisone, a glucocorticoid, would not be given. These clients also have hyperglycemia, not hypoglycemia. The client with Cushing's syndrome has fluid retention, which would necessitate a limitation in fluid intake.
NP = Pl
CN = He/3
CL = Ap
SA = 1

14. 1, 5, 6. Clients with primary aldosteronism have an excessive secretion of aldosterone, which causes signs and symptoms of hypokalemia. In hypokalemia, the client experiences muscle weakness, fatigue, and leg cramps. In primary aldosteronism, the serum sodium levels are high or unchanged, resulting in normal blood pressure or hypertension, not hypotension. These clients experience polyuria, not scanty urine output, and polydipsia, not decreased thirst.
NP = As
CN = Ph/8
CL = Ap
SA = 1

15. 2. Addison's disease, adrenocortical insufficiency, is a deficiency in both mineralocorticoids and glucocorticoids. With deficient mineralocorticoids, the client experiences a decrease in serum sodium. The client would need to increase salt intake at times when sodium requirements are increased, such as illness, hot weather, and stress. Edema or weight gain indicates the dosage of hormone replacement is too high. Postural hypotension indicates insufficient fluid volume. Solu-Cortef may be given IM or IV but should never be given subcutaneously.
NP = Pl
CN = Ph/8
CL = Ap
SA = 1

16. 1, 5, 6. Addison's disease is an endocrine condition in which there is a deficiency in both glucocorticoids and mineralocorticoids, which gives a wide range of symptoms related to the deficiency of both hormones. An insufficient amount of mineralocorticoids is characterized by persistent gastrointestinal symptoms, such as vomiting and diarrhea, and hypotension. Bronze-like pigmentation of the skin is also characteristic of

Addison's disease. An insufficient amount of glucocorticoids is characterized by weight loss and anorexia. Pedal edema would be a symptom of an increase in glucocorticoids and mineralocorticoids.
NP = Ev
CN = Ph/8
CL = Ap
SA = 1

17. 1. A client with pheochromocytoma has a tumor that secretes excessive amounts of epinephrine and norepinephrine. During an adrenalectomy to remove the tumor, there is a possibility that excessive amounts of these two hormones will be released, causing the blood pressure to go dangerously high. Respiratory obstruction, hemorrhage, and paresthesia are not caused by excessive secretion of these hormones.
NP = As
CN = Ph/8
CL = Ap
SA = 1

18. 2. The client with type 2 diabetes mellitus has insulin resistance or insufficient insulin production. Since insulin resistance is associated with obesity, weight reduction is the single most important action to take for the client with type 2 diabetes to achieve glucose control. Clients with type 2 diabetes do not normally require insulin injections except in periods of stress. Blood glucose monitoring should be done periodically before a meal. Clients with type 2 diabetes rarely have ketonuria because they usually have sufficient insulin to prevent the breakdown of fat.
NP = Ev
CN = Ph/8
CL = An
SA = 1

19. 4. It is recommended that the fat content in the diabetic diet be no more than 30% of the total calories and that saturated fats be limited to 10% of the total calories. Carbohydrate foods convert 100% to glucose but 50% of protein foods convert to glucose as well. Simple carbohydrates are not preferred for the major percentage of carbohydrates because many of the foods in that category are also high in fat content. It is recommended that the highest percentage of calories should be from carbohydrate foods (50 to 60%) with fat providing 20 to 30% of calories and proteins providing 10 to 20% of calories.
NP = Pl
CN = Ph/5
CL = An
SA = 1

20. 3. Clients with diabetes mellitus who are NPO for short-term procedures should not be given insulin until they are able to eat to prevent a hypoglycemic reaction. Therefore, insulin is withheld until the client returns to the division and is no longer NPO. Insulin is not usually rescheduled for a specific time but is given as soon as the client returns to the nursing unit. Most x-ray procedures require only a short period of time away from the nursing unit so it is not necessary to decrease the insulin dosage ordered for that day.
NP = Pl
CN = Ph/7
CL = Ap
SA = 1

21. 3. A client in diabetic ketoacidosis has a breathing pattern called Kussmaul breathing, which is rapid and deep and is often accompanied by acetone (fruity odor) breath. Hypotension would be noted as the body experiences intravascular volume depletion. The skin becomes warm and dry as the client becomes dehydrated from the metabolic acidosis.
NP = An
CN = Ph/8
CL = Ap
SA = 1

22. 2. Diabetic ketoacidosis (extreme hyperglycemia) results from an increased need for insulin, which could occur when an insufficient amount of insulin is taken, doses are omitted, or one experiences periods of stress such as surgery, infection, or trauma. Taking more than the prescribed insulin dose, exercising after a dose of insulin, or skipping a meal would result in hypoglycemia rather than hyperglycemia.
NP = An
CN = Ph/8
CL = An
SA = 1

23. 3. The main purpose for performing hourly blood glucose readings for a client in diabetic ketoacidosis is to monitor the client's response to measures to lower the high blood glucose levels. The insulin dose is then adjusted according to the reading. Blood glucose determinations will not give an estimate of fluid retention, identify symptoms of kidney damage, or determine the severity of liver damage.
NP = An
CN = Ph/8
CL = An
SA = 1

24. 1. A client with diabetes mellitus needs to perform blood glucose monitoring more frequently when ill because blood sugar levels are elevated during periods of stress such as illness, surgery, or trauma. Alcohol use is not restricted totally but moderation is recommended. The meals each day need to have approximately the same amount of calories and carbohydrates to maintain consistent blood sugar levels. Acetone in the urine indicates a need for more insulin rather than less.
NP = Im
CN = He/3
CL = An
SA = 1

25. 3. A pumice stone should be used to smooth corns and calluses when performing foot care to avoid injury to the foot. Lotion can be used on the top and bottom of the foot but should not be used between the toes where it could cause retention of moisture and skin breakdown. Walking barefoot should not be done at any time including walking on the beach. Feet should be examined every day.
NP = Pl
CN = Ph/8
CL = Ap
SA = 1

26. 4. A client with diabetic ketoacidosis is in a crisis state and needs to be stabilized and the blood glucose level brought down to a safe level. A client in an Addisonian crisis is also in a crisis state to reverse shock, restore blood circulation, and replace steroids. Severe hypotension is a cardinal feature that needs to be monitored by a registered nurse. Unlicensed assistive personnel do not have the knowledge to assist a client to select a diet low in calories, carbohydrates, and sodium. If the initial diet has been planned, a licensed practical nurse may assist in the marking of the diet. Unlicensed assistive personnel may walk a client who had the parathyroid gland removed three days ago.
NP = Im
CN = Sa/1
CL = An
SA = 8

27. 4,1,2,3. Hyperglycemic hyperosmolar nonketotic syndrome is a state of severe hyperglycemia (serum glucose from 600 to 1200 mg/dl) and hyperosmolarity (above 350 mOsm/kg). Diabetic ketoacidosis is a state of extreme hyperglycemia (800 to 1000 mg/dl), which occurs when there is an absence of insulin or markedly inadequate amounts of insulin. A client with myxedema has the most severe form of hypothyroidism. A client with Cushing's syndrome is the client with the least severe disease. Cushing's

syndrome is a disorder characterized by excessive secretion of the glucocorticoid cortisol from the adrenal cortex.
NP = Im
CN = Sa/1
CL = An
SA = 1

28. **Calcium gluconate.** Calcium gluconate in saline given parenterally is the drug used to treat tetany in a client who has hypoparathyroidism.
NP = Im
CN = Ph/6
CL = An
SA = 5

29. **2.** Treatment for diabetic ketoacidosis includes treating the acidosis with an IV administration of insulin generally ordered as units per hour. Hyperglycemic hyperosmolar nonketotic syndrome is usually treated in the same way as diabetic ketoacidosis except that insulin does not play a role because acidosis is not present. The goals of emergency care for Addisonian crisis are to reverse shock, restore blood circulation, and replace needed steroids. The pituitary tumor may be removed in a client with Cushing's syndrome.
NP = An
CN = Ph/8
CL = An
SA = 1

30. **2.** Type 1 diabetes mellitus is characterized by the inability to produce insulin because the beta cells are destroyed. A second blood glucose test is necessary to verify that the glucose is elevated before the diagnosis of diabetes mellitus can be made.
NP = An
CN = Ph/8
CL = An
SA = 1

NEUROLOGICAL DISORDERS - COMPREHENSIVE EXAM

1. When comparing neurological diseases that cause alterations in neurotransmission, the nurse identifies which of the following diseases that cause a decrease in the available amount of a neurotransmitter? Select all that apply:

[ ] **1.** Multiple sclerosis

[ ] **2.** Huntington's chorea

[ ] **3.** Guillain-Barré syndrome

[ ] **4.** Amyotrophic lateral sclerosis

[ ] **5.** Myasthenia gravis

[ ] **6.** Epilepsy

2. Which of the following changes in a client with myasthenia gravis should the nurse report as a critical sign of myasthenic crisis?

1. Dilated pupils and blurred vision

2. Difficulty swallowing and breathing

3. Progressive muscle weakness in the trunk and limbs

4. Confusion and aphasia

3. The nurse is admitting a client suspected of having multiple sclerosis. Which of the following is the most common initial clinical manifestation the nurse assesses?

1. Diarrhea

2. Headache

3. Visual disturbances

4. Skin infections

4. The nurse is caring for a client following a cerebrovascular accident. The nurse assesses what clinical manifestation to be the first indication of an increased ischemia to the brain?

1. Emotional instability

2. Spatial perception deficit

3. Increase in blood pressure

4. Decrease in consciousness

5. When providing care to a client in the acute stage after a cerebrovascular accident, the nurse should include which of the following interventions?

1. Administer a tube feeding within 24 hours

2. Administer an enema to prevent constipation

3. Provide 1500 to 2000 ml of fluids per day

4. Position the client in a high-Fowler's position

6. A family member of a client who had a cerebrovascular accident asks the nurse why her spouse cries easily and has extreme mood swings. Which of the following is the most appropriate response by the nurse?

1. "Your husband can only remember depressing events from the past."
2. "This is a way of getting attention, and the behavior should be ignored."
3. "This behavior is a common response over which he has little control."
4. "Your husband feels guilty about the extra demands he is making on the family."

7. Ongoing nursing measures for a client in the rehabilitative phase following a cerebrovascular accident should include
   1. Administer a bisacodyl (Ducolax) suppository daily
   2. Insert an indwelling Foley catheter
   3. Place a footboard at the end of the bed
   4. Perform daily range of motion exercises
8. A client has sustained a spinal cord injury. Which of the following emergency measures should receive priority in the client's plan of care?
   1. Monitor vital signs and assess the extent of the client's injuries
   2. Immobilize the client with a cervical collar and apply sand bags around the body
   3. Hyperextend the neck to establish and maintain a patent airway
   4. Observe for nausea and vomiting and offer emotional support
9. Which of the following is a priority for the nurse providing care to a client who sustained a concussion?
   1. Provide a safe environment so the client does not sustain additional injuries
   2. Assess the client's ability to swallow and avoid any situation that can lead to aspiration
   3. Monitor for signs of change in the level of consciousness or increased intracranial pressure
   4. Assess for irregular breathing, which indicates a deterioration in neurologic status
10. A client sustains a vertebral fracture at the T1 level as a result of diving into shallow water. During an emergency neurological assessment, the nurse finds
    1. an inability to move the lower arm.
    2. a normal biceps reflex in the arms.
    3. a loss of pain sensation in the hands.
    4. a difficulty in breathing and a flaccid diaphragm.

11. Which of the following assessments provide the nurse with the most accurate information for a client with a spinal cord injury who is developing autonomic dysreflexia?
Select all that apply:

[ ] **1.** Marked hypertension

[ ] **2.** Bradycardia

[ ] **3.** Dyssynergia

[ ] **4.** Absence of sweating

[ ] **5.** Constipation

[ ] **6.** Flaccid paralysis

12. A client's family member asks the nurse what the physician meant when he said the client had a transient ischemic attack (TIA). The appropriate response by the nurse is that a TIA is

1. "a transient attack caused by multiple small emboli."

2. "a period of alternating exacerbations and remissions."

3. "an ischemic attack that results in progressive neurologic deterioration."

4. "a temporary episode of neurologic dysfunction."

13. The nurse is admitting a client with tetanus. Which of the following nursing interventions should be included in the plan?

1. Cover the client with a warm blanket

2. Administer penicillin, laxatives, and enemas

3. Place the client in a quiet, dark room and avoid movement

4. Massage the client's joints and muscles

14. The nurse collects data on a client suspected of having Parkinson's disease. Which of the following findings should be reported?
Select all that apply:

[ ] **1.** Increased muscle tonus

[ ] **2.** Agnosia

[ ] **3.** Difficulty chewing and swallowing

[ ] **4.** Scotomas

[ ] **5.** Masked facies

[ ] **6.** Festination

15. The nurse should include which of the following in the teaching given to a client with multiple sclerosis?

1. Low-fat, gluten-free diet with megavitamin therapy

2. Discontinue taking baclofen (Lioresal) when the spasticity disappears

3. Avoid fatigue and extremes of heat and cold
4. Restrict the fluid intake to 1500 ml per day

16. The nurse is caring for a client with Huntington's disease. Which of the following measures should receive priority in the plan of care?
    1. Increase calories to 2000 calories per day
    2. Encourage genetic counseling
    3. Assist with bathing and dressing
    4. Offer diversional activities

17. The nurse identifies which of the following phases of the nursing process as the priority when planning the nursing care during the acute phase of Guillain-Barré syndrome? ______________

18. The nurse is assessing a client following a cerebrovascular accident due to a thrombus. The nurse observes an improvement in the client's condition within two weeks as a result of
    1. the reabsorption of the thrombus.
    2. the formation of new nerve pathways.
    3. displaced brain tissue.
    4. subsiding edema.

19. Cerebrovascular accidents may lead to loss or impairment of sensory-motor functions on the side of the brain that is damaged. The nurse documents this as what type of deficit? ______________

20. A client is scheduled to be evaluated for transient ischemic attacks (TIAs). The nurse correctly informs the client that which of the following studies will evaluate the flow of blood through the carotid arteries to provide information about partial or complete obstruction?
    1. Computed axial tomography (CT)
    2. Magnetic resonance imaging test (MRI)
    3. Positron emission tomography (PET)
    4. Transcranial doppler

21. When preparing a client who has been experiencing transient ischemic attacks (TIAs) for a computed axial tomography (CT) scan, the nurse should explain which of the following aspects of the procedure?
    1. There are no food or fluid restrictions prior to the procedure
    2. A contrast dye may be administered intravenously, leaving a metallic taste in the mouth
    3. The total procedure lasts 10 to 20 minutes
    4. The procedure is painful and an analgesic will be given if needed

22. The nurse is caring for a client who is dysphagic following a cerebrovascular accident. Which of the following interventions should the nurse include in the plan of care?
Select all that apply:

[ ] **1.** Serve food and fluids that are cold

[ ] **2.** Add Thick-It to liquids

[ ] **3.** Offer pureed foods

[ ] **4.** Inspect affected side of the mouth after eating

[ ] **5.** Place food on the unaffected side when eating

[ ] **6.** Elevate the head of bed 20° for 10 minutes after eating

23. A client who experienced a spinal cord trauma following a gunshot wound is exhibiting decreased reflexes, a loss of sensation, and flaccid paralysis. It is critical that the nurse reports this as ____________

24. The nurse assesses that one of the pins in a halo external fixation device is loose in a client who has a cervical spinal injury. The most appropriate action by the nurse is

1. Tighten the pin with a screwdriver
2. Report the loose pin to the physician
3. Tape the screw down so it does not fall out
4. Inform the physician when he makes rounds

25. The nurse observes a client with Parkinson's disease exhibiting involuntary, short, rapid shuffling movements. The nurse documents the finding as ____________

26. The nurse is caring for a client with myasthenia gravis. Which of the following would indicate to the nurse that the client's condition is deteriorating?

1. Frequent urinary tract and skin infections
2. Fatigue of muscles during activity which is worse at night
3. Muscle atrophy and contractures
4. Aspiration and respiratory insufficiency

27. The nurse assesses which of the following to be characteristic of amyotrophic lateral sclerosis?
Select all that apply:

[ ] **1.** Fever

[ ] **2.** Muscles wasting

[ ] **3.** Fasciculations

[ ] **4.** Headache

[ ] 5. Weakness of upper extremities

[ ] 6. Shuffling gait

28. The nurse should include which of the following interventions in the plan of care for a client with Guillain-Barré syndrome?

1. Provide a quiet room with low lighting to prevent environmental stimuli
2. Develop an active exercise program
3. Monitor the blood pressure and prevent sudden changes in posture
4. Instruct the client to consciously focus on walking

29. A client with multiple sclerosis asks the nurse if following a special diet will slow down the disease. The most appropriate response by the nurse is

1. "You should eat a high-calorie and high-protein diet."
2. "There is no special diet but eat well-balanced meals."
3. "It is best to avoid a diet high in saturated fat."
4. "You should eat a diet low in tyramine."

30. The nurse is caring for a client with myasthenia gravis. Which of the following would indicate to the nurse that the client is experiencing a cholinergic crisis?
Select all that apply:

[ ] 1. Decreased blood pressure

[ ] 2. Severe muscle weakness

[ ] 3. Increased salivation

[ ] 4. Difficulty swallowing

[ ] 5. Difficulty speaking

[ ] 6. Difficulty breathing

31. A client with myasthenia gravis presents to the emergency room with dysphagia, weakness, slurred speech, rhonchi, a blood pressure of 180/110, and a pulse of 120. Which of the following is the priority nursing action?

1. Foley catheter insertion
2. Nasogastric tube insertion
3. Peritoneal dialysis
4. Endotracheal intubation

32. The nurse is obtaining a history from a client with Guillain-Barré syndrome. The most significant finding is

1. a recent viral infection.
2. a family history of the disease.

3. a long, insidious onset of symptoms.
4. an intoxication of certain chemicals.

33. During the acute phase of Guillain-Barré syndrome, which of the following nursing activities should the nurse give priority?
    1. Keep suction equipment nearby
    2. Active range of motion
    3. Help the client to eat
    4. Alternative methods of communication

34. The nurse correctly tells a client with a T8 spinal cord injury that which of the following activities is possible?
    1. Maintain balance when sitting
    2. Stand with full leg braces
    3. Ambulate with short leg braces
    4. Climb stairs

35. The nurse is caring for a client with Huntington's disease. Which of the following nursing diagnoses should have priority in the plan of care?
    1. Acute pain
    2. Risk for aspiration
    3. Impaired verbal communication
    4. Disturbed body image

36. The nurse is caring for a client with bacterial meningitis. Which of the following indicates to the nurse that the client's condition is deteriorating?
    1. Nuchal rigidity
    2. Hearing loss
    3. Fever
    4. Headache

37. The nurse identifies which syndrome in a client who has an incomplete left-sided spinal cord injury and is experiencing left-sided motor paralysis, loss of vibratory and position sense, and right-sided loss of pain and temperature sensation? ______________

38. The nurse assesses which of the following to be present in a client who sustained a spinal cord injury and is experiencing poikilothermism?
    1. Lack of coordination between the urethral relaxation and detrusor contraction
    2. A decrease in sweating

3. Flaccid muscles
4. Distended bowel and bladder

39. The nurse is caring for a client admitted to the emergency room after sustaining facial trauma. Which of the following nursing measures should receive priority in the client's plan of care?
    1. Control the hemorrhage
    2. Assess the level of consciousness
    3. Maintain a patent airway
    4. Evaluate the extent of the injury

40. The nurse is admitting a client after a right-sided cerebrovascular accident. Which of the followin'g assessments would the nurse expect to find?
    1. Paralysis of the left side of the body and impulsive behavior
    2. Paralysis of the right side of the body and language deficits
    3. Speech deficit and slow, cautious behavior
    4. Anxiety and depression in relation to the disability

41. The nurse is caring for a client after an anterior craniotomy for a large brain tumor. Which of the following nursing interventions should be in the plan?
    1. Elevate the head of the bed 10°
    2. Ensure the client remains flat on the back
    3. Maintain the neck in a flexed position
    4. Avoid placing the client on the operative side

42. The nurse assesses the gag reflex in a client who has a decreased level of consciousness by assessing which of the following nerves?
    1. Cranial nerve IX
    2. Cranial nerve VII
    3. Cranial nerve II
    4. Cranial nerve V

43. The nurse is performing a cranial nerve assessment. Which of the following is the correct method of assessing cranial nerve I?
    1. Ask the client to close one eye, look directly at the bridge of the nurse's nose, and indicate when the object appears in the periphery of the visual fields
    2. Ask the client to close the eyes and indicate when a ticking watch is heard as it is brought closer to the ear

3. Ask the client to follow the nurse's finger as it moves horizontally and vertically and diagonally
4. Ask the client to close one nostril, close the eyes, and sniff from a bottle containing a spice

44. The nurse assesses which of the cranial nerves by asking the client to shrug the shoulders against resistance and to turn the head to either side against resistance? ______________

45. The nurse is caring for a client who becomes very frustrated and sometimes angry, after understanding what is said but not being able to communicate verbally. Using a diagram to illustrate the area of the brain affected, the nurse points to which area of the brain responsible for verbal communication? ______________

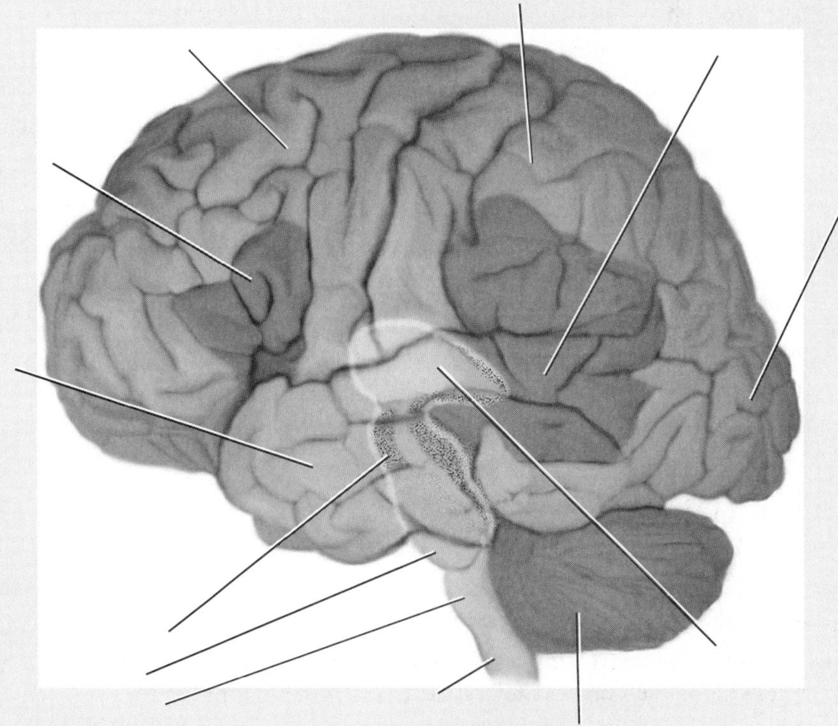

46. The registered nurse appropriately delegates which of the following nursing tasks to a licensed practical nurse?
    1. Develop a teaching plan for a client admitted following a spinal cord trauma
    2. Perform a complete head-to-toe assessment on a client suspected of having multiple sclerosis

3. Obtain a health history from a client with Huntington's disease
4. Assist a client who sustained a stroke to perform the activities of daily living

ANSWERS AND RATIONALES

1. 2, 5. Myasthenia gravis is a disease that causes a reduction in the body's ability to utilize the neurotransmitter acetylcholine. Huntington's disease is associated with a decrease in the amount of two neurotransmitters: gamma-aminobutyric acid (GABA) and acetylcholine (Ach). Multiple sclerosis, Guillain-Barré syndrome, amyotrophic lateral sclerosis, and epilepsy are not associated with decreased amounts of neurotransmitters.
NP = An
CN = Ph/8
CL = Ap
SA = 1

2. 2. The primary complication of myasthenic crisis is difficulty swallowing and breathing as a result of a severe muscle weakness.
NP = An
CN = Ph/7
CL = An
SA = 1

3. 3. The most common clinical manifestations of multiple sclerosis are sensory, motor, cerebellar, and emotional. Visual disturbances including diplopia, blurred vision, and a patchy blindness are most common. When the bowel is affected, it is generally constipation.
NP = As
CN = Ph/8
CL = Ap
SA = 1

4. 4. A decrease in consciousness following a cerebrovascular accident is the first indication of an increased ischemia to the brain.
NP = As
CN = Ph/8
CL = Ap
SA = 1

5. 3. One goal in the nursing care of a client in the acute stage of a cerebrovascular accident is to maintain tissue perfusion by keeping the client hydrated and preventing further brain damage. Fluids should be given orally or intravenously.
A daily oral intake of 1500 to 2000 ml should be encouraged.

NP = Pl
CN = Ph/8
CL = Ap
SA = 1

6. 3. As a result of the stroke, clients have a difficult time controlling their emotions. Their emotions are extremely unpredictable and exaggerated. For example, the client may cry one moment and express anger the next.
NP = An
CN = Ph/8
CL = An
SA = 1

7. 4. After stabilizing a client who sustained a cerebrovascular accident, generally during the first 12 to 24 hours, the goal of care changes from preserving life to lessening the resulting disability and maximizing function. Administering bisacodyl (Ducolax), inserting a Foley catheter, and placing a footboard at the end of the bed are interventions that should be implemented in the acute stage of stroke management care.
NP = Pl
CN = Ph/8
CL = Ap
SA = 1

8. 2. The priority intervention in the care of a client with a spinal card injury is to immediately immobilize the client by applying a cervical collar and sand bags around the client until the extent of the injury can be evaluated.
NP = Pl
CN = Sa/1
CL = An
SA = 1

9. 3. The priority nursing intervention for a client who had a concussion is to monitor the client for an altered level of consciousness and increased intracranial pressure. A decrease in the level of consciousness and an increased intracranial pressure occur from the bruising to the brain. Areas of hemorrhage, infection, necrosis, and edema may result.
NP = Pl
CN = Sa/1
CL = An
SA = 1

10. 2. An injury to the T1 level preserves the innervation of the upper extremities and back. The client has use of the hands and arms.
NP = As
CN = Ph/8

CL = Ap
SA = 1

11. 1, 2. Autonomic dysreflexia is a widespread cardiovascular uncompensated reaction created by the sympathetic nervous system. Two classic features of autonomic dysreflexia include severe hypertension and severe bradycardia. The systolic blood pressure may be as high as 300 mm Hg and the pulse as low as 30 beats per minute. Dyssynergia is an absence of coordination between urethral relaxation and detrusor contraction, which may be present in a neurogenic bladder. An absence of sweating occurs below the level of injury and is a common manifestation of a traumatic injury to the spinal cord. This leaves the temperature control external to the client. Constipation is the result of a neurogenic bowel because innervation to the bowel is lost as a result of the injury to the spinal cord. Flaccid paralysis is an anticipated finding below the site of injury to the spinal cord.
NP = As
CN = Ph/8
CL = Ap
SA = 1

12. 4. A transient ischemic attack (TIA) is a temporary neurological dysfunction of the vascular structures of the brain. They may be due to microemboli impairing the blood flow temporarily. A TIA may be an indication of a pending cerebrovascular accident.
NP = An
CN = Ph/8
CL = An
SA = 1

13. 3. An overstimulation of the sympathetic nervous system could potentially result in a seizure. Sudden jarring movements, noise, bright lights, or massage may bring on a seizure. Therefore, it is essential to place the client in a dark room and avoid sudden movements.
NP = Pl
CN = Ph/8
CL = Ap
SA = 1

14. 1, 5, 6. Clinical manifestations of Parkinson's disease include tremor, masked facies, and festination. The tremor often manifests itself in the hand as a "pill rolling" behavior. Masked facies and festination occur in bradykinesia as a result of the loss of autonomic movement.
NP = An
CN = Ph/8
CL = Ap
SA = 1

15. 3. Clients with multiple sclerosis should conserve their strength and avoid fatigue. Extremes of heat and cold should be avoided to decrease the risk of the client becoming ill.
NP = Pl
CN = He/3
CL = Ap
SA = 1

16. 2. Huntington's disease is an autosomal dominant disorder. Clients with this disorder have a 50% chance of transmitting the disease to their children. Genetic counseling should be encouraged so that the client becomes knowledgeable about testing options as well as transmission of the disease. Offering diversional activities would not be a priority intervention and would not discourage the client from dealing with concerns that may be more immediate. Calorie intake in Huntington's disease is often significantly increased to over 4000 calories per day. Assisting with bathing and dressing would not be a priority nursing intervention.
NP = Pl
CN = Ph/8
CL = Ap
SA = 1

17. **Assessment.** The most life-threatening and serious complication of Guillain-Barré syndrome is respiratory failure. Assessment of the respiratory system is vital in order to prevent death from respiratory failure. Planning of the client's care, implementation of appropriate interventions, and evaluation of the nursing care provided can only occur after the client has been adequately assessed for care needs.
NP = An
CN = Sa/1
CL = An
SA = 1

18. 4. Thrombus is the most common cause of cerebrovascular accidents. Within 72 hours, the affected area becomes edematous. When the edema begins to subside, an improvement in the client's condition will be noted.
NP = Ev
CN = Ph/8
CL = An
SA = 1

19. **Ipsilateral deficit.** Ipsilateral deficit is a loss of motor function and sensation on the same side as the site of the injury to the brain.
NP = Im
CN = Ph/8

CL = Ap
SA = 1

20. 4. A transcranial doppler study evaluates the blood flow through the cerebral arteries. A computed tomography (CT) is a computer-assisted x-ray that cross-sections parts of the body to detect areas of hemorrhage or infarct. A magnetic resonance imaging (MRI) process uses magnetic energy to image the brain and spinal cord. A positron emission tomography (PET) is a scan that measures the metabolic activity of the brain to evaulate cellular damage or death.
NP = Im
CN = Ph/7
CL = Ap
SA = 1

21. 2. A client does not need to be NPO prior to a computed tomography (CT) scan. A contrast medium may be administered, leaving a metallic taste in the mouth. The procedure is not painful and no analgesic is administered. The procedure does take longer than 10 to 20 minutes.
NP = Pl
CN = Ph/7
CL = Ap
SA = 1

22. 2, 4, 5. Interventions for a client who is dysphagic include adding Thick-It to liquids, placing food on the unaffected side, and elevating the head of the bed to 30° for 30 minutes after eating. Foods should be served at room temperature and the affected side of the mouth should be inspected after eating. Pureed foods are not tolerated well.
NP = Pl
CN = Ph/8
CL = Ap
SA = 1

23. spinal shock. Approximately 50% of clients who sustain a spinal cord injury experience spinal cord shock. Spinal shock is the loss of sensation, flaccid paralysis, and decreased reflexes. It may mask the neurological function following the injury.
NP = An
CN = Ph/8
CL = An
SA = 1

24. 2. It is most appropriate for the nurse to immediately notify the physician if a screw becomes loose on a halo device to prevent it from falling out and allowing further injury. The nurse should never tighten it.

NP = Im
CN = Ph/8
CL = Ap
SA = 1

25. bradykinesia. Bradykinesia is the slowed movement that occurs in Parkinson's disease as a result of the alterations that occur in the basal ganglia and extrapyramidal tract. This results in a stooped posture, masked facies, drooling, and shuffled gait (festination).
NP = Im
CN = Ph/8
CL = Co
SA = 1

26. 4. A client with myasthenia gravis who develops a respiratory infection or insufficiency or who aspirates is deteriorating. All of these indicate myasthenic crisis, an exacerbation of the weakness in the muscles controlling swallowing and breathing.
NP = An
CN = Ph/7
CL = An
SA = 1

27. 2, 3, 5. The client with amyotrophic sclerosis typically presents with weakness of the upper extremities in conjunction with muscle wasting and fasciculations. Fever, severe headache, and nuchal rigidity are associated with meningitis. Muscle fatigue with activity and difficulty swallowing are associated with myasthenia gravis. Mild tremors, loss of postural reflexes, and shuffling gait are associated with Parkinson's disease.
NP = As
CN = Ph/8
CL = Ap
SA = 1

28. 3. A client with Guillain-Barré syndrome may experience orthostatic hypotension as a result of the autonomic dysfunction. Monitoring the client's blood pressure and preventing sudden changes in posture are essential interventions.
NP = Pl
CN = Ph/8
CL = Ap
SA = 1

29. 2. There is no special diet that has been proven effective in the treatment of multiple sclerosis. A well-balanced diet is sufficient.

NP = An
CN = Ph/5
CL = Ap
SA = 1

30. 1, 3. Cholinergic crisis occurs in myasthenia gravis as a result of an overdose of anticholinesterase and results in nausea, vomiting, diarrhea, abdominal cramps, dyspnea, hypotension, increased salivation, papillary miosis, and blurred vision. Difficulty in swallowing and speaking are indications of myasthenic crisis. Severe muscle weakness and difficulty breathing occur in Guillain-Barré syndrome.
NP = An
CN = Ph/7
CL = An
SA = 1

31. 4. A client with myasthenia gravis who presents with difficulty speaking, breathing, swallowing, tachycardia, and hypertension is experiencing myasthenic crisis. A priority nursing action is to insert an endotracheal tube because of the difficulty breathing. The goal is to prevent respiratory distress.
NP = Im
CN = Sa/1
CL = An
SA = 1

32. 1. Guillain-Barré syndrome is associated with a preceding viral upper respiratory or gastrointestinal infection. The syndrome is acute and typically progresses rapidly. Guillain-Barré syndrome is not associated with genetic transmission or exposure to chemical substances.
NP = An
CN = Ph/8
CL = An
SA = 1

33. 1. It is essential that suction equipment be readily available when caring for a client in the acute phase of Guillain-Barré syndrome to ensure airway patency.
NP = Pl
CN = Sa/1
CL = Ap
SA = 1

34. 2. A spinal cord injury to the T8 affects the vagus nerve particularly innervating the gastrointestinal and genitourinary organs. Stabilization of the thoracic and back muscles remains, allowing the client to stand with

full leg braces or ambulate with crutches. The potential to maintain balance generally occurs in an injury at the L1 level.
NP = Im
CN = Ph/8
CL = An
SA = 1

35. **2.** Huntington's disease is an autosomal dominant genetic disorder that results in an excess of dopamine. In addition to the chorea movement, the facial movements are involved. A difficulty in chewing and swallowing increases the potential for aspiration. Risk for aspiration would be the priority nursing diagnosis.
NP = An
CN = Sa/1
CL = An
SA = 1

36. **2.** Nuchal rigidity, fever, and headache are classic signs of meningitis. Cranial nerve irritation is the most common complication of meningitis. Irritation of the eighth cranial nerve (vestibulocochlear) may cause deafness, which may be a permanent deficit.
NP = An
CN = Ph/7
CL = An
SA = 1

37. **Brown-Sequard's syndrome.** Brown-Sequard's syndrome occurs as a result of an incomplete spinal cord lesion. There is an ipsilateral (same side) injury causing a loss of motor function and position and a vasomotor paralysis on the same side as the injury. There is also contralateral (opposite side) pain and altered temperature sensation on the side opposite the point of injury.
NP = An
CN = Ph/8
CL = Ap
SA = 1

38. **2.** Poikilothermism is an interruption of the sympathetic nervous system preventing temperature sensations from reaching the brain in a client who sustained a spinal cord injury. The client would have a decrease in the ability to sweat. Dyssynergia is a lack of coordination between the urethral relaxation and detrusor contraction. Autonomic dysreflexia is an uncompensated cardiovascular reaction caused by the sympathetic nervous system. The most common cause is a distended bowel and bladder.
NP = As
CN = Ph/8

CL = An
SA = 1

39. 3. The nurse's first intervention is to establish a patent airway, and if one is not present, to prepare for emergency tracheotomy or cricothyroidotomy. After maintaining airway patency, the nurse assesses the bleeding and the extent of the injury.
NP = Pl
CN = Sa/1
CL = Ap
SA = 1

40. 1. A stroke on one side of the brain will affect the motor function on the opposite side because of the crossing over of the pyramidal pathways in the medulla. Damage to the right side of the brain is also associated with impulsive behavior. Because motor deficits are associated with contralateral brain lesions, paralysis of the right side would not occur. Language deficits are associated with damage to the left side of the brain, as the left hemisphere is dominant for language in most clients. Distress and depression are not specific to either right- or left-sided brain damage.
NP = As
CN = Ph/8
CL = An
SA = 1

41. 4. The appropriate position for a client who had an anterior craniotomy for a large tumor is on the nonoperative side. This prevents displacement of the cranial contents by gravity. The head of the bed should be elevated to 30° to facilitate venous drainage.
NP = Pl
CN = Ph/8
CL = Ap
SA = 1

42. 1. Cranial nerves IX (glossopharyngeal) and X (vagus) innervate the pharynx. Assessment of CN IX and X evaluates the presence of the gag reflex. Cranial nerve VII is the facial nerve. Cranial nerve II is the optic nerve. Cranial nerve V is the trigeminal nerve.
NP = As
CN = Ph/7
CL = Ap
SA = 1

43. 4. Cranial nerve I is the olfactory nerve and responsible for the sense of smell.
NP = Ev
CN = Ph/8
CL = An
SA = 1

44. **Cranial nerve XI.** Cranial nerve XI is the spinal accessory nerve and is assessed by asking the client to shrug the shoulders against resistance and to turn the head to the side against resistance.
NP = As
CN = Ph/8
CL = An
SA = 1

45. **Broca's area.**

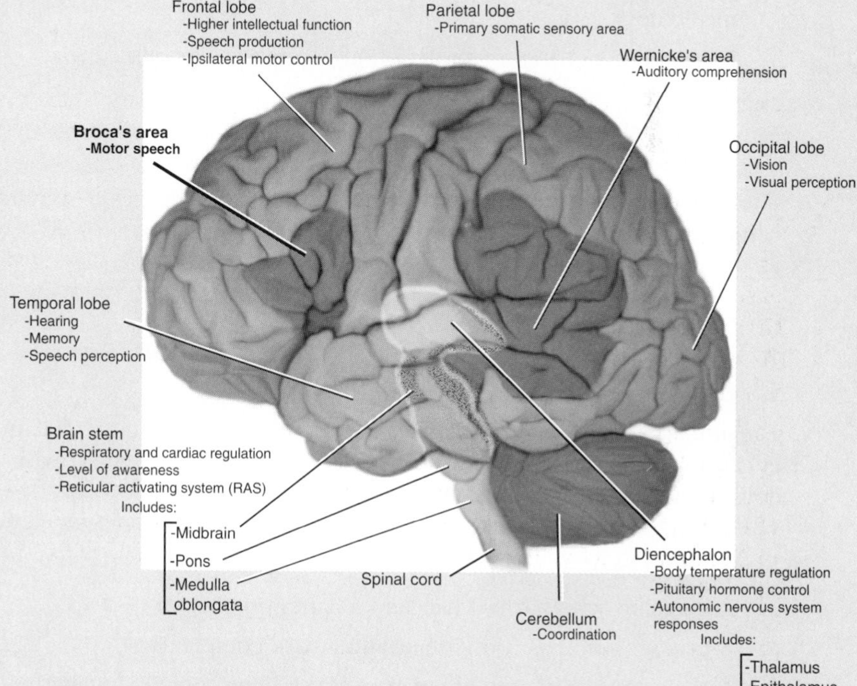

Broca's area of the frontal lobe of the brain is responsible for motor speech. Expressive aphasia or aphasia in which the client can understand what is said but cannot communicate verbally results. A client with expressive (Broca's or motor) aphasia is aware of the impairment and often becomes frustrated or angry at the inability to communicate.
NP = An
CN = Ph/8
CL = Ap
SA = 1

INTEGUMENTARY DISORDERS - COMPREHENSIVE EXAM

1. The nurse is caring for an adolescent client with acne who is very depressed because the acne treatment has been unsuccessful. Which of the following nursing diagnoses is the priority for this client?

1. Risk for impaired skin integrity related to comedones on the back and shoulders
2. Anxiety related to the long-term effects and benefits of antiacne medicines
3. Imbalanced nutrition: less than body requirements related to prescribed dietary changes
4. Situational low self-esteem related to cosmetic effects of acne lesions and scarring

2. The nurse observes and reports which of the following as a significant complication of untreated impetigo?

1. Dehydration
2. Diarrhea
3. Hematuria
4. Hypotension

3. The nurse is conducting a skin cancer screening workshop. The nurse evaluates which of the following clients to be at greatest risk for developing skin cancer?

1. A construction worker who has black hair and a dark complexion
2. A lifeguard who has red hair and a light complexion
3. A teacher who has brown hair and a dark complexion
4. A sales clerk who has blond hair and a light complexion with freckles

4. The nurse is discharging a client with atopic dermatitis. Which of the following measures would be essential to include in this client's discharge instructions?

1. Wash daily with a superfatted soap and warm water
2. Bathe in the hottest water that is tolerable
3. Limit bathing or showering to three times a week
4. Use bubble bath or bath oil when bathing

5. The nurse is preparing to teach a class to clients with psoriasis. Which of the following should the nurse include in the class?

1. Psoriasis cannot be cured but can be controlled with treatment

2. The lesions are regular shaped, flat, or slightly red macules with indistinct red borders

3. Psoriasis will improve in cold weather climates

4. The most common site for the lesions is the face

6. A client with herpes zoster asks the nurse how the disease was contracted. The appropriate response by the nurse would be

1. "I will ask your doctor because each case is individualized."

2. "It is caused by sexual contact with an infected person."

3. "The exact cause is unknown but generally it is the result of an infection."

4. "You must have had chickenpox because it is the reactivation of the virus that causes chickenpox."

7. The nurse is admitting a client with a known venous insufficiency. Which of the following assessments support a diagnosis of stasis dermatitis?
Select all that apply:

[ ] **1.** Itching

[ ] **2.** Localized reddened vesicles

[ ] **3.** Brown-stained skin

[ ] **4.** Oozing, crusty rash

[ ] **5.** Dry skin

[ ] **6.** Maceration between skin surfaces

8. Which of the following does the nurse instruct a client with contact dermatitis to avoid?
Select all that apply:

[ ] **1.** Pollens from weeds

[ ] **2.** Caffeine

[ ] **3.** Rubber compounds

[ ] **4.** Dyes

[ ] **5.** Fatigue

[ ] **6.** Detergents

9. The nurse is admitting a client with matted, crusted hair that has a foul odor. The scalp has erythema and scratching marks. The nurse should notify the physician of what disease? ______________

10. A client has received teaching about intertrigo. Which of the following statements by the client would indicate that the client has understood the instructions?
    1. "I will use talc but not cornstarch products on my skin."
    2. "I will stay away from my grandchildren until my lesions are healed."
    3. "I will use topical Benadryl to dry up the lesions."
    4. "I will avoid using fabric softener in the laundry."

11. The nurse is discharging a client with herpes simplex. Which of the following should the nurse include in the discharge instructions for this client?
    Select all that apply:
    [ ] 1. Eat a high-protein diet
    [ ] 2. Wear cotton underwear
    [ ] 3. Keep the lesions moist
    [ ] 4. Take sitz baths
    [ ] 5. Avoid sexual activities with lesions
    [ ] 6. Drink at least 2000 ml of fluid daily

12. The nurse is teaching a class on preventive measures to delay the signs of aging.Which of the following is a priority for the nurse to include in the class?
    1. Avoid chronic exposure to sunlight
    2. Maintain an adequate intake of protein
    3. Use superfatted, alkaline soaps
    4. Take a dietary supplement of vitamin E

13. While caring for a client with impetigo, the nursing priority is
    1. Apply warm saline soaks to the crusty areas
    2. Use meticulous handwashing
    3. Monitor for hematuria
    4. Administer the prescribed oral penicillin

14. Which of the following is the priority intervention in the emergency management of a client with a chemical burn?
    1. Establish and maintain an airway
    2. Assess for associated injuries

3. Remove clothing containing the chemical

4. Wash the chemical off with cool water

15. A client has sustained deep partial-thickness burns of both legs in a house fire and received 100% oxygen via face mask. Which of the following would be appropriate outcomes related to respiratory status?

1. $SaO_2 > 95\%$, respiratory rate 16–24/minute, unlabored

2. $SaO_2 > 85\%$, clear breath sounds, ability to cough

3. $PaCO_2 < 35$ mm Hg, respiratory rate 20 to 28/minute

4. $PaCO_2 > 45$ mm Hg, clear breath sounds, 16 to 20/minute

16. The nurse evaluates a client who is 12 hours postburn and has a urinary output of 200 ml since the injury. The nurse prepares for which of the following?

1. Increase the oral intake to 30 ml/hr

2. Increase the rate of intravenous fluids

3. Administer the prescribed furosemide (Lasix)

4. Reposition the Foley catheter

17. A client four days postburn injury has a nursing diagnosis of pain related to full-thickness burns of both arms. The priority nursing intervention for this client is to

1. Instruct the client in the use of guided imagery to manage pain between medication doses

2. Instruct the client on the importance of asking for pain medication before the onset of the pain

3. Administer an analgesic medication on a regular schedule before the client requests it

4. Arrange for a psychiatrist to speak with the client about pain management

18. The nurse is caring for a client with vitiligo. The nurse uses a picture illustrating the cross section of the skin to explain to the client what part of the skin is responsible for the vitiligo. Which of the following structures should the nurse point to as being responsible for the condition? ______________

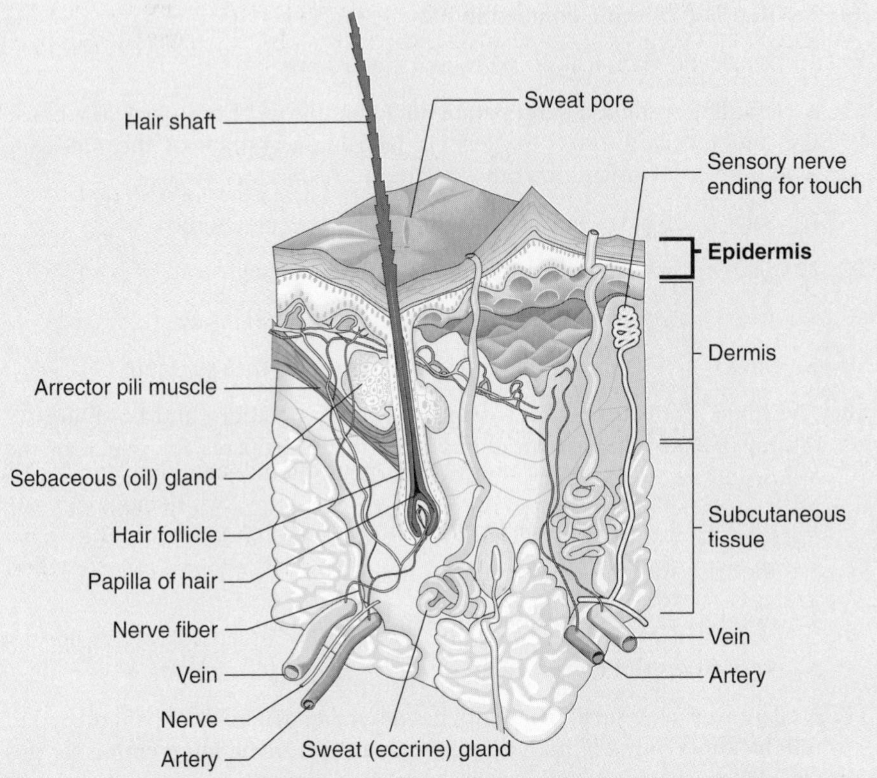

19. The nurse is concerned about the tissue perfusion in a client who has full-thickness burns of the right arm. Which of the following interventions is an appropriate intervention to enhance circulation?
    1. Assess the peripheral pulses with a Doppler stethoscope
    2. Elevate the injured extremity
    3. Limit blood pressure measurements to once a day
    4. Remove constrictive jewelry or clothing
20. The client, who has partial-thickness burns on the face, asks about skin care after discharge. Which of the following should be included in discharge teaching?
    1. Avoid sunlight for the next three months
    2. Continue to eat 8000 calories daily for the next month
    3. Wear a pressure garment daily for one year
    4. Avoid facial makeup for at least a year

21. The client with a serious burn injury is receiving wound care via the open method. Which of the following explanations by the nurse of the open method is most accurate?

1. "It allows for greater movement."

2. "It is less painful than other wound care methods."

3. "It is used only in those clients who have impaired circulation."

4. "It is used to reduce infection."

22. When admitting a client, the nurse observes a tick. The nurse should

1. shave the hair from the affected area.

2. twist the tick out with the fingers.

3. place the client in isolation.

4. cover the area with a lubricating oil.

23. The nurse is caring for a client in the early emergent phase of a burn injury. The nurse assesses the following laboratory data: hemoglobin 13.2 g/100 ml, hematocrit 50%, serum sodium 130 mEq/L. The nurse evaluates which of the following as the best explanation for these laboratory values?

1. They are the result of a loss of serum and interstitial fluid through the burn wound

2. They are the result of hemodilution from rapid replacement of intravenous fluids

3. All of the laboratory tests are within normal ranges

4. They are slightly abnormal but will return to normal once intravenous fluids have been started

24. The nurse assesses a ringlike rash in the groin and should notify the physician of what? ______________

25. The nurse is caring for a child with chickenpox who has multiple elevated areas each approximately 0.3 cm, which are accumulations of fluid between the upper layers of the skin containing serous fluid. Which of the following terms should the nurse use when documenting these areas?

1. Vesicles

2. Bullae

3. Papules

4. Macules

26. The registered nurse appropriately delegates which of the following client assignments?

1. Admit a client with cellulitis
2. Develop a plan of care for a client with a pressure ulcer on the coccyx
3. Assess the laboratory data on a client with partial-thickness burns
4. Apply a topical cream for itching in a client with herpes zoster

ANSWERS AND RATIONALES

1. 4. Situational low self-esteem related to cosmetic effects of acne lesions and scarring is the priority for a client with acne. Remember the majority of these clients are adolescents and body image and self-esteem issues are paramount.
NP = An
CN = Ph/8
CL = An
SA = 1

2. 3. Impetigo is caused by group A beta-hemolytic streptococci, staphylococci, or both and results in thick, honey-colored crusted lesions classically located on the face with erythemic borders. These lesions are also pruritic. Impetigo is generally treated with penicillin and localized treatments of warm saline or aluminum acetate compresses. If left untreated, glomerulonephritis and hematuria may result.
NP = An
CN = Ph/7
CL = An
SA = 1

3. 2. Although all people are at risk for development of skin cancer, those with light complexions, red hair, and freckles and who burn easily in the sun are at greatest risk. Those with exposure to the sun because of their occupation are also at increased risk. A person with dark hair and dark complexion is less susceptible to developing skin cancer even when exposed to sun through daily work. Having freckles and light complexion are risk factors, but employment as a teacher implies less sun exposure. Blond hair and freckles increase risk but employment as a sales clerk suggests less sun exposure than a lifeguard who has an occupation that requires being in the sun.
NP = Ev
CN = Ph/7
CL = Ap
SA = 1

4. 1. Warm water and superfatted soap are advised to hydrate and lubricate the skin in a client with atopic dermatitis. Hot water is irritating to the skin

and clients are advised to avoid extremely hot water. Bathing is advised on a daily basis. Perfumes contained in bubble bath and bath oil products may aggravate atopic dermatitis, which is usually an allergic reaction.
NP = Pl
CN = Ph/8
CL = Ap
SA = 1

5. 1. Psoriasis is a chronic dermatitis that cannot be cured but can be controlled with treatment. It is characterized by thick, scaly plaques affecting the scalp, elbows, trunk, knees, and extensor surfaces of the extremities. The fingernails are the most common site. Psoriasis generally improves in warm weather.
NP = Pl
CN = Ph/8
CL = Ap
SA = 1

6. 4. Herpes zoster is an activation of the varicella-zoster virus. Clients who have not had chickenpox but have been exposed to the open lesions of a client with herpes zoster may contract herpes zoster. Clients who have had chickenpox and have partial immunity to it are also susceptible.
NP = An
CN = Ph/7
CL = An
SA = 1

7. 1, 3, 5. Stasis dermatitis is commonly associated with venous insufficiency. Dilated veins, itching, and brown-stained skin are common. There are shallow ulcers that are slow to heal. A feeling of heaviness in the legs may also be present. Localized reddened vesicles occur in contact dermatitis. Red oozing, crusty rash is characteristic in the acute phase of atopic dermatitis. Maceration between skin surfaces is an assessment finding in intertrigo.
NP = As
CN = Ph/8
CL = Ap
SA = 1

8. 3, 4, 6. Rubber compounds, dyes, fragrances in skin care products, detergents, fabric softeners, and nickel and mercury products are to be avoided in contact dermatitis. Pollen from trees, weeds, and grasses are triggers in rhinitis. Caffeine, alcohol, and spicy foods are to be avoided in acne rosacea. Fatigue and emotional stress are triggers in asthma and urticaria.
NP = Im
CN = Ph/7

CL = An
SA = 1

9. **Pediculosis capitis.** Pediculosis capitis is head lice manifested by a matted, crusty appearance to the hair that has a foul odor. The scalp has the classic erythema and scratching marks.
NP = An
CN = Ph/8
CL = Co
SA = 1

10. **1.** Intertrigo is redness, maceration, itching, and burning between two skin surfaces that rub together. The most important interventions for this condition focus on drying and aeration of body skin folds. Talc is preferred, since use of cornstarch promotes the growth of *Candida albicans*. Intertrigo is not contagious. Topical diphenhydramine is useful for itching but will not accelerate the healing process. Additionally, topical corticosteroids or antifungals are the drugs of choice for reducing inflammation in this condition. The use of fabric softener is unrelated to intertrigo.
NP = Ev
CN = Ph/8
CL = An
SA = 1

11. **2, 4, 5.** Herpes simplex is a highly contagious disorder. Therefore, all sexual contact with an infected client with lesions present must be avoided. Sitz baths and cotton underwear are recommended interventions for comfort measures. The lesions should be kept dry.
NP = Pl
CN = He/3
CL = Ap
SA = 1

12. **1.** Limiting exposure to the sun is the most important preventive measure in reducing premature aging of the skin. The effects of the UV rays are cumulative. Maintaining an adequate intake of protein and calories is important but not a priority. Poor nutrition does contribute to aging skin. Using superfatted alkaline soap is helpful if the client has dry skin. Research indicates that taking a dietary supplement of vitamin E, an antioxidant, is effective in slowing the aging process.
NP = Pl
CN = Ph/8
CL = Ap
SA = 1

13. 2. Although applying warm saline soaks to the crusty areas and administering oral penicillin to a client with impetigo are appropriate nursing interventions, the priority is meticulous handwashing. Impetigo is highly contagious and not only can the nurse get it but it can also be spread from client to client when the nurse does not practice strict handwashing. Hematuria is a complication that occurs in untreated impetigo and should be monitored.
NP = Im
CN = Sa/1
CL = An
SA = 1

14. 4. Establishing and maintaining an airway is important but can be done only after stopping the burning process. In the case of a chemical burn, this is done by washing off the chemical with cool water. Assessing for associated injuries would come after stopping the burning process and establishing an airway. Removing the chemical-soaked clothing is important but not the priority. The chemical-soaked clothing is a continual source of the burning process.
NP = Ev
CN = Sa/1
CL = Ap
SA = 1

15. 1. Oxygen saturation must be at least 95%, with an unlabored respiratory rate of 16 to 24/minute. Breath sounds should be clear. An oxygen saturation of 85% corresponds to a PaO_2 of approximately 60% (too low). A $PaCO_2$ of less than 35 mm Hg indicates a potential for respiratory alkalosis. A $PaCO_2$ of greater than 45 mm Hg indicates the potential for respiratory acidosis.
NP = Ev
CN = Sa/1
CL = An
SA = 1

16. 2. Success of fluid resuscitation is based on urine output of at least 30 ml/hr or 0.5 mg/kg/hr. Based on this client's urine output, it appears that the rate of IV fluids is not fast enough to replace the volume lost in the burn injury. An increase in the rate of IV infusions would be expected. A client should have all oral intake withheld, since the risk of paralytic ileus is great postburn. Diuretics will not be useful until adequate fluid replacement has occurred. Repositioning the Foley catheter ensures that there are no kinks obstructing the flow of urine drainage.
NP = Im
CN = Ph/8

CL = Ap
SA = 1

17. 3. Control of pain is crucial. In the early days postburn, it is important that the nurse anticipate the client's need for pain relief and provide medication before the previous dose has worn off. It is especially important to provide additional medication before painful procedures. Later in the healing process, guided imagery may be useful to augment medications. It is not the client's responsibility to assume control of the administration of medications. Pain medication should be given regularly and before the client asks for it. A psychiatrist is not an appropriate intervention because it implies that there is something "wrong" with the client who experiences pain and that it can be "talked" away.
NP = Im
CN = Sa/1
CL = An
SA = 1

18. **Epidermis.**

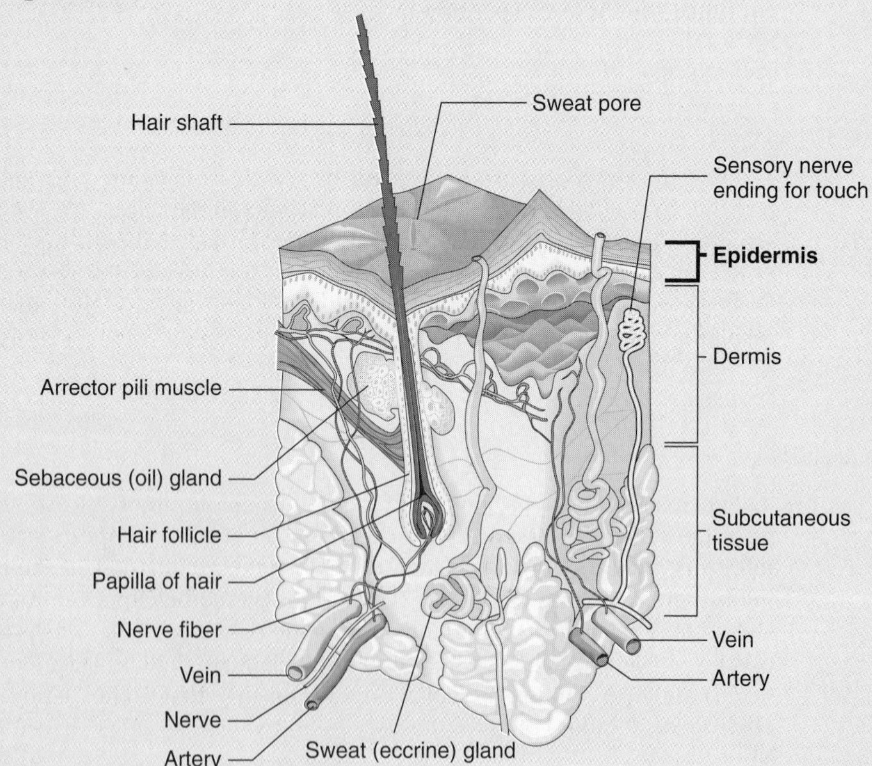

Vitiligo is aoo disorder characterized by a destruction of the melanocytes. The epidermis contains the melanocytes that produce the melanin. It is the melanin that gives the skin its color. In vitiligo, the melanocytes are destroyed and the client is left with milky white patches of skin surrounded by normal skin.
NP = Im
CN = Ph/8
CL = Ap
SA = 1

19. 4. Removal of any constricting jewelry or clothing on the affected extremity is the priority to enhance circulation. Positioning the arm in a dependent position may also be helpful. Assessing peripheral pulses with a Doppler stethoscope is an effective method to determine the presence of peripheral pulses but does not necessarily enhance circulation and should be done only after removing restrictive clothing. It is inappropriate to elevate the extremity because it makes it more difficult for arterial circulation to reach the periphery. The client will need frequent blood pressure readings. However, the affected arm should not be used.
NP = Ev
CN = Ph/8
CL = Ap
SA = 1

20. 3. Pressure garments flatten scar tissue, giving the client more mobility and better cosmetic appearance. They should be worn for one to two years. Clients following a burn injury are advised to avoid sunlight for a full year. Encouraging a client to eat 8000 calories is too many calories after discharge and will promote weight gain. The use of makeup, after wounds are healed, may help the client feel more normal. Alcohol-free moisturizers may be used.
NP = Pl
CN = He/3
CL = Ap
SA = 1

21. 1. The open method allows the client to have greater freedom of movement and the nurse to have better visibility of the burn wounds. The open method is not necessarily less painful than other methods. In fact, exposure of burn wounds to the air may cause pain. It is a useful method for any client with a burn injury and is not limited to those with circulatory difficulties. Prevention of infection is not a rationale associated with only the open method; it is an overall goal in burn wound care.
NP = An
CN = Ph/8

CL = Ap
SA = 1

22. 4. The appropriate nursing intervention for a client who has a tick is to cover the area with a lubricating oil or jelly. Never remove the tick with the fingers and never twist it. Shaving the area and placing the client in isolation are not appropriate interventions.
NP = Im
CN = Ph/8
CL = Ap
SA = 1

23. 1. In the early emergent phase of burn care, there is an increased capillary permeability, and water, sodium, and plasma proteins leave plasma to move into the interstitial spaces, thus decreasing serum sodium and albumin. Serum potassium goes up because injured cells and hemolyzed RBCs release potassium into the bloodstream. Because of water loss from the vascular compartment, the hematocrit looks artificially elevated (hemoconcentration not hemodilution). The lowered serum sodium is not a result of rapidly infused IV fluids but is a result of actual sodium loss through the burn wounds. The lab values will not automatically return to normal. The client requires vigilant monitoring of fluid and electrolyte replacement during the emergent phase of injury.
NP = Ev
CN = Ph/8
CL = An
SA = 1

24. **Tick bite.** A tick bite is a ringlike rash most frequently noted in the groin, buttocks, axillae, trunk, legs, and arms.
NP = As
CN = Ph/8
CL = Co
SA = 1

25. 1. Vesicles are an accumulation of fluid between the upper layers of the skin, forming an elevated mass containing serous fluid less than 0.5 cm in size. Bullae are the same as vesicles but greater than 0.5 cm. Papules are solid elevated lesions less than 0.5 cm in size. Macules are localized changes in the skin color of less than 1 cm in diameter.
NP = Ev
CN = Ph/8
CL = Co
SA = 1

26. 4. It would be appropriate for a registered nurse to delegate to a licensed practical nurse the application of a topical cream for itching in a client with herpes zoster. Admitting a client, developing a plan of care, and assessing the laboratory data on a client are all job functions reserved for the registered nurse.
NP = Im
CN = Ph/8
CL = An
SA = 8

MUSCULOSKELETAL DISORDERS - COMPREHENSIVE EXAM

1. The nurse is caring for a client who has a cast for a fracture of the proximal tibia. Which of the following clinical manifestations would the nurse interpret as indicative of compartment syndrome?
   1. Pain distal to the injury that is not relieved by analgesics
   2. Distended bladder and inability to void
   3. Chest pain, dyspnea, confusion, fever, and petechia
   4. Bleeding into tissues, strong rapid pulse, and feeling of impending doom
2. A client's family member asks the nurse why the client's cast feels warm immediately after application. The most appropriate response by the nurse is
   1. "I will notify the physician. It is possible that infection has set in."
   2. "It is normal for the cast to be warm for a short period of time after application."
   3. "I will cover the cast with a blanket to facilitate drying."
   4. "It is possible that it is an allergic reaction to the material used in making the cast."
3. The nurse is discharging a client after a total hip replacement. Which of the following measures would be essential to include in the client's discharge instructions?
   1. Teach the client how to bend down correctly to put on shoes and socks
   2. Encourage the client to maintain the hip in an adducted position
   3. Instruct the client to sit in chairs with arms
   4. Teach the client the importance of daily active range of motion exercises

4. The client returns from surgery for an amputation with a compression dressing in place. The client asks the nurse why the dressing has to be so snug. The appropriate response by the nurse is to
   1. "Prevent injury to the stump."
   2. "Promote drainage of secretions."
   3. "Prevent suture line infection."
   4. "Promote stump shrinkage."
5. The nurse is caring for a client with Bryant's traction. Which of the following should the nurse include in the plan of care for this client?
   1. Check the pelvic belt for security
   2. Place a foot board at the end of the bed
   3. Assess the knee sling for smoothness
   4. Maintain the buttocks free of the bed
6. The nurse is caring for a client in a body cast. Which of the following would indicate the client is experiencing cast syndrome?
   Select all that apply:
   [ ] **1.** Leukocytosis
   [ ] **2.** Abdominal pressure
   [ ] **3.** Vomiting
   [ ] **4.** Restricted elbow motion
   [ ] **5.** Nausea
   [ ] **6.** Fever
7. A client with a body cast developed cast syndrome. The client's family asks the nurse what the treatment is. The appropriate response by the nurse is
   1. "A pain pill will be administered."
   2. "The skin around the cast will be massaged."
   3. "The cast syndrome will get better when the cast is completely dry."
   4. "A tube will be inserted through the nose and into the stomach and connected to suction."
8. The client asks the nurse what a comminuted fracture is. The appropriate response by the nurse is
   1. "The bone is broken into two parts, and the skin may or may not be broken."
   2. "It is an incomplete fracture with one side splintered and the other side bent."
   3. "The bone has broken into several fragments, but the skin is intact."
   4. "There is a break in the skin, and the bone is protruding."

9. The nurse is discharging a client following a total hip replacement. Which of the following measures is a priority to include in the client's discharge instructions?
   1. Encourage the client to turn on the affected side in bed
   2. Instruct the client to maintain the hips in an internally rotated position
   3. Encourage the client to take short walks every day
   4. Instruct the client to notify the dentist of a prosthesis before having dental work

10. The nurse is admitting a client with persistent skeletal pain when ambulating and diarrhea of a nine-month duration. The nurse suspects which of the following diagnoses?
    1. Osteosarcoma
    2. Rheumatoid arthritis
    3. Osteoarthritis
    4. Osteomalacia

11. The nurse is teaching a class on fracture healing to a group of nursing students. Which of the following stages of fracture healing should the nurse include in the class?
    1. Granulation tissue is an unorganized conglomeration of bone that is mixed about the fracture parts
    2. Ossification begins two to three weeks after the fracture and continues until healing is complete
    3. Callus formation begins with bleeding, edema, and the formation of a hematoma
    4. Consolidation is the final stage of bone healing

12. The nurse is admitting an 18-year-old male after he sustained a football injury. The client is experiencing pain and swelling of the distal femur. The nurse suspects which of the following diagnoses?
    1. Osteoclastoma
    2. Osteosarcoma
    3. Ewing's sarcoma
    4. Multiple myeloma

13. Based on an understanding of uric acid in the urine, the nurse caring for the client should
    1. teach a diet including citrus fruits, juices, and milk and milk products.
    2. encourage voiding at more frequent intervals.

3. encourage increased activity such as walking.
4. discourage the dietary intake of grains and pasta.

14. The client is admitted with a fracture in which the bone has been forced through the tissue and skin overlying the fracture site. On initial assessment the nurse would classify this as an ______________

15. When teaching a client with osteoarthritis, which of the following would the nurse include?
    1. It is a chronic systemic inflammatory disease of the connective tissue
    2. It is a disease of young people
    3. It usually affects weight-bearing joints
    4. It has multisystem organ involvement early

16. The nurse is caring for a client with a cast. Which of the following nursing interventions should the nurse include in the plan of care?
    1. Remove small amounts of padding from the cast if the client complains the cast is tight
    2. Dry the cast with a hair dryer on a low setting after it becomes wet
    3. Keep the cast covered with plastic for a minimum of 12 hours a day to prevent soiling
    4. Teach the client that scratching inside the cast is permitted only with small blunt objects

17. The nurse is caring for a client after a hip arthroplasty. Which of the following interventions should the nurse include in the client's plan of care?
    1. Flex the operative hip 90°
    2. Abduct the operative hip
    3. Adduct the operative hip
    4. Turn 45° onto operative side

18. The nurse is admitting a client to the hospital. The nurse assesses the client's finger joints to be swollen. The nurse reports the most likely cause of this finding is the result of
    1. inflammation of the joint's synovial tissue.
    2. the presence of urate crystals in the synovial tissue.
    3. an infection of the bone and surrounding tissues.
    4. the formation of bony spurs on the joint surfaces.

19. Balanced suspension traction has been prescribed for a client. Based on an understanding of the principles of this traction, the nurse caring for the client should

1. position the client toward the end of the bed.
2. elevate the head of the bed 45°.
3. maintain 90° angle of shoulder and elbow joints.
4. administer skin care with client raising the buttocks off the bed.

20. The nurse is admitting a client with osteoporosis and a hip fracture. The nurse identifies this fracture as ______________

21. The nurse correctly assists a client following a hip arthroplasty to get out of bed into which of the following chairs?
   1. Wheelchair with footrest
   2. Recliner chair with both legs elevated
   3. Low, soft lounge chair
   4. Straight-back arm chair

22. The nurse caring for a client with gout should review which of the following diagnostic tests as most reliable?
   1. 24-hour urine for uric acid
   2. Erythrocyte sedimentation rate
   3. Serum uric acid
   4. Aspiration of the synovial fluid from a joint

23. The nurse is discharging a client with lupus erythematosus. Which of the following measures would be essential to include in the client's discharge instructions?
   1. Small frequent meals
   2. Avoid chilling
   3. Avoid sunlight
   4. Increase fluids

24. The nurse should include which of the following in the teaching provided to a client with osteoarthritis?
   Select all that apply:
   [ ] 1. Never take both aspirin and a nonsteroidal anti-inflammatory drug
   [ ] 2. Use correct posture and body mechanics
   [ ] 3. Follow a high-protein, high-calorie diet
   [ ] 4. Systemic organ involvement occurs late in the disease
   [ ] 5. Anemia is a common manifestation
   [ ] 6. Wear supportive shoes

25. The nurse is teaching a class on osteoporosis. Which of the following should the nurse include in the class?
Select all that apply:
[ ] 1. An oophorectomy decreases the risk of osteoporosis
[ ] 2. Physical activity decreases the risk of osteoporosis
[ ] 3. Cigarette smoking
[ ] 4. Women have a lower calcium intake than men throughout their lives
[ ] 5. African-American women have a higher incidence of osteoporosis
[ ] 6. History of anorexia nervosa

26. The nurse assesses which of the following clients to be at greatest risk for an amputation?
1. A 70-year-old client with osteoarthritis
2. A 80-year-old client with rheumatoid arthritis
3. A 40-year-old client with gout
4. A 55-year-old client with diabetes mellitus

27. Because a client has a left ankle sprain, plans for nursing intervention should include
1. application of warm moist heat for 20 minutes at a time during the first 48 hours.
2. application of a compression dressing left in place until healing has occurred.
3. active range of motion to left ankle to maintain mobility following injury.
4. administration of an analgesic and rest.

28. The nurse is admitting a client suspected of a right intertrochanteric fracture. Which of the following are priority findings for the nurse to report supporting this diagnosis?
1. External rotation of the right hip and a shorter right leg
2. Fever of 101°F and erythema of the right hip
3. Muscle spasms and pain of the right leg
4. Weakness of the right leg and hip when ambulating

29. The nurse is discharging a client with osteomalacia. What is a priority to include in the discharge instructions for this client? ______________

30. The nurse assesses which of the following musculoskeletal changes to be present in older adults?
Select all that apply:

[ ] 1. Decreased bone mass

[ ] 2. Increased muscle tonicity

[ ] 3. Increased glycogen stores

[ ] 4. Decreased coordination

[ ] 5. Decreased Achilles reflex

[ ] 6. Decreased nerve conduction

31. A client is being prepared by a nurse to have an MRI study completed in 30 minutes. The nurse should cancel the MRI after which of the following assessments is made?

1. The client has a knee prosthesis
2. The client had a large meal 30 minutes ago
3. The client is dehydrated
4. The client's reflexes are slow

32. The nurse is collecting a health history for a client before surgery. Which of the following is a priority for the nurse to include in the health history?

1. Family history of arthritis
2. Use of assistive devices
3. Medications
4. Lifestyle history

33. Which of the following procedures should the nurse include when assessing a client's ability to tandem gait walk? Instruct the client to walk across the room

1. normally.
2. heel to toe.
3. on the toes.
4. on the heels.

34. When preparing a client for a bone scan, it would be essential for the nurse to plan to explain which of the following aspects of the procedure?

1. NPO for two to three hours before the procedure
2. A radioactive isotope medication will be administered with a full glass of water 30 minutes before the procedure
3. A radioactive substance will be administered two to three hours before the procedure
4. Avoid contact with people for 24 hours due to the radioactivity

35. The nurse caring for a client following an arthroplasty evaluates which of the following as normal muscle strength and movement against gravity and against minimal resistance?

1. 3
2. 4
3. 5
4. 6

36. A client has received teaching regarding why the residual limb should not be elevated following an above-the-knee amputation. Which of the following misunderstandings would indicate to the nurse that the client needs further instruction?

1. Elevation has no bearing on the incidence of phantom pain
2. Elevation will result in wound dehiscence
3. The flexed position will promote hip flexion contractures
4. The flexed position will promote clot formation at the incision site

37. Which of the following assessments would provide the nurse with the most accurate information regarding the client's activity tolerance?

1. Breath sounds
2. Degree of flexibility
3. Muscle strength and coordination
4. Vital signs before, during, and after an activity

38. The nurse monitors a client's range of motion exercises and watches as the client moves his limb away from the body's midline. What term should the nurse use when documenting this movement? ______________

39. Which of the following clients would be appropriate to delegate to a licensed practical nurse?

1. A client with an amputation admitted with a dehiscence
2. A client with a full-body cast suspected of having compartment syndrome
3. A client with a leg fracture who has an order for instructions on crutch walking
4. A client with a hip fracture who needs reinforcement of range of motion exercises

40. Which of the following should the nurse include when instructing a student nurse on the appropriate use of a mobility aid?

1. A standard walker should be used by a client whose balance is too limited to use a four-wheeled walker
2. The axillary crutch is the most useful substitute for a cane
3. A quad cane is the type of cane that provides the most support of all types of cane
4. The Canadian crutch is the most common type of crutch used for a client who has strong extensor muscles of the arm

41. The nurse includes which of the following when instructing a client on the swing-to gait?
    1. Move both crutches forward together followed by bringing the body beyond the crutches
    2. Move the right crutch forward followed by the left leg, then move the left crutch forward followed by the right leg
    3. Move the left crutch and right foot forward together, then move the right crutch and left leg forward
    4. Move both crutches and the weaker leg forward, then move the stronger leg forward

ANSWERS AND RATIONALES

1. 1. Pain distal to the fracture site that is not relieved by analgesics is the classic feature of compartment syndrome. Compartment syndrome is a complication associated with fractures, specifically fractures of the proximal tibia or distal humerus. Compartment syndrome occurs when structures are compressed within a closed structure in the affected extremity from fascial sheaths or bone. It can also occur from an external device such as a cast or splint. Chest pain, dyspnea, confusion, fever, petechia, tachycardia, and sense of impending doom are all indications of a fat embolism syndrome.
   NP = An
   CN = Ph/8
   CL = Ap
   SA = 1

2. 2. It is normal for the cast to feel warm immediately following application and for a short period of time (generally 24 to 72 hours). This is especially true with a plaster of paris cast. During this time, an increase in edema may be noted. A fresh cast should never be covered with a blanket. This would cause a buildup of heat within the cast.
   NP = An
   CN = Ph/8

CL = An
SA = 1

3. 3. It is essential, or the priority, for the nurse to instruct a client following a total hip replacement to sit in a chair with arms to aid in rising to a standing position. Bending over to put on socks and shoes and placing the hip in an adducted position are contraindicated following a total hip replacement. All predispose the client to dislocation. A client following a total hip replacement would not perform active range-of-motion exercises.
NP = Pl
CN = Ph/8
CL = Ap
SA = 1

4. 4. The purpose of the compression dressing postoperatively is to be snug enough to promote stump shrinkage and facilitate the fitting of an appropriate prosthesis.
NP = An
CN = Ph/8
CL = An
SA = 1

5. 4. The buttocks should be free of the bed to facilitate nursing care. Bryant's traction is used with children who sustained a fracture of the femur or to stabilize the hip joint of children who weigh less than 30 lb (14 kg) or are under 2 years of age.
NP = Pl
CN = Ph/8
CL = Ap
SA = 1

6. 2, 3, 5. Cast syndrome is characterized by abdominal pressure, nausea, and vomiting and occurs when the abdomen compresses the superior mesenteric artery against the duodenum.
NP = Ev
CN = Ph/7
CL = Ap
SA = 1

7. 4. Cast syndrome results when a body jacket cast has been applied too tightly over the chest and abdomen, compressing the superior mesenteric artery against the duodenum. Nausea, vomiting, and abdominal pain result. The appropriate treatment is to insert a nasogastric tube to facilitate gastric decompression and suction. The cast may need to be splinted or removed.
NP = An
CN = Ph/8

CL = An
SA = 1

8. 3. A comminuted fracture occurs when the bone is broken into several fragments but the skin remains intact. A bone that is broken into two parts with the skin either broken or not is a fracture either communicating or noncommunicating with the external environment. An incomplete fracture, when one side of the bone is splintered and the other side bent, is a greenstick fracture. When the bone is protruding through broken skin, it is an open fracture.
NP = An
CN = Ph/8
CL = Co
SA = 1

9. 4. It is a priority for a client who had a total hip replacement to notify the dentist of a prosthesis before dental work so that prophylactic antibiotics can be administered.
NP = Pl
CN = Sa/1
CL = An
SA = 1

10. 4. Osteomalacia is an uncommon bone disorder found in adults resulting from a vitamin D deficiency. The disorder is characterized by persistent pain when bearing weight such as with ambulation. Osteomalacia may occur as a result of chronic diarrhea. Osteosarcoma is a rapidly metastasizing bone cancer generally found in young adults with a history of a minor injury. Rheumatoid arthritis is a chronic and systemic disease generally affecting diarthrodial joints. Joint stiffness in the morning is a classic feature. Osteoarthritis is a degenerative joint disease affecting weight-bearing joints. In addition to systemic manifestations such as fatigue and fever, clinical manifestations such as pain on motion or weight bearing relieved by rest is characteristic.
NP = An
CN = Ph/8
CL = Ap
SA = 1

11. 2. Ossification is the period of fracture healing generally between two to three weeks after the initial injury. Although the fracture is still apparent on an x-ray, the callus (area of cartilage, osteoblasts, calcium, and phosphorus formed within the first week after the fracture) prevents movement of the fracture site under gentle stress. The client will either be progressed from skeletal traction to a cast or have the cast removed to permit limited movement.

NP = Pl
CN = Ph/8
CL = Ap
SA = 1

12. 2. Osteosarcoma is the most common and malignant neoplasm commonly found in young adult males after sustaining a minor injury, such as a football injury, that brings them into the health care system. The clinical manifestations include a slow onset of pain and edema generally around the knee associated with involvement of the distal femur, proximal humerus, or tibia. Osteoclastoma, or giant cell tumor, is a highly destructive tumor affecting the long bones in young adults. Common clinical manifestations include localized pain, edema, and impaired mobility. It is generally not associated with a history of injury. Ewing's sarcoma is a long bone cancer occurring in young adult males but, like osteoclastoma, is not associated with an injury. It has clinical manifestations of localized pain, edema, a palpable mass, fever, and leukocytosis. It is much less common than osteosarcoma. Multiple myeloma, or plasma cell myeloma, is the most common primary bone neoplasm in older adults. Clinical manifestations include back pain, anemia, and thrombocytopenia.
NP = An
CN = Ph/8
CL = Ap
SA = 1

13. 1. Although research indicates a diet high in purines alone has little effect on the hyperuricemia found in gout, a diet low in purines, such as citrus fruits, juices, milk and milk products, is still encouraged.
NP = Im
CN = Ph/8
CL = Ap
SA = 1

14. **open fracture.** An open fracture is a fracture in which the bone has been forced through the tissue and skin over the fracture site.
NP = As
CN = Ph/8
CL = Co
SA = 1

15. 3. Osteoarthritis is a degenerative joint disease primarily affecting the weight-bearing joints. It affects older adults and involvement is limited to the joints and surrounding tissues. Rheumatoid arthritis is a chronic systemic inflammatory disease with multisystem involvement affecting the connective tissue.

NP = Pl
CN = He/3
CL = Ap
SA = 1

16. 2. The nurse should check with the physician before permitting a synthetic cast to become wet. If the cast does become wet, it should be patted dry with a towel or dried with a hair dryer on a low setting. The padding inside the cast should never be removed. Covering the cast is to be avoided. A client should also be instructed to avoid scratching inside the cast.
NP = Pl
CN = Ph/8
CL = Ap
SA = 1

17. 2. Following a hip arthroplasty, the hips should be abducted with an abductor pillow to prevent dislocating the hip. The hip should not be allowed to flex greater than 90° or to adduct. Both of these actions and incorrectly turning a client on the operative side predispose a client to a dislocation.
NP = Pl
CN = Ph/8
CL = Ap
SA = 1

18. 1. Swollen finger joints are a predominant clinical manifestation in rheumatoid arthritis as a result of an inflammation of the synovial tissue. The presence of urate crystals in the synovial fluid is gout. An infection of the bone and surrounding tissues is osteomyelitis. Bony spurs may occur on joint surfaces.
NP = An
CN = Ph/7
CL = Ap
SA = 1

19. 4. Balanced suspension traction is a form of skeletal traction that uses the Thomas splint and Pearson attachment, which allows raising the buttocks off the bed and facilitates skin care. The head of the bed should not be elevated because it may cause the client to migrate toward the end of the bed. Maintaining a 90° angle of the shoulder and elbow joints is a function of overhead arm (skeletal) traction.
NP = An
CN = Ph/8
CL = Ap
SA = 1

20. pathological. A pathological fracture is a fracture that occurs spontaneously as a result of a disease. A hip fracture can occur as a result of osteoporosis.
NP = An
CN = Ph/8
CL = Co
SA = 1

21. 4. A straight-back arm chair is the appropriate type of chair for a client who had a hip arthroplasty to facilitate rising to a standing position and preventing a dislocation.
NP = Im
CN = Ph/8
CL = Ap
SA = 1

22. 4. The most reliable diagnostic test for gout is the aspiration of synovial fluid from a tophus or an inflamed joint to detect the presence of monosodium urate monohydrate crystals. A 24-hour urine for uric acid is used to detect fluctuations in the daily concentrations. Erythrocyte sedimentation rate is a serological test that may be elevated in any inflammatory disorder. Serum uric acid is not a reliable diagnostic test for gout because hyperuricemia may occur as a result of other factors, such as drugs, or may be present in the general population.
NP = An
CN = Ph/7
CL = An
SA = 1

23. 3. Sunlight or exposure to other forms of ultraviolet radiation may precipitate a flare-up in a client with systemic lupus erythematosus who is photosensitive.
NP = Pl
CN = He/3
CL = Ap
SA = 1

24. 1, 2, 6. Although aspirin is not commonly used in the treatment of osteoarthritis, some clients continue to use it. Clients should be advised to avoid using both aspirin and nonsteroidal anti-inflammatory drugs, because the combination may prolong bleeding time and inhibit platelet function. Correct posture, body mechanics, and supportive shoes are important in the management of osteoarthritis. No specific diet is beneficial in osteoarthritis. Weight reduction and maintenance may be

encouraged to reduce the stress on the joints. Systemic organ involvement is absent in osteoarthritis. Unlike rheumatoid arthritis, anemia is uncommon in osteoarthritis.
NP = Pl
CN = He/3
CL = Ap
SA = 1

25. 2, 3, 4, 6. Significant risk factors for osteoporosis include being female, Caucasian, Asian, having a sedentary lifestyle, having had an oophorectomy, cigarette smoking, and a history of anorexia nervosa or bulimia.
NP = Pl
CN = He/3
CL = An
SA = 1

26. 4. Although middle-aged and older adults have a higher incidence of amputations, amputations are not associated with osteoarthritis, rheumatoid arthritis, or gout. A client who is middle age (55 years) and has diabetes mellitus is more prone to having an amputation because of the vascular changes that occur in diabetes.
NP = As
CN = Ph/7
CL = An
SA = 1

27. 4. A sprain is generally a twisting or wrenching injury to the ligamentous structures around a joint. Immediately following the injury, application of ice, rest, limited movement, and an analgesic are appropriate treatments.
NP = Pl
CN = Ph/8
CL = Ap
SA = 1

28. 1. Primary clinical manifestations associated with intertrochanteric (area between the greater and lesser trochanter) fracture are external rotation and shortening of the affected leg. Muscle spasms, pain, and weakness may occur but are not the classic features because they may occur in many fractures or disorders.
NP = An
CN = Ph/7
CL = Ap
SA = 1

29. **Vitamin D supplement.** Osteomalacia is an uncommon disorder in adults resulting from a vitamin D deficiency. It is a priority to place vitamin D in the plan of care for this client.
NP = Pl
CN = He/3
CL = Ap
SA = 1

30. **1, 4, 6.** Speed and coordination are slower in the older client because muscle tone and nerve conduction decrease with age. Bone mass also decreases in the older client. The Achilles reflex usually does not change throughout the lifespan. There is a decreased ability to release and store glycogen during stress.
NP = As
CN = Ph/8
CL = Ap
SA = 1

31. **1.** Metal devices, such as a prosthetic knee or a pacemaker, cannot be placed into an MRI. There are no special preparations such as restriction of food or fluids for an MRI. Hydration status is not affected by an MRI. The client lies on a flat bed with the MRI procedure; therefore, having slow reflexes will have no effect on the procedure.
NP = Im
CN = Ph/7
CL = An
SA = 1

32. **3.** Medication use is the highest priority because some medications interfere with anesthesia medications by making them more potent, require medical management prior to surgery (methotrixate, anticoagulants), and require additional medications during surgery (steroids). Family history, use of assistive devices, and lifestyle history are important data in the health history, but medication use is the highest priority in a client going to surgery.
NP = Pl
CN = He/3
CL = An
SA = 1

33. **2.** Assessment of the client's gait is important because the use of assistive devices may be required in the client's course of treatment and the type of assistive device is determined by the stability of the gait and upper body strength. Plantar and dorsiflexion weaknesses can be detected early in the assessment of the client's gait. Walking on the toes determines plantar flexion. Weakness and walking on the heels assesses dorsiflexion

weakness. Walking across the room normally determines posture and other gait problems, not tandem gait walking. Tandem gait walking is assessed by having the client walk heel to toe across the room.
NP = Im
CN = Ph/8
CL = Ap
SA = 1

34. 3. There are no dietary restrictions prior to a bone scan. Radioactive isotopes used in a bone scan procedure are not oral preparations. An injection of a radioactive substance will be done two to three hours before the procedure; however, this will not render the client radioactive for any time period. Postprocedure the nurse should be alert for an allergic reaction to the radioactive substance.
NP = Pl
CN = Ph/7
CL = Ap
SA = 1

35. 2. Active movement and some resistance is expected after a hip arthroplasty and is referred to as a muscle strength score of 4. A score of 3 would indicate the client has no strength for resistance. A score of 5 would indicate full muscle strength and that is not achieved until at least six weeks after an arthroplasty. There is no 6 on the scale of muscle strength.
NP = Ev
CN = Ph/8
CL = An
SA = 1

36. 3. Phantom pain occurs in 80% of clients with an amputation; however, there is no evidence that phantom pain is increased with elevation. Dehiscence is defined as the separation of previously joined wound edges; elevation does not cause wound dehiscence. Contributing factors in dehiscence include infection, granulation tissue that is not strong enough to withstand the force placed on the wound, and obesity, which interferes with healing. The most common contracture in a client with an amputation is a hip flexion contracture and can be avoided in three ways: restrict sitting in a chair to 30 minutes at a time, avoid elevating the residual limb on pillows, and have the client lie on his or her abdomen with hips extended at least three times a day for 30 minutes at a time. Clotting of blood is a normal process of healing that occurs with or without elevation of the residual limb.
NP = Ev
CN = Ph/7

CL = An
SA = 1

37. 4. Breath sounds assess the lungs. Degree of flexibility and muscle strength and coordination are required for ambulation; these need to be assessed to determine the ability to ambulate. Vital signs taken before, during, and after an activity will indicate how the client tolerated the activity. Increased heart rate, breathlessness, increased blood pressure, and intolerable pain indicate intolerance to the activity.
NP = As
CN = Ph/8
CL = An
SA = 1

38. Abduction. Movement toward the body's midline is adduction and away from midline is abduction.
NP = An
CN = Ph/8
CL = Co
SA = 1

39. 4. A client who had an amputation and has experienced a dehiscence requires the assessment skills of a registered nurse. A client with a full-body cast who is suspected of having compartment syndrome needs the assessment skills of the registered nurse to detect the appropriate clinical manifestations of a compartment syndrome. A licensed practical nurse cannot develop a teaching plan as needed in the case of crutch walking after a client has sustained a leg fracture. Developing a teaching plan is a skill reserved for a registered nurse. A licensed practical nurse may reinforce teaching that is already developed, as in the case of a client who has been receiving range of motion teaching.
NP = Im
CN = Sa/1
CL = An
SA = 1

40. 3. A client whose balance is too limited to pick up and move a standard walker should use a four-wheeled walker. An axillary crutch is not a substitute for a cane. An axillary crutch is used for short-term therapy. A cane may be a permanent or long-term therapy. A Canadian crutch may be used for a client who has a permanent disability and has the additional cuff for the upper arm to give added support.
NP = Pl
CN = He/3
CL = An
SA = 1

41. 1. In the swing-to gait, both crutches are moved forward together followed by bringing the legs through beyond the crutches. This gait is used by clients who have a paralysis of their lower extremities. When using the two-point gait, the left crutch and right foot are moved forward together followed by moving the right crutch and left foot together. The crutch walk requires some weight bearing on each foot. During the four-point gait, the right crutch is moved forward followed by the left foot, then the left crutch forward followed by the right foot. This is the most stable of all crutch walks. It provides the most support while requiring weight bearing on both legs. It may be used for some types of paralysis, such as in children with cerebral palsy. In the three-point gait, both crutches are moved forward with the weaker leg followed by moving the stronger leg forward. In this gait, the client is required to bear all weight on the unaffected leg.
NP = Pl
CN = He/3
CL = An
SA = 1

GENITOURINARY DISORDERS - COMPREHENSIVE EXAM

1. The nurse is evaluating a client's laboratory results. Which of the following should the nurse report as indicative of kidney dysfunction?
   1. Inorganic phosphorus of 6 mg/dl
   2. Potassium of 4 mEq/L
   3. Creatinine of 0.8 mg/dl
   4. Blood urea nitrogen of 18 mg/dl

ANSWERS AND RATIONALES

1. 1. Normal phosphorus is 3 to 4.5 mg/dl so 6 mg/dl is elevated and indicative of renal failure. The potassium, creatinine, and blood urea nitrogen levels are all within normal ranges.
NP = An
CN = Ph/7
CL = An
SA = 1

Practice Test 3

GENITOURINARY DISORDERS - COMPREHENSIVE EXAM

1. The nurse correctly collects which of the following to obtain a urine culture?
   1. First voided specimen in the morning
   2. 24-hour specimen
   3. Mid-stream specimen
   4. Double-voided specimen

2. A client is admitted with calcium oxalate calculi. The nurse instructs the client that which of the following dietary selections would contribute to calcium oxalate calculi?
   Select all that apply:
   [ ] **1.** Tomato soup
   [ ] **2.** Fried eggs
   [ ] **3.** Bran muffin
   [ ] **4.** Rhubarb pie
   [ ] **5.** Cocoa
   [ ] **6.** Orange juice

3. The nurse is discharging a female client with cystitis. Which of the following discharge instructions should the nurse include?
   1. Bathe frequently using a bubble bath
   2. Avoid caffeine-containing beverages
   3. Drink 1500 to 2000 ml of fluids daily
   4. Use contraceptive jelly with sexual intercourse

4. The nurse is discharging a female client with urethritis. Which of the following would be most important for the nurse to include in this client's discharge instructions?
   1. Daily application of a vaginal deodorant spray
   2. Avoid sexual intercourse until symptoms subside
   3. Warm sitz baths with bath salts
   4. Eliminate phosphorus-rich foods
5. The nurse is caring for a client in acute renal failure and correctly administers which of the following fluid replacements?
   1. 400 ml of fluids replaced on Saturday for 200 ml of urine excreted on Friday with no other losses
   2. 800 ml of fluids replaced on Wednesday for 300 ml of urine excreted on Tuesday with no other losses
   3. 1000 ml of fluids replaced on Monday for 400 ml of urine excreted and 300 ml of diarrhea
   4. 1500 ml of fluids replaced on Tuesday for 200 ml of urine excreted and 100 ml of emesis
6. The nurse is admitting a client suspected of having pyelonephritis. Which of the findings support the diagnosis?
   1. A history of diabetes and hypertension
   2. A history of gastroenteritis
   3. A white blood cell count of 8000
   4. A creatinine level of 0.8 mg/dl and a BUN of 20 mg/dl
7. The nurse is caring for a client who sustained a knife wound to the right flank area. Which of the following would indicate to the nurse that the client's condition is deteriorating?
   Select all that apply:
   [ ] **1.** Increased urinary output
   [ ] **2.** Tachycardia
   [ ] **3.** Tachypnea
   [ ] **4.** Decreased thirst
   [ ] **5.** Hypotension
   [ ] **6.** Muscle weakness
8. The nurse is teaching a client receiving dialysis how to self-monitor at home between dialysis treatments. Which of the following should the nurse include as the priority?
   1. Take the pulse and respiratory rate daily
   2. Obtain a daily weight

3. Perform a daily blood glucose
4. Maintain a daily activity diary

9. A client with chronic renal failure is about to begin hemodialysis and asks the nurse about the frequency of the treatments. The appropriate response by the nurse is
   1. five hours of treatment two days a week.
   2. three to four hours of treatment three days a week.
   3. two to three hours of treatment five days a week.
   4. two hours of treatment seven days a week.

10. The nurse is caring for a client in chronic renal failure. Which of the following would indicate to the nurse that the client's condition is critical?
    1. BUN of 23 mg/dl
    2. Potassium of 7 mEq/L
    3. Uremic fector
    4. Renal osteodystrophy

11. The nurse is caring for a client with uric acid calculi. Which of the following dietary selections should the nurse include in the dietary instructions?
    Select all that apply:
    [ ] 1. Red wine
    [ ] 2. Apples
    [ ] 3. Whole grain bread
    [ ] 4. Corn
    [ ] 5. Catfish
    [ ] 6. Milk

12. Which of the following is the most appropriate nursing action when the nurse has inserted a urinary catheter in a male client but there is no return of urine?
    1. Advance the catheter farther
    2. Remove the catheter
    3. Tape the catheter in place and encourage fluids
    4. Report signs of urinary infection

13. A client scheduled for a cystoscopy asks the nurse to explain the test. The appropriate response by the nurse is that a cystoscopy is
    1. "A noninvasive procedure capable of distinguishing minor differences in tissue density."
    2. "An invasive procedure in which a lighted instrument is passed through the urethra for direct visualization."

3. "A noninvasive procedure that uses reflected sound waves to visualize the kidneys."
4. "An invasive procedure in which a contrast medium is injected directly into the renal artery to examine the renal blood flow."

14. The nurse is removing an indwelling catheter. Which of the following nursing measures should receive priority?

1. Deflate the balloon of the catheter
2. Cleanse the perineal area with antiseptic swabs
3. Maintain an accurate intake and output
4. Wrap the catheter in a towel or waterproof drape

15. The nurse is discharging a client who has had recurrent urinary infections. Which of the following common signs of a urinary infection should the nurse instruct a client to report to the physician?
Select all that apply:

[ ] **1.** Dysuria
[ ] **2.** Urgency
[ ] **3.** Polyphagia
[ ] **4.** Enuresis
[ ] **5.** Cloudy urine
[ ] **6.** Nocturnal incontinence

16. The nurse is caring for a client with an arteriovenous fistula who is receiving hemodialysis treatments three times a week. Which of the following observations indicate to the nurse that the client is experiencing arterial steal syndrome?

1. The client is complaining of nausea, vomiting, and a headache
2. The presence of redness, warmth, and edema at the site of the fistula
3. The client appears pale and complains of numb fingers that are cool to the touch
4. The abdomen is distended and tender upon palpation

17. A client's family member asks the nurse why the client on hemodialysis developed dialysis disequilibrium syndrome. The nurse's response should be based on the understanding that dialysis disequilibrium syndrome occurs as a result of

1. a contaminated connection site between the catheter and machine.
2. a rapid change in the sodium and water levels.
3. the presence of residual blood left in the dialysis machine.
4. too rapid a decrease in the blood urea nitrogen levels.

18. Which of the following is the priority nursing action when a urinary catheter has been inserted in a female client with no urine return?
    1. Insert the catheter another four inches
    2. Secure the catheter tubing to the inside of the thigh
    3. Encourage the client to increase fluid intake
    4. Leave the catheter in the vagina and insert another catheter
19. Which of the following menu selections indicates that a newly diagnosed client in acute renal failure needs further instructions on appropriate dietary choices?
    1. Baked potato with salt substitute and margarine
    2. Turkey sandwich with white bread and mayonnaise
    3. Scrambled eggs, bacon, and coffee
    4. Applesauce with cinnamon and sugar
20. The nurse caring for a client with a urinary catheter is planning to clamp the catheter for specimen collection. Which of the following catheters would the nurse be able to clamp?
    1. Ureteral catheter
    2. Foley catheter
    3. Suprapubic catheter
    4. Nephrostomy catheter
21. The nurse should include which of the following in the male urinary catheterization procedure?
    1. With the nondominant gloved hand, cleanse the tip of the penis
    2. Hold the catheter four inches from the tip for insertion
    3. Lift the penis to a 45° angle for insertion
    4. Insert the catheter a total of six inches into the urethra
22. When preparing a client for an electrohydraulic lithotripsy, it is essential for the nurse to explain which of the following aspects of the procedure?
    1. Electrohydraulic lithotripsy is an invasive procedure in which an interaction between a wavelength and dye fragment large calculi
    2. There is no pain during or after an electrohydraulic lithotripsy
    3. Electrohydraulic lithotripsy involves the use of an endoscope to remove small calculi lodged in the bladder or ureter
    4. The urine may be bright red initially followed by a dark red or smoky colored urine

23. The nurse is assisting a client with struvite calculi to make which of the following menu selections?
Select all that apply:
[ ] **1.** Roast beef
[ ] **2.** Asparagus
[ ] **3.** Tea
[ ] **4.** Cottage cheese
[ ] **5.** Strawberries
[ ] **6.** Whole wheat bread

24. When considering a renal transplantation as a treatment option for chronic renal failure, the nurse should consider which of the following?
Select all that apply:
[ ] **1.** Renal transplantation is a cure for chronic renal failure.
[ ] **2.** Acute rejection occurs within 48 hours of transplantation.
[ ] **3.** Renal transplantation is the preferred treatment in advanced cardiac disease.
[ ] **4.** Most cadaver donors are young, in good health, and the victim of a trauma.
[ ] **5.** The recipient must receive dialysis within 24 hours of transplantation.
[ ] **6.** Removal of the donor kidney takes three to four hours.

25. The nurse is preparing the client assignments for the day. Which of the following client assignments would be appropriate for the registered nurse to assign to a licensed practical nurse?
   1. A client who has developed an infection at the vascular access route used for hemodialysis
   2. A client with acute pyelonephritis who is to receive IV antibiotics
   3. A client experiencing urinary retention and needing intermittent catheterization for a residual urine of less than 50 ml
   4. A client in chronic renal failure with a serum potassium of 7 mEq and a blood pressure of 140/90

26. The nurse is caring for a client who had a cystoscopy. Which of the following measures should the nurse include in the client's plan of care?
   1. The nurse assesses the client for abdominal distention, flatulence, and cramping
   2. The nurse restricts the client's fluid intake until after the first voided specimen

3. The nurse instructs the client to empty the bladder and measures residual urine
4. The nurse monitors the client for fever, dysuria, and a drop in blood pressure

27. The nurse evaluates a client's hourly output to be less than 15 ml. Which of the following is the priority nursing intervention for this client?
   1. Call the physician
   2. Document the output
   3. Encourage fluids
   4. Ensure privacy for voiding

28. The nurse is observing another nurse secure an indwelling catheter drainage bag on a client in bed. Which of the following indicates the nurse understands the correct procedure?
   1. Place the drainage bag on the bed
   2. Secure the drainage bag to the side rail of the bed
   3. Place the drainage bag on the floor
   4. Hook the drainage bag to the bed frame

29. The nurse is caring for a group of clients and reports which of the following clients as having an abnormal daily urinary output?
   1. A 10-day-old newborn with a daily urinary output of 250 ml
   2. A 2-month-old infant with a daily urinary output of 400 ml
   3. A 5-year-old child with a daily urinary output of 700 ml
   4. A 35-year-old adult with a daily urinary output of 1000 ml

ANSWERS AND RATIONALES

1. **3.** The purpose of a mid-stream specimen is to confirm the presence of a urinary tract infection and identify the offending organism.
   NP = Im
   CN = Ph/7
   CL = Ap
   SA = 1

2. **1, 4, 5.** The goal of dietary management for calcium oxalate calculi is to reduce dietary oxalate. Tomatoes, rhubarb, and cocoa are all foods that are high in dietary oxalate and should be avoided. Fried eggs, bran muffin, and orange juice are all acid-ash foods that are permitted and do not contribute to the development of calcium oxalate calculi.

NP = Im
CN = Ph/5
CL = Ap
SA = 1

3. 2. Because caffeine-containing beverages irritate the mucosa of the bladder, they should be avoided. Taking bubble baths and using contraceptive jelly with intercourse promote the development of cystitis. Drinking 1500 to 2000 ml of fluids a day is not increasing fluids; 2500 to 3000 ml of fluids are encouraged daily.
NP = Pl
CN = Ph/8
CL = Ap
SA = 1

4. 2. Instructing a female client to avoid sexual intercourse until the symptoms of urethritis subside is important because a common infecting organism is *Trichomonas.* The use of perineal deodorant sprays and sitz baths with bath salts are to be avoided because they will exacerbate the symptoms. Avoiding phosphorus-rich foods has no effects on urethritis.
NP = Pl
CN = Ph/8
CL = Ap
SA = 1

5. 2. Fluids replacement in a client in acute renal failure should be restricted to equal urinary output plus 500 to 600 ml for insensible loss. Replacing 400 ml on Saturday for 200 ml of urine excreted on Friday with no other losses is not a sufficient amount of fluid replacement. Replacing 1000 ml of fluids on Monday for 400 ml of urine excreted and 300 ml of diarrhea or replacing 1500 ml on Tuesday for 200 ml of urine excreted and 100 ml of emesis both are incorrect because they indicate fluid overload.
NP = Im
CN = Ph/7
CL = An
SA = 1

6. 1. A history of diabetes mellitus puts a client at a greater risk for urinary tract infection. For the client with diabetes, a diagnosis of pyelonephritis should be suspected when a client presents with clinical manifestations of a UTI.
NP = An
CN = Ph/7
CL = An
SA = 1

7. 2, 3, 5. Tachypnea, tachycardia, and hypotension are all clinical manifestations of shock that indicate the client who sustained a renal trauma is experiencing a deteriorating condition that could be life threatening.
NP = An
CN = Ph/7
CL = An
SA = 1

8. 2. Instructing a client to take daily weights between dialysis treatments is the priority to monitor fluid loss. A client should not gain more than 1.5 kg between dialysis treatments to avoid severe hypertension that may occur from losing large volumes of fluid.
NP = Pl
CN = Sa/1
CL = An
SA = 1

9. 2. Hemodialysis treatments generally last three to four hours three times a week.
NP = An
CN = Ph/8
CL = Ap
SA = 1

10. 2. A potassium level of 7 mEq is very critical because fatal arrhythmias may occur. Although the BUN is elevated in renal failure, 23 mg/dl is not critically elevated. A slightly elevated BUN may be the result of dehydration. Uremic fector (urine-smelling breath) and renal osteodystrophy (skeletal changes) are clinical manifestations that may occur in renal failure but are not life threatening.
NP = An
CN = Ph/7
CL = An
SA = 1

11. 2, 4, 6. An alkali-ash diet including tea, milk, vegetables, fruits (except plums, prunes, and cranberries) is permitted. Whole grains, fish with bones, pastries, and red wine are to be avoided.
NP = Pl
CN = Ph/5
CL = Ap
SA = 1

12. 1. It is most appropriate to advance a urinary catheter further after catheterizing a male client to determine if the catheter was inserted seven to nine inches. Removing the catheter, taping the catheter in

place, encouraging fluids, and reporting signs of urinary infection do not determine correct placement. Removing a catheter would result in another catheter being inserted and increasing the risk of a urinary infection.
NP = Ev
CN = Ph/7
CL = Ap
SA = 1

13. 2. An invasive procedure in which a lighted instrument is passed through the urethra for direct visualization is the definition of a cystoscopy. A noninvasive procedure distinguishing minor differences in tissue density is the definition of a CT scan. A noninvasive procedure that uses reflected sound waves to visualize the kidneys is the definition of an ultrasound. An invasive procedure in which a contrast medium is injected directly into the renal artery to examine renal blood flow is the definition of a renal arteriogram.
NP = An
CN = Ph/7
CL = Ap
SA = 1

14. 1. When removing an indwelling catheter, deflating the balloon of the catheter is the priority to facilitate easy removal of the catheter and to prevent trauma to the bladder and urethra.
NP = An
CN = Sa/1
CL = An
SA = 1

15. 1, 2, 5. An increased urgency and frequency of urination, dysuria, foul-smelling cloudy urine, and pyuria are all clinical manifestations of a urinary tract infection. Polyphagia is a clinical manifestation of diabetes mellitus. Enuresis and nocturnal incontinence are not common clinical manifestations.
NP = Pl
CN = He/3
CL = Ap
SA = 1

16. 3. A client with a vascular access site who is receiving hemodialysis is experiencing arterial steal syndrome if the client is pale with cold and numb fingers. If prompt treatment is not initiated, the fingers may become gangrenous. Nausea, vomiting, and headache occur from a rapid decrease in the blood urea nitrogen level during hemodialysis and indicate dialysis disequilibrium syndrome. Redness, warmth, and edema at the site of the fistula indicate the presence of an infection at the vascular access route. A distended abdomen and an abdomen tender upon palpation indicate the

presence of abdominal pain that may occur as a result of a complication of peritoneal dialysis.
NP = Ev
CN = Ph/7
CL = An
SA = 1

17. 4. Although the exact cause of dialysis disequilibrium syndrome is unknown, the theory is that it is caused by too rapid a decrease in the blood urea nitrogen level during hemodialysis. A contaminated connection site between the machine and catheter may occur in peritoneal dialysis. A rapid change in sodium and water levels results in muscle cramps. The presence of residual blood left in the dialysis machine indicates bleeding is occurring.
NP = Ev
CN = Ph/7
CL = An
SA = 1

18. 4. The most likely reason there is no urine after catheterizing a female client is that the catheter was accidentally placed in the vagina. Leaving the catheter in the vagina when inserting another sterile catheter ensures correct placement.
NP = Pl
CN = Sa/1
CL = Ap
SA = 1

19. 1. A baked potato is very high in potassium and although salt substitute is a good choice for salt restriction, it is a significant source of potassium. Dietary potassium should be restricted because the ability of the kidney to excrete potassium is impaired.
NP = Ev
CN = Ph/5
CL = An
SA = 1

20. 2. Foley catheters may be clamped. Care must be taken to avoid kinking, clamping, or obstructing a ureteral, suprapubic, or nephrostomy catheter. Obstructing a ureteral or nephrostomy catheter will result in increased pressure in the renal pelvis, causing tissue damage. Suprapubic catheters will not drain well if mechanically obstructed.
NP = Ev
CN = Ph/7

CL = Ap
SA = 1

21. 2. The catheter should be held three to four inches from the catheter tip to have control of the catheter and prevent contamination during insertion. The penis should be cleansed with the gloved dominant hand. The penis should be held perpendicular to the client's body so the urethra is straight to facilitate easy insertion. The catheter is inserted seven to nine inches in the male urethra.
NP = Im
CN = Ph/7
CL = Ap
SA = 1

22. 4. The initial few voidings after an electrohydraulic lithotripsy may be bright red followed by a dark red or smoky colored urine, with a gradual return to normal. A persistent bright red urine indicates hemorrhage. Laser lithotripsy is an invasive procedure in which there is an interaction between a wavelength and dye to fragment large calculi. Colicky pain is experienced postprocedure after an electrohydraulic lithotripsy. An endoscope to remove small calculi lodged in the bladder or ureter indicates a cystoscopy.
NP = Pl
CN = He/3
CL = Ap
SA = 1

23. 2, 3, 5. Red meats, dairy products, and whole grains are foods high in phosphate and are to be avoided. Fruits, vegetables, and tea may be permitted in the dietary management of struvite calculi.
NP = Im
CN = Ph/5
CL = Ap
SA = 1

24. 4, 5, 6. While most live donors are related to the recipient and in good health, most cadaver donors are young and the victim of a trauma. The renal transplantation recipient must have dialysis within 24 hours of receiving the kidney. It does take three to four hours to remove the donor kidney. Although renal transplantation is not a cure, it may reverse pathophysiological changes in the diseased kidney and eliminate the need for dialysis. Hyperacute rejection is the rejection that occurs within 48 hours. Acute rejection occurs six weeks to two years after transplantation. Renal transplantation is contraindicated in advanced cardiac disease.
NP = An
CN = Ph/8

CL = Ap
SA = 1

25. 3. The licensed practical nurse cannot administer IV medications or assess an infected vascular access route used for hemodialysis. The licensed practical nurse cannot care for a client who is not stable, as is the case of the client with a potassium of 7 mEq and the potential of fatal arrhythmias in chronic renal failure.
NP = Pl
CN = Sa/1
CL = An
SA = 1

26. 4. The nurse observes for fever, dysuria, or a drop in blood pressure postcystoscopy. All indicate complications or problems. Complications that may result from cystoscopy include urinary retention, urinary tract hemorrhage, bladder infection, and perforation.
NP = Pl
CN = Ph/7
CL = Ap
SA = 1

27. 1. The priority nursing intervention when a client has an hourly urine output of 15 ml is to call the physician. An hourly urine output of 15 ml for 24 hours is 360 ml. Oliguria is a urine output of 100 to 400 ml in a 24-hour period and may be an indication of dehydration, kidney disease, or end-stage renal disease. Anuria is a urine output of less than 100 ml. Normal urinary output is generally estimated to be 30 ml per hour. After notifying the physician of a severely compromised urinary output, it may be appropriate to encourage fluids and ensure privacy for voiding. Documenting any output is important.
NP = Pl
CN = Sa/1
CL = Ap
SA = 1

28. 4. The correct position for a urinary drainage bag on a client in bed is to hook the drainage bag to the bed frame. The bed frame is a nonmovable part of the bed that will not cause the bag to be raised or lowered or pull on the client. Placing the catheter bag on the floor predisposes the client to a urinary infection.
NP = Ev
CN = Ph/8
CL = Ap
SA = 1

29. 4. A daily urinary output of 1000 ml for an adult client is abnormal. Normal daily urinary adult output is 1500 ml. The normal daily urinary output for a newborn 10 days to 2 months is 250 to 400 ml. Normal daily urinary output for a child 2 months old to 1 year old is 400 to 500 ml. The normal daily urinary output for a child 1to 3 years old is 500 to 600. The normal daily urinary output for a child 3 to 5 years old is 600 to 700 ml. The normal daily urinary output for a child 5 to 8 years old is 700 to 1000 ml. The normal daily urinary output for a child 8 to14 years old is 800 to 1400 ml.
NP = An
CN = Ph/8
CL = An
SA = 1

ONCOLOGY DISORDERS - COMPREHENSIVE EXAM

1. A client's family member asks the nurse whether cancer is contagious. The nurse's response is based on the understanding that
   1. cancer cells cannot travel through the air.
   2. cancer is the unregulated growth of a person's own cells.
   3. cancer is only contagious shortly after diagnosis.
   4. clients with cancer should not share drinking glasses with others.
2. The nurse is teaching a class to a group of nursing students on the factors in the various types of cancers. Which of the following should the nurse include in the class?
   1. Breast cancer is the leading cause of cancer death in women
   2. Skin cancer is most common in dark-skinned persons
   3. Lung cancer is the leading cause of cancer death in women
   4. Colon cancer is more prevalent in men
3. A client asks the nurse, "Why did I get breast cancer?" Which of the following is the most appropriate response by the nurse?
   1. "Breast cancer risk is primarily related to a woman's diet."
   2. "There are very few risk factors for breast cancer."
   3. "Breast cancer is most often inherited from one's mother."
   4. "Breast cancer is more common in women over age 50."
4. A client asks the nurse what the physician meant when stating the client's cancer was stage I. Which of the following is the appropriate response by the nurse?

1. "The cancer is localized to where it began."
2. "The cancer has spread to other organs."
3. "The cancer has spread to lymph nodes near the area where the cancer began."
4. "The cancer cannot metastasize."

5. While taking a nursing history from a client, the client describes a sore that will not heal. The priority nursing action is to
   1. obtain an order for an antibiotic.
   2. monitor the sore until it begins to heal.
   3. report this as one of the seven warning signs of cancer.
   4. instruct the client on proper wound dressing.
6. A client asks, "How can I reduce my risk of cancer?" Which of the following is the appropriate response of the nurse?
   1. "There is no way to reduce the risk of cancer."
   2. "Regular exercise can reduce cancer risk."
   3. "Limiting alcohol has no impact on cancer risk reduction."
   4. "Becoming a vegetarian is the best way to reduce cancer risk."
7. A 20-year-old woman asks the nurse if she should be screened for breast cancer. Which of the following is the most appropriate response by the nurse?
   1. "Only women with a family history of breast cancer need to be screened."
   2. "Women your age do not need to worry about breast cancer screening."
   3. "Annual mammograms should begin at age 20."
   4. "Women should begin monthly breast self-exam at age 20."
8. Which of the following should the nurse include in the plan of care for a client who has cancer and is having a CT scan?
   1. Observe the client for flushing, itching, or nausea
   2. Stay with the client to provide support
   3. Administer p.r.n. pain medication
   4. Inform the client to move all extremities every few minutes
9. The nurse is caring for a client going through a workup for cancer who is very depressed and saying, "There is no hope when you have cancer. You always die." Which of the following statements would be most appropriate for this client?

1. "Surgery is rarely used to treat cancer."
2. "Bone marrow transplant is only used to treat blood-related cancers."
3. "Gene therapy is widely used outside of clinical trials."
4. "Many cancers are treated with a combination of surgery, chemotherapy, and radiation."

10. Based on an understanding of safety precautions related to brachytherapy, the nurse should consider which of the following?

1. The client will be radioactive for a month after returning home
2. A dislodged implant should be picked up immediately after becoming dislodged
3. Pregnant nurses may care for this client without concern
4. Body fluids of clients with radioactive implants are radioactive

11. The nurse is caring for a client who is complaining of cancer-related pain. Which of the following is the priority nursing action?

1. Confirm the client's report with a close family member
2. Give a limited amount of narcotics to avoid addiction
3. Believe the client's report of pain
4. Avoid administering nonnarcotic and narcotic pain medication together

12. The nurse is caring for a client diagnosed with cancer who is currently between cycles of chemotherapy. The nurse should assess this client for what most common adverse reaction to chemotherapy? ______________

13. The nurse is caring for a client 14 days after the first administration of chemotherapy. Which of the following is the first indication that the client has an infection and action must be taken?

1. Pain
2. Foul-smelling drainage from a surgical site
3. At least a 2° elevation in body temperature for 24 hours
4. A 1° elevation in body temperature for 24 hours

14. The nurse should implement which of the following in the plan of care to prevent an infection in a client receiving chemotherapy?

1. Instruct the client to always wear a mask when leaving the room
2. Limit the number of invasive procedures performed
3. Instruct the client's family that hand washing is only minimally effective in infection prevention
4. Instruct the client to eat fresh fruits and vegetables as often as possible

15. Which of the following interventions is a priority to include in a plan of care for a client with thrombocytopenia?
    1. Assist the client to shave with a straight-edged razor
    2. Administer an enema for constipation
    3. Avoid the use of aspirin and nonsteroidal anti-inflammatory medications
    4. Administer meperidine (Demerol) if shaking chills occur

16. The client asks the nurse, "What should I eat after receiving chemotherapy to decrease nausea?" What type of diet should the nurse instruct the client is best tolerated during chemotherapy? ______________

17. Because a client receiving chemotherapy is at risk for developing mouth sores, the nurse instructs the client to
    1. eat citrus fruits or juices several times a day.
    2. rinse the mouth with saline solution several times a day.
    3. brush the teeth and gums vigorously to remove plaque.
    4. rinse the mouth with an over-the-counter mouthwash several times a day.

18. One day after receiving chemotherapy, the client is nauseous and has vomited. The nurse should implement which of the following as the priority nursing intervention?
    1. Encourage the client to drink fluids to replace volume losses
    2. Spray the room with air freshener to cover nauseating smells
    3. Assess whether antiemetic medication has been given as ordered
    4. Contact the client's physician because nausea and vomiting should only occur immediately after chemotherapy

19. The nurse should monitor a client receiving both chemotherapy and narcotic pain medication for what most common adverse reaction?
    1. Headache
    2. Constipation
    3. Skin rash
    4. Depression

20. A client with stage IV cancer is deteriorating and asks the nurse, "Am I going to die?" Based on the nurse's understanding of promoting coping in clients with cancer, the priority response is
    1. "You'll have to discuss that with your physician."
    2. "Don't worry about dying, your physician has ordered very effective chemotherapy."

3. "You should go to a support group -- I'll give you a brochure."
4. "That may happen--would you like to talk about this?"

21. When assessing the emotional well-being of a client newly diagnosed with cancer, it is a priority for the nurse to ask
    1. "Do you cry a lot?"
    2. "Who do you usually turn to for support in times of stress?"
    3. "Do you want the physician to prescribe an antidepressant for you?"
    4. "Are you worried about dying of cancer?"

22. A client with metastasis to the bone displays clinical manifestations of confusion, muscle weakness, and nausea. Based on an understanding of oncology emergencies, which of the following is the priority for the nurse to assess?
    1. Pain
    2. Input and output
    3. Serum calcium and ECG
    4. Glucose and potassium

23. A nurse is discharging a client following a mastectomy and axillary lymph node dissection. Which of the following is a priority to include in the plan of care for this client?
    1. Instruct the client on surgical drain care and range of motion exercises
    2. Instruct the client to wear a sling on the surgical side until the first return physician appointment
    3. Instruct the client to follow a low-fat diet
    4. Instruct the client on preparation for radiation therapy that is required after mastectomy

24. The nurse is assessing a client being treated for ovarian cancer. Which of the following would the nurse expect to be the primary assessment finding?
    1. Malaise
    2. Abdominal ascites
    3. Hypertension
    4. Elevated serum creatinine

25. The nurse is teaching a client to perform a testicular self-examination and should inform the client that what finding should be reported immediately as the first and primary sign of testicular cancer? ____________

26. The registered nurse is delegating nursing tasks to a licensed practical nurse. Which of the following may the nurse delegate?

1. Assess a client's nutritional status following a Billroth II
2. Administer prescribed chemotherapy to a client with leukemia
3. Develop a screening program for colon cancer
4. Assist a client to ambulate following a lobectomy

27. The nurse is caring for a client suspected of having cancer of the kidney. Which of the following clinical manifestations support the diagnosis? Select all that apply:

[ ] 1. Dull, aching pain
[ ] 2. Changes in memory
[ ] 3. Gross hematuria
[ ] 4. Headache
[ ] 5. Abdominal mass
[ ] 6. Loss of appetite

28. The nurse is evaluating the following four clients for their risk of breast cancer. Which of the following clients does the nurse conclude is at highest risk?

1. A client who had three children before the age of 30 years
2. A client who is under the age of 50 years
3. A client who took estrogen hormones
4. A client who had menarche after the age of 16 years

29. The nurse is caring for a client following a head and neck surgery. Which of the following is the priority role for the nurse to assume?

1. Assist the client in coping with dysfunction and body image changes
2. Provide oral care with saline and peroxide solution
3. Assess the client's ability to eat
4. Encourage the client to engage in support groups

30. Which of the following nursing tasks does the registered nurse delegate to a licensed practical nurse?

1. Prepare the client with an osteosarcoma for an amputation
2. Provide education to a group of clients on skin cancer prevention
3. Monitor a client with leukemia for signs of bleeding from thrombocytopenia
4. Assess a client with lung cancer for superior vena cava syndrome

ANSWERS AND RATIONALES

1. 2. Cancer is not contagious, nor is it transmitted to other persons via the air or the oral route. Cancers develop from genetic errors that occur in a person's own cells, which leads to unregulated cell growth.
NP = An
CN = Ph/8
CL = Ap
SA = 1

2. 3. Lung cancer is the leading cause of cancer death in women. Breast cancer is the second-leading cause of women's cancer death. Skin cancer most commonly occurs in fair-skinned persons. Colon cancer is equally likely to affect both men and women.
NP = Pl
CN = Ph/7
CL = Ap
SA = 1

3. 4. While diet is believed to be responsible for contributing to cancer development, it is not the primary cause of breast cancer. There are many risk factors for breast cancer, including the possibility of inheriting a genetic mutation from either one's mother or father. Breast cancer, like many cancers, is more common in older persons, and in many cases age is one of the only risk factors a woman has.
NP = An
CN = Sa/1
CL = Ap
SA = 1

4. 1. In general, cancers that cannot metastasize are called stage 0. Those that have the capability of spreading, but have not, are stage I. Cancers which have spread to regional lymph nodes are often referred to as stage II or III. Once cancer has spread to other organs, it is stage IV.
NP = An
CN = Ph/8
CL = Ap
SA = 1

5. 3. A sore that will not heal is one of the seven warning signs of cancer and, therefore, further examination by the physician is needed. Monitoring the wound, using an antibiotic, and appropriate wound dressing may all be appropriate after it has been determined by the physician that this does not represent a cancer, or after a biopsy of the area is obtained.

NP = Im
CN = Sa/1
CL = Ap
SA = 1

6. 2. There are several ways to reduce the risk of getting cancer. Regular exercise several times per week is recommended to reduce the risk of most types of cancer. Reducing the amount of red meat and increasing the amount of fruits and vegetables is also a way to reduce cancer risk. However, becoming a vegetarian is not necessary. Alcoholic beverages should be reduced to no more than two per day in order to reduce the cancer risk.
NP = An
CN = Ph/7
CL = Ap
SA = 1

7. 4. All women, regardless of their family history, should be screened for breast cancer. Screening mammograms are typically not recommended before age 40; however, women should begin monthly breast self-exam at age 20. Breast cancer is typically a disease of women over age 50; however, even women in their twenties have been diagnosed.
NP = An
CN = Ph/8
CL = Ap
SA = 1

8. 1. An allergic reaction to the contrast media administered during CT scans can produce symptoms of flushing, itching, or nausea. Clients should hold very still during the scan. CT scans are painless, and therefore, pain medication is generally not needed. Since this scan involves x-ray, the nurse cannot stay with the client, but would have to remain in a protected area.
NP = Pl
CN = Ph/8
CL = Ap
SA = 1

9. 4. Surgery is the primary treatment for many cancers, and is often combined with chemotherapy and radiation therapy. Gene therapy is primarily experimental and, therefore, used within clinical trials. Bone marrow transplants are used for some solid tumor cancers as well as blood-related cancers.
NP = An
CN = Ph/8

CL = Ap
SA = 1

10. 2. Brachytherapy involves temporarily implanting a radioactive source in the client in order to destroy nearby cancer cells. Therefore, the client is radioactive while the implant is in place and pregnant nurses should not be assigned to care for this client. The client will not be radioactive once the implant is removed and there are no concerns related to returning home. Body fluids of this client are not radioactive and should be handled with standard universal precautions. If the radioactive implant becomes separated from the client, it must only be handled with forceps and placed in a special container maintained at the bedside.
NP = An
CN = Ph/7
CL = An
SA = 1

11. 3. The client's report of pain should always be believed to exist when and how it is described. According to the World Health Organization's analgesic ladder for pain management, nonnarcotic and narcotic pain medications should be used together to provide better pain relief than either provides alone. Fewer than 1% of clients become addicted to narcotic pain medication when used appropriately, so this is not a reason to limit treatment of a client's pain.
NP = Im
CN = Sa/1
CL = An
SA = 1

12. Fatigue. Fatigue is the most common adverse reaction to chemotherapy, affecting almost 100% of clients. Nausea may not occur with all chemotherapy, and occurs to a more or lesser degree depending on the chemotherapy administered. Skin and emotional problems can occur, but are more rare and very individualized to the client.
NP = As
CN = Ph/8
CL = Ap
SA = 1

13. 4. Fourteen days postchemotherapy is a typical time for the neutrophil count to be very low (nadir), making the client most susceptible to infection. Due to the client's immunocompromised state, the nurse must be alert to very subtle changes that indicate infection, such as a mild temperature elevation. Pain is usually not a primary sign of infection. Foul-smelling drainage and a significant temperature elevation may be

signs of infection, but the nurse should not wait for these more obvious signs before taking action in such a client.
NP = Ev
CN = Ph/8
CL = Ap
SA = 1

14. 2. Hand washing is one of the most effective ways to prevent infection in clients immunocompromised by chemotherapy. The nurse would not want to discourage this practice among the client's family members. Masks do not need to be worn by clients receiving chemotherapy unless they have had a bone marrow transplant. Fresh fruits and vegetables should be washed very well, if eaten at all. Many institutions encourage clients to avoid fresh produce when their white blood cell counts are low. Minimizing invasive procedures, such as number of blood draws and avoiding urinary catheters, is a very effective way to reduce the chance of infection.
NP = Im
CN = Ph/7
CL = Ap
SA = 1

15. 3. Thrombocytopenia (low platelets) increases the client's risk of bleeding. Clients should be discouraged from using a straight-edged razor, invasive procedures such as enemas, and taking medications with anticoagulant properties (such as aspirin and nonsteroidal anti-inflammatory medications). Administering meperidine (Demerol) for shaking chills is appropriate during administration of a platelet transfusion.
NP = Pl
CN = Sa/1
CL = An
SA = 1

16. **Bland.** Sweet, fried, and spicy foods can contribute to nausea if eaten the first few days after chemotherapy administration. A bland diet is usually recommended.
NP = Pl
CN = Ph/5
CL = Ap
SA = 1

17. 2. Rinsing the oral mucosa with saline (or a salt and soda solution) helps to cleanse and protect the tissue from breakdown. Brushing vigorously and eating citrus products can irritate the oral mucosa. Over-the-counter mouthwashes containing alcohol can be drying and are usually discouraged.

NP = Im
CN = Ph/7
CL = Ap
SA = 1

18. 3. Depending upon the chemotherapy administered, nausea and vomiting may not occur at all or may occur several hours to several days after treatment. While it is important to assure that the client remains properly hydrated and that nausea triggers (such as smells) are removed, the nurse's first priority is to assess whether antiemetic medication has been administered as ordered.

NP = Im
CN = Sa/1
CL = An
SA = 1

19. 2. A primary adverse reaction of narcotic pain medication is constipation. Many chemotherapy agents cause constipation. The nurse should monitor this client for this assessment finding. Headache, skin rash, and depression are possible adverse reactions in a wide range of situations. They are not a common finding in the majority of clients receiving chemotherapy and narcotic pain medications.

NP = As
CN = Ph/6
CL = Ap
SA = 5

20. 4. The nurse should be honest with the client and provide opportunities for the client to express concerns openly, taking the time to listen in order to promote effective coping. Telling clients to not worry or to discuss their concerns with someone else closes communication, shows lack of respect, and minimizes the client's feelings.

NP = An
CN = Sa/1
CL = An
SA = 1

21. 2. It is important to assess the client's support system and usual ways of coping with stress, since people usually rely on these same systems and coping mechanisms when faced with a crisis like cancer. Asking who the client turns to in times of stress is an open-ended question, which invites discussion between the client and nurse. Asking if the client cries a lot, wants the physician to order an antidepressant, or is afraid of dying are closed-ended questions, which can be answered by a yes or no response. These questions show the nurse is making presumptions about the client's emotional state and they do not invite open discussion.

NP = As
CN = Ph/8
CL = Ap
SA = 1

22. 3. Clients with bony metastases are at the greatest risk for hypercalcemia, which displays clinical manifestations of confusion, muscle weakness, and nausea, as well as an elevated serum calcium and ECG changes. Assessing the client's pain, intake and output, glucose, and potassium are assessments that are important for clients in general but not specific to the client described.
NP = As
CN = Sa/1
CL = An
SA = 1

23. 1. Following a mastectomy, clients are typically discharged to home with a surgical drain. Instruction in the care of the surgical drain is essential. In addition, to regain range of motion and prevent lymphedema of the arm on the operated side, clients should be instructed in range of motion exercises to begin upon physician order. Clients should be instructed to use the arm for usual activity postoperatively, as ordered by the physician. The arm does not have to be kept in a sling. While everyone should eat a diet low in fats to reduce the risk of a variety of diseases, this is not essential to this client's plan of care. Radiation therapy is typically not required following mastectomy as it is after lumpectomy.
NP = Pl
CN = Sa/1
CL = An
SA = 1

24. 2. All clients with cancer may at some time have malaise or elevated blood pressure. The major assessment finding for clients with ovarian cancer is abdominal ascites. This may cause discomfort, shortness of breath, and emotional distress. Daily abdominal girth measurements are often performed while the client is hospitalized. Elevated serum creatinine is not an assessment finding typically found in clients with ovarian cancer.
NP = As
CN = Ph/8
CL = Ap
SA = 1

25. **A small, hard mass in the scrotum.** Clients performing testicular self-examination should palpate the scrotum for a small, hard mass, which is the most common sign of testicular cancer. Low back pain may be a

symptom of many things, including late testicular cancer that has spread to lymph nodes. This will not be found on testicular self-examination.
NP = Im
CN = Sa/1
CL = Ap
SA = 1

26. 4. A licensed practical nurse cannot assess or develop a screening program. Administering chemotherapy is a nursing task reserved for specially trained registered nurses. A licensed practical nurse may assist a client to ambulate following a surgery.
NP = Im
CN = Sa/1
CL = Ap
SA = 1

27. 1, 3, 5. Clinical manifestations of kidney cancer include dull, aching pain, gross hematuria, and an abdominal mass. Headaches and changes in memory are clinical manifestations of a central nervous system tumor. Loss of appetite is a clinical manifestation of gastric cancer.
NP = An
CN = Ph/8
CL = Ap
SA = 1

28. 3. Although the majority of women with breast cancer have no identifiable risk factors, the woman at greatest risk is the woman who took estrogen hormones. Women who are over the age of 50 years, have no children, or had children after the age of 30 years are also at a greater risk for breast cancer.
NP = Ev
CN = Ph/7
CL = An
SA = 1

29. 1. Although providing oral care with a saline and peroxide solution, assessing the client's ability to eat, and encouraging the client to engage in support groups are important interventions, the nurse's primary role is to assist the client in coping with issues of dysfunction, losses, and body image changes associated with difficult and disfiguring treatments.
NP = Im
CN = Sa/1
CL = An
SA = 1

30. 3. A licensed practical nurse can monitor a client with leukemia for signs of bleeding from thrombocytopenia. A licensed practical nurse should not

prepare a client with osteosarcoma for an amputation. Providing education to a group of clients on skin cancer prevention and assessing a client with lung cancer for superior vena cava syndrome are nursing tasks that should be performed by a registered nurse.
NP = Im
CN = Sa/1
CL = An
SA = 8

HEMATOLOGICAL DISORDERS - COMPREHENSIVE EXAM

1. A client who has received two units of packed red blood cells complains of shortness of breath, a headache, and a cough. The nurse should implement which of the following nursing interventions for this client?

1. Position the client in Trendelenburg position

2. Increase the IV fluid rate and contact the physician

3. Position the client in an upright position with feet in a dependent position

4. Discontinue the oxygen because the client has too much hemoglobin

2. The nurse caring for a client having an allergic reaction to a transfusion of blood should have what medication available for immediate administration? ______________

3. During an admission, the nurse assesses which of the following clinical manifestations to be present in a client with thrombocytopenic thrombotic purpura (TTP)?
Select all that apply:

[ ] **1.** Confusion

[ ] **2.** Polyuria

[ ] **3.** Multiple petechiae

[ ] **4.** Ecchymosis

[ ] **5.** Anorexia

[ ] **6.** Epistaxis

4. The nurse, caring for a client with several IV catheters, increases the heparin infusion for lower extremity deep vein thrombosis to maintain a therapeutic PTT level. The client develops tarry stools, hypotension, and faint peripheral pulses. Which of the following is the priority intervention?

1. Discontinue heparin

2. Monitor for bleeding and thrombosis

3. Maintain IV access
4. Inform the client of the treatments provided

5. The nurse is preparing a client with von Willebrand's disease for an elective dental procedure. Based on an understanding of this disorder, which of the following drugs should the nurse administer to this client?
   1. Heparin
   2. Desmopressin acetate (DDAVP)
   3. Hydroxyurea (Hydrea)
   4. Melphalan (Alkeran)

6. The nurse is admitting a client in an outpatient clinic for a routine history and physical. The client has a temperature of 38 °C or 100.5 °F orally, a low normal blood pressure, dry cough, and a rash. The nurse anticipates the physician will order which of the following blood work?
   1. CBC and differential
   2. Liver function tests
   3. Thyroid function profile
   4. Coagulation panel

7. A client being phlebotomized for polycythemia vera asks the nurse what the purpose is. The nurse should give this client which explanation of the purpose of removing blood?
   1. "To help treat the anemia."
   2. "To decrease blood volume."
   3. "To decrease the coagulation factors."
   4. "To increase viscosity of the blood."

8. The nurse is discharging a client with essential thrombocytosis. Which of the following should the nurse include in the discharge instructions?
   1. Smoking cigarettes may continue in moderation
   2. Avoid driving a car
   3. Treatments received in the hospital will cure the disorder
   4. Home visits will occur to teach self-injection of interferon

9. The nurse is caring for a client with hemoglobin sickle C disease who is complaining of abdominal pain and has not been able to eat much at meals. With these clinical manifestations, the nurse anticipates which of the following findings?
   1. Splenomegaly
   2. Cardiomyopathy

3. Pneumonia
4. Neutropenia

10. A client is admitted with sickle cell anemia who is complaining of severe bone pain. The nurse observes the client is tachycardic with a heart rate of 108 beats/min and the sclera is yellow-tinged. Which of the following is the appropriate nursing intervention?
    1. Phlebotomize one unit of blood
    2. Administer morphine sulfate 5 mg IV every 30 minutes until relief
    3. Give nitroglycerin sublingually
    4. Give dexamethasone 10 mg orally

11. A nurse is admitting a client to the hospital for anemia. Which of the following statements by the client would indicate to the nurse a diagnosis of extrinsic hemolytic anemia?
    1. "I have G6PD deficiency and I'm always tired."
    2. "I got malaria last year on a trip to Africa."
    3. "The doctor told me I don't eat the right food and gave me iron pills."
    4. "I have sickle cell anemia."

12. Which of the following should the nurse include when preparing to give a client with iron deficiency anemia parenteral iron?
    1. Apply ice to the injection site afterward
    2. Use the Z-track method
    3. Avoid giving the injection in the gluteus muscle
    4. Massage the skin after the injection

13. The nurse is caring for a client with a chronic bleeding ulcer. Which of the following drugs should the nurse administer to this client for the iron deficiency anemia?
    1. Ferrous sulfate
    2. Zinc
    3. Vitamin B_{12}
    4. Filgrastim (Neupogen)

14. Which of the following statements should the nurse include when explaining acute leukemia and disseminated intravascular coagulation (DIC) to another nurse?
    1. "Treatment should be initiated for the leukemia, which is the underlying cause of the DIC."
    2. "Treatment of the leukemia will be delayed until the DIC is under control."

3. "Anticoagulants will not be used in the treatment because the client is already at risk of bleeding."
4. "Provide supportive care and initiate a referral to hospice."

15. The nurse is caring for a client who has developed a deep vein thrombosis with bed rest. Which of the following should the nurse implement in this client's plan of care?
    1. Encourage participation in daily physical therapy treatments
    2. Instruct all visitors to wash hands and wear masks in the room
    3. Fit the client for antithrombosis stockings
    4. Administer morphine sulfate

16. A client is admitted to the hospital with a hemoglobin level of 7 g/dl. The nurse should assess the client for which of the following manifestations indicating a diagnosis of acute anemia?
    1. Blood pressure of 180/90
    2. Oral temperature of 37.2 °C or 99.1 °F
    3. Apical pulse of 120 beats/min
    4. Respiratory rate of 12 breaths/min

17. During an admission of a client with a platelet count of less than 20,000/mm^3 and after removing the blood pressure cuff from the client's arm, the nurse notices a new red rash in the area where the cuff had been. The nurse should report this rash as what? ______________

18. A nurse is preparing to transfuse two units of red blood cells to a client with a hemoglobin level of 7.5 g/dl. The blood bank has indicated that the blood has been filtered to reduce leukocytes. The nurse understands the rationale for filtering of blood products as which of the following?
    1. Filtering does not reduce the transmission of cytomegalovirus to the recipient
    2. Filtering donated blood fails to protect the donor from infection
    3. Filtering blood reduces the incidence of febrile and nonhemolytic transfusion reactions
    4. Filtering leukocytes from blood increases recipient immunization to leukocyte antigens

19. The nurse admitted a client with hemophilia A to the hospital after a waterskiing accident. The client is experiencing pain and a large ecchymosis on the lower back. The nurse evaluates which of the following laboratory data supporting this finding?
    1. An increase in the coagulation time
    2. A decreased hemoglobin/hematocrit level

3. Neutropenia
4. Basophilia

20. Which of the following is a priority for the nurse to implement in a client presplenectomy?
    1. Administer analgesics
    2. Carefully position the client, promoting lung expansion
    3. Encourage several small meals a day
    4. Administer pneumococcal vaccine

21. The nurse is assessing the educational needs of a client with anemia. Which of the following nursing interventions will best facilitate the client's learning?
    1. Choose a time for teaching when the client is well rested and least fatigued
    2. Choose a time when the client's family is not around to distract the client from learning
    3. Arrange a seminar for the client and family to attend
    4. Any time is appropriate as long as the teaching takes place

22. The nurse is planning the daily nursing care assignments. Which of the following nursing tasks may the nurse delegate to a licensed practical nurse?
    1. Administer immunoglobulin and glucocorticoids to a client who has immune thrombocytopenic purpura (ITP)
    2. Administer low molecular weight heparin to a client who is prone to a venous thrombosis
    3. Assess and report clinical manifestations of an infection in a client with neutropenia
    4. Maintain venous access for plasma exchange in a client with thrombotic thrombocytopenic purpura (TTP)

23. The nurse is planning the care for a client with a diagnosis of anemia due to acute blood loss associated with a motor vehicle accident. Which of the following nursing diagnoses is a priority for this client?
    1. Risk for injury
    2. Activity intolerance
    3. Imbalanced nutrition: less than body requirements
    4. Ineffective therapeutic regimen management

24. The nurse is teaching a client with anemia about maximizing iron intake. Which statement from the client represents a good understanding of oral iron replacement therapy?

1. "The iron pill could turn my skin brown."
2. "I should take my iron pill before meals with orange juice."
3. "It is best to take my iron pill with an antacid to decrease the stomach upset."
4. "I could notice some blood in my stool after taking the iron pill."

25. A client with a blood clot has been receiving heparin and warfarin sodium and begins to bleed. What drug should the nurse administer to counteract the effects of the warfarin? ______________

26. The nurse is teaching a class on thrombocytopenia. The nurse indicates an understanding of the difference between thrombotic thrombocytopenic purpura (TTP) and hemolytic uremic syndrome (HUS) by stating that hemolytic uremic syndrome occurs in

1. the elderly client.
2. children.
3. the client with thrombocytopenia.
4. the young adult client.

27. When working with a client with aplastic anemia, the nurse should include which of the following considerations in planning the goals of care?

1. The client is at risk for infection and bleeding
2. The client's nutritional intake is low with an associated weight loss
3. The client has pain and will need pain management
4. The client may need a splenectomy

28. The nurse evaluates a client with polycythemia to have which of the following clinical manifestations?
Select all that apply:

[ ] **1.** Headache
[ ] **2.** Purpura
[ ] **3.** Tinnitus
[ ] **4.** Paresthesias
[ ] **5.** Abdominal fullness
[ ] **6.** Nosebleeds

29. The nurse is preparing clinical assignments for the day. Which of the following would be appropriate for the nurse to delegate to unlicensed assistive personnel?

1. Walk a client who has aplastic anemia and neutropenia
2. Monitor the circumference of a limb on a client with a blood clot

3. Assess a client with thrombotic thrombocytopenic purpura for signs of bleeding
4. Take the vital signs of a client with sickle cell anemia

30. Which of the following is a priority for the nurse to include in the plan of care for a client with hemochromatosis?
    1. Instruct the client to avoid contact sports
    2. Instruct the client to limit the dietary intake of iron
    3. Prepare the client for a phlebotomy
    4. Assess the client's hematocrit level

ANSWERS AND RATIONALES

1. 3. The client is experiencing circulatory overload and will have less respiratory distress in an upright position. The head is down in the Trendelenburg position and would increase blood pressure and add pressure to the heart and lungs, making the client more symptomatic. Oxygen may be used as a treatment for circulatory overload.
   NP = Im
   CN = Ph/8
   CL = Ap
   SA = 1

2. **Epinephrine.** Epinephrine may be ordered to treat an allergic reaction.
   NP = Pl
   CN = Ph/6
   CL = Ap
   SA = 5

3. 1, 3, 4, 6. Clinical manifestations of thrombocytopenic thrombotic purpura include mental changes, multiple petechiae, ecchymosis (bruising), and epistaxis (nosebleeds). Other clinical manifestations include very heavy menses, blood in the stool and vomit, and decreased urine output.
   NP = As
   CN = Ph/8
   CL = Ap
   SA = 1

4. 1. A client receiving IV heparin who develops tarry stools, hypotension, and faint peripheral pulses is experiencing heparin-induced thrombocytopenia and thrombosis syndrome (HITTS). The priority intervention is to discontinue the heparin, followed by monitoring the client for bleeding and thrombosis, maintaining IV access, and informing

the client of the treatment prescribed. The client has increased needs for heparin in order to be therapeutic, which indicates the metabolism of the drug has changed. This change could be caused by antibodies to the drug. Bleeding occurs because of the destruction of platelets, but also may be caused by the heparin. The faint peripheral pulses could indicate arterial occlusion from the thrombotic nature of HITTS.
NP = An
CN = Sa/1
CL = An
SA = 1

5. 2. Von Willebrand's disease is a hereditary bleeding disorder caused by the deficiency of the von Willebrand coagulation protein and platelet dysfunction. Desmopressin acetate (DDAVP) is given intravenously or as a nasal spray to increase factor VIII and von Willebrand factor concentration. Heparin would not be used because it would increase bleeding. Hydroxyurea (Hydrea) and melphalan (Alkeran) are myelosuppressive agents used in the treatment of polycythemia.
NP = An
CN = Ph/6
CL = An
SA = 5

6. 1. The client's clinical manifestations of a temperature of 38 °C or 100.5 °F, low blood pressure, dry cough, and a rash indicate infection. The CBC and differential are the most appropriate tests for the nurse to order in this situation. The CBC can help determine immune status of the client and the differential may show a predominance of neutrophils in some infections. The liver function tests, coagulation tests, and a thyroid profile are not indicated for these signs.
NP = An
CN = Ph/7
CL = Ap
SA = 1

7. 2. Polycythemia vera causes an increase in blood cells. The blood volume and increase in blood viscosity are treated by phlebotomy. A phlebotomy would remove blood that can cause anemia, but it does not treat anemia. The client with polycythemia vera should also be hydrated to decrease the viscosity of the blood. Removing blood does not increase blood thickness.
NP = An
CN = Ph/7
CL = Ap
SA = 1

8. 4. Interferon alfa-2a is one of several available treatments for thrombocytosis. Thrombocytosis is not curable and treatments may continue for years, depending on the platelet count. Smoking adds to the risk of complications and cessation should be encouraged. Driving a car is not discouraged unless the client has a stroke or other severe complication of the disease.
NP = Pl
CN = Ph/8
CL = Ap
SA = 1

9. 1. Splenomegaly is common in hemoglobin sickle C disease. The clinical manifestations of abdominal pain and early satiety also are consistent with splenomegaly.
NP = An
CN = Ph/8
CL = An
SA = 1

10. 2. The client has sickle cell anemia and is experiencing a painful hemolytic episode. It is typical to require opioids for pain relief. Phlebotomy alone would not help the client who already has anemia unless it was followed by a transfusion of normal blood. Nitroglycerin and dexamethasone are not used in the treatment of this client's condition.
NP = Pl
CN = Ph/8
CL = Ap
SA = 1

11. 2. Extrinsic causes of hemolytic anemia include infections like malaria. Intrinsic causes, such as G6PD and sickle cell anemia, have been present since birth. If the client has low iron from a dietary deficiency that is likely not a hemolytic anemia.
NP = An
CN = Ph/8
CL = An
SA = 1

12. 2. The Z-track method of administering parenteral iron prevents leakage of the iron into subcutaneous tissues. Applying ice would slow absorption, and massaging the skin could spread the iron into the subcutaneous tissues. The upper lateral quadrant of the gluteus muscle is favored for deep injection because it is a large muscle.
NP = Pl
CN = Ph/6

CL = Ap
SA = 5

13. 1. Chronic bleeding from an ulcer can lead to iron deficiency anemia. Iron replacement could be accomplished with oral or parenteral therapy. Vitamin B_{12} deficiency is administered to people with poor dietary intake or pernicious anemia. Neupogen is used to regulate the production of neutrophils in the bone marrow. Zinc is a mineral supplement of no value in iron deficiency anemia.
NP = Im
CN = Ph/6
CL = Ap
SA = 5

14. 1. Treating the underlying etiology of disseminated intravascular coagulation (DIC), in this case, the acute leukemia, is appropriate. Chemotherapy for the leukemia and heparin for the DIC can be initiated together. The use of anticoagulants can reduce the risk of thrombosis in DIC. It would be inappropriate to discontinue treatments because both leukemia and DIC are treatable.
NP = Pl
CN = Ph/8
CL = An
SA = 1

15. 3. The client on bed rest is at risk for further development of the deep vein thrombosis. Support stockings or other compression devices can aid in clot prevention. The client would not be attending physical therapy until the clot is resolved. The affected limb should be elevated without any weight bearing initially. Morphine sulfate would not be used in deep vein thrombosis.
NP = Im
CN = Ph/8
CL = Ap
SA = 1

16. 3. An acute drop in hemoglobin results in the body's attempt to reestablish equilibrium. A diminished blood volume causes the heart to beat faster in order to circulate the smaller volume. The blood pressure would decrease acutely and the respiratory rate would increase. The body temperature would not fluctuate to indicate a change in hemoglobin unless from shock, in which case it would decrease.
NP = An
CN = Ph/8
CL = An
SA = 1

17. **Small pinpoint petechiae.** Thrombocytopenia of less than 20,000 /mm^3 can result in petechial hemorrhage into the skin from very little pressure on the limb. The blood pressure cuff most likely caused this. Other typical sites of petechiae are in lower extremities that have been in a dependent position.
NP = An
CN = Ph/8
CL = An
SA = 1

18. 2. Filtering blood products does reduce the incidence of febrile nonhemolytic reactions. Filtering does reduce the transmission of cytomegalovirus, does protect the donor, and filtering the leukocytes reduces the recipient's immunization to leukocyte antigens.
NP = An
CN = Ph/6
CL = An
SA = 5

19. 2. The hemophiliac, unable to clot blood effectively, is most likely suffering from internal organ or muscle bleeding as a result of the accident. This would be reflected in a decrease in the hemoglobin/hematocrit level. The white cell count and differential would not be affected unless there were another, unrelated condition occurring simultaneously.
NP = Ev
CN = Ph/7
CL = An
SA = 1

20. 4. A priority to implement in the plan of care for a client scheduled to undergo a splenectomy is to administer a pneumococcal vaccine. Administering analgesics, carefully positioning the client to facilitate optimum lung expansion, and encouraging small frequent meals are all interventions for splenomegaly but not specifically for a client presplenectomy.
NP = Im
CN = Sa/1
CL = An
SA = 1

21. 1. Fatigue is a major complication of anemia. The client will need to have short sessions after periods of rest in order to learn effectively. Inclusion of family members in the educational process is ideal, especially in the teaching of the fatigued client.

NP = Pl
CN = He/3
CL = Ap
SA = 1

22. 2. Low molecular weight heparin is administered subcutaneously to a client who is prone to a venous thrombosis and may be administered by a licensed practical nurse. Immunoglobulin and glucocorticoids are administered intravenously to a client with immune thrombocytopenic purpura (ITP) and must be administered by a registered nurse.
Assessing a client with neutropenia for an infection and reporting that infection is a nursing task reserved for the registered nurse. Maintaining a venous access for plasma exchange in a client with thrombotic thrombocytopenic purpura (TTP) is also a job function reserved for a registered nurse.
NP = Pl
CN = Sa/1
CL = An
SA = 8

23. 1. The priority nursing diagnosis in a client with anemia due to acute blood loss from a motor vehicle accident is risk for injury related to a decrease in circulating blood volume.
Other less important nursing diagnoses related to an acute blood loss are activity intolerance, imbalanced nutrition: less than body requirements, and ineffective therapeutic regimen management.
NP = An
CN = Sa/1
CL = An
SA = 1

24. 2. Iron is best absorbed on an empty stomach and in an acidic environment such as orange juice. Taking an antacid would decrease the absorption of iron. Oral iron therapy will not alter the skin color. IM iron can stain the site of injection brown. Stool color can change to a darker brown color as the result of oral iron replacement.
NP = Ev
CN = Ph/6
CL = An
SA = 5

25. Vitamin K. Warfarin sodium given orally may be initiated after heparin infusion and overlapping with the warfarin until the INR is 2.0 to 3.0. Vitamin K interferes with warfarin and can be used to counteract its effect if bleeding occurs.
NP = An

CN = Ph/6
CL = An
SA = 5

26. 2. Thrombotic thrombocytopenic purpura (TTP) is a syndrome of thrombocytopenia and other manifestations such as mental status changes, bleeding, fever, and kidney failure occurring in adults of any age. When it occurs in children, its main effects are on the kidneys and it is called HUS.
NP = An
CN = Ph/8
CL = An
SA = 1

27. 1. Aplastic anemia is a life-threatening stem cell disorder with many possible etiological mechanisms characterized by a hypoplastic, fatty bone marrow and pancytopenia. Pancytopenia plan of care is a priority to prevent complications like infection and bleeding (private room, strict handwashing, and minimizing invasive procedures). A client who has a poor nutritional intake and associated weight loss is most likely suffering from some form of nutritional anemia. Pain medication for a client who has pain would be an appropriate intervention for a client with sickle cell anemia. A client who has an enlarged spleen may need a splenectomy.
NP = Pl
CN = Ph/8
CL = An
SA = 1

28. 1, 3, 5. Clinical manifestations of polycythemia include headaches, dizziness, tinnitus, visual disturbances, and gastrointestinal pain and fullness. Paresthesia is a clinical manifestation of thrombocytosis. Purpura (purple patches on the skin) and nosebleeds are found in thrombotic thrombocytopenic purpura.
NP = Ev
CN = Ph/8
CL = Ap
SA = 1

29. 4. Unlicensed assistive personnel may take the vital signs of a client with sickle cell anemia. It would not be appropriate to delegate walking a client with aplastic anemia and neutropenia because this client must be in a private room away from all sources of infection and may have special filtration. Measuring the circumference of a limb in a client with a blood clot would not be appropriate for unlicensed assistive personnel to do because it requires the knowledge to know how to move a limb to safely

obtain the measurement. Unlicensed assistive personnel should not assess the presence of any condition. This is a skill reserved for the nurse.
NP = Pl
CN = Sa/1
CL = An
SA = 8

30. 3. The goal of treatment for a client with hemochromatosis is to remove iron from the body. Periodic phlebotomy of 500 ml of blood weekly is scheduled, followed by a maintenance schedule of every three to six months.
NP = Im
CN = Sa/1
CL = An
SA = 1

FLUID, ELECTROLYTE, AND ACID-BASE DISORDERS - COMPREHENSIVE EXAM

1. A client has a sodium level of 125 mEq/L. Which of the following nursing assessments would support the diagnosis that this client is also hypovolemic?
Select all that apply:
[ ] **1.** Flushed skin
[ ] **2.** Abdominal cramps
[ ] **3.** Decreased bowel sounds
[ ] **4.** Orthostatic hypotension
[ ] **5.** Dry mucous membranes
[ ] **6.** Low grade fever

2. The physician orders a urine specific gravity and a urine sodium for a client who was admitted with a serum sodium of 121 mEq/L. Which of the following is the best response by the nurse when asked by a nursing student what is the purpose of the test?

1. "The tests are designed to determine which drug is causing the client's low sodium levels."

2. "An elevated urine specific gravity and urine sodium would indicate the client has syndrome of inappropriate antidiuretic hormone, or SIADH."

3. "If the results show a urine specific gravity of less than 1.010, the client may have syndrome of inappropriate antidiuretic hormone, or SIADH."
4. "A low urine sodium level may indicate that the client has syndrome of inappropriate antidiuretic hormone, or SIADH."

3. A client with ascites secondary to liver failure has a supine blood pressure of 79/40 and complains of dizziness. Which of the following is the priority nursing intervention for the nurse to implement?
   1. Place the client in Trendelenburg position
   2. Increase oral intake of fluids
   3. Measure the abdominal girth
   4. Place the client in supine position with legs elevated 45°
4. After successful diuresis, a client in heart failure admitted for fluid volume overload is ready for discharge. Which of the following statements by the client demonstrates an understanding of a 1000 ml per day fluid restriction ordered by the physician?
   1. "I must restrict my fluids in order to decrease the number of times I have to urinate during the night."
   2. "I can have 50 ounces of fluid each day."
   3. "When I feel thirsty, I can suck on hard candy."
   4. "I can have all the ice chips I want if my mouth gets dry."
5. The nurse is caring for a client with a serum magnesium level of 1.2 mEq/L and a serum potassium of 3.4 mEq/L. The nurse administers which of the following drugs initially?
   1. Calcium carbonate
   2. Potassium chloride
   3. Magnesium sulfate
   4. Sodium bicarbonate
6. The nurse is evaluating the medical records of four clients. Which client does the nurse evaluate to be at greatest risk for syndrome of inappropriate antidiuretic hormone (SIADH)?
   1. Client with a thyroidectomy
   2. Client with oat cell carcinoma of the lung
   3. Client with a fractured hip
   4. Client with polycystic kidney disease
7. When planning the care of a client with a phosphorus level of 1.1 mEq/L, the nurse should perform which of the following interventions?

1. Maintain strict aseptic technique when performing procedures
2. Restrict fluid intake to 1500 ml per day
3. Administer intravenous saline solution as ordered
4. Teach the client to avoid eggs, whole grains, and nuts

8. The nurse anticipates finding which of the following electrolyte imbalances in a client who has a phosphorus level of 3.2 mg/dl?

1. Hypokalemia
2. Hypermagnesemia
3. Hypernatremia
4. Hypocalcemia

9. The nurse is caring for a client who had a thyroidectomy. Which of the following would indicate to the nurse that the client's condition is deteriorating?

1. Serum sodium of 135 mEq/L
2. Serum potassium of 3.5 mEq/L
3. Serum phosphorus of 1.8 mg/dl
4. Serum calcium of 7.0 mg/dL

10. The nurse is planning the care of a client with hyperaldosteronism. Which of the following nursing diagnoses does the nurse conclude to be the priority?

1. Imbalanced nutrition: more than body requirements
2. Excess fluid volume
3. Self-care deficit
4. Deficient knowledge

11. When administering magnesium sulfate intravenously, the nurse should monitor the client for which of the following clinical manifestations of hypermagnesemia?
Select all that apply:

[ ] **1.** Hypotension
[ ] **2.** Hyperactive deep tendon reflexes
[ ] **3.** Chvostek's sign
[ ] **4.** Impaired swallow ability
[ ] **5.** Somnolence
[ ] **6.** Vomiting

12. A client with congestive heart failure is admitted with hypokalemia secondary to diuresis with loop diuretics. Which of the following client statements indicates the client has misunderstood the discharge instructions?

1. "I will treat leg cramps with a warm heating pad."
2. "I will try to increase my intake of melon and bananas."
3. "I will take my potassium supplements with meals."
4. "I will weigh myself every morning."

13. The nurse receives an order to give potassium chloride 20 mEq over one hour intravenously through a PICC line to treat a serum potassium level of 3.0 mEq/L. Which of the following should be the nurse's next action?
    1. Question the order, because the rate is too fast
    2. Administer the potassium over two hours
    3. Give the potassium as ordered
    4. Question the order, because the potassium level is normal
14. The nurse caring for a client with hyperphosphatemia and chronic renal failure assists the client to make which of the following low phosphorus menu selections?
    1. Scrambled eggs and whole wheat toast
    2. Chicken sandwich
    3. Milkshake
    4. Fresh fruit plate
15. Which of the following nursing measures would be appropriate for a client with a serum sodium level of 125 mEq/L and a serum osmolality of 270 mOsm/kg?
    1. Teach the client to avoid antacids such as sodium bicarbonate
    2. Teach the client to limit fluid intake as indicated by the physician
    3. Monitor for constipation and abdominal distention
    4. Strain the urine for calculi
16. Which of the following instructions on how to take calcium supplements should the nurse include in the discharge plan?
    1. Take the calcium supplements 30 minutes before meals
    2. Take all calcium supplements at one time in the morning
    3. Take the calcium supplement with meals to avoid gastric upset
    4. Take the calcium supplement alone with other prescribed medications
17. The nurse is observing a staff member preparing to give a client a potassium chloride bolus. Which of the following is the priority intervention by the nurse?
    1. Encourage the staff nurse to ensure that no precipitates are formed in the drug
    2. Assist the staff nurse in monitoring vital signs during and after the drug is given

3. Tell the staff member that potassium chloride is never given as a bolus
4. Instruct the staff nurse to flush the IV line to ensure patency

18. A client with congestive heart failure is receiving furosemide (Lasix) 80 mg IV BID. The nurse should monitor for which of the following electrolyte imbalances?
Select all that apply:
[ ] 1. Hypokalemia
[ ] 2. Hypocalcemia
[ ] 3. Hypermagnesemia
[ ] 4. Hyponatremia
[ ] 5. Hyperphosphatemia
[ ] 6. Hyperchloremia

19. The nurse receives an order to initiate total parenteral nutrition (TPN) for a client with alcoholism. Before hanging the solution, the nurse should monitor for which electrolyte imbalance?
1. Hypophosphatemia
2. Hypocalcemia
3. Hyponatremia
4. Hypomagnesemia

20. The nurse is caring for a client with metabolic acidosis. Which of the following should the nurse include in the plan of care for this client?
1. Initiate seizure precautions
2. Review the client's drugs for antacids and loop diuretics
3. Relieve anxiety with sedatives as ordered
4. Position the client to facilitate breathing and promote chest expansion

21. The nurse is caring for a client with respiratory acidosis secondary to pneumonia. Which of the following would indicate the client's condition is deteriorating?
1. PCO_2 increasing from 46 to 50 mm Hg
2. PCO_2 decreasing from 50 to 44 mm Hg
3. HCO_3 increasing from 26 to 29 mEq/L
4. pH increasing from 7.33 to 7.36

22. The nurse is assessing a client with hypokalemia. Which of the following assessments is a priority for the nurse to report to the physician immediately?

1. Leg cramps
2. Abdominal pain and vomiting
3. Strong, bounding pulse
4. Weight gain and headache

23. The nurse is caring for a client with hypovolemic hyponatremia secondary to prolonged diuresis. The physician orders 3% normal saline at 50 ml per hour for 12 hours. Which nursing action would receive priority when carrying out this order?
    1. Carefully monitor the drip rate without a pump
    2. Question the physician's order
    3. Monitor for dyspnea and crackles in lung bases
    4. Review medication list for drugs that may exacerbate hyponatremia

24. A client admitted with pneumonia and fever has a respiratory rate of 32 and is complaining of lightheadedness and tingling in the fingers. ABG values are pH of 7.50, $PaCO_2$ of 30, HCO_3 of 24, and PO_2 of 90. What is an appropriate independent nursing intervention?
    1. Administer sedatives
    2. Encourage the client to increase activity
    3. Encourage deep breathing exercises every hour
    4. Stay with the client and maintain a calm environment

25. A client with acute pancreatitis complains of numbness and tingling around the mouth. The nurse should assess which of the following for hypocalcemia?
    1. Tap the facial nerve adjacent to the ear and observe for a brief contraction of the upper lip
    2. Check urine osmolality
    3. Monitor ECG for peaked T waves
    4. Inflate a blood pressure cuff around the upper arm and observe for increased numbness in the extremity

26. The nurse is caring for a client exhibiting irritability, diarrhea, irregular pulse, and paresthesias and who has a serum potassium level of 5.8 mEq/L. The nurse notifies the physician that the client is experiencing what fluid and electrolyte imbalance? _______________

27. The nurse should monitor a client with a potassium of 2.8 mEq/L for which of the following clinical manifestations?
    Select all that apply:

    [ ] 1. Anxiety
    [ ] 2. Soft, flabby muscles

[ ] 3. Decreased reflexes

[ ] 4. Diarrhea

[ ] 5. Muscle weakness

[ ] 6. Polyuria

28. The nurse is evaluating a client who is experiencing thirst, restlessness, weakness, postural hypotension, and weight loss. The client has a serum sodium level of 150 mEq/L. The nurse reports that this client is experiencing what fluid and electrolyte imbalance? ______________

29. Which of the following clinical manifestations should the nurse monitor for in a client with a serum sodium of 130 mEq/L?
Select all that apply:

[ ] 1. Twitching

[ ] 2. Rapid, thready pulse

[ ] 3. Dry swollen tongue

[ ] 4. Tremors

[ ] 5. Vomiting

[ ] 6. Bradycardia

30. The nurse is caring for a client who becomes confused and stuporous, has decreased reflexes, is dehydrated, and starts vomiting. The nurse should assess what electrolyte for an imbalance? ______________

31. Which of the following nursing clients may the nurse delegate to a licensed practical nurse?
    1. A client with a pH of 7.33, PCO_2 of 35, and HCO_3 of 17
    2. A client who is confused, has decreased deep tendon reflexes, and a serum calcium of 12.8 mg/dl
    3. A client who has a rapid, weak, thready pulse, postural hypotension, and a serum sodium of 128 mEq/L
    4. A client with a serum sodium of 133 mEq/l, phosphorus of 1.8 mg/dl, and a potassium of 4.6 mEq/L

32. The nurse is reviewing the blood chemistry results of a client. Which of the following findings should the nurse report?
    1. Serum calcium level of 9.6 mg/dl
    2. Glucose tolerance of 110 mg/dl
    3. Total protein of 7.0 g/dl
    4. Serum magnesium level of 3.6 mEq/L

33. The nurse evaluates which of the following factors to have an effect on body fluid and electrolytes?

1. An infant kidney conserves more fluid with less loss than an adult kidney
2. An obese woman has a larger proportion of body fluid than a lean man
3. Excessive alcohol intake results in decreased calcium, magnesium, and phosphate levels
4. Stress decreases production of antidiuretic hormone and increases blood volume

34. A client had the following lunch that the nurse needs to total. What is the correct total milliliters the nurse should record? Six ounces of coffee, eight ounces of water, two ounces of jello, four ounces of pureed meat, and three ounces of sherbet. ____________

35. The nurse is evaluating the serum laboratory results on the following four clients. It is a priority that the nurse report the laboratory results on which of the following clients first?

1. A client with multiple myeloma and a calcium level of 12 mg/dl
2. A client who has experienced episodes of vomiting and has a chloride level of 95 mEq/L
3. A client who denies drinking milk and has a phosphorus level of 3.0 mg/dl
4. A client who perspires profusely and has a sodium level of 137 mEq/L

ANSWERS AND RATIONALES

1. 4, 5. Hypovolemic hyponatremia occurs when both water and sodium are lost, but the sodium loss is greater than the water loss. Flushed skin and a low grade fever are clinical manifestations of hypernatremia. Abdominal cramps and decreased bowel sounds indicate hypokalemia.
NP = An
CN = Ph/8
CL = An
SA = 1

2. 2. A client with syndrome of inappropriate antidiuretic hormone (SIADH) retains water and excretes sodium in the renal tubules. This results in more concentrated urine and an increased urine sodium level. Many drugs can cause hyponatremia, but a urine specific gravity and urine sodium will not specify which ones.
NP = An
CN = Ph/8
CL = An
SA = 1

3. 4. A client who has ascites secondary to liver failure, a supine blood pressure of 79/40, and complains of dizziness is hypovolemic due to third spacing of fluids. This client is symptomatic, and the nurse must intervene to improve perfusion to the brain. Placing the client in a Trendelenburg position will place extra pressure on the diaphragm and inhibit respirations. Increasing the oral intake and measuring the abdominal girth are not the priority interventions. Fluid volume that moves out of the vascular space into the extravascular space is third spacing.
NP = Pl
CN = Sa/1
CL = An
SA = 1

4. 3. Ice is a good choice to relieve thirst, but the volume must be recorded as liquid intake. 1000 ml is approximately 33 ounces. The client can take diuretics before 4 p.m. if nighttime urination is a problem, but the fluid restriction is ordered to decrease the potential for fluid overload. Sucking on hard candy often brings relief of thirst for persons on fluid restrictions.
NP = Ev
CN = Ph/8
CL = An
SA = 1

5. 3. It is often necessary to replace magnesium before addressing other electrolyte imbalances, because magnesium is necessary for the transport of electrolytes such as potassium across cell membranes. if the serum magnesium is low, potassium may be lost through the urine.
NP = Im
CN = Ph/6
CL = An
SA = 1

6. 2. Conditions associated with syndrome of inappropriate antidiuretic hormone (SIADH) include oat cell carcinoma of the lung, trauma or tumors of the CNS, stroke, asthma, and COPD and drugs such as psychotropics, oral hypoglycemic, and chemotherapeutic agents. Polycystic kidney disease is a risk factor for diabetes insipidus. SIADH is a condition of an oversecretion of ADH. Diabetes insipidus is an undersecretion of ADH.
NP = An
CN = Ph/7
CL = An
SA = 1

7. **1.** Normal serum phosphorus is 2.8 to 4.5 mg/dl. Clients with low phosphorus levels (less than 1.8 mg/dl) are more susceptible to infection because of the resulting lack of ATP that causes a decreased functioning of leukocytes. Fluid restriction is appropriate for hyponatremia. Eggs, whole grains, and nuts are a good source of phosphorus and their intake should be encouraged.
NP = Im
CN = Ph/8
CL = Ap
SA = 1

8. **4.** When phosphorus levels are high, calcium levels are low. Many clinical manifestations of hyperphosphatemia are also clinical manifestations of hypocalcemia.
NP = An
CN = Ph/7
CL = An
SA = 1

9. **4.** Hypoparathyroidism and subsequent hypocalcemia can result after a thyroidectomy. Laryngeal muscles are prone to spasm in the presence of hypocalcemia. A calcium level of 7.0 mg/dl must be addressed immediately. A serum sodium of 135 mEq/L, potassium of 3.5 mEq/L, and phosphorus of 1.8 mg/dl are lab values all within normal limits.
NP = An
CN = Ph/7
CL = An
SA = 1

10. **2.** Aldosterone causes sodium and water retention in the kidneys leading to increases in fluid volume. The client may require education about the condition, but this is a secondary intervention. Self-care deficit and imbalanced nutrition are not appropriate nursing diagnoses for hyperaldosteronism.
NP = Ev
CN = Ph/8
CL = An
SA = 1

11. **1, 5, 6.** Hypermagnesemia is usually caused by an increased magnesium intake and accompanies renal failure. Products such as milk of magnesia result in an increased magnesium intake. Normal serum magnesium is 1.5 to 2.5 mEq/L. Clinical manifestation of hypermagnesemia initially include lethargy, drowsiness, nausea, and vomiting. Later manifestations include hypotension and somnolence. Cardiac arrest can occur.

NP = As
CN = Ph/8
CL = Ap
SA = 1

12. 1. Leg cramps are a clinical manifestation of hypokalemia. This client should be aware of and report clinical manifestations of hypokalemia to the physician rather than treat them independently. Low potassium can lead to arrhythmias.
NP = Ev
CN = Ph/8
CL = An
SA = 1

13. 3. Potassium may be given 20 mEq/hr through a centrally placed catheter. A PICC line is a central line.
NP = P1
CN = Ph/8
CL = Ap
SA = 1

14. 4. Eggs, poultry, whole grains, and dairy products are all foods high in phosphorus. A fresh fruit plate is low in phosphorus.
NP = Im
CN = Ph/5
CL = Ap
SA = 1

15. 2. A client who has a serum sodium level of 125 mEq/L and a serum osmolality of 270 mOsm/kg is experiencing mild hypervolemic hyponatremia, which is treated with fluid restriction. Teaching the client to avoid antacids is a treatment for hypernatremia. Monitoring the client for constipation and abdominal distention is indicated in hypokalemia. Straining the urine for calculi is indicated in hypercalcemia.
NP = Pl
CN = Ph/8
CL = Ap
SA = 1

16. 1. A calcium supplement should be taken on an empty stomach to promote absorption. Calcium supplements can interfere with the absorption of other drugs. The best time to take calcium is 30 minutes before meals.
NP = Pl
CN = He/3
CL = Ap
SA = 1

17. 3. If potassium is given as a bolus, it may cause fatal arrhythmias. It would be appropriate to ensure that no precipitates are formed in the drug, to monitor vital signs, and to flush the IV line to ensure patency only when the potassium is given as an intravenous piggyback.
NP = Im
CN = Ph/6
CL = Ap
SA = 1

18. 1,2,4. Potassium, calcium, and sodium are depleted through the urine when loop diuretics are administered.
NP = As
CN = Ph/8
CL = An
SA = 1

19. 1. Alcoholics often have low phosphorus levels. As solutions high in glucose are administered, insulin is produced by the body, which causes glucose and phosphorus to move into the cells. Serum levels of phosphorus are subsequently lowered. Hypocalcemia, hyponatremia, and hypomagnesemia would not be advertently affected by total parenteral nutrition.
NP = As
CN = Ph/7
CL = Ap
SA = 1

20. 4. A compensatory response to metabolic acidosis is the elimination of carbon dioxide through rapid, deep respirations. The nurse should promote this response through proper positioning of the client. Sedation may inhibit respiratory compensation. Seizures are more likely in metabolic alkalosis..
NP = P1
CN = Ph/8
CL = Ap
SA = 1

21. 1. A PCO_2 that increases from 46 to 50 mm Hg is respiratory acidosis and is caused by hypoalveolar ventilation and carbon dioxide retention in the lungs. The increased carbon dioxide levels would indicate that the client's condition is deteriorating. A HCO_3 increasing from 26 to 29 indicates that renal compensation is occurring. A PCO_2 decreasing from 50 to 44 mm Hg and a pH increasing from 7.33 to 7.36 would indicate improvement in the client's condition.
NP = An
CN = Ph/8

CL = An
SA = 1

22. 2. Abdominal pain and vomiting may be clinical manifestations of paralytic ileus, a serious complication of hypokalemia. Leg cramps are a sign of hypokalemia, but they do not require urgent intervention. A strong, bounding pulse is a sign of hypervolemia. Weight gain and headaches are symptoms of hyponatremia with increased extracellular volume.
NP = An
CN = Ph/8
CL = An
SA = 1

23. 3. Hypertonic saline solutions may cause fluid overload and pulmonary edema. All hypertonic saline solutions should be administered with a pump to ensure sodium levels do not rise too quickly and cause brain injury. 3% saline is commonly ordered for treatment of hyponatremia. Reviewing the drugs is important, but it is not a priority action.
NP = Im
CN = Ph/8
CL = Ap
SA = 1

24. 4. A client who has a pH of 7.50, $PaCO_2$ of 30, HCO_3 of 24, and PO_2 of 90 is in respiratory alkalosis. Staying with the client and maintaining a calm environment will assist the client to slow breathing and retaining more CO_2, thus bringing the pH back into normal range. Deep breathing exercises would most likely worsen the client's condition. Encouraging deep breathing is contraindicated because clients are often exhausted and require rest after expending so much energy breathing. Administering sedatives is not an independent nursing intervention.
NP = Im
CN = Ph/8
CL = An
SA = 1

25. 1. Tapping the facial nerve adjacent to the ear and observing for a brief contraction of the upper lip is the correct method for testing for Chvostek's sign, a test for hypocalcemia. Inflating a blood pressure cuff around the upper arm and observing for increased numbness in the extremity is not correct because the nurse would observe for carpopedal spasm 1 to 4 minutes after applying the cuff. This is called Trousseau's sign. Peaked T waves are present in hyperkalemia.
NP = As
CN = Ph/8
CL = Ap
SA = 1

26. **Hyperkalemia.** Clinical manifestations of hyperkalemia include irritability, abdominal cramps, diarrhea, weakness of lower extremities, paresthesias, and an irregular pulse. Normal serum potassium is 3.5 to 5.5 mEq/L.
NP = An
CN = Ph/8
CL = An
SA = 1

27. **2, 3, 5, 6.** Clinical manifestations of hypokalemia include soft, flabby muscles, decreased reflexes, muscle weakness, polyuria, fatigue, paresthesias, and an irregular pulse. Normal serum potassium is 3.5 to 5.5 mEq/L.
NP = As
CN = Ph/8
CL = Ap
SA = 1

28. **Hypernatremia.** Normal serum sodium is 135 to 145 mEq/L. Clinical manifestations of hypernatremia include thirst, weakness, postural hypotension, weight loss, and restlessness.
NP = An
CN = Ph/8
CL = Ap
SA = 1

29. **2, 4, 5.** Normal serum sodium is 135 to 145 mEq/L. Clinical manifestations of hyponatremia include rapid, thready pulse, tremors, weight loss, vomiting, and postural hypotension.
NP = As
CN = Ph/8
CL = Ap
SA = 1

30. **Calcium.** A client who is lethargic and weak, has decreased reflexes, is confused, vomiting, and dehydrated, and becomes stuporous is experiencing hypercalcemia. Normal serum calcium is 9 to 11 mg/dl.
NP = As
CN = Ph/8
CL = Ap
SA = 1

31. **4.** A serum sodium of 133 mEq/L, phosphorus of 1.8 mg/dl, and potassium of 4.6 mEq/L are all normal electrolytes and this client may be delegated to a licensed practical nurse. A client with a pH of 7.33, PCO_2 of 35, and HCO_3 of 17 is in metabolic acidosis and should be cared for by a registered nurse. Both the client with a rapid, weak, thready pulse, postural

hypotension, and a serum sodium of 128 mEq/L and the client who is confused, has decreased deep tendon reflexes, and a serum calcium of 12.8 mg/dl merit close monitoring. The first client is hyponatremic and the second client has hypercalcemia.
NP = Pl
CN = Sa/1
CL = An
SA = 8

32. 4. Normal serum calcium is 9 to 11 mg/dl. Normal glucose tolerance is 70 to 120 mg/dl. Normal total protein is 6.0 to 8.0 g/dl. Normal serum magnesium is 1.5 to 2.5 mEq/L. A high magnesium level may be the result of hypothyroidism, Addison's disease, renal failure, or an excessive intake of magnesium-based antacids.
NP = An
CN = Ph/8
CL = An
SA = 1

33. 3. Excessive alcohol intake does decrease calcium, magnesium, and phosphate levels. The infant kidney loses more fluid with a greater loss than an adult kidney. An obese woman has a greater proportion of body fat and a smaller proportion of body fluid than a lean man. Stress increases production of the antidiuretic hormone and decreases blood volume.
NP = Ev
CN = Ph/8
CL = An
SA = 1

34. 570. Six ounces of coffee is equal to 180 ml. Eight ounces of water is equivalent to 240 ml. Two ounces of jello is equivalent to 60 ml. Three ounces of sherbet is equal to 90 ml. Four ounces of pureed meat is not a fluid food. The total ml for this diet is 570 ml.
NP = Im
CN = Ph/8
CL = Ap
SA = 1

35. 1. Normal serum calcium is 9 to 11 mg/dl. A client with multiple myeloma has hypercalcemia. Although vomiting may result in a low chloride level, normal serum chloride is 95 to 105 mEq/L. Normal serum phosphorus is 2.8 to 4.5 mg/dl. A client who does not drink milk or has a decreased intake of vitamin D foods may be at risk for a phosphorus deficiency. Normal serum sodium is 135 to 145 mEq/L. A client who perspires a lot may develop hyponatremia.
NP = Ev
CN = Sa/1
CL = An
SA = 1

PERIOPERATIVE NURSING - COMPREHENSIVE EXAM

1. The nurse informs another nurse that the primary purpose of preoperative education is to ______________

2. A client experiences a severe anaphylactic reaction to the preoperative antibiotic. The nurse's priority intervention is to
   1. assess the client's airway.
   2. initiate cardiopulmonary resuscitation.
   3. manage the client's anxiety.
   4. elevate the client's bed to 45°.

3. During admission to the postanesthesia care unit (PACU), the priority nursing assessment for a client who has received a general anesthetic is to assess
   1. the client's motor and sensory function.
   2. the client's blood pressure and pulse.
   3. for a patent airway.
   4. the level of consciousness.

4. The nurse is caring for a client with type 1 diabetes who is planning elective surgery. Preoperatively, the nurse anticipates that the client's insulin dosage will be
   1. determined by the anesthesia provider.
   2. changed to a longer-acting type.
   3. increased to cover the stress of surgery.
   4. changed to an oral hyperglycemic agent.

5. The nurse is caring postoperatively for a client who experienced a significant amount of blood loss intraoperatively. When assessing for hypovolemic shock, the nurse is most concerned about
   1. hypertension.
   2. cyanosis.
   3. tachypnea.
   4. oliguria.

6. A client is experiencing a paralytic ileus in the PACU (postanesthesia care unit). A priority nursing assessment would be to
   1. check for gastric distention.
   2. auscultate for bowel sounds.
   3. assess the client's temperature.
   4. monitor for respiratory effort.

7. The nurse caring for the client preoperatively would notify the surgical and anesthetic teams if the client experiences
   1. a white blood cell count of 7 million.
   2. hemoglobin of 15 g.
   3. oral temperature of 37.2° or 99.1°F.
   4. urinalysis with positive HCG.
8. Preoperatively, a client complains of severe anxiety related to the planned surgical procedure. Which of the following is the priority intervention for the nurse to implement?
   1. Encourage the client to discuss what is causing the fearfulness
   2. Explain to the client that surgical procedure is safe and that complications are rare
   3. Explain to the client that the surgical team is very experienced in performing the scheduled procedure
   4. Ask the client if a referral to social services or pastoral care would appeal
9. During preoperative education, the nurse teaches the client postoperative measures that decrease the likelihood of deep vein thrombosis. What is the priority nursing intervention that would accomplish this goal?______________
10. The nurse is reviewing the medication history of a client scheduled for an outpatient surgical procedure next week. Which of the following drugs would necessitate verbal notification of the surgical team prior to admitting the client to the outpatient surgical area?
    1. Captopril (Capoten)
    2. Warfarin sodium (Coumadin)
    3. Erythromycin
    4. Oral contraceptive pills
11. A client receives preoperative sedation prior to the surgical team obtaining the client's signature on the surgical permit. What is the priority nursing intervention? ______________
12. In the postanesthesia care unit, a client who has had an outpatient surgical procedure complains of intense thirst. Postoperative orders state: "advance diet as tolerated." Prior to offering the client fluids, the nurse should first assess ______________ .
13. A client presents preoperatively for an elective umbilical hernia repair. The nurse notes in the medical history that the client has an arteriovenous (A-V) fistula in the right arm. Which of the following is a priority for the nurse to assess after intraoperative positioning of the client?

1. Pulse distal to the A-V fistula
2. Presence of a thrill over the fistula site
3. Client's blood pressure
4. Capillary refill distal to A-V fistula

14. Perioperatively, the nurse notes that a client is paraplegic. The perioperative nurse should include which of the following in planning care for this client?
 1. Monitor fluid and electrolyte balance
 2. Position the client to decrease pressure on coccyx
 3. Assess pupil response
 4. Assess vital signs

15. A client is scheduled for a left orchiectomy. When assessing the client's understanding of the planned surgical procedure, the nurse realizes that the client does not understand that his left testicle will be removed. What is the nurse's priority nursing action? ______________

16. The nurse is planning preoperative care for a client with asthma. The nurse anticipates that preoperatively the client will be told to
 1. administer inhaler drugs as ordered.
 2. withhold all drugs ordered.
 3. increase the dose of inhalers.
 4. change inhaled drugs to longer-acting bronchodilators.

17. When preparing to delegate nursing tasks to unlicensed assistive personnel, which of the following may be delegated?
 1. Assess the vital signs of a client returning from surgery
 2. Inform a client on the importance of coughing, turning, and deep breathing postoperatively
 3. Assist a client following surgery to select a high-protein diet
 4. Walk a client postoperatively 20 feet

18. The nurse is caring for a client after surgery for cancer of the esophagus. The client experiences a decreased air exchange as a result of pooling of secretions in the dependent areas of the bronchiole. The nurse notifies the physician that the client has mostly likely suffered ______________ .

19. A client with a history of ongoing anorexia nervosa presents preoperatively for an ORIF (open reduction, internal fixation) of the right ankle. The nurse would anticipate that which of the following laboratory tests would be a priority to assess preoperatively?

1. Hemoglobin and hematocrit
2. Total cholesterol and triglycerides
3. Fasting glucose level
4. Serum electrolytes

20. A client is scheduled for an elective right knee arthroscopy. Preoperatively, the nurse notes that the surgical consent has been obtained for a left knee arthroscopy. The nurse should

1. notify the surgical team.
2. correct the surgical consent form.
3. write on the client's right knee the word "correct."
4. review the history and physical form.

21. A client notes an allergy to iodine and shellfish. The perioperative nurse anticipates that

1. the client may experience hives intraoperatively.
2. the client will receive a dose of intravenous antihistamine.
3. Betadine prep solution will not be utilized.
4. the surgical procedure may be cancelled.

22. Preoperatively, a client's order reads "NPO after midnight." When assessing the client preoperatively, the client verbalizes that a small glass of orange juice was consumed at 5 a.m. Which of the following is the most appropriate intervention?

1. Document the time of orange juice consumption on the preoperative checksheet
2. Notify the anesthesia team of the time of last oral fluid intake
3. Explain the definition of NPO to the client
4. Call the surgical team for cancellation of the surgical procedure

23. Intraoperatively, a client has an estimated blood loss of 1200 ml. The nurse's priority assessment postoperatively in the postanesthesia care unit (PACU) would be

1. blood pressure.
2. skin color.
3. level of consciousness.
4. peripheral pulses.

24. Postoperatively, a client is difficult to arouse. Which of the following is the priority nursing intervention?

1. Assess the client for eye opening
2. Give simple commands to the client in a loud voice
3. Perform a sternal rub on the client
4. Reposition the client

25. The postanesthesia care nurse administers opioid analgesia intravenously in small amounts for a client who has had an exploratory laparotomy. The priority nursing intervention after administering the opioid analgesic is to assess the client's
    1. abdominal dressing
    2. respiratory rate
    3. blood pressure
    4. pain response

ANSWERS AND RATIONALES

1. **increase the client's knowledge to positively affect health status.** The primary purpose of preoperative client education is to increase the client's knowledge of interventions that may be performed to enhance the client's health status and to reduce the risk of postoperative complications.
   NP = Im
   CN = Ph/8
   CL = Co
   SA = 1

2. **1.** Emergent management of a client's airway is critical during an anaphylactic reaction because edema may increase markedly with time. Initiation of cardiopulmonary resuscitation may be instituted based upon nursing assessment of airway, breathing, and circulation. Although management of the client's anxiety and elevation of the head of the bed may be appropriate, these would not be the priority nursing responses.
   NP = Im
   CN = Ph/8
   CL = Ap
   SA = 1

3. **3.** Upon admission to the PACU (postanesthesia care unit), the nurse immediately assesses for a patent airway. A client's airway may be obstructed after a general anesthetic due to relaxation of the musculature surrounding the airway. Blood pressure, pulse, and level of consciousness would be assessed after the airway is assessed and maintained. The A (airway), B (breathing), and C (circulation) always come first.

NP = As
CN = Sa/1
CL = Ap
SA = 1

4. 1. Members of the anesthesia team determine preoperative insulin orders. Typically, insulin doses are decreased preoperatively due to a client's NPO status. Insulin is not changed to a longer-acting type. Type 1 diabetics cannot take oral hyperglycemic agents, as they produce no endogenous insulin. While insulin needs do increase because of physiologic stress, administering increased doses of insulin preoperatively to a client who is NPO will predispose the client to hypoglycemia.
NP = An
CN = Ph/8
CL = An
SA = 1

5. 4. The renal system compensates in hypovolemic shock by conserving volume. In hypovolemic shock, urinary output decreases. Hypertension, cyanosis, and tachypnea are not clinical manifestations of hypovolemic shock.
NP = As
CN = Ph/8
CL = Ap
SA = 1

6. 2. Postoperatively, the PACU nurse assesses for the return of peristaltic function by auscultation of bowel sounds. Gastric distention may occur with decreased peristalsis, but is less specific for paralytic ileus than absent or decreased bowel sounds. Temperature and respiratory effort are unrelated to a paralytic ileus.
NP = As
CN = Sa/1
CL = Ap
SA = 1

7. 4. A positive HCG result indicates that the client is pregnant, which mandates notification to the anesthetic and surgical teams. A white blood cell count of 7 million, a hemoglobin of 15 g, and an oral temperature of 37.2 °C or 99.1°F are all within normal limits.
NP = Im
CN = Ph/8
CL = Ap
SA = 1

8. 1. The most appropriate nursing intervention is to assess the cause of the client's anxiety. Discussing complication rates and the surgical team may

offer false assurance and may limit the client's ability to express concerns. Prior to referring a client to social services, it is important that the nurse assess the client's needs.

NP = Im
CN = Sa/1
CL = An
SA = 1

9. **Encourage the client to ambulate soon after surgery.** Ambulation as soon as possible after surgery promotes venous return and decreases venous pooling.

NP = Pl
CN = Sa/1
CL = An
SA = 1

10. **2.** The use of Coumadin puts the client at risk for intraoperative bleeding and would necessitate notifying the surgical team. The use of ACE inhibitors, antibiotics, or oral contraceptive pills would warrant written notation in the client's chart, but would not mandate verbal notification.

NP = An
CN = Ph/8
CL = An
SA = 1

11. **Notify the surgical team.** The surgeon is responsible for obtaining informed consent for the surgical procedure prior to the administration of preoperative sedation. The nurse is not responsible for informing the client about the procedure.

NP = Im
CN = Sa/1
CL = An
SA = 1

12. **the client's gag reflex.** Prior to the administration of any fluids, the client must have recovered the gag reflex in order to prevent aspiration. It is a priority that the nurse assess for the return of the gag reflex prior to the administration of any oral fluids.

NP = As
CN = Sa/1
CL = An
SA = 1

13. **2.** The perioperative nurse is responsible for assisting in the positioning of the client for the surgical procedure in order to decrease risk of injury. The presence of a thrill over the fistula site is an indication that the A-V fistula remains patent.

NP = As
CN = Sa/1
CL = An
SA = 1

14. 2. The client who is paraplegic is at risk for skin breakdown, particularly over the coccyx. It is the nurse's responsibility to assess the skin for evidence of skin breakdown and to provide padding to areas that are under pressure, in order to prevent ulcer formation. Monitoring intake and output and assessing pupil response and vital signs are appropriate postoperative interventions.
NP = Pl
CN = Ph/8
CL = Ap
SA = 1

15. **Notify the physician.** As a client advocate, it is the nurse's responsibility to notify the surgical team of the client's lack of understanding of the proposed surgical procedure. It is the surgeon's responsibility to obtain informed consent.
NP = Im
CN = Sa/1
CL = An
SA = 1

16. 1. Preoperatively, asthmatic clients should be taught to continue using their inhaled bronchodilators as needed. In addition, clients should be instructed to bring their inhalers to their preoperative appointments so that the nurse can accurately identify the drugs and dosages.
NP = An
CN = Ph/6
CL = An
SA = 1

17. 4. Unlicensed assistive personnel may walk a client postoperatively 20 feet. A nurse is required to assess a client's vital signs upon returning to the room postoperatively. Unlicensed assistive personnel do not have the knowledge to assist a client to select a high-protein diet or cough, turn, or deep breathe.
NP = Im
CN = Sa/1
CL = An
SA = 8

18. **atelectasis.** Atelectasis is a decreased ventilation that occurs as a result of pooling of secretions in dependent areas of the bronchiole.

NP = An
CN = Ph/8
CL = Ap
SA = 1

19. 4. A client with anorexia nervosa has an increased risk of electrolyte imbalance. In order to provide safe anesthetic and surgical care, the nurse can anticipate that the client would have preoperative serum electrolytes drawn.
NP = As
CN = Ph/7
CL = An
SA = 1

20. 1. The surgical team is notified of the discrepancy between the surgical consent and the client's report of anticipated surgery. The discrepancy must be clarified with the surgical team prior to the initiation of the client's surgical procedure.
NP = Im
CN = Ph/8
CL = Ap
SA = 1

21. 3. A client who reports an allergy to iodine and shellfish should not have prep solutions with Betadine applied because a severe allergic reaction may result. A different pre-op solution will be chosen by the surgical team.
NP = An
CN = Ph/8
CL = Co
SA = 1

22. 2. Clients are ordered to be NPO prior to surgery in order to decrease the risk of aspiration. The anesthesia team is notified of an NPO violation for determination of the next action to take. The anesthesia team, in consultation with the surgical team, determines if the case will progress as scheduled.
NP = Pl
CN = Ph/8
CL = Ap
SA = 1

23. 1. A client who has experienced a large estimated blood loss (EBL) is at risk for hypovolemic shock.Blood pressure should be closely monitored for hypotension.
NP = As
CN = Ph/8

CL = Ap
SA = 1

24. 3. The application of noxious stimuli, such as a sternal rub, may increase the client's level of consciousness and decrease the risk of airway occlusion by relaxation of the tongue.
NP = Pl
CN = Sa/1
CL = An
SA = 1

25. 2. The nurse should carefully monitor the client for adverse reactions related to the administration of an opioid analgesia. The main adverse reaction is respiratory depression. A respiratory rate of less than 12 per minute may indicate respiratory depression and the need for the administration of an antidote.
NP = As
CN = Sa/1
CL = An
SA = 1